HEALTH INFORMATION EXCHANGE

SECOND EDITION

HEALTH INFORMATION EXCHANGE

NAVIGATING AND MANAGING A NETWORK OF HEALTH INFORMATION SYSTEMS

SECOND EDITION

Edited by

BRIAN E. DIXON

Department of Epidemiology, Richard M. Fairbanks School of Public Health, Indiana University, Indianapolis, IN, USA; Center for Biomedical Informatics, Regenstrief Institute, Inc., Indianapolis, IN, USA; Department of Veterans Affairs, Health Services Research & Development Service, Center for Health Information and Communication, Indianapolis, IN, USA

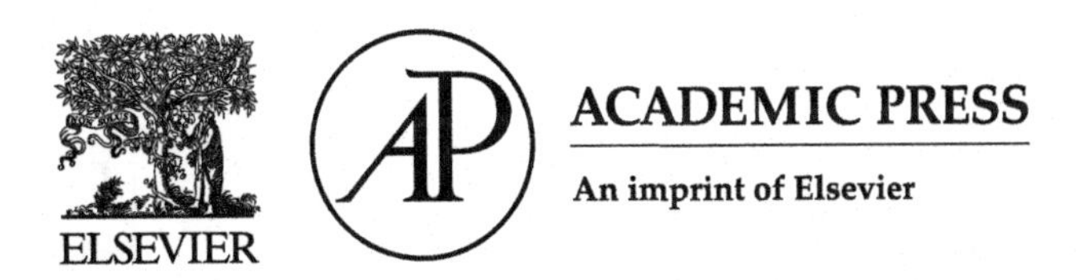

Academic Press is an imprint of Elsevier
125 London Wall, London EC2Y 5AS, United Kingdom
525 B Street, Suite 1650, San Diego, CA 92101, United States
50 Hampshire Street, 5th Floor, Cambridge, MA 02139, United States
The Boulevard, Langford Lane, Kidlington, Oxford OX5 1GB, United Kingdom

ISBN: 978-0-323-90802-3

For Information on all Academic Press publications
visit our website at https://www.elsevier.com/books-and-journals

Publisher: Stacy Masucci
Acquisitions Editor: Linda Versteeg-Buschman
Editorial Project Manager: Pat Gonzalez
Production Project Manager: Omer Mukthar
Cover Designer: Harris Greg

Typeset by MPS Limited, Chennai, India

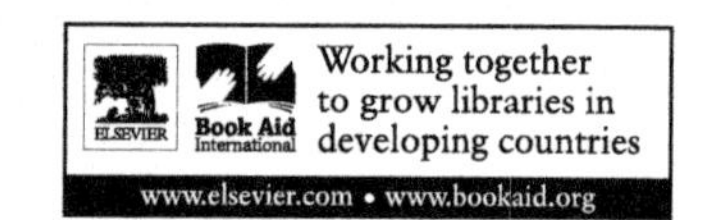
ELSEVIER
Book Aid International
Working together
to grow libraries in
developing countries
www.elsevier.com • www.bookaid.org

Contents

List of contributors

Kelly J. Abrams Master of Health Administration in Health Informatics and Information Management (MHA-HIIM) Program, Johnson-Shoyama Graduate School of Public Policy, University of Regina, Regina, SK, Canada

Julia Adler-Milstein Center for Clinical Informatics and Improvement Research, University of California, San Francisco, CA, USA

Atif Al Braiki Malaffi, Abu Dhabi, United Arab Emirates

Hamed Al Hashemi Department of Health – Abu Dhabi, Abu Dhabi, United Arab Emirates

Katie S. Allen Center for Biomedical Informatics, Regenstrief Institute, Inc., Indianapolis, IN, USA; Department of Epidemiology, Richard M. Fairbanks School of Public Health, Indiana University, Indianapolis, IN, USA

Chinedu Aniekwe US Centers for Disease Control and Prevention, Center for Global Health, Office of the Director, Atlanta, GA, USA

Eyasu Ashebier John Snow, Inc., Addis Ababa, Ethiopia

Gonfa Ayana Ethiopian Public Health Institute, Addis Ababa, Ethiopia

Robert F. Bailey RTI International Translational Health Sciences Division, Research Triangle Park, NC, USA

Cristina Barboi Department of Epidemiology, Richard M. Fairbanks School of Public Health, Indiana University, Indianapolis, IN, USA; Center for Biomedical Informatics, Regenstrief Institute, Inc., Indianapolis, IN, USA

Adebobola Bashorun Federal Ministry of Health, Abuja, Nigeria

Ofir Ben-Assuli Faculty of Business Administration, Ono Academic College, Kiryat Ono, Israel

Paul G. Biondich Center for Biomedical Informatics, Regenstrief Institute, Inc., Indianapolis, IN, USA; Indiana University School of Medicine, Indianapolis, IN, USA

Kenneth S. Boockvar Department of Veterans Affairs, James J. Peters VA Medical Center, Bronx, NY, USA; Icahn School of Medicine at Mount Sinai, New York, NY, USA

Jack Bowie Apelon, Inc., Ridgefield, CT, USA

David Broyles Marion County Public Health Department, Indianapolis, IN, USA

Ryan Crichton Jembi Health Systems, Cape Town, South Africa

Caitlin M. Cusack Insight Informatics, Washington, DC, USA

Ibrahim Dalhatu US Centers for Disease Control and Prevention, Abuja, Nigeria

Ahmed Deeb Earlham College, Richmond, IN, USA

Yaron Denekamp Clalit Health Services, Tel Aviv, Israel; School of Public Health, Haifa University, Haifa, Israel

Brian E. Dixon Department of Epidemiology, Richard M. Fairbanks School of Public Health, Indiana University, Indianapolis, IN, USA; Center for Biomedical Informatics, Regenstrief Institute, Inc., Indianapolis, IN, USA; Department of Veterans Affairs, Health Services Research & Development Service, Center for Health Information and Communication, Indianapolis, IN, USA

Luke Duncan PATH, Seattle, WA, USA

Sue S. Feldman Department of Health Services Administration, School of Health Professions, University of Alabama at Birmingham, Birmingham, AL, USA; Informatics Institute,

Keersink School of Medicine, University of Alabama at Birmingham, Birmingham, AL, USA

Ammon R. Fillmore Indiana Health Information Exchange, Indianapolis, IN, USA

Carl Fourie Program for Appropriate Technology in Health (PATH), Seattle, WA, USA

Emily Franzosa Department of Veterans Affairs, James J. Peters VA Medical Center, Bronx, NY, USA; Icahn School of Medicine at Mount Sinai, New York, NY, USA

Candace J. Gibson Department of Pathology & Laboratory Medicine, Schulich School of Medicine & Dentistry, Western University, London, ON, Canada

Nora J. Gilliam Department of Epidemiology, Richard M. Fairbanks School of Public Health, Indiana University, Indianapolis, IN, USA

Rahul Goyal Malaffi, Abu Dhabi, United Arab Emirates

Shaun J. Grannis Indiana University School of Medicine, Indianapolis, IN, USA; Center for Biomedical Informatics, Regenstrief Institute, Inc., Indianapolis, IN, USA

Randall W. Grout Center for Biomedical Informatics, Regenstrief Institute, Inc., Indianapolis, IN, USA; School of Medicine, Indiana University, Indianapolis, IN, USA

Saira N. Haque North America Medical Affairs, Pfizer Inc., New York, NY, USA; Pfizer Medical Outcomes and Analytics, New York, NY, USA

David Horrocks Chesapeake Regional Information System for Our Patients (CRISP), Baltimore, MD, USA

Bob Jolliffe Department of Informatics, University of Oslo, Oslo, Norway

Pallavi Jonnalagadda The Center for the Advancement of Team Science, Analytics, and Systems Thinking in Health Services and Implementation Science Research (CATALYST), The Ohio State University College of Medicine, Columbus, OH, USA

John P. Kansky Indiana Health Information Exchange, Indianapolis, IN, USA

Andrew S. Kanter Department of Biomedical Informatics and Epidemiology, Columbia University, New York, NY, USA; Intelligent Medical Objects, Inc., Northbrook, IL, USA

James M. Kariuki US Centers for Disease Control and Prevention, Center for Global Health, Division of Global HIV and TB, Atlanta, GA, USA

David C. Kendrick MyHealth Access Network, Tulsa, OK, USA; Department of Medical Informatics, University of Oklahoma, Norman, OK, USA

Hadi Kharrazi Center for Population Health IT (CPHIT), Department of Health Policy and Management, Johns Hopkins School of Public Health, Baltimore, MD, USA; Biomedical Informatics and Data Science Section, Johns Hopkins School of Medicine, Baltimore, MD, USA

Ramona Kyabaggu Master of Health Administration in Health Informatics and Information Management (MHA-HIIM) Program, Johnson-Shoyama Graduate School of Public Policy, University of Regina, Regina, SK, Canada

Bisera Lakinska Malaffi, Abu Dhabi, United Arab Emirates

Li-Hui Lee Department of Health Care Management, National Taipei University of Nursing and Health Sciences, Taipei, Taiwan

Burke W. Mamlin Center for Biomedical Informatics, Regenstrief Institute, Inc., Indianapolis, IN, USA; School of Medicine, Indiana University, Indianapolis, IN, USA

Eric-Jan Manders US Centers for Disease Control and Prevention, Center for Global Health, Office of the Director, Atlanta, GA, USA

J. Marc Overhage Enterprise Analytics Core, Elevance Health, Indianapolis, IN, USA

Erika G. Martin Rockefeller College of Public Affairs and Policy, University at Albany, Albany, NY, USA

Timothy D. McFarlane Family and Social Services Agency, State of Indiana, Indianapolis, IN, USA

Carl D. McKinley Regenstrief Institute, Inc., Indianapolis, IN, USA

Melissa McPheeters RTI International, Research Triangle Park, NC, USA

Nir Menachemi Health Policy and Management, Richard M. Fairbanks School of Public Health, Indiana University, Indianapolis, IN, USA

Teryn P. Morgan Center for Biomedical Informatics, Regenstrief Institute, Inc., Indianapolis, IN, USA; Department of BioHealth Informatics, School of Informatics and Computing, Indiana University, Indianapolis, IN, USA

Bedri Ahmed Mumme ICAP at Columbia University, Addis Ababa, Ethiopia

Lisa A. Murie US Centers for Disease Control and Prevention, Center for Global Health, Division of Global HIV and TB, Atlanta, GA, USA

Kalechristos Abebe Negussie Clinton Health Access Initiative, Addis Ababa, Ethiopia

Christian Nøhr Department of Planning, Aalborg University, Aalborg, Denmark

Charles Nzelu Federal Ministry of Health, Abuja, Nigeria

Martin Osumba Global Public Health Impact Center, RTI International, Nairobi, Kenya

Mitchell Parker Indiana University Health, Indianapolis, IN, USA

Asaminew Petros US Centers for Disease Control and Prevention, Addis Ababa, Ethiopia

Saurabh Rahurkar The Center for the Advancement of Team Science, Analytics, and Systems Thinking in Health Services and Implementation Science Research (CATALYST), The Ohio State University College of Medicine, Columbus, OH, USA; Department of Epidemiology, Richard M. Fairbanks School of Public Health, Indiana University, Indianapolis, IN, USA

Drew Richardson Indiana Health Information Exchange, Indianapolis, IN, USA

Todd M. Rogow Healthix, New York, NY, USA

Katie S. Allen Center for Biomedical Informatics, Regenstrief Institute, Inc., Indianapolis, IN, USA; Department of Epidemiology, Richard M. Fairbanks School of Public Health, Indiana University, Indianapolis, IN, USA

Johan Ivar Sæbø Department of Informatics, University of Oslo, Oslo, Norway

Thomas Schmidt Center for Health Informatics and Technology, University of Southern Denmark, Odense, Denmark

Minen Sead Ethiopian Public Health Institute, Addis Ababa, Ethiopia

Rita Sembajwe Global Public Health Impact Center, RTI International, Atlanta, GA, USA

Dykki Settle PATH, Seattle, WA, USA

Jennifer Shivers Center for Biomedical Informatics, Regenstrief Institute, Inc., Indianapolis, IN, USA; Global Health Informatics, Regenstrief Institute, Inc., Indianapolis, IN, USA

Catherine J. Staes College of Nursing, University of Utah, Salt Lake City, UT, USA; Department of Biomedical Informatics, School of Medicine, University of Utah, Salt Lake City, UT, USA

Eileen F. Tallman Department of Epidemiology, Richard M. Fairbanks School of Public Health, Indiana University, Indianapolis, IN, USA

Willi L. Tarver The Center for the Advancement of Team Science, Analytics, and Systems Thinking in Health Services and Implementation Science Research (CATALYST), The Ohio State University College of Medicine, Columbus, OH, USA; Richard M. Fairbanks School of Public Health, Indiana University-Purdue University Indianapolis, Indianapolis, IN, USA

Scott Teesdale Resolve To Save Lives, New Orleans, LA, USA

Japjit Kaur Tutt Center for Biomedical Informatics, Regenstrief Institute, Inc., Indianapolis, IN, USA

Elizabeth E. Umberfield Department of Epidemiology, Richard M. Fairbanks School of Public Health, Indiana University, Indianapolis, IN, USA; Center for Biomedical Informatics, Regenstrief Institute, Inc., Indianapolis, IN, USA; Division of Nursing Research, Mayo Clinic, Rochester, MN, USA

Nimish Valvi Center for Biomedical Informatics, Regenstrief Institute, Inc., Indianapolis, IN, USA

Joshua R. Vest Department of Health Policy and Management, Richard M. Fairbanks School of Public Health, Indiana University, Indianapolis, IN, USA; Center for Biomedical Informatics, Regenstrief Institute, Inc., Indianapolis, IN, USA

Jonathan Weiner Center for Population Health IT (CPHIT), Department of Health Policy and Management, Johns Hopkins School of Public Health, Baltimore, MD, USA

Hsyien-Chia Wen School of Healthcare Administration, College of Management, Taipei Medical University, Taipei, Taiwan

Dereje Woldehanna US Centers for Disease Control and Prevention, Addis Ababa, Ethiopia

Chantal Worzala Alazro Consulting LLC, Takoma Park, MD, USA

Foreword*

I was tickled by Dr. Dixon's invitation to write the foreword for this new edition of *Health Information Exchange: Navigating and Managing a Network of Health Information Systems*. It brought back memories of the halcyon days at Regenstrief Institute when we developed the world's first Health Information Exchange (HIE). We launched in 2003 with two tranches of funding from the U.S. National Library of Medicine and called it the Indianapolis Network for Patient Care (INPC). The initial version served three Indianapolis emergency rooms [1] and a few clinics. It then grew to include five independent health care organizations with a total of 13 hospitals and many smaller entities [2]. I remember thinking, as I walked into one of the CEO's offices to ask him to send all of his hospital's medical data to INPC, "there is no way they will say yes." But he and the other CEOs did say yes. Dr. Donald A.B. Lindberg remarked, "Clem has been there a long time. They trust him" [3]. However, I think they agreed because they were good people who sincerely wanted to provide Indianapolis care providers with the best patient care information they could. With the leadership, we developed a legal agreement [4] that specified what care, research, and public health purposes the INPC data could serve and under what circumstances, which eliminated many hospital concerns.

INPC carried data from all sources on one central system. This design was important, because it let us detect and fix errors as messages arrived and enabled us to support full-time experts who knew how to fix them. We developed algorithms to link all the registration records for given patient within, and across hospitals, and we mapped tests and measurement codes from each hospital to standard codes. With these two capabilities, INPC could present all medical data for a given patient in one unified display, as though the hospitals had merged. Readers will find the more complete story of Indiana's and two other successful HIEs in Chapters 22, 25, and 26, respectively.

We installed many hundreds of interfaces during the early years. Each interface between a source and INPC took 1–2 days, including the time to create a VPN connection over a T1 line and to fix problems in the structure and content of the incoming V2 HL7 message (Chapter 9), which was made easier as we switched to standard internet connections. In contrast, the semantic standardization (Chapter 10) of laboratory test codes required significant labor, typically 8–12 months of human effort. In an ideal world, we would deliver standard observation codes as part of the electronic results message, but with the exception of a few large, reference laboratories hospital systems, this has not yet happened. Everyone is keenly interested in having clinical data, but they ignore the importance of the coding standards required to make the data usable. Finally, I would add to the advice in Chapter 3 that policy makers should focus more closely on the need for inclusion of standard observation codes in test results messages, investigation of issues that prevent their inclusion, and assess the degree to which such codes are present and accurate.

The content in this book should serve as a strong reference text and guiding principles for those working to implement HIE in their state or nation. Hopefully with the knowledge in these pages, others will have similar success in the adoption and use of HIE networks that meaningfully transform care and outcomes around the world.

Clement J. McDonald
National Library of Medicine, Bethesda, MD, USA; Indiana University School of Medicine, Indianapolis, IN, USA

References

[1] Overhage JM, Tierney WM, McDonald CJ. Design and implementation of the Indianapolis Network for Patient Care and Research. Bull Med Libr Assoc 1995;83 (1):48–56.
[2] McDonald CJ, Overhage JM, Barnes M, Schadow G, Blevins L, Dexter PR, et al. INPC Management Committee The Indiana network for patient care: a working local health information infrastructure. Health Aff 2005;24(5):1214–20.
[3] McDonald CJ, Humphreys BL. The U.S. National Library of Medicine and Standards for Electronic Health Records: one thing led to another. Stud Health Technol Inform 2022;288:90. Available from: https://doi.org/10.3233/SHTI210984.
[4] Sears C, Prescott VM, McDonald CJ. The Indiana network for patient care: a case study of a successful healthcare data sharing agreement. American Bar Association Health eSource; 2005.

Preface

The world needs you. Individuals who understand the principles and best practices in health information exchange (HIE) are necessary to fix the flaws in modern health information systems, strengthen interoperability, and lead the organizations that manage HIE networks. It will take hundreds of HIE professionals and many thousands of HIE-savvy health professionals to design, develop, implement, and leverage future HIE networks and functionality to improve patient care and population health outcomes around the world. I hope this book plays a role in making that vision a reality.

I am pleased (and relieved) to offer the world the Second Edition of this book. Originally designed to meet my needs as a professor at Indiana University in my course on Health Information Exchange (which later became part of the AMIA 10 × 10 program), the book has been lauded by students as well as institutions around the globe. For example, the Health Information Management Systems Society (HIMSS) named the First Edition as its "Book of the Year" at its global conference in 2017. In 2019 a colleague texted me a photo of the book from East Africa where it was featured in a small library in a Centers for Disease Control and Prevention (CDC) field office. Feedback from readers over the past 6 years has filled me with pride and joy. I am delighted the First Edition made such an impact.

Comments from readers, including students, colleagues, and peers, also fueled my passion to update and strengthen the book. Upon reflection during the 2018 OpenHIE Community Meeting in Arusha, Tanzania, it became clear that the First Edition focused too much on HIE in the context of the United States. There were only a handful of examples from other nations, especially nations that possessed more robust HIE infrastructures than most areas of the United States. Moreover, technological advances, greater use of mobile devices, market consolidations, expansion of vendor-based HIE networks, and new policies passed by governments around the world focused on health IT and HIE necessitated more than a cosmetic update to the book. For these reasons, in 2019, I began in earnest to formulate a plan for updating the book for publication 5 years after its initial release. My goal was to take a sabbatical from the university during the second half of 2020 and focus my efforts solely on the refresh with an eye toward international collaboration involving travel to multiple destinations where HIE exists or was in progress. Just as I was finalizing plans for some of my travels, the COVID-19 pandemic emerged and changed the world forever, including the planned revisions for this book. The plan evolved multiple times during 2020 and 2021 with a new goal of publishing the Second Edition in summer or fall of 2022 coinciding with 6 years after the book's initial release.

I did not make it to all my originally planned destinations, and some international content could not be incorporated. However,

I was able to visit some sites and work (via Zoom) with many wonderful international collaborators on this edition. The pandemic further provided strong case examples and evidence on why HIE is so important. HIE networks rapidly responded to support their communities, especially providers and health professionals as well as public health workers on the frontlines of the COVID-19 pandemic who required information on those infected, hospitalized, and vaccinated. This was true in the United States and globally. These stories have been incorporated into the Second Edition as much as possible, and there are many references to numerous articles and websites that detail how HIE networks and organizations responded to provide data and information when needed at a time when information was scarce, and misinformation was rampant. Thus the pandemic only delayed production and publication; it did not permanently prevent the project from reaching fruition. It is unfortunate, however, that so many people had to suffer, die, or become burned out for nations to realize that our public health information infrastructure, including HIE networks, were deficient and need to be strengthened in preparation for global health phenomena like an emerging infectious disease.

Now more than ever, as the world emerges from the COVID-19 pandemic, HIE is essential for the future of health systems and the populations they serve. This edition builds upon a strong foundation but expands the breadth and depth of knowledge with respect to HIE networks. New case studies from multiple nations provide examples of working, robust information infrastructures that can be emulated around the globe. New chapters explore emerging areas in HIE that provide hope for the future. With robust HIE networks, a health system can deploy dashboards and data integrations that enable coordinated, accountable management of patients, populations, health workers, and resources under normal circumstances and in times of crisis. HIE networks can further support advancements in patient safety, quality, and person-centered care. Moreover, at the population level, HIE networks can facilitate achievement of universal health care, public health intelligence, and well-being for communities. I hope that the theories, approaches, and practices detailed in this text support health system leaders and students in confronting the challenges of today and the future.

Brian E. Dixon

Acknowledgments

I am delighted the group of authors represented in this book responded to my call to action on updating the text. Most are HIE organizational leaders or researchers who are internationally recognized experts in HIE theory, approaches, or practice. Others are health system leaders who helped develop and implement HIE approaches in their health system, or they are leaders who leverage HIE networks to facilitate clinical or public health decision-making in their community. Each of them is highly regarded and respected in their field by colleagues and peers. They dedicated many hours preparing and revising the content in this book, and I am honored to serve as the editor for their content. I could not have updated this text without their assistance in this journey, so I heartily thank them for their time and effort.

In addition, I wish to recognize and acknowledge multiple colleagues at the Regenstrief Institute who supported the development of this edition. Donna Schildbach supported my travel logistics, and she assisted in editing several final drafts. Jessica Halterman and Ashley Wiensch, MPH, from the Center for Biomedical Informatics helped manage the students working with me on research and drafting of content. They also managed research teams and projects I had to neglect while on sabbatical to finish this edition. I also thank Jennifer Shivers, MFA, and Jamie Thomas of the Global Health Informatics team for their help in recruiting and communicating with authors from the OpenHIE Community. I am indebted to the entire OpenHIE Community for not only agreeing to help cocreate multiple chapters but also in freely and graciously sharing their collective wisdom and resources on HIE, including many of the images readers will find throughout the book. In this edition, many of the OHIE authors are local experts who share their experiences in implementing HIE technologies in their countries—knowledge sharing critical to supporting the global HIE community.

Finally, I cannot express fully my love and gratitude for my wife, Kathryn Dixon, MEd, and sons who supported me as there were several occasions when I had to miss out on family time to write or edit a chapter. Thank you for your endless love and support!

SECTION 1

Health information exchange fundamentals

CHAPTER

1

Introduction to health information exchange

Brian E. Dixon[1,2]

[1]Department of Epidemiology, Richard M. Fairbanks School of Public Health, Indiana University, Indianapolis, IN, USA [2]Center for Biomedical Informatics, Regenstrief Institute Inc., Indianapolis, IN, USA

LEARNING OBJECTIVES

By the end of the chapter, the reader should be able to:

- Define the concept of health information exchange (HIE);
- Differentiate between the use of HIE as a noun and a verb;
- Differentiate between EHR and HIE systems;
- Discuss the evolution of HIE and lessons from early HIE efforts;
- Describe various archetypes and terminologies of HIE found around the world;
- List and describe the four core components of HIE; and
- Identify the roles that HIE plays in supporting health care and public health.

1.1 Introduction

Medicine, nursing, pharmacy, dentistry, and allied health professions are information-centric occupations [1,2]. Clinicians must navigate a large corpus of knowledge from the biomedical sciences and an endless stream of new facts, new treatments, and new diagnostic tools. Clinicians must further deal with information from an array of disparate sources, which they must process into decisions and prioritized tasks for the clinical team and patient [3–6]. Nonclinical roles must also review and input information about patients and populations to administer health care processes and organizations.

To support health care professionals in managing the array of information available about patients and populations, health systems have adopted and continue to incorporate a variety of information and communications technologies

Health Information Exchange
DOI: https://doi.org/10.1016/B978-0-323-90802-3.00013-7

(ICT) into the delivery and administration of health care. Over the last two decades, there has been a significant increase in the adoption and use of health ICT systems across the globe. In the United States, electronic health record (EHR) systems are ubiquitous in hospitals with 96% of non-Federal acute care hospitals reporting use of a certified system as of 2015 [7], and EHR systems are present in 86% of office-based practices [8]. Most nations in Europe, including Germany, Denmark, and Sweden, as well as Australia, New Zealand, and Canada report primary care practice access to EHR systems above 85%. Rates are lower in low- and middle-income countries, yet research shows that many nations in Asia, Africa, South America, and the Middle East have made progress in implementing EHR systems in the last 5–10 years [9–14]. Growth in adoption has been fueled by both policies, such as the Health Information Technology for Economic and Clinical Health (HITECH) Act [15,16] in the United States; Canadian federal investment in Canada Health Infoway and various provincial e-health initiatives [17]; and the belief that ICT systems can improve the quality, safety, and efficiency of health services and delivery [18–20].

Although EHR systems and other forms of health ICT have been demonstrated to be effective at improving health care delivery and outcomes, isolated ICT systems cannot maximize health outcomes because health care delivery occurs within the context of a highly complex system. Patients receive care in a variety of care settings. While there exist a number of health systems that organize (and sometimes manage under an umbrella corporation) primary care, inpatient, laboratory, radiology, and pharmacy services, patients have flexibility in where they receive care. Researchers at the Regenstrief Institute found high levels of patient crossover among emergency departments within and between health system networks [21]. Using data from 96 emergency departments representing over 7.4 million visits and 2.8 million patients over a 3-year period, the researchers found that on average 40% of visits involved patients with data at more than one emergency department. At 15 emergency departments, more than half of their encounters involved patients with data in other health system EHR systems. Similar studies find that providers can only access some of their patients' information via their EHR system and therefore ICT systems need to be better connected [22,23]. Such fragmentation of information can occur during specific episodes of care, say when a Veteran is discharged from a non-Veterans hospital to a Veterans home, or over the course of the lifetime as patients receive health care for a wide variety of acute and chronic illness.

Because information exists within ICT "silos" managed by various actors within the health system, patients often become the primary method of information transfer between providers [24]. Paper records as well as phone calls between hospital and clinic staff are also used to share information about a patient's status. These methods are undesirable for many reasons, including but not limited to inefficiency and the likelihood for error. For example, a study that validated parents' knowledge of their child's vaccination history found discrepancies in 13% of cases between what parents reported and what was recorded in an immunization information system [25]. Poor verbal information exchange between providers can often lead to medical errors [26,27]. To alleviate the burden placed on patients and improve efficiency in accessing information critical to care delivery, health systems establish information exchange between ICT systems. Health information exchange (HIE) enables more complete and timely sharing of data and information among ICT systems used in health care delivery, supporting provider and patient access to information when and where it is needed.

The purpose of this book is to provide a robust description of HIE, its various forms, its use around the world, its governance, and its technical design. Because HIE is critical to the success of health care improvement and reform around the world, this book aims to inform those in clinical practice, health care administration, public health, and information technology about HIE and its role in supporting health systems. This chapter defines HIE then describes the evolution of it within the US health system. This chapter further discusses the rise of HIE in other countries and describes the various forms of HIE found in health systems around the world. The end of the chapter describes the goals and structure of the book, arming the reader with tools for applying the information to their profession.

1.2 Health information exchange

HIE is defined as the electronic transfer of patient-level health-related data or information across diverse and often competing organizations across the health ecosystem. Note that the term transfer can denote either an active push of data or the retrieval (pull) of data, and it can also denote viewing information that might reside in a virtual environment (e.g., app, web browser). The key differentiator for HIE is that a health worker in a hospital can send, receive, or view data from another clinic or hospital that likely uses a different information system to store information about patients or populations. In practice, the term HIE is often used both as a *verb* and a *noun*.

1.2.1 HIE as a verb

As a verb, or action word, HIE refers to movement of data or information electronically among stakeholders in the health system. The stakeholders are many in size and shape, including doctors' offices, hospitals, laboratories, payors (e.g., insurance companies), pharmacies, urgent care centers, retail-based clinics, home health agencies, long-term postacute care facilities (e.g., nursing homes), public health departments (e.g., ministries of health), federally qualified health centers, and/or mental health providers. The methods for sharing or moving data also vary, and they can include pushing information to the next care providers, retrieving data from a medical record system managed by another organizations, or viewing information managed centrally by a governmental agency (e.g., immunization registry). The information exchanged can range too, from a care plan to a summary of a visit to a laboratory result to a medical history. And while faxes are electronic forms of ICT thus technically HIE, most people tend to conceive of HIE as supporting efforts to move health care organizations away from faxing analog, unstructured documents toward the exchange of digital, structured information that can be readily consumed and acted upon by computer systems (e.g., semantic interoperability). Yet, as you will come to find out from information and examples in this book, many current forms of HIE occurring all over the world involve the transmission of largely unstructured information in the form of an electronic fax, PDF (Portable Document Format), or a dictated clinical report. Indeed, health systems are in a state of transition toward completely digital health data and information that can be readily exchanged using HIE techniques, but this transition is a work-in-progress for most nations.

1.2.2 HIE as a noun

The noun use of HIE refers to an organization, usually a legal corporation, that facilitates information exchange (the verb form) within a network of facilities or at the level of a community, state, or region. While the exact form and composition of the entity or corporation varies [28], as you will note from reading the case studies, many communities and nations are organizing HIE activities under an entity that can facilitate the trust, governance, and technical aspects of information sharing within an enterprise, community, state, or nation. This is because HIE involves sharing or transferring sensitive information about a person and most societies in the world value an individual's right to privacy. Therefore HIE occurs within a complex frame of not only multiple health care providers but also legal and regulatory policies that govern how health information should be protected as it is captured, stored, and shared.

Organizations that facilitate the technical services and legal/regulatory governance necessary for HIE are referred to as *Health Information Organizations* or HIOs. Often a third-party nonprofit corporation is best suited to manage the human, regulatory, and technical aspects of data sharing as opposed to diffusing these responsibilities across each health care provider that participates in the exchange of data. In other instances, an HIO may be a division of a hospital or network of health care facilities that need to facilitate the exchange of information among disparate, standalone ICT systems within an enterprise [e.g., large tertiary care hospital, integrated delivery network (IDN), group of federally qualified health centers]. The various types of HIOs that exist are defined further in this chapter.

1.2.2.1 How HIE is used in this book

In this book, we consider HIE principally as a verb, emphasizing the electronic exchange of data or information among various stakeholders within the health system. However, because HIE is often facilitated in a community, state, or nation by an organization, we will refer to *HIO* when speaking about the noun form of HIE. In putting the book together, we try to be consistent in the use of these two acronyms: HIE and HIO. However, we may occasionally get it wrong or mixed up. Sometimes, we use HIE network instead of HIO. Spotting such mix-ups will be good practice for the real-world as you will encounter a variety of uses and terms when reading the sources referenced in the book as well as many other documents that discuss HIE in both the academic and gray literature.

Several synonyms and, quite frankly, confusing alternative terms used to describe HIE on websites and published documents are summarized in Table 1.1. Please note that alternative terms are not always true synonyms, although their use is common enough many people perceive them to be synonyms. Preferred terms used in this book are suggested for your use as well when writing or speaking about HIE.

1.2.3 Typology of Health Information Organizations

While HIE as a verb can exist in a wide variety of forms (e.g., secure email of a document from a primary care physician to a specialist, secure file transfer from a hospital to a public health department containing preclinical diagnosis information for patients showing up at an emergency department), organized HIE activities by an HIO generally take one of the following forms: (1) enterprise HIE, (2) government-facilitated HIE, (3) community-based HIE, (4) vendor-facilitated HIE, or (5) health record banking (e.g., patient-mediated exchange). In the following subsections, we examine each form of HIE.

1.2.3.1 Enterprise HIE

While there still exist "independent" hospitals and physician practices (e.g., management of the hospital or practice is solely performed by the physicians or CEO), many hospitals, physician practices, nursing homes, and even public health clinics operate as part of a larger for-profit, public, or nonprofit organization, referred to often as health systems, hospital systems, or IDNs. The differences in labels

TABLE 1.1 Terms, synonyms, and alternatives commonly used to describe the fundamentals of HIE.

Preferred terms associated with HIE in practice	Description of term	Commonly used alternatives and synonyms
Send	Action in which health data or information is transferred from one information system to another information system managed by a different organization. For example, a hospital sends a discharge summary to the primary care physician responsible for follow up care.	Push and directed exchange
Retrieve	Action in which one information system queries health data or information from another information system managed by a different organization. For example, a physician uses their EHR system to retrieve a radiology report stored in an emergency department information system.	Pull and query-based exchange
View	Action in which a health information system user in one organization looks at health data or information managed by a different organization. A nurse practitioner in a primary care clinic uses a web browser to view a list of medications prescribed to the patient by providers at the hospital upon discharge.	Access and portal-based exchange
Network	A set of information systems that use communication protocols over digital interconnections to communicate with one another.	Data network, wide area network, and local area network
Document	A written, printed, or typed electronic record that summarizes medical care (e.g., diagnoses, treatment, outcomes) provided to a patient. For example, a hospital might scan a printed discharge summary from another hospital into a PDF that becomes a document stored in the local EHR.	PDF, report, CCD, CDA, and scan
HIO	Nonprofit or for-profit legal corporation, or division of a health system, that facilitates the technical services and governance necessary for HIE to occur among providers, health systems, cities, regions, states, or a nation or nations.	RHIO, QHIN, NHIN, and Community HIO

depend on the governance structure or the composition of the organization (i.e., inclusion of hospitals, outpatient practices, insurance plans). Notable examples include Kaiser Permanente, Geisinger Health, Mayo Clinic, the MD Anderson Cancer Network, and the Veterans Health Administration (VHA). Because these health systems are composed of two or more hospitals, physician practices, or other care facilities, they have a need to exchange data and information among the network or group of affiliate organizations. Additionally, individual hospitals or practices, or even systems may be part of an accountable care organizations (ACOs). ACOs are not individual organizations themselves, but they are more of an arrangement of services around payment methods [29]. An individual health system may offer an ACO itself, or partner with other provider organizations (e.g., specialists) in an ACO arrangement. In this respect, ACOs also need to exchange data and information interorganizationally.

When a health system fosters information exchange among its affiliates, we refer to this as *Enterprise HIE* because the exchange is only within a narrowly defined network of organizations [28]. For example, the VHA, part of the US Department of Veterans Affairs, operates 171 medical centers as well as 1283 ambulatory care and community-based outpatient clinics across the United States and its territories. In the early 2000s, the VHA connected its facilities using a software program referred to as VistaWeb (now referred to as the Joint Legacy Viewer or JLV). The software is an Internet-based viewer in which clinicians at the VHA medical center in Indianapolis, Indiana can access documents such as the discharge summary from the VHA medical center in Palo Alto, California for a veteran who had a surgery in Palo Alto last year while visiting his grandchildren. This is enterprise HIE because the VHA medical center cannot look up information on facilities outside VHA (although this is changing as described elsewhere in the book), only those facilities managed by VHA. Vest and Simon [30] refer to this form of HIE as *intrasystem exchange*.

1.2.3.2 Community-based HIE

Community-based HIE involves exchange of data and information among providers and health care organizations located in a geographic region that may be marketplace competitors or otherwise unaffiliated, meaning they have no ownership relationship with each other. For example, an academic medical center, large hospital system, and group of federally qualified health centers might agree to exchange data for better serving low-incoming populations in an urban area. While they compete in the marketplace, these organizations recognize they are better served through HIE because they routinely observe patient crossover, which can lead to repeating tests and procedures for patients who receive uncompensated care. If each organization became more aware of these patients' history, they might be able to save money while sparing patients from unnecessary care. Vest and Simon [30] refer to community-based HIE as *intersystem exchange*.

Typically, community-based HIE efforts are facilitated by an HIO that operates within a specific geographic area (e.g., city, county, state, region). Vest and Menachemi [28] also refer to community HIOs as "public" exchanges because these entities are often managed by nonprofit community corporations that are transparent and public facing. Examples of community-based HIOs include the Indiana Health Information Exchange in Indianapolis, IN (ihie.org, see Chapter 22), CRISP (crisphealth.org, see Chapter 25), and DHIN (dhin.org). A key distinguishing feature of community-based HIE is that the HIO is driven by priorities set by its Board or governance group, which is often composed of Chief Information Officers (CIOs), ICT Directors, HIE Managers, or Chief Medical Informatics Officers (CMIOs) at the various organizations that participate in the HIO. Sometimes HIOs can also have Board members from the larger community, including community foundation directors, elected officials, large employers, and patients.

1.2.3.3 Government-facilitated HIE

The HITECH Act provided not only eligible US hospitals and providers with incentives for adopting EHR systems but also funding for the Office of the National Coordinator for Health Information Technology (ONC) to stimulate HIE. Since March 2010, ONC has invested over $500 million in state-based HIE programs [31]. To apply for funding from ONC, each state needed to identify a state-designated entity to receive and manage HIE efforts within the state. While some states designated entities such as quality improvement organizations or a single HIO within the state, most states elected to designate a state government agency (e.g., Governor's office, Medicaid office) to receive and manage the funding given the close ties between HIE and the state's efforts to encourage EHR adoption among Medicaid providers. Although some state government agencies redistributed funds to HIOs within the state to support local HIE efforts, many states created a state-level HIE organization. For example, in Michigan, the state created the Michigan Health Information Network (MiHIN) Shared Services which is a collection of shared software and professional services at the state level. Qualified organizations, state agencies, and community HIEs that demonstrate technical capability and execute the appropriate legal agreements can connect to MiHIN for several statewide HIE services such as public health reporting.

Thus, when state governments or other municipal organizations act as either a statewide HIO or primary facilitator of HIE within state boundaries, we refer to this as *government-facilitated HIE*. This designation distinguishes these activities, which are driven by public policy and agency priorities (e.g., alignment with Medicaid programs), from the efforts of enterprise HIE, which are usually driven by the priorities of a private health system. Likewise, the control of the HIO by a government agency distinguishes government-facilitated HIE from community-based HIE, even though both types of HIOs work with health care providers on HIE initiatives. Furthermore, community HIOs may be receive public funding for their services. Government-facilitated HIE efforts are unique in that they typically operate at a technical level that supports a "network of networks" in which data and information are "pushed" or "pulled" from provider A to provider B at a single point in time. However, the information pushed or pulled is typically not stored in a central data repository or retained by the municipal HIE network. Such a model allows each state to have multiple HIOs and other entities that operate independently of the statewide network and focus on community-level HIE activities.

The former Nationwide Health Information Network (now referred to as the eHealth Exchange) is an example of a government-facilitated HIE. The network was initiated by the US Federal government, which established a set of HIE services that could be leveraged to enable exchange of information among networks including enterprise HIE networks (e.g., the VHA) and community-based HIE networks [32]. Often one of the organizations involved in the HIE was a federal agency, such as the Social Security Administration (SSA; see Chapter 26). However, the network was also used for exchange of data that did not involve the federal government. In 2012, the network became a public–private partnership as the number of nongovernment networks expanded.

Although the eHealth Exchange is a public–private partnership, it simply connects other networks to one another and establishes "rules of the road" for information as it travels from Boston to San Francisco. Furthermore, much of the network focuses on meeting the needs of federal health partners such as the SSA and VHA. Because of its focus and technical methods for exchange, the network continues to be viewed as government-facilitated HIE rather than as community-based HIE.

1.2.3.4 Vendor-facilitated HIE

HIE that is facilitated by an EHR system vendor such as the Cerner Corporation (Kansas City, MO) is referred to as *vendor-facilitated HIE*. Like the Enterprise form, the vendor layers a set of HIE services on top of its EHR infrastructure, enabling its customers to send or receive information to other customers of that vendor's EHR system. And like the community-based form, many vendor HIE services enable exchange of information with hospitals and facilities outside a given IDN. Each vendor network establishes rules for exchange and controls which outside entities are connected for data sharing. Yet, unlike the other HIE forms, vendor-based HIE solutions are driven by company priorities not public agencies or community-driven consensus. Although customers may make requests to the company, influencing decisions are more challenging than in other forms of HIE. Furthermore, new capabilities may come with a price tag when vendors control the network.

An example of this form of HIE is Care Everywhere from Epic Systems (Verona, WI). End users can click an "outside records" button while viewing a patient's chart. The clinician then searches for another institution part of the network (e.g., another Epic customer). Once an institution is selected, the provider then searches for the patient within the EHR system of that institution. The provider then enters a reason for the query and completes an authorization form attesting to the need for the release of medical information. Finally, the information from the other EHR is available for viewing.

Initially, vendor-facilitated HIE networks only connected customers of the single vendor's EHR platform to one another. Even though the other customers might be across the state or located in another state, the network did not connect to health systems that used another vendor's EHR. In recent years, this is changing with the growth of multivendor networks. Examples of multivendor networks include Car*e*quality and the CommonWell Health Alliance from the Cerner Corporation (Kansas City, MO). Like the government-facilitated HIE model, multivendor networks often allow clinicians to view documents from another health system using a different EHR platform, but the data are not retained once the clinician closes the document. The information available might also be more limited than that available through a community-based HIO.

1.2.3.5 Health record banking

Health record banking consists of an organization (e.g., nonprofit, commercial business) that offers consumers a secure, digital repository into which electronic medical records from various providers can be deposited. As consumers seek care from other providers, information can be withdrawn when the patient provides consent. In essence, health record banks (HRBs) act as vendor-agnostic patient portals or personal health record (PHR) applications [33]. Consumers control what information is deposited and when information can be withdrawn. According to the health record banking alliance, consumers can also use tools to clean up and reconcile the information stored in their account. This type of HIE could therefore be classified as *patient-mediated exchange* as the consumer is in the driver's seat.

Unlike vendor-facilitated HIE, HRBs are typically offered by a community organization rather than a PHR tethered to a specific EHR vendor's platform. As opposed to community-based HIEs in which all provider participants contribute data about a patient, consumers can choose whether or not records from a given provider are deposited into the account. For example, a patient might choose to not deposit records from their mental health counselor or primary care provider. Advocates for HRBs argue that banks should be decentralized and operated by local organizations as opposed to statewide entities [34]. Advocates further argue that HRBs promote consumer engagement, error correction, and data for population health management and research [35].

An example of an HRB is the Lower Saxony Bank of Health (LSBH), founded in 2011 [36]. Health care providers were connected to the bank, which maintained a list of all patients (customers) and providers. Instead of centralizing data at the bank, the bank identified patients' records at the various health care providers, maintaining a list of where patients' records were stored. Patients authorized providers to access documents from other providers using standards developed by the international Integrating the Healthcare Enterprise (IHE) organization. The bank was incorporated in Germany as an "entrepreneurial company" and marketed as a "neutral third-party information broker." Unfortunately, the website for LSBH cannot be found, and whether it remains operational could not be verified at the time of publication.

Moreover, the publication which describes LSBH [36] identifies a dozen other HRB initiatives, including Microsoft Vault and the Oregon HRB. Operational status could only be verified for only one entity: NoMoreClipboard [37], which markets itself as a PHR.

A challenge for HRBs is financing [38]; many of them desired for providers to pay for operations while making the services free to consumers. Today there are multiple efforts to develop patient-facing application programming interfaces (APIs) in which patients can access their health data to become mediators of their information. For example, Apple Inc. uses the SMART on FHIR (Fast Healthcare Interoperability Resources) standard to allow patients to download their medical records from providers' EHR systems. Downloadable data types include allergies, conditions, immunizations, lab results, medications, and vitals. Currently the development of patient-facing APIs rests on providers who essentially pay for these services that benefit patients (for free). It is too early to tell whether this model may face similar challenges to HRBs or disrupt existing HRB efforts.

1.2.4 Fundamental components of HIE

Although there exist various forms and types of HIE, fundamentally there are just a few core components to any type of HIE. At a basic level, to conduct HIE, there must exist two health system actors with an established relationship that have a need to send or receive information about a patient or population. These components are illustrated in Fig. 1.1 and discussed as follows.

1.2.4.1 Health system actors and relationships

In order for information to be exchanged, there needs to be a reason for conducting the exchange. Therefore every form of HIE requires at least two actors who have an established

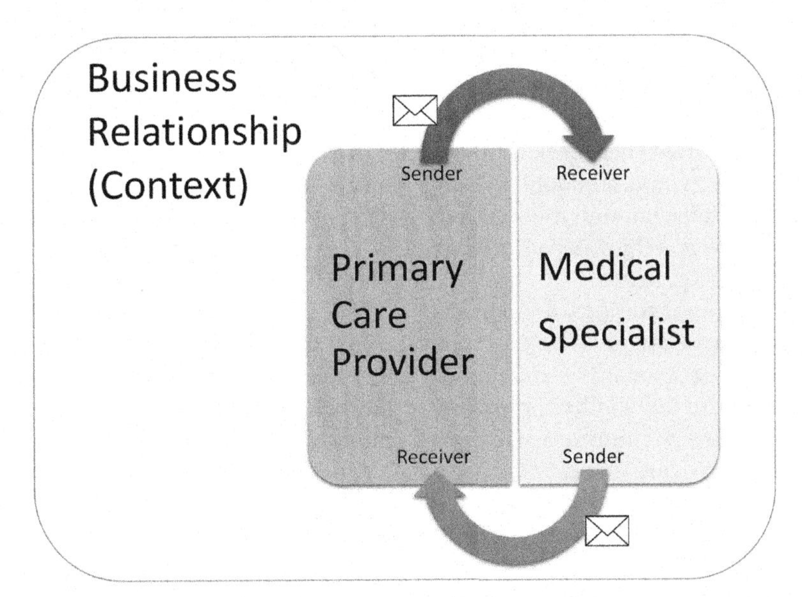

FIGURE 1.1 Graphical representation of the fundamental components of health information exchange. Information is exchanged in transactions between a sender and a receiver, and the exchange of information takes place within the context of a business relationship that governs the sharing of information between the two entities.

relationship that facilitates HIE. Organizations have numerous, complex relationships to people and other organizations. For example, organizations employ people which creates a social contract in which employees perform duties in exchange for remuneration and other compensation (e.g., health benefits, 401(k) plan). When organizations have relationships with other organizations, they often codify these through contracts or business associate agreements. Physician practices can have relationships with a hospital or health system that outlines things such as patient referrals and physician admitting privileges. Public health agencies have relationships with hospitals and clinics, which are often obligated to report cases of communicable disease to the agencies.

In many cases, the existing relationships between actors in the health system provide a foundation for HIE. Suppose that Dr. Smith works in his private physician practice on Mondays and Wednesdays and at the hospital outpatient clinic on Tuesdays and Thursdays. When a nurse at the practice calls Dr. Smith while he is at the hospital clinic, he can relay information about a patient to the nurse and he might be accessing via the hospital EHR system. Now if the nurse at the practice were to access the hospital EHR data directly from her desk without involving Dr. Smith, this would probably be facilitated by private HIE, either through a portal into the hospital EHR system or a third-party software that connects the two ICT systems.

In other instances, organizations negotiate a specific data usage agreement whereby one organization releases or exchanges data with another organization for an explicit purpose. Consider, for example, a community health system with four acute care hospitals and a long-term care provider with eight nursing homes. Although these organizations perform different health services in the community, they may wish to work together to create efficiencies during transfers of care (e.g., which a patient is discharged from the hospital to a nursing home). The organizations may enter into a transfer agreement that allows for the general transfer of patients and information when medical needs necessitate a transfer of care. However, to improve efficiency, the organizations may wish to connect their respective ICT systems for HIE instead of rely upon paper-based transfer documents. These organization may now need to execute a business associate agreement pursuant to HIPAA regulations, which govern the disclosure of protected health information. In doing so, the organizations make explicit what detailed patient-level information each organization will share through HIE between their respective ICT systems.

In either scenario, two or more actors have a relationship that underlies the need for exchange of information about patients or populations. Executing agreements and codifying relationships becomes more complex when there are greater than two actors, and managing many two-way relationships can be challenging. Managing relationships, agreements, and multiple actors is therefore a core function of HIE and HIOs, and the complexities often overshadow the technological methods by which data are exchanged between two or more actors. These challenges and models for facilitating multiple organization HIE are covered in greater detail later in this book.

1.2.4.2 ICT Systems

HIE as we have defined it necessitates electronic transfer between ICT systems. Therefore ICT systems need technical methods for facilitating exchange of information. In ICT speak, there must be a *sender* and a *receiver*. For example, a laboratory information system (LIS) *sends* laboratory test results to an EHR system to record the results in a patient's records. Yet, an LIS can also *receive* an order to perform a laboratory test from an EHR system. These electronic transactions provide the technical foundation for HIE. Almost any ICT system in health care can be either a sender or a receiver depending on the scenario. Therefore the potential configuration of technical networks involving ICT are many. Regardless of which ICT systems are involved in HIE or the direction in which information flows, there will be senders and receivers. Several chapters in this book describe in greater detail the technologies that support sending and receiving health information among networks of ICT systems.

1.2.4.3 *Transactions or messages*

Electronic transactions in health care can be conceived of as messages between two people or organizations. In the physical world, messages take the form of envelopes and packages. Envelopes and packages come in all shapes, sizes, and weights, so do electronic transactions. For example, electronically transmitting information that a particular patient has arrived at the clinic and is waiting to see the doctor is akin to putting a single, small piece of paper into a small envelope. Exchanging a discharge summary is like sending a multiple page document in a large envelope. This transaction requires additional "overhead" or structure so that the receiving ICT system can interpret the information inside the envelope. Still greater requirements are needed for the exchange of a magnetic resonance imaging (MRI) scan that includes large, detailed images. A special envelope would be necessary to protect the image from getting bent or damaged in transit. Similarly, ICT systems would require a specialized, structured message and sufficient storage as well as transport capacity for transferring the MRI images. Specialized, structured messages are referred to in the HIE world as technical standards. When ICT systems can send and receive messages, we say they can interoperate or possess interoperability. This book contains several chapters that explain the technical standards that enable the various kinds of messages to be sent and received by health ICT systems.

1.2.4.4 *Content or payload*

Inside of messages are contents—patient demographics, laboratory results, and images. ICT speak sometimes refers to contents as payloads. While in transit from one ICT system to another, the technologies that facilitate the transport do not care about the contents inside the message. However, for the information exchanged to be stored and used by the receiving ICT system (as well as the system's users—humans), ICT systems need methods for understanding the message contents. In HIE, we refer to these methods as data standards, which we say create semantic interoperability between ICT systems. This book is full of examples and a couple of chapters that illustrate the importance of data standards and the need for semantic interoperability.

1.3 Evolution of health information exchange in the United States

The concept of HIE has been around for more than 30 years. In the 1990s, the John A. Hartford Foundation began a Community Health Management Information System (CHMIS) initiative aimed at improving access to data in support of cost and quality improvement [39]. The idea was to support IDNs' access to information by engaging health care stakeholders (the members of the network) to electronically exchange transactions that would feed central data repositories. Large investments were made in several states to form what became known as Community Health Information Networks (CHINs). Despite many intellectually supporting the notion of a CHIN [40], most CHINs failed due to a number of reasons, including:

1. Lack of Stakeholder Engagement—Most CHINs did not create shared mission that all stakeholders could rally around. In many markets, the competitive nature

overshadowed the weak or poorly conceived mission of the CHIN.
2. Command and Control—Stakeholders, especially providers outside the IDN, often perceived the IDN or health system to be in control of the centralized repository, which bred fear in highly competitive markets. Vendors also "pushed" their proprietary technology platform from the beginning, creating skepticism among the health care executives. A general lack of control ensued and thus no one was really in charge.
3. Unclear Value Proposition—From the beginning, CHIN developers asserted that stakeholders would see benefits after the development and usage of the CHIN. However, stakeholders were not provided with clear evidence or information on the value-add of the CHIN. Quickly the stakeholders lost interest in continuing to finance the CHIN when they could not perceive value to their organization.
4. Infrastructure Woes—Many CHINs aimed to create a large, common data repository into which stakeholders would put claims, encounter data, problem lists, medications, etc. However, the Internet did not yet exist so it was difficult (and expensive) to "wire" all of the stakeholders and create a sufficient infrastructure. Furthermore, the politics of a single data "pot" further exacerbated fears over control.

On the heels of the CHINs, a number of communities began to develop a Local Health Information Infrastructure (LHII). Whereas the CHINs focused on supporting exchange of data to meet the needs of IDNs facilitating managed care, LHIIs focused on clinician-driven, community-wide initiatives focused in scope. For example, providers in the Indianapolis area desired to share information among emergency departments in support of transitions of care [40]. In addition, LHIIs focused on first developing stakeholder engagement rather than jumping directly into discussions around the design of the technical architecture. Emphasis was placed on building trust and establishing a strong, shared vision for what services the LHII would provide and for whom they would be provided. In addition, LHIIs seemed to incorporate a few other factors that resulted in greater success over their CHIN predecessors:

1. Clear Control from a Neutral Third Party—Successful LHIIs engaged a neutral, respected organization to take ownership of community engagement activities. In Indianapolis, it was a health services research organization affiliated with the medical school. In Santa Barbara, California, it was a regional health plan. These parties helped facilitate dialogue, establish trust among the partners, and mobilize leaders without appearing biased toward a particular vendor, platform, or the IDN.
2. Involvement of Public Health—Early LHIIs engaged public health authorities. Sometimes the health department served as the trusted neutral party. In other instances, the LHII simply brought knowledge and experience in coalition building around a health issue to the group.
3. Communication and Change Management—The LHIIs paid particular attention to keeping stakeholders "in the loop," even though it meant many hours of meetings and phone calls for the leadership and managing partner. However, strong communication allowed for reiteration of reasonable expectations and kept committees and volunteers focused.
4. Attention to Legal and Financial Barriers—LHII leadership spent significant time discussing and developing strategies for overcoming both legal issues as well as the plan for sustaining data exchange after a period of initial investment.

Although arguably more successful than the CHINs, many LHIIs also failed to become fully operational or sustain operations [41]. Yet, their failures and successes proved to be excellent lessons for the next generation of HIE organizations—the Regional Health Information Organizations (RHIOs). RHIOs emerged about 10 years ago to tackle the very thorny issue of sustainability. Whereas the LHIIs emphasized "local" by engaging stakeholders in a city or county, RHIOs aimed to become regional HIE authorities. The idea was that HIE might not be sustainable on a small scale but would be sustainable with economies of scale across an entire state or group of states. Several RHIOs were funded through grants by the Agency for Healthcare Research and Quality [42–44]. Using the funding, the RHIOs aimed to not only become operational but also develop the business case for HIE [45]. Surveys from the late 2000s by the eHealth Initiative found that over 100 communities reported, they were in various stages of developing an RHIO [46,47]. Yet, like many LHIIs, many RHIOs failed for similar reasons as their antecedents [48,49]. As many as 25% of efforts identified in the previous year's survey would simply vanish when community efforts were surveyed the following year.

Since the passage of the HITECH Act, HIE in the United States has received a large investment from the government. Funding to create statewide HIE efforts pushed the industry to drop the "R" from RHIO. Furthermore, emerging HIOs began to diversify with respect to form (e.g., centralized data repository), technology platform (e.g., push, pull), and governance. While some focused on supporting IDNs, others focused on creating "networks of networks" in which HIE could be performed by a wider array of local-, regional-, and national-level stakeholders. National-level HIE efforts emerged, including the eHealth Exchange [50] that connects state and regional HIE initiatives with federal government agencies as well as national data networks such as SureScripts, LLC. In 2019, the Meaningful Use program transition into the Promoting Interoperability program, spurring additional focus on HIE [51]. The landscape of HIE changed dramatically over the last decade, yet the core lessons or principles of the CHINs and LHIIs remain. HIOs must establish value to stakeholders to generate sustainable revenue streams in order to grow toward achieving a shared vision. This point is well illustrated in a recent study [52] that showed the total number of operational HIE networks in the United States declined between 2014 and 2019, yet the number of HIE networks self-reported to be financially viable remained relatively stable.

The COVID-19 pandemic demonstrated the value of HIE to many stakeholders in health systems around the world. In the United States, it became abundantly clear that data on laboratory results, hospitalizations, emergency department visits, and vaccinations all need to be captured digitally and shared with others in order to coordinate care and monitor population health [53]. HIE organizations across the United States created valuable services quickly in the wake of COVID-19 [54], and hospital systems previously reluctant to participate in HIE chose to join due to valuable services offered by entities with an available infrastructure ready to support the health system during a crisis. Moreover, nations with robust HIE were able to leverage their capabilities to deploy solutions for vaccine passports and test results quickly. Other nations struggled to implement workarounds during the pandemic. Perhaps a silver lining of the pandemic was a clear demonstration to the world that HIE is a necessary component of every nation's digital health infrastructure.

1.4 HIE outside the United States

The concept of HIE is not uniquely American [55]. Nations such as Denmark (see Chapter 28) and Israel (see Chapter 31) have more advanced health data integration than most US states. Over the last decade, a significant number of HIE efforts emerged all over the world [56–59], including several in low- and middle-income countries (LMICs, see Chapter 29). Perceptions and conceptualization of HIE as well as the maturity of HIE efforts differ by region as well as nation.

What distinguishes international HIE activities from those in the United States is often the definition or perception of what constitutes HIE. For example, most HIOs in the United States conceive HIE often as a broad set of services or functions that facilitate specific transactions in which information is exchanged for a defined purpose (e.g., results delivery, referral, discharge summary). In many countries, HIE is conceived more as a national-level, patient-centric EHR or a longitudinal record of care received by a person over his or her lifetime [60]. Thus many of the HIE functions defined and discussed in the United States occur in other countries through provincial or national health authorities rather than private health systems, and rarely are they defined explicitly as HIE. Yet, when emergency department clinicians from five different countries were interviewed about obtaining information from outside of his or her hospital, their experiences and challenges with HIE were quite similar [59].

In 2012, the World Health Organization (WHO) published a National eHealth Strategy Toolkit [61] that supports national-level establishment of a roadmap and action plan for the adoption of health ICT as well as HIE. Although the explicit term HIE is only mentioned a couple of times in the "Infrastructure" section, the report nonetheless guides ministries of health toward planning for the exchange of data and information between ICT systems they implement. For example, the WHO suggests that the critical components of a national eHealth environment [61] include:

1. Infrastructure—The foundations for electronic information exchange across geographical and health-sector boundaries. This includes physical infrastructure (e.g., networks), core services, and applications that underpin a national eHealth environment.
2. Standards and Interoperability—ICT standards that enable consistent and accurate collection and exchange of health information across health systems and services.

The toolkit and subsequent follow-up from the WHO eHealth Technical Advisory Group [62] are driving creation and adoption of national eHealth strategies. Moreover, several nations have explicitly called out HIE and interoperability in their national e-Health strategies. Activities in multiple nations supported the development of a Community of Practice in which members share knowledge as well as standards-based approaches and reference technologies for facilitating HIE. This initiative, known as OpenHIE (ohie.org), seeks "to improve the health of the underserved through the open collaborative development and support of country driven, large scale health information sharing architectures." Currently multiple nations are using the OpenHIE framework and community to implement HIE infrastructures, including Haiti, Ethiopia, West Africa, Kenya, Tanzania, and Rwanda.

Because there are now many working HIE infrastructure around the world, this edition of the book features multiple case studies that examine HIE networks outside the US Instructors are encouraged to use these case studies in their classrooms, and health system leaders are encouraged to read them for application of lessons to the development, implementation, and use of HIE.

1.5 Purpose and structure of this book

The purpose of this book is to cover the landscape of HIE for those in health administration, health policy, health ICT (clinical informatics), and public health. While there exist many peer-reviewed articles, whitepapers, and webinars on HIE, there are few comprehensive resources on HIE. As already alluded in this chapter, HIE is much more than simply connecting ICT systems together using hardware and software. The various information sources on HIE to date provide snapshots of these dimensions, analyzing a technical method, legal framework, or governance model. In this book, we put the dimensions together as a reference for those studying or practicing HIE. In this second edition of the book, we expand the breadth and depth of HIE information by incorporating recent developments from the field and international efforts toward broad adoption of interoperability.

This book is divided into multiple sections that provide in-depth coverage of HIE and its dimensions. This first section provides an overview of HIE as a specialized field of study and practice within the larger profession of health (clinical) informatics. It further examines policies and other drivers that encourage the adoption and use of HIE. The next section introduces readers to the organizational and managerial aspects of HIE, including privacy as well as cybersecurity of health information. Then the book examines the technical architectures and building blocks of HIE, critical to enabling data sharing across the health care ecosystem. The fourth section reviews how HIE impacts health care delivery processes as well as patient and population outcomes. Increasingly there is emphasis on HIE to leverage the growing volumes of health care data for informing ways to streamline delivery, reduce costs, and strengthen the quality of care. This section further looks ahead at where HIE and HIOs seek to go in the future. The final section contains a collection of case studies in HIE from HIOs around the world that illustrate the various dimensions, forms, and aspects of HIE. At the end of the book, the reader should have a firm grasp on both the complexities involved in HIE and information critical for forging a strategy for developing, implementing, and/or managing HIE activities in their own nation, health system, or community.

1.6 Summary

A growing evidence base and the COVID-19 pandemic make it apparent that HIE is necessary to realize the full value of health ICT. Yet, HIE is complex and challenging, requiring not only robust technical infrastructure and standards but also legal, regulatory, governance, and policy frameworks that facilitate the adoption and use of HIE. Exchange of information also requires trust and strong relationships among health system organizations and their leaders. This book provides information on the foundations and nature of HIE as well as guidance on how to manage HIE within a complex environment, be that a regional health system or nation.

Questions for discussion

1. Compare and contrast the various types of HIE. Which type of HIE might afford the greatest value to a critical access hospital? What about a large physician practice?
2. What is the role of an HIO? Why might a community wish to use an HIO rather than just ask the largest hospital system IT department to manage HIE for the region?
3. Which lesson from the CHINs and LHIIs is most important to modern HIE initiatives?
4. Why might a global pandemic like COVID-19 change attitudes toward HIE?
5. How do the definitions of HIE vary around the world? Why might HIE be implemented differently in a country outside the United States?

References

[1] Krumholz HM. Big data and new knowledge in medicine: the thinking, training, and tools needed for a learning health system. Health Aff (Proj Hope) 2014;33 (7):1163–70. Available from: https://doi.org/10.1377/hlthaff.2014.0053.

[2] McGowan JJ, Passiment M, Hoffman HM. Educating medical students as competent users of health information technologies: the MSOP data. Stud Health Technol Inform 2007;129(Pt 2):1414–18.

[3] Singh H, Spitzmueller C, Petersen NJ, Sawhney MK, Sittig DF. Information overload and missed test results in electronic health record-based settings. JAMA Intern Med 2013;173(8):702–4. Available from: https://doi.org/10.1001/2013.jamainternmed.61.

[4] Markman M. Information overload in oncology practice and its potential negative impact on the delivery of optimal patient care. Curr Oncol Rep 2011;13 (4):249–51. Available from: https://doi.org/10.1007/s11912-011-0179-7.

[5] Zeldes N, Baum N. Information overload in medical practice. J Med Pract Manage MPM 2011;26(5):314–16.

[6] Bernard E, Arnould M, Saint-Lary O, Duhot D, Hebbrecht G. Internet use for information seeking in clinical practice: a cross-sectional survey among French general practitioners. Int J Med Inf 2012;81 (7):493–9. Available from: https://doi.org/10.1016/j.ijmedinf.2012.02.001.

[7] Henry J, Pylypchuk Y, Searcy T, Patel V. Adoption of electronic health record systems among U.S. Non-Federal Acute Care Hospitals: 2008–2015. Washington DC: Office of the National Coordinator for Health Information Technology; 2016 [updated May 2016; cited 2021 Oct 28]. ONC Data Brief No. 35. Available from: https://www.healthit.gov/data/data-briefs/adoption-electronic-health-record-systems-among-us-non-federal-acute-care-1.

[8] Office of the National Coordinator for Health Information Technology. Office-based Physician Health IT Adoption and Use: US Department of Health and Human Services; 2019 [updated May 17, 2019; cited 2019 Oct 3]. Available from: https://dashboard.healthit.gov/datadashboard/documentation/physician-health-it-adoption-use-data-documentation.php.

[9] Liang J, Li Y, Zhang Z, Shen D, Xu J, Zheng X, et al. Adoption of Electronic Health Records (EHRs) in China during the past 10 years: consecutive survey data analysis and comparison of sino-American challenges and experiences. J Med Internet Res 2021;23(2):e24813. Available from: https://doi.org/10.2196/24813.

[10] Kose I, Rayner J, Birinci S, Ulgu MM, Yilmaz I, Guner S. Adoption rates of electronic health records in Turkish Hospitals and the relation with hospital sizes. BMC Health Serv Res 2020;20(1):967. Available from: https://doi.org/10.1186/s12913-020-05767-5.

[11] Alanazi B, Butler-Henderson K, Alanazi M. Perceptions of healthcare professionals about the adoption and use of EHR in Gulf Cooperation Council countries: a systematic review. BMJ Health Care Inf 2020;27(1). Available from: https://doi.org/10.1136/bmjhci-2019-100099.

[12] Kanakubo T, Kharrazi H. Comparing the trends of electronic health record adoption among hospitals of the United States and Japan. J Med Syst 2019;43(7):224. Available from: https://doi.org/10.1007/s10916-019-1361-y.

[13] Vazquez MV, Palermo C, Islas MB, Zapata M, Giussi Bordoni MV, Esteban S, et al. Adoption factors related to electronic vaccine record in the public primary care network of Buenos Aires City. Stud Health Technol Inform 2019;264:2001–2. Available from: https://doi.org/10.3233/shti190755.

[14] Odekunle FF, Odekunle RO, Shankar S. Why sub-Saharan Africa lags in electronic health record adoption and possible strategies to increase its adoption in this region. Int J Health Sci (Qassim) 2017;11(4):59–64.

[15] Centers for Medicare and Medicaid Services. Meaningful use. Baltimore, MD: Centers for Medicare & Medicaid Services; 2013 [updated August 23; cited 2013 Aug 27]. Available from: https://www.cms.gov/Regulations-and-Guidance/Legislation/EHRIncentivePrograms/Meaningful_Use.html.

[16] Furukawa MF, Poon E. Meaningful use of health information technology: evidence suggests benefits and challenges lie ahead. Am J Managed Care 2011;17(12 Spec No.):SP76a-SP.

[17] Canada Health Infoway. Progress in Canada [cited 2014 Jun 13]. Available from: https://www.infoway-inforoute.ca/index.php/progress-in-canada.

[18] Whipple EC, Dixon BE, McGowan JJ. Linking health information technology to patient safety and quality outcomes: a bibliometric analysis and review. Inf Health Soc Care 2013;38(1):1–14. Available from: https://doi.org/10.3109/17538157.2012.678451.

[19] Blaya JA, Fraser HS, Holt B. E-health technologies show promise in developing countries. Health Aff (Proj Hope) 2010;29(2):244–51. Available from: https://doi.org/10.1377/hlthaff.2009.0894.

[20] Bates DW, Gawande AA. Improving safety with information technology. N Engl J Med 2003;348(25):2526–34. Available from: https://doi.org/10.1056/NEJMsa020847.

[21] Finnell JT, Overhage JM, Grannis S. All health care is not local: an evaluation of the distribution of emergency department care delivered in Indiana. AMIA Annu Symp Proc 2011;2011:409–16.

[22] Schoen C, Osborn R, Squires D, Doty M, Pierson R, Applebaum S. New 2011 survey of patients with

complex care needs in eleven countries finds that care is often poorly coordinated. Health Aff (Proj Hope) 2011;30(12):2437–48. Available from: https://doi.org/10.1377/hlthaff.2011.0923.

[23] Hammond WE, Bailey C, Boucher P, Spohr M, Whitaker P. Connecting information to improve health. Health Aff (Proj Hope) 2010;29(2):284–8. Available from: https://doi.org/10.1377/hlthaff.2009.0903.

[24] Gaglioti A, Cozad A, Wittrock S, Stewart K, Lampman M, Ono S, et al. Non-VA primary care providers' perspectives on comanagement for rural veterans. Military Med 2014;179(11):1236–43. Available from: https://doi.org/10.7205/milmed-d-13-00342.

[25] MacDonald SE, Schopflocher DP, Golonka RP. The pot calling the kettle black: the extent and type of errors in a computerized immunization registry and by parent report. BMC Pediatr 2014;14:1. Available from: https://doi.org/10.1186/1471-2431-14-1.

[26] Troyer L, Brady W. Barriers to effective EMS to emergency department information transfer at patient handover: a systematic review. Am J Emerg Med 2020;38(7):1494–503. Available from: https://doi.org/10.1016/j.ajem.2020.04.036.

[27] Huth K, Stack AM, Chi G, Shields R, Jorina M, West DC, et al. Developing standardized "receiver-driven" handoffs between referring providers and the emergency department: results of a multidisciplinary needs assessment. Jt Comm J Qual Patient Saf 2018;44 (12):719–30. Available from: https://doi.org/10.1016/j.jcjq.2018.05.003.

[28] Vest JR, Menachemi N. A population ecology perspective on the functioning and future of health information organizations. Health Care Manage Rev 2019;44 (4):344–55. Available from: https://doi.org/10.1097/hmr.0000000000000185.

[29] Berwick DM. Launching accountable care organizations — The proposed rule for the medicare shared savings program. N Engl J Med 2011;364(16):e32. Available from: https://doi.org/10.1056/NEJMp1103602.

[30] Vest JR, Simon K. Hospitals' adoption of intra-system information exchange is negatively associated with inter-system information exchange. J Am Med Inform Assoc 2018;25(9):1189–96. Available from: https://doi.org/10.1093/jamia/ocy058.

[31] Office of the National Coordinator for Health Information Technology. State health information exchange cooperative agreement program. Washington, DC: U.S. Department of Health & Human Services; 2014 [updated April 14, 2014; cited 2015 May 7]. Available from: http://healthit.gov/policy-researchers-implementers/state-health-information-exchange.

[32] Department of Health & Human Services US. Nationwide Health Information Network (NwHIN) 2013 [cited 2013 Feb 21]. Available from: http://www.healthit.gov/policy-researchers-implementers/nationwide-health-information-network-nwhin.

[33] Health Record Banking Alliance. What is a health record bank? HRBA; 2018 [cited 2021 Nov 4]. Available from: https://www.healthbanking.org/.

[34] Mantravadi S. Future of health record banking in hospital referral regions. Am J Managed Care; 2016 [updated September 15; cited 2021 Nov 4]. Available from: https://www.ajmc.com/view/future-of-health-record-banking-in-hospital-referral-regions.

[35] Gibson RF. Benefits of electronic medical record banks. JAMA Intern Med 2017;177(9):1398. Available from: https://doi.org/10.1001/jamainternmed.2017.2716.

[36] Plischke M, Wagner M, Haarbrandt B, Rochon M, Schwartze J, Tute E, et al. The lower saxony bank of health. rationale, principles, services, organization and architectural framework. Methods Inf Med 2014;53 (2):73–81. Available from: https://doi.org/10.3414/me13-02-0003.

[37] NoMoreClipboard. About 2020 [cited 2021 Nov 4]. Available from: https://www.nomoreclipboard.com/patients/about.

[38] Yasnoff WA, Shortliffe EH. Lessons learned from a health record bank start-up. Methods Inf Med 2014;53 (2):66–72. Available from: https://doi.org/10.3414/me13-02-0030.

[39] Rubin RD. The community health information movement: where it's been, where it's going. In: O'Carroll PW, Yasnoff WA, Ward ME, Ripp LH, Martin EL, editors. Public Health Informatics and Information Systems. Springer-Verlag; 2002. p. 595–616.

[40] Lorenzi NM. Strategies for creating successful local health information infrastructure initiatives. In: U.S. Department of Health and Human Services, editor. Washington, DC: Assistant Secretary for Policy and Evaluation; 2003.

[41] Miller RH, Miller BS. The Santa Barbara County care data exchange: what happened? Health Aff (Proj Hope) 2007;26(5):w568–80. Available from: https://doi.org/10.1377/hlthaff.26.5.w568.

[42] Nocella KC, Horowitz KJ, Young JJ. Against all odds: designing and implementing a grassroots, community-designed RHIO in a rural region. J Healthc Inf Manage 2008;22(2):34–41.

[43] Frisse ME, King JK, Rice WB, Tang L, Porter JP, Coffman TA, et al. A regional health information exchange: architecture and implementation. AMIA Annu Symp Proc 2008;212–16.

[44] Dixon BE, Welebob EM, Dullabh P, Samarth A, Gaylin D. Summary of the status of regional health information exchanges (RHIOs) in the United States. Rockville, MD: Agency for Healthcare Research and

Quality; 2007 [May 15, 2009]. Available from: http://healthit.ahrq.gov/portal/server.pt/gateway/PTARGS_0_3882_813237_0_0_18/Summary%20of%20the%20Status%20of%20Regional%20Health%20Information%20Exchanges.pdf.

[45] Poon EG, Cusack CM, McGowan JJ. Evaluating healthcare information technology outside of academia: observations from the national resource center for healthcare information technology at the Agency for Healthcare Research and Quality. J Am Med Inf Assoc 2009;16(5):631–6. Available from: https://doi.org/10.1197/jamia.M3033.

[46] eHealth Initiative. Results of 2009 Survey on Health Information Exchange: State of the Field. Washington, DC: eHealth Initiative; 2009 [cited 2010 Mar 22]. Available from: http://www.ehealthinitiative.org/results-2009-survey-health-information-exchange.html.

[47] eHealth Initiative. The State of Health Information Exchange in 2010: Connecting the Nation to Achieve Meaningful Use. Washington, DC: ehealth Initiative; 2010 [cited 2010 Sep 29]. Available from: http://ehealthinitiative.org/uploads/file/Final%20Report.pdf.

[48] Adler-Milstein J, Bates DW, Jha AK. U.S. Regional health information organizations: progress and challenges. Health Aff (Proj Hope) 2009;28(2):483–92. Available from: https://doi.org/10.1377/hlthaff.28.2.483.

[49] Adler-Milstein J, McAfee AP, Bates DW, Jha AK. The state of regional health information organizations: current activities and financing. Health Aff (Proj Hope) 2008;27(1):w60–9. Available from: https://doi.org/10.1377/hlthaff.27.1.w60.

[50] Healtheway. Home 2012 [cited 2013 Feb 6]. Available from: http://www.healthewayinc.org/.

[51] Centers for Medicare and Medicaid Services. Promoting Interoperability Programs. Baltimore, MD: Centers for Medicare & Medicaid Services; 2020 [updated February 11, 2021; cited 2021 Feb 21]. Available from: https://www.cms.gov/Regulations-and-Guidance/Legislation/EHRIncentivePrograms.

[52] Adler-Milstein J, Garg A, Zhao W, Patel V. A survey of health information exchange organizations in advance of a nationwide connectivity framework. Health Aff 2021;40(5):736–44. Available from: https://doi.org/10.1377/hlthaff.2020.01497.

[53] Dixon BE, Caine VA, Halverson PK. Deficient response to COVID-19 makes the case for evolving the public health system. Am J Prev Med 2020;59(6):887–91. Available from: https://doi.org/10.1016/j.amepre.2020.07.024.

[54] Dixon BE, Grannis SJ, McAndrews C, Broyles AA, Mikels-Carrasco W, Wiensch A, et al. Leveraging data visualization and a statewide health information exchange to support COVID-19 surveillance and response: application of public health informatics. J Am Med Inf Assoc 2021;28(7):1363–73. Available from: https://doi.org/10.1093/jamia/ocab004.

[55] Vest JR. Health information exchange: national and international approaches. Adv Health Care Manage 2012;12:3–24.

[56] Park H, Lee SI, Hwang H, Kim Y, Heo EY, Kim JW, et al. Can a health information exchange save healthcare costs? Evidence from a pilot program in South Korea. Int J Med Inf 2015. Available from: https://doi.org/10.1016/j.ijmedinf.2015.05.008.

[57] Geissbuhler A. Lessons learned implementing a regional health information exchange in Geneva as a pilot for the Swiss national eHealth strategy. Int J Med Inf 2013;82(5):e118–24. Available from: https://doi.org/10.1016/j.ijmedinf.2012.11.002.

[58] Nirel N, Rosen B, Sharon A, Blondheim O, Sherf M, Cohen AD. OFEK virtual medical records: an evaluation of an integrated hospital-community system. Harefuah 2011;150(2):72–8 209.

[59] Klapman S, Sher E, Adler-Milstein J. A snapshot of health information exchange across five nations: an investigation of frontline clinician experiences in emergency care. J Am Med Inf Assoc 2018;25(6):686–93. Available from: https://doi.org/10.1093/jamia/ocx153.

[60] Adler-Milstein J, Ronchi E, Cohen GR, Winn LA, Jha AK. Benchmarking health IT among OECD countries: better data for better policy. J Am Med Inf Assoc 2014;21(1):111–16. Available from: https://doi.org/10.1136/amiajnl-2013-001710.

[61] World Health Organization. National eHealth Strategy Toolkit. Geneva, Switzerland: World Health Organization and International Telecommunication Union; 2012.

[62] World Health Organization. eHealth Technical Advisory Group 2015 [cited 2015 March 29]. Available from: http://www.who.int/ehealth/tag/en/.

CHAPTER

2

Health information exchange as a profession

Candace J. Gibson[1], *Kelly J. Abrams*[2] *and Ramona Kyabaggu*[2]

[1]Department of Pathology & Laboratory Medicine, Schulich School of Medicine & Dentistry, Western University, London, ON, Canada [2]Master of Health Administration in Health Informatics and Information Management (MHA-HIIM) Program, Johnson-Shoyama Graduate School of Public Policy, University of Regina, Regina, SK, Canada

LEARNING OBJECTIVES

By the end of the chapter the reader should be able to:

- Describe the different types of professionals needed to establish and work with interoperable electronic health records and link them in a health information exchange.
- Describe the specific roles and functions of health information and health information exchange professionals.
- Understand the current supply and demand for individuals in the eHealth/digital health information workforce.
- Describe the routes for education, training, and credentialing of these various health information professionals.

2.1 Introduction

2.1.1 Implementation and adoption of electronic health records and health information exchange

Significant strides have been made in deploying and implementing electronic medical/health records (EMR/EHR) within physicians' offices [1–6] and health facilities [7–11] over the past 15 years. Since 2008, office-based physician adoption of any EMR/EHR has more than doubled and as of 2017, nearly 9 in 10 office-based physicians had adopted an EHR, and nearly 4 in 5 (80%) had adopted a certified[1] EHR [6]. The most recent figures available (for 2019) from

[1] The Office of Interoperability and Standards within the Office of the National Coordinator for Health IT (ONC) oversees certification programs for health information technology providing assurance to purchasers and users that an EHR system offers the necessary technological capability, functionality, and security to maintain data confidentially and work with other systems to share data securely. Eligible providers who seek to qualify for incentive payments under the Medicare and Medicaid Promoting Interoperability/EHR Incentive Programs are required by statute to use Certified EHR Technology. See description and criteria at https://www.healthit.gov/topic/certification-ehrs/about-onc-health-it-certification-program.

Health Information Exchange
DOI: https://doi.org/10.1016/B978-0-323-90802-3.00007-1

the National Electronic Health Records Survey[2] of primary care physicians report that 90% of physicians use an EHR [12]. About 98% of US hospitals now report the implementation and use of electronic records [10,11].

In these studies and surveys, physicians were deemed to have adopted a "basic EHR" (vs a fully functional or comprehensive electronic record) if they reported their practice performed all of the following computerized functions: provided patient demographics, patient problem lists, electronic lists of medications taken by patients, clinician notes, orders for medications, viewing laboratory results, and viewing imaging results [13]. The principal differences between a fully functional or comprehensive system and a basic system were the absence of certain order-entry capabilities (e.g., for lab and radiology tests) and clinical decision support (e.g., warnings of drug interactions; reminders of screening and necessary tests) in a basic system.

Practices that are part of an integrated delivery system or share resources with other clinicians had higher rates of EMR/EHR adoption, and use of multifunctional health information technology (IT), electronic health information exchange (HIE), and electronic access for patients [14]; yet a high percentage of primary care physicians still reported that they did not routinely receive timely information from specialists or hospitals [1,2]. In 2012 nearly 6 in 10 hospitals actively exchanged electronic health information with providers and hospitals outside their organization, an increase of 41% since 2008 [9]. EHR adoption and HIE participation were associated with significantly greater hospital exchange activity, but exchanges with providers outside the organization and exchanges of clinical care summaries and medication lists remained limited [9].

In 2015 64% of physicians had an EHR with the capability to exchange secure messages with patients, an over 50% increase since 2013 [15]. Sixty-three percent of physicians had the capability for their patients to electronically view their medical record, 41% had the capability for patients to download their medical record, and 19% had the capability for patients to electronically send or transmit their medical record to a third party. Together, 16% of all physicians could provide all three functions—view, download, and transmit—to their patients [15,16]. Beginning in 2015, healthcare professionals participating in the Medicare or Medicaid EHR Incentive Programs were required to demonstrate all three capabilities: view, download, and transmit. By 2019 three-quarters of hospitals reported electronically finding (or querying) patient health information from sources outside their health system; but still only about half of all hospitals (55%) performed all four domains of interoperability (e.g., send, receive, find, integrate data) [16].

Despite the broad EMR/EHR adoption across all US hospitals, there is concern that an "advanced use" digital divide exists between critical access hospitals (CAHs)[3] and non-CAHs [11,17]. Looking at 10 advanced EHR functions related to performance measurement

[2] NEHRS is a nationally representative, mixed-mode survey of US office-based physicians that collects information on the adoption, use, and interoperability of EHR systems. Information on physician and practice characteristics is also collected. NEHRS is sponsored by the ONC-HIT and conducted by CDC's National Center for Health Statistics annually as a sample survey of nonfederally employed, office-based physicians who are primarily engaged in direct patient care and are located in the 50 US states or the District of Columbia.

[3] Critical access hospital (CAH) is a designation conferred by the CMS to eligible rural hospitals that provide high quality limited outpatient and inpatient services. They represent more than two-third of all rural hospitals and are vital for ensuring the health of communities that may not have access to larger facilities. Critical access hospitals. CMS.gov. https://www.cms.gov/Medicare/Provider-Enrollment-and-Certification/CertificationandComplianc/CAHs.

(PM) (such as monitoring patient safety with adverse event alerts, supporting continuous quality improvement, use of dashboards to measure organizational and individual performance, adherence to clinical guidelines, identification of patients at risk) there was substantial variation in hospitals surveyed with only 23.8% of hospitals with all 10 functions. Similarly, for 10 parameters of patient engagement (PE), hospital adoption ranged from 95% of patients having the ability to view their health data online to only 37% able to submit patient-generated data, 42% able to electronically request prescriptions refills or schedule appointments online. Only 15% had adopted all 10 PE functions. CAHs significantly lagged in advanced use functions critical to improving care quality. In an update on progress, even though virtually all hospitals regardless of status have adopted EHRs and increased the use of some of the advanced functions related to PE (up to 59%) and PM/clinical data analytics (CDA) (up to 56% with at least 8 of the 10 measures), this digital divide has persisted and even widened for CDA functions (only 32% use in CAHs) [11]. This may be due to different advanced use needs among CAH patients but also to a "lack of access to the necessary technical expertise" [11]. Three functions in PE demonstrated the largest gap: importing records from other organizations, sending electronic care summaries to third parties, and allowing online refill requests—all functions that rely on interoperable health networks and HIE and in some cases, the use of application programming interfaces (APIs) that are mandated in the 21st Century Cures Act [11]. The authors suggested "that the IT and organizational capabilities necessary to support advanced use may be distinct from those required for EHR adoption" and these providers may be struggling to obtain them [17]. The necessary technical expertise and knowledge may be missing at both the clinician level and the availability of technical support staff (i.e., health information professionals).

2.1.2 Incentives promoting use of electronic health records and increasing the health information technology workforce

Adoption of EHRs in the United States has been driven by the Health Information Technology for Economic and Clinical Health (HITECH) Act of 2009, intended to promote the adoption of "meaningful use"[4] of health information technology (HIT) by providing resources to build the national HIT infrastructure [18]. To a certain extent, this funding was also intended to increase the HIT workforce through the HITECH Workforce Development program, or at least provide additional training resources for those working to implement these systems and for the healthcare workforce that would be using them [19–22]. In 2011 the Centers for Medicare & Medicaid Services (CMS) established the Medicare and Medicaid EHR Incentive Programs to encourage medical

[4] The term "meaningful use" came into use with the HITECH Act of 2009 in an attempt to promote the adoption and use of EHRs, particularly certified EHRs that defined standards for clinical data use and exchange intended to improve quality, safety, efficiency, care coordination, and reduce health disparities; increase patient engagement; and ensure adequate privacy and security protection for personal health information. The criteria were introduced in three stages—stage 1 in 2011–12 (data capture and sharing), stage 2 in 2014 (advanced processes, health information exchange), and stage 3 in 2016 and beyond (improved outcomes). Unfortunately, the criteria to meet were cumbersome and unpopular among providers and the incentive program was revised in 2018 and renamed the Interoperability Program. HealthIT.gov—Promoting Interoperability—https://www.healthit.gov/topic/meaningful-use-and-macra/promoting-interoperability.

and eligible professionals, eligible hospitals, and critical care access hospitals to "adopt, implement, upgrade, and demonstrate meaningful use of certified electronic health record technology (CEHRT)" [23]. Historically, the incentive program consisted of three stages and incentive payments for EHR funding were dependent on meeting the meaningful use criteria outlined in the three stages [24]. The program was successful in driving both EHR adoption and in increasing, to some extent, the necessary health IT force needed to implement and work with them [19–22,25].

The 21st Century Cures Act,[5] passed in 2016 further promotes the use of EHRs overall; it also requires that all healthcare providers make electronic copies of patient records available to patients. CMS regulations that came into effect in 2021 include policies that require or encourage payers to implement APIs[6] via computer and smartphone applications to improve the electronic exchange of healthcare data—sharing information with patients or exchanging information between a payer and provider or between two payers or providers often through a HIE network. FHIR-based[7] APIs can connect to mobile apps or to a provider's EHR or practice management system to enable a more seamless method of exchanging information. The Cures Act final rule "supports seamless and secure access, exchange, and use of electronic health information" [26].

Thus, just as the HITECH Act accelerated and facilitated the deployment of electronic health information systems, the 21st Century Cures Act and its rules and requirements concerning "information blocking" and FHIR-based APIs to promote data exchange between patients and providers will drive the next generation of HIE networks and health system data use to address advanced use functions and improve quality of care and health outcomes. The information "blocking" rule actually requires the reverse or the *absence* of information blocking, that is, that information not be blocked by the health facility/provider, nor patient access delayed to any eligible information that is entered and stored in their EHR. As of April 5, 2021, the following eight categories of clinical notes created in an EHR must be immediately available to patients through a secure online portal: consultation notes, discharge summary notes, history and physicals, imaging narratives, lab report narratives, pathology report narratives, procedure notes, and progress notes.

[5] H.S. 34: 21st Century Cures Act. Introduced in 2015 and came into law in December 2016. An act to accelerate the discovery, development, and delivery of 21st century cures, and for other purposes. https://www.congress.gov/bill/114th-congress/house-bill/34.

[6] API or application programming interface provides the "front end" for the tools that are developed for passing information between providers, providers and payers, or providers and patients, that allows a computer program or system to access the features and data of a different program or system. This entry point defines how data must be formatted and the types of interactions supported, such as how data can be searched. To be successfully exchanged and ready for an operation, data must be formatted in the same way. Many modern applications, both desktop and mobile, use APIs to retrieve, store, and update data. The FHIR API mainly involves the access and exchange of data. https://www.healthit.gov/sites/default/files/page/2021-04/FHIR%20API%20Fact%20Sheet.pdf.

[7] Fast Healthcare Interoperability Resources, or FHIR, is an interoperability rule that will enable seamless, on-demand information exchange of clinical records among providers and data systems and will result in coordinated, cost-efficient care. FHIR is the global standard for passing data between systems developed by Health Level-7 (HL7). The information models and APIs developed using this standard provide a means of sharing health and care information between providers and their systems no matter what setting care is delivered in.

2.1.3 Promoting use of electronic health records and health information exchange globally

Driven by the potential to significantly impact the practice of healthcare by improving quality of care, reducing costs, increasing patient safety, and improving health outcomes many other countries have provided funding or incentives to encourage the widespread adoption and use of EHRs and development of HIE. Worldwide, in the Organisation for Economic Co-operation and Development (OECD) countries, on average, 82% of primary care physicians' offices and 73% of medical specialists' offices use EMR [27,28]. The OECD study reporting on 38 countries, found widespread use of electronic clinical records at the point of care; however, the exchange of electronic clinical records across healthcare organizations was less common, similar to what is seen in the United States. There were also large variations in the availability and use of telehealth services across countries and, in many countries, patients were not able to access their test results online, book appointments or renew prescriptions electronically, or exchange secure messages with their healthcare providers [29].

HIE is currently limited in many low- and middle-income countries (LMICs), often reflecting the many barriers to its successful implementation. In some countries, efforts have progressed further than in others and in certain regions, HIE efforts extend across national borders [30]. In a comparison of HIE in six countries (China, England, Scotland, India, Switzerland, and the United States) the differences in accomplishing HIE are seen as "differences in progress along a comparable pathway, with similar barriers being identified" [30]. In countries that have successfully achieved HIE, the impetus has come from the government and the changes in the digitization of health records and the infrastructure, policies, and processes needed were reinforced with economic incentives to healthcare providers (e.g., in the United States, England, China). Akhlaq and coauthors [31] undertook a systematic review of the literature (63 studies across 24 countries) to understand the barriers and facilitators to implementation and use of HIEs and identified seven key categories/factors including social-political, financial, infrastructure (equipment, power, telecommunications), organizational (lack of training, lack of human resources), technical (system design issues), individual, and data management (lack of timely reporting, poor data quality) that affected implementation either negatively or positively [31, see Figure 3, p. 1322]. Concerning human resources, "training of staff and healthcare professionals was found to be the most essential facilitator" under the theme of organizational factors. Hiring more staff, involving key health personnel for new policies, and defining new roles and career structures to facilitate the management of health information systems were also identified as facilitators.

Globally the World Health Organization (WHO) through its resolutions on eHealth and digital health have urged member states to develop national strategies that identify priority areas where efforts can be focused and where key lessons, frameworks, and guidelines can be shared among nations [32]. The next set of 17 sustainable development goals[8] promote the goals of good health and well-being for all, no poverty, zero hunger, quality education,

[8] https://www.undp.org/sustainable-development-goals and https://sdgs.un.org/goals. The Sustainable Development Goals (SDGs), or Global Goals, were adopted by the United Nations in 2015 as a universal call to action to end poverty, protect the planet, and ensure that by 2030 all people enjoy peace and prosperity. The 17 SDGs are integrated— action in one area will affect outcomes in others; and development must balance social, economic, and environmental sustainability. The SDGs are designed to end poverty, hunger, AIDS, and discrimination against women and girls. The creativity, knowhow, technology, and financial resources from all of society are necessary to achieve the SDGs.

gender equality, and others and strongly rely on the potential of information and communications technology (ICT), quality health data, and HIE [33] to accelerate progress and achieve these goals by 2030 and to meet the WHO's "triple billion" targets by 2023. The latter targets to ensure that 1 billion more people benefit from universal health coverage, that 1 billion more people are better protected from health emergencies, and that 1 billion more people enjoy better health and well-being [34].

We are still a long way from the goal of a truly interactive learning healthcare system in which many of our currently siloed systems become interoperable and fully able to exchange information securely and efficiently. To continue promoting and prioritizing interoperability and exchange of healthcare data, CMS renamed the EHR Incentive Programs to the Promoting Interoperability Programs in April 2018. This change moved the programs beyond the requirements of meaningful use to a new phase with an increased focus on interoperability, improving patient access to health information, and the increased use of advanced functions enabled by access to health data.

2.2 Human resource needs—digital health information professionals

As we have moved past the tipping point and simple replacement of the paper record to a critical mass of electronic records and users and the value-added or more meaningful use of the record and the data which it contains, we increasingly run into a barrier due to the lack of adequately trained personnel. To realize fully operational and integrated EHRs and HIE and their benefits, industry requires health professionals who are familiar with technology and information systems; data and information standards and interoperability across platforms; human factors and process engineering; technology adoption and user-supporting mechanisms; methods of re-engineering and project management; privacy and security of personal health information; the management of health information through its lifecycle; and the use and analysis of health data for optimization of healthcare delivery [19,20,22,35,36].

Experience through the COVID-19 pandemic has also accelerated the advanced use of many digital technologies, most notably in telehealth and virtual care, and in the need for rapid access and sharing of data between health facilities and public health agencies. The implementation of virtual care, long seen as a potential solution to an urban-rural divide and the oversight and management of chronic diseases, similar to early EHR use lagged in implementation but experienced a surge during the restrictions imposed by quarantine and isolation [37–40]. Early in the COVID-19 pandemic, in-person ambulatory healthcare visits declined by 60% across the United States, while telehealth visits increased, accounting for up to 30% of total care provided in some locations [38]. Almost all physicians (95%) reported that they had undertaken some form of video or teleconsultation after March 2020, compared to only 15% of physicians before March 2020 [37,38]. During the first quarter of 2020, the number of telehealth visits increased by 50%, with a whopping 154% increase in visits noted in the week of March 27, 2020, compared with the same period in 2019 [37]. These rates have seen some decline [40] as we move back to normal and ease restrictions of social distancing and quarantine, but the convenience for patients and necessary policy changes in technology infrastructure, licensure, geographic location (barriers eliminated), and reimbursement (increased) (if continued!) now ensure that this is part of modern 21st century practice.

This chapter outlines the human resources and competencies needed to put an HIE network in place to ensure that data are available for patient access, quality assurance, and health system improvement, that is, the health information human resources needed within any future fully integrated health system. The chapter will provide an overview of the various types of digital health workers and health information professionals needed, explain each profession's skill set and knowledge base, and define new roles that support HIE networks. Learning outcomes or competencies for health information, health informatics (HI), and health information management (HIM) have been delineated by various professional associations and/or credentialing bodies. These competencies will be briefly presented along with the current credentials and their certifying bodies. A national digital health human resources strategy and investigation of the existing health information workforce is suggested to address the current shortage of skilled workers and to develop a long-term strategy for education and training of the necessary personnel, including clinical professionals, to ensure the quality of health data collected, its security and confidentiality, interoperability of health information systems, and to manage and maintain health information organizations and HIEs in the future.

2.2.1 The nature of eHealth/digital health information professionals: their competencies, roles, and work

Eysenbach [41] defined eHealth as "an emerging field in the intersection of medical informatics, public health and business, referring to health services and information delivered or enhanced through the Internet and related technologies." He further described the term as not only the ICT, but the way of thinking and commitment to a networked community (be it local, regional, or global) to improve healthcare. Thus eHealth refers to the application of informatics concepts, methods, and tools to the health system and the people (providers, administrators, patients, families) involved in it. As such, eHealth refers to the work of health informaticians, health information managers, health information technologists (HITs), and HIE professionals, as well as others [41].

As more technologies are added and evolve (e.g., telehealth), the term "**digital health**" is being used to broadly define "the field of knowledge and practice associated with the development and use of digital technologies to improve health" [42]. The term digital health is based in eHealth and has been introduced as "a broad umbrella term encompassing eHealth (which includes mHealth), as well as emerging areas, such as the use of advanced computing sciences in 'big data', genomics and artificial intelligence" [42].

As digital health systems are implemented there is a shift of emphasis on the need for technology proficient individuals to those who have the expertise and competencies to work *with* the data and information contained within an interoperable health information system or exchanged via HIE. There is also an increasing need for all health professionals to understand both HI and HIM principles. With the implementation of the final rules of the 21st Century Cures Act, two changes, in particular, will impact the need for HIE professionals and skills: the first the use of FHIR-based[7] APIs[6] to facilitate health data exchange and patient access to their health information and hence the need for API developers who may be in house or third-party developers (or mobile health app developers), and second the provisions for so-called information blocking or open notes.

Within an HIE network, professionals with multiple skills are needed in the areas of computer science, systems engineering, informatics and information management, business, and project management, and the need for teams to work together collaboratively to institute and implement complex systems and use them optimally. Several of these key health information professionals are discussed briefly below considering their main functions and areas of expertise along with their education and competencies. Many of these professionals are trained through specific programs at the college and university level (within both undergraduate and graduate programs), certified within a given specialty, and are members of a representative professional organization. Increasingly as technology changes more rapidly and new demands and problems are encountered the usefulness of micro-credentialing or the provision of specific skills to address particular challenges is becoming more readily available and acceptable [43]. Many of these additional competencies are included in short training programs that are offered by educational institutions (e.g., Conestoga College) and/or industry/vendors (e.g., IBM, Google, Epic) or government (e.g., ONC Workforce Program HI training modules) as postgraduate certificates, badges, or micro-credentials. Many of these programs are adapted for adult, life-long learners who may still be in the workforce and are often offered online through online learning platforms such as Coursera, EdX, or FutureLearn, to accommodate these constraints and often in partnership with industry or university.

2.2.2 Who are the eHealth/digital health information professionals?

2.2.2.1 *Health informaticians (HI professionals)*

Health informatics (HI) is the discipline that researches, formulates, designs, develops, implements, and evaluates information-related concepts, methods, and tools (e.g., ICT) to support clinical care, research, health services administration, and education. Health informaticians are digital health professionals who have become competent in the discipline of HI and thus deploy and use methods (e.g., planning, management, analytic, procedural) and tools (e.g., information and communications systems) in support of health system processes. Generally speaking, health informaticians qualify for this designation by completion of a bachelor's degree in HI or another field, and/or an advanced degree in HI, or by achieving professional certification [e.g., Certified Professional in Healthcare Information and Management Systems (CPHIMS)] (see Table 2.1). Samplings of HI job roles include health application designer or developer, change manager/workflow re-designer, data analyst, chief informatics officer, and program evaluation specialist [35,44].

HI professionals also exist within clinical specialties (e.g., medicine, public health, nursing, dentistry, pharmacy) and may have completed advanced informatics training following clinical education and/or several years of clinical practice.

2.2.2.2 *Residency and fellowship training—clinical informatics subspecialty*

The American Medical Informatics Association (AMIA) and internationally the International Medical Informatics Association (IMIA) led the charge for the introduction of a "clinical informatics" (CI) subspecialty setting out core competencies which included fundamentals (i.e., information systems, the flow of data, information, and knowledge through the healthcare system); clinical decision-making and care process improvement; health information systems; and leadership and management of change [45–47]. In 2013 the first certification examination that could be taken within any board specialty (approved by the American Board of Medical Specialties) and open to graduates of both American and Canadian schools was offered. Slightly over 2000 physicians have taken the certification examinations to date [47,48]. Beginning in 2023, only candidates trained in an Accreditation Council for Graduate Medical Education-accredited fellowship program will be eligible for the CI board examination (about three dozen clinical fellowships have been accredited in the United States and internationally).

TABLE 2.1 Health information certifications—credentials offered.

Credential designation	Competency areas	Curriculum standard/accreditation	Training or degree required
HIM certifications through CCHIIM[a]			
Registered Health Information Technician (RHIT)	See **2018 AHIMA Health Information Management Curricula Competencies** (six domains outlined below)[c]. At the associate-level programs can choose one or both specialty tracks which include Data Management and Revenue Management	Standards and Interpretations for Accreditation of Associate Degree Programs in Health Information Management (CAHIIM[b]); program meets or exceeds 2018 AHIMA HIM curriculum competencies for associate programs	Completion of a 2-year academic program that prepares students for a career in health information; offered by a CAHIIM-accredited program (see https://www.cahiim.org/accreditation)
Registered Health Information Administrator (RHIA)	Each academic level comprises six common domains representing the areas of mastery important for all HIM students and practitioners. I. Data Structure, Content, and Information Governance; II. Information Protection: Access, Use, Disclosure, Privacy, and Security; III. Informatics, Analytics, and Data Use; IV. Revenue Cycle Management; V. Health Law & Compliance; VI. Organizational Management & Leadership	Standards and Interpretations for Accreditation of Baccalaureate Degree Programs in Health Information Management (CAHIIM); program meets or exceeds 2018 AHIMA HIM curriculum competencies for baccalaureate degree programs	Completion of a 4-year baccalaureate degree or masters level requirements from a CAHIIM-accredited program that prepares students for a career in health information. (Candidates with a bachelor's degree from an accredited college or university AND a postgrad certificate from a CAHIIM-accredited HIM program are eligible to sit for the RHIA exam.)
Certified Coding Associate (CCA)	Self-study, entry-level coding certification. Coding professionals who hold the CCA credential have demonstrated coding competency across all settings, including hospitals and physician practices	AHIMA-approved coding certificate program	Entry level; minimum high school level diploma + 6 months experience or completion of an AHIMA-approved coding certificate program
Certified Coding Specialist (CCS)	The CCS credential demonstrates a professional's tested skills in data quality and accuracy as well as mastery of coding proficiency	Focus on more experienced coder in inpatient setting	Two or more years of coding experience
Certified Coding Specialist (CCS-P)	Self-study, comprehensive physician's office coding certification	Focus on more experienced coder in ambulatory care and outpatient setting	Two or more years of coding experience
Certified Health Data Analyst (CHDA)	CHDA establishes competence in big data for both organization and analysis	Knowledge to acquire, manage, analyze, interpret, and transform healthcare data into accurate, consistent, and timely information and to communicate with individuals and groups at multiple levels	Associate degree + 5 years experience; RHIT + 3 years experience or a baccalaureate or master's degree + 1 year experience

(*Continued*)

TABLE 2.1 (Continued)

Credential designation	Competency areas	Curriculum standard/accreditation	Training or degree required
Clinical Documentation Improvement Practitioner (CDIP)	Individuals earning the CDIP credential demonstrate expertise in clinical documentation within patient health records	Experience in CDI guidance, knowledge of documentation requirements relative to compliant coding and billing, in addition to EHR functionality to support documentation capture	RHIA or RHIT or CCS/CCS-P or RN, MD, DO + 2 years experience in CDI OR associate degree + 3 years experience
Certified Healthcare Privacy and Security (CHPS)	Competence in designing, implementing, and administering comprehensive privacy and security protection programs in all types of healthcare organizations	Privacy and Security certification that documents Health Insurance Portability and Accountability Act (HIPAA) and Information Security expertise	Baccalaureate + 4 years experience; RHIA + 2 years experience or advanced grad degree + 2 years experience; RHIT + 4 years experience; associate + 6 years experience
HIM certifications through CCHIM			
Certified Health Information Management Professional (CHIM)	Health Information Management (includes coding & classifications; HIM standards; privacy, security, and confidentiality; and analysis & business intelligence) Health Information Fundamentals Curricular Standards include the following practice areas: information governance, data quality, clinical knowledge, analytics, privacy, and technology (CCHIM—Oct 2020)	Learning Outcomes in HIM (LOHIM -Version 3) 2015 Designates learning outcomes required in eight domains (biomedical sciences; Canadian healthcare system; HIM; analysis & business intelligence; privacy, confidentiality, and access; information systems and technology; management; ethics and practice)—covers the health information fundamentals	College/Diploma Diploma, Baccalaureate degree, or Master's degree From a CCHIM-accredited program
Certified Terminology Standards Specialist (CTSS)	The curriculum is grouped according to the following core domains: • Foundations of Controlled Terminologies • Management of Controlled Terminologies • Application of Controlled Terminologies • Foundations of Interoperability Standards • Application of Interoperability Standards	Canadian Terminology Standards Certification Curricular Competencies (2016) Designates learning outcomes in five domains (as noted in Column 2, Competency areas)	Postgraduate certificateFrom a CCHIM-accredited program
	Clinical documentation improvement specialists impact the accuracy of medical	No published competency document	Eligibility for CCDIS certification includes:

Certified Clinical Documentation Improvement Specialist (CCDIS)	documentation and coding in the healthcare system. A strong, highly respected clinical documentation improvement (CDI) specialist program can make a difference in achieving the goals of enhancing quality care, improving case mix, and ensuring the appropriate utilization of resources through quality information		Nurses and physicians with a minimum of three years of experience working in a healthcare setting Other regulated health professionals who have worked in clinical documentation improvement for a minimum of 3 years Certified HIM professionals or international equivalent with a minimum of 3 years of current HIM work experience in coding-related area
Certified Classification and Coding Specialist (CCCS)	The Certified Classification and Coding Specialist designation was developed for CHIM professionals with 5 + years of classification and coding experience in acute inpatient settings	No published competency document	Must be a certified HIM professional and: • Be currently working in the field of classification and coding with 5 or more years of experience; or • Be a graduate from a preparatory CCS program that is recognized by the CCHIM
HI certification through HIMSS			
Certified Associate in Healthcare Information and Management Systems (CAHIMS)	Health Informatics Health Information Systems	Knowledge of health IT and management systems. The CAHIMS credential is designed to be a career pathway to the CPHIMS credential. Content outlined in: CAHIMS Candidate Handbook, April 2021[e]	Undergraduate degree with <5 years related experience
Certified Professional in Healthcare Information and Management Systems (CPHIMS)	Health Informatics Health Information Systems	Covers general healthcare and technology areas as well as in-depth knowledge of health IT systems, including analysis, design, selection, implementation, support, maintenance, testing, evaluation, privacy, and security. Content outlined in: CPHIMS Candidate Handbook, April 2021[f]	Undergraduate degree with 5 years related IM experience (3 in healthcare); graduate degree with 3 years' experience (2 in healthcare) or 10 years' related experience (8 in healthcare)
CPHIMS-CA Administered by Digital Health	Core competencies in: • Health Sciences	Competency and the skills, knowledge, and abilities to perform safely and	Undergraduate degree with 5 years related experience (3 in HI);

(*Continued*)

TABLE 2.1 (Continued)

Credential designation	Competency areas	Curriculum standard/accreditation	Training or degree required
(Canada); developed in conjunction with HIMSS—Canadian version	◦ Canada's Health System ◦ Clinical & Health Services • Information Sciences ◦ IT and IM • Management Science ◦ Analysis and Evaluation ◦ Project Management ◦ Organizational & Behavioral Management	effectively in a broad range of Canadian practice settings. Core competencies defined in HIP Core Competencies, V3.0, November 2012[g]	graduate degree with 3 years' experience (2 in HI)
HI Certification through AMIA and the Health Informatics Certification Commission			
AMIA Certified Health Informatics Professional (ACHIP)	Competencies based on practice analysis and cover five domains: Foundational knowledge (in information technology, informatics, the healthcare system); decision-making processes and outcomes; health information systems (HIS); data governance, management, and analytics; and leadership, professionalism, strategy, and transformation.	Education and work experience in HI and certification examination – see AHIC Certification Guide, April 2021[d]	Master's or doctoral degree in health informatics or a degree with a focus in informatics from an accredited program, college, or university plus 4 to 6 years of health informatics experience; OR Master's or doctoral degree in a health informatics related field from an accredited program, college, or university (e.g., dentistry, nursing, pharmacy, computer science, public health, medicine) plus 6–8 years of experience
Other HI-related credentials and certification organizations			
Computing Technology Industry Association (CompTIA)—Healthcare IT Technician	Healthcare IT Systems	Skills and knowledge needed to implement, deploy, and support healthcare IT systems in clinical settings that range from individual practices to healthcare facilities. Covers a variety of topics, including regulatory rules and requirements, organizational behavior, IT best practices and operations, medical business operations and security topics	
HealthCare Information Security and Privacy Practitioner (HCISPP) (Administered	Healthcare Industry Regulatory Environment Privacy and Security	Fundamental knowledge and experience in security and privacy	Must have a minimum of 2 years of experience in one domain of the HCISPP credential that includes

through ISC^2—membership body of certified information and software security professionals worldwide)	Information Governance and Risk Management Information Risk Assessment Third Party Risk Management	controls that protect personal health information	security, compliance & privacy. Legal experience may be substituted for compliance. Information management experience may be substituted for privacy. One year of the 2 years of experience MUST be in the healthcare industry

[a] *Commission on Certification for Health Informatics and Information Management (CCHIIM) is a standing commission of AHIMA dedicated to assuring the competency of professionals practicing health informatics and information management (HIIM). CCHIIM provides strategic oversight of all AHIMA certification programs.*

[b] *Commission on Accreditation for Health Informatics and Information Management Education (CAHIIM)—In 2018 CAHIIM released new standards for Associate and Baccalaureate Health Information Management (HIM) programs. Additionally, AHIMA released new curricular competencies for Associate, Baccalaureate, and Master's HIM programs.*

[c] *American Health Information Management Association (AHIMA)/Council for Excellence in Education (CEE)—https://www.ahima.org/who-we-are/governance/cee/cee/; https://ahima.org/him-curricula/.*

[d] *American Medical Informatics Association (AMIA) Health Informatics Certification—AMIA Health Certification Guide—approved by the AMIA Health Informatics Certification Commission and AMIA Certification Department in April 2021. Available from: https://brand.amia.org/m/111c459e7f6c0c0b/original/AMIA_AHIC_Certification_Guide_April_2021_wo_appendicies.pdf.*

[e] *Healthcare Information and Management Systems Society (HIMSS). CAHIMS Candidate Handbook. Effective April 2021. https://www.himss.org/sites/hde/files/media/file/2021/04/05/cahims-handbook.pdf.*

[f] *HIMSS. CPHIMS Candidate Handbook. Effective April 2021. https://www.himss.org/sites/hde/files/media/file/2021/04/05/cphims-handbook.pdf.*

[g] *Digital Health Canada (formerly COACH) Health Information Professional Core Competencies, V 3.0. November 2012. Available from: https://digitalhealthcanada.com/wp-content/uploads/2019/07/Health-Informatics-Core-Competencies.pdf.*

ACHIP, AMIA Certified Health Informatics Professional; *CCHIM*, Canadian College of Health Information Management; *EHR*, electronic health record; *HI*, health informatics; *HIMSS*, Healthcare Information Management Systems Society.

2.2.2.3 Health informatics for nonclinicians

AMIA also established the AMIA Health Informatics Certification (AHIC) program to address the needs created by the growing number and expanding role of health informaticians beyond the clinical informaticists and their increased impact on healthcare delivery, public health, and consumer health. AHIC and the HI credential enable HI professionals to demonstrate competence, commitment to excellence, mastery of HI knowledge, and the ability to apply this knowledge to real-world healthcare challenges. A health informatics committee provides HI practice benchmarking and competency criteria that support HI professionals and the organizations that hire them [49].

Certification is intended for professionals who come from a range of educational and training pathways including dentistry, medicine, nursing, pharmacy, public health, HI, and computer science, and who have HI experience that includes critical thinking and analysis; independent decision-making; project management; managing personnel, resources, or partner relationships; leading or supporting teams; policy development; or strategic planning. An individual who meets the AHIC eligibility criteria, passes the AHIC exam, and fulfills recertification requirements is known as an *AMIA Certified Health Informatics Professional* or ACHIP (see Table 2.1).

2.2.2.4 Health information management professionals

Health information management (HIM) professionals are members of the digital health team trained in the discipline of health information management. The Canadian Health Information Management Association (CHIMA) defines HIM as the discipline that focuses on healthcare data and the management of healthcare information, regardless of the medium and format [50]. The American Health Information Management Association (AHIMA) defines health information management as the body of knowledge and practice that ensures the availability of health information to facilitate real-time healthcare delivery and critical health-related decision-making for multiple purposes across diverse organizations, settings, and disciplines [51].

Research and practice in HIM address the nature, structure, and translation of data into usable forms of information for the advancement of health and healthcare of individuals and populations. HIM roles are described as health information managers, clinical data specialists, patient information coordinators, data quality managers, information security managers, data resource administrators, research and decision support specialists. The HIM practice domains also broadly include planning (administration, policy development, information governance, strategic planning), informatics, and health IT [35,50–52].

An analysis of job postings globally for HI and HIM fell into four discrete categories related to (1) health IT (technology-focused), (2) health research (clinically focused), (3) health leadership and health project management (sales/marketing/management-focused), and (4) health compliance (compliance-focused) [53]. The majority of jobs focused on project management, health leadership, and health IT with fewest, interestingly, on HI. This may be due to a lack of standardized HI job titles that may have been missed in the analysis. The United Kingdom, Canada, Australia, and India had a higher number of data analysis jobs compared with the United States which had a higher number in consumer engagement, clinical documentation improvement, and information governance [53].

AHIMA in emphasizing the expanding and future roles for HIM professionals [54–56], has updated its curriculum to include some of these competencies (i.e., data analytics and information governance) [57] and within its Career Map application (https://my.ahima.org/careermap) has broken down current and future emerging roles/careers into four job families related to—coding and revenue cycle, informatics, data analytics, and information governance. Senior positions for HIM professionals include roles within HIE networks such as *Project Manager of Health Information Exchange* (responsible for managing the HIE budgeting, planning, organization and community relations, and implementation of projects), *Director, Health Information Exchange* (responsible for developing and implementing the policies and overall administration and management of the organization), and *Integration Analyst, Health Information Exchange* (responsible for the design, development, testing, support, and maintenance of application integration supporting both clinical and business processes). In all of these positions, the career trajectory is seen as building on a background of proficiency and experience in health information management through an undergraduate degree and Registered Health Information Administrator (RHIA) or Registered Health Information Technician (RHIT) credential (AHIMA certifications, see Table 2.1) with additional qualifications in Health Administration, Information Technology, or Informatics.

2.2.2.5 Health information technologists or health information and communications technologists

HITs may have a computer science or engineering background and are familiar with ICT (including hardware and software), information systems and networks, and programming. HIT professionals are trained in one or more technical areas that may include systems (e.g., operating system, database, programming languages, software engineering and development) and applications software (e.g., productivity tools, departmental information systems, office systems), hardware, communications and networking, biomedical engineering, and in a variety of methods or procedures such as project management, security, risk management, and process engineering [35,44,58]. Health IT programs include specific knowledge of the health system and medical sciences; computer sciences/engineering usually does not and those individuals with knowledge of the health system (such as HIs or HIMs) can provide the liaison function within a collaborative team to "translate" the needs and workflow requirements of the provision of healthcare. Computer and information research scientists design innovative uses for new and existing technology to solve complex computing problems for business, science, medicine, and other fields [59].

Most computer and information research scientists need a master's or higher degree in computer science or a related field, such as computer engineering. The employment of computer and information research scientists is projected to grow 22% from 2020 to 2030, much faster than the average for all occupations, as is the employment of software developers, quality assurance analysts, and testers. About 189,200 openings for software developers, quality assurance analysts, and testers are projected each year, on average, over the next decade [60]. With the introduction of the information-sharing requirement of the Cures Act largely enabled through FHIR-based API applications more software developers with these skills are required.

Most standards (e.g., Health Level-7) and terminologies (e.g., SNOMED, ICD-10) used in EHRs and HIE are international, supporting the need for a defined set of competencies for HIM, HI, and HIT/health information and communications technologists (HICT) workers globally. Knowledge about standards is typically acquired on the job or through learning academies facilitated by international standards organizations, including OpenHIE, HL7, and SNOMED.

To address the need for a skilled workforce, the US Department of Commerce supported AHIMA and International Federation of Health Information Management Associations (IFHIMA) in a collaborative effort to establish a global health information professional curricula and competency standard that provides a framework for healthcare and education systems worldwide to build a workforce strategy. No single, individual health information profession owns the full spectrum of skills and competencies for health information generation, use, management, and exchange. The health information professions addressed in the curricula outlined are HI, HIM, and HIT/HICT with the recognition of the interdisciplinary nature and collaborative environment of health information practices to support patient, provider, and population needs and "these professions are fluid and overlapping, and that hybrid roles are becoming increasingly common" [61].

2.2.2.6 Health information security specialists

The security of health data and health information can be considered from both information technology and information management perspective, the former with an emphasis on cybersecurity and ensuring a resistant network and the latter from the perspective of maintaining data integrity, privacy, and quality. The number and cost of cyber breaches in all industries have been steadily increasing; the costliest country in the 2021 IBM "Cost of a Data Breach" report was the United States and the costliest industry was healthcare [62].

Globally, the healthcare industry has seen some of the largest and most costly cyber and ransomware attacks. For example, Anthem, Inc. the second-largest health insurer in the United States was the victim of one of the largest healthcare hacks in history; in February 2015; hackers stole the personal information from up to 80 million records which included full names, addresses, social security numbers, birthdates, employment histories, and income data [63]. The global *WannaCry* ransomware attack in May 2017 demonstrated the widespread vulnerability of older operating systems within health facilities involving about 200,000 computers in over 150 countries. This "worm" infected computers and the encrypted data held on them. Within the United Kingdom, normal operations of the National Health Service (NHS) were brought to a standstill [64,65]. No NHS organization paid the ransom, but the true cost of disrupted services is unknown. Costs included thousands of canceled appointments, additional IT support and IT consultants provided to local NHS trusts and services, the cost of restoring data and systems affected by the attack, and overtime costs for national and local NHS staff who worked to resolve and prevent problems [64]. For more information on the importance of security for HIE networks and the ability to maintain the confidentiality of data and its integrity for use, please see Chapter 7.

HIM professionals can provide expertise to an organizational security team or committee or act as members of a cyber incident response team. Future career options for health information professionals, in general, include those related to cybersecurity (e.g., Chief Information Security Officer or Security Manager; Security Analyst) usually after taking additional cybersecurity courses or programs. Positions requiring the *Certified in Healthcare Privacy and Security* (CHPS, administered through AHIMA) or *Healthcare Information Security and Privacy Practitioner* credential [HCISPP, administered through the International Information Systems Security Certification Consortium $(ISC)^2$] have increased by more than 1400% since 2014! [53]. The US Bureau of Labor Statistics projects an increase of 33% or 47,100 jobs from the current 141,200 jobs (2020–30), mostly related to the replacement of current workers [66]. Most information security analyst positions require a bachelor's degree in a computer-related field, but employers usually prefer to hire analysts with experience in a related occupation. In a survey to understand why health information security breaches keep occurring, researchers found that talent shortage in the sector could be a huge contributor. The findings also show that these IT roles take 70% longer to fill on average than in other industries [67]. The healthcare industry invests less than 6% of its budget on cybersecurity; for comparison, the United States spends 16% of its federal budget on cybersecurity.

2.2.2.7 *Health data analysts*

As the volume and variety of health data within EHR and HIE networks increase there is an increasing need for individuals who can utilize, analyze, and transform that data into actionable information for decision-making within a healthcare organization or ultimately a learning health system. Health data analysts (HDA) assist in data acquisition, data analysis, data management, data interpretation and reporting, and data governance. AHIMA offers a CHDA credential to those with a prior RHIA or RHIT or bachelor's degree or 3–5 years of experience (see Table 2.1) [68]. Knowledge of healthcare practices is important for HDA. Those trained in math and data science may also work in healthcare [69]. These workers must understand disease classification systems, medical terminology, and healthcare reimbursement methods so that they can interpret data and understand how it relates to improving costs and patient care; thus many come from a background in HIM or healthcare administration. HDA decide what data are needed to answer specific questions or problems; may design surveys, experiments, or opinion polls to collect data; develop or use mathematical or statistical models and software to analyze, interpret, and create visualizations to communicate these analyses to technical and nontechnical audiences.

Those who perform more sophisticated analyses often overlap with the work of statisticians or epidemiologists. The Bureau of Labor Statistics does not keep statistics on HDAs but in looking at information for Math and Data Scientists and Statisticians [70] and Epidemiologists [71] jobs are expected to grow by 30% or more over the next decade (i.e., by 15,000 for biostatisticians and by 2300 for epidemiologists). Employment growth is expected to result from the more widespread use of statistical analysis to inform business, healthcare, and policy decisions and the rapid increase in digitally stored data within the EHR and from transactions conducted online through social media, smartphones, and other mobile devices.

2.2.2.8 *Health information exchange professionals*

HIE, as defined in Chapter 1, is "the electronic transfer of patient-level health-related data or information across diverse and often competing organizations across the health ecosystem." The nature and size of these organizations are quite variable (e.g., hospitals, physician's offices, laboratory systems, community care centers, mental health centers) as well as the information transmitted (e.g., a discharge summary, care plan, laboratory results, medication lists). A health information organization (HIO) refers to "an organization that facilitates information exchange within a network of facilities, community, state or region" ensuring the protection and security of personal health information as it is shared across multiple healthcare providers.

Although several professionals already discussed may possess the skills and knowledge to work in an HIO or HIE, specific certification programs for HIE professionals did not succeed. These former efforts tried to extend certification beyond the technical, legal, and regulatory requirements for data and information governance. These programs included content specific to HIE planning; information architecture and stewardship; the use of new technologies to integrate and exchange data between and among organizations; personal health records; telehealth and home monitoring; and other exchanges of electronic information among organizations (e.g., CPHIE through Health IT Certification [72]). Previous Health IT Certification, LLC certifications in health IT (CPHIT), electronic health records (CPEHR), and health information exchange (CPHIE) were transferred to the Healthcare Information Management Systems Society (HIMSS) in September 2016 (Margret Amatayakul, personal communication). HIMSS agreed to maintain the CPHIT, CPEHR, and CPHIE professional certifications through December 31, 2018, and offered certification holders the opportunity to transition to the HIMSS CPHIMS certification (see Table 2.1). Currently, HIE and interoperability knowledge and skills are distributed across certifications, including CPHIMS as well as the CI subspeciality in medicine.

2.2.3 Other key personnel—clinical healthcare professionals

2.2.3.1 *Medical and clinical trainees*

As the integration of IT within healthcare has changed the face of the clinical environment, it is also essential to prepare medical trainees and other health professionals (i.e., nurses, pharmacists, epidemiologists) for the current and future digital health environment to ensure safe and effective use of these technologies. Few medical schools within the United States and Canada have formally introduced training in informatics, information management, information governance, or data analytics into undergraduate trainee programs [73]. At the postgraduate or residency-level greater progress has been made, particularly in those subspecialties where digital technologies have made the greatest inroads as a part of modern practice (e.g., radiology, pathology, emergency medicine, surgery).

Within Canada, Canada Health Infoway (the organization charged with overseeing the introduction of digital technologies across the country), in partnership with three professional associations, the Association of Faculties of Medicine of Canada, the Canadian Nursing Association, and the Association of Faculties of Pharmacy in Canada have defined ehealth competencies for each profession and developed teaching resources, curricular materials, case studies, and clinical examples to support faculty in preparing future clinicians to understand and practice in a digital environment [73–77] (e.g., see Modules for Health Professional Students at https://elearnhcp.ca/).

Within an HIE there may be health informaticians, health information managers, as well as additional support staff providing the necessary business, financial, public relations, and privacy and security skills. Thus as we will see in this and other healthcare organizations the concept of the *health information professional* in general is gaining ground and defined as those individuals who have key responsibilities for use of health data, information, and knowledge in roles that range from the managers, policymakers, clinicians, educators, researchers, and leaders "who are tasked with analysing, designing, developing, implementing, maintaining, operating, evaluating, and governing the formats, technologies, systems, and services that mobilise health data, information, and knowledge" [36], p. 5].

2.3 Digital health information professionals—supply and demand

Health information workers are essential to modern medical practice and to ensuring quality healthcare outcomes, but finding them and delineating their competencies, roles, and functions is often difficult and often not clearly articulated as a specific component of the modern healthcare workforce and healthcare organization [36]. There is no uniform competency-based educational curriculum or credential required for most of those who are working as health information professionals. In Canada and the United States and globally, health information managers are the only "profession" that have a recognized college or accrediting/credentialling body for programs and practitioners and a professional association, for example, the Canadian College of Health Information Management (CCHIM) and the Commission on Accreditation for Health Informatics and Information Management Education (CAHIIM) and their affiliated professional associations, CHIMA and AHIMA, respectively (Table 2.1) [50,52].

An increasing number of HI programs are also now accredited through a joint effort of AHIMA and AMIA through CAHIIM [78]. These bodies mapped out specific curricular competency requirements (see Table 2.1) and accreditation requirements for HI programs, for example, HI curricular competencies [79] and/or HIM, for example, HIM curricular competencies [80]. These efforts have been echoed or supported on a global level through the corresponding international associations—IFHIMA through its Global Academic Curricular Competencies for Health Information Professionals [61] and IMIA [81]; each of these bodies, in turn, have developed curricular competencies for health information professionals.

The lack of uniformity and increasing complexity in digital health and HIE networks has serious implications and "flow-on effects" including "shortages of skilled workers, inadequate skills training opportunities, and ultimately suboptimal health ICT implementation and scaling up" [36], p. 5]. In the recent work by Australian HI and HIM practitioners Butler-Henderson, Day, and Gray, this essential digital workforce supporting the efficient and effective management of health and healthcare is called the "HIDDIN" workforce—comprising the professionals who have key responsibilities for work in **H**ealth **I**nformatics, **D**igital, **D**ata, **I**nformation, and **K**nowledge roles—a clever play on words that highlights the invisibility ("hidden") of these various key/essential workers.

Labor statistics for digital health or health information positions, in general, are difficult to come by. The US Bureau of Labor Statistics collects specific information for "medical records and health information specialists" that are largely the RHIA and RHIT positions related to HIM; coding and categorizing patient information for insurance reimbursement purposes, and for databases and registries; and to maintain patients' medical and treatment histories mainly within health facilities [82]. These jobs are expected to grow at a rate of 9% between 2020 and 2030 or 37,100 individuals. An estimated 416,400 people are currently employed in the "medical records and health information specialists" category. Additional HI and HIM expertise are also part of a separate category, "medical and health services managers." The medical and health services managers' category includes labor statistics representing those employed as managers of HIM or HIT services, health information analysis or decision support, and healthcare administrators defined as those "who plan, direct, and coordinate medical and health services." They may manage an entire facility, a specific clinical area or department, or a group medical practice. This category is expected to experience a far greater growth rate than the average for all job categories. Medical and health services managers held about 429,850 jobs in 2020 and a growth rate of 32% or 139,600 jobs is expected [83]. Medical and health services managers must adapt to changes in healthcare laws, regulations, and technology. Health information managers, for example, are responsible for the maintenance and security of all patient records and data and must stay up to date with evolving information technology, current or proposed laws about health information systems, and trends in managing large amounts of complex data. They ensure that databases are complete, accurate, and accessible only to authorized personnel. Medical and health services managers typically need at least a bachelor's degree to enter the occupation; however, master's degrees are common and sometimes preferred by employers [83].

Employment in computer and IT occupations, in general, is projected to grow 13% from 2020 to 2030 [58], adding about 667,600 new jobs. Demand for these workers will stem from the greater emphasis on cloud computing, the collection and storage of big data, and information security needs across all industries. Categories within the area of IT such as information security analysts (33%); software developers, quality assurance analysts, and testers (22%); web developer and digital designers (13%); and computer and information systems managers (11%), are all expected to grow at rates well above the average (% growth indicated in brackets) [58–60]. Demand for computer and information systems managers is expected to grow as firms increasingly expand their operations to digital platforms or as health information systems and HIEs are further implemented and integrated. Employment growth will result from the need to bolster cybersecurity in these computer and information systems. However, some of the other computer technology roles such as computer network architect (5%), database administrator (8%), and computer systems support specialist (9%), will show only average or modest growth or note in the case of computer programmers are expected to decline in numbers over the next 10 years [58].

The only available Canadian figures come from a 2014 Canadian HI-HIM human resource sector study that forecast a shortfall of up to 12,000 skilled individuals in the eHealth/digital health field over the next five years (at that time to 2019) [84]. The two areas of major concern were IT and HIM. Within the HIM profession alone, 44.5% of all certified HIM professionals in Canada were 50 years of age or older and expected to retire within the next 5–10 years necessitating a minimum replacement demand of 718 HIM professionals. Based on the current replacement rate of HIM professionals in Canada (approximately 300 per year become certified), Canada is already falling short of new entrants to the profession. When both the growth and skills shortage numbers are included, the number of HIM professionals required increases to 1124 per annum, a projected shortage of 824 people per year. Unless the forecast job vacancies are filled and the existing workforce retrained, the report painted a dire picture of unexpected delays, cost overruns, and risks to patient safety and care [84,85].

A target figure for eHealth/digital health professional needs/supply in the United States was based on rough estimates of implementation of electronic records within hospitals and physicians' offices using an analysis of about 5000 hospitals in the HIMSS Analytics Database [86–88]. Hersh and Wright found an overall staffing ratio of 0.142 IT full-time equivalents (FTE) per hospital bed and extrapolating to all hospital beds in the United States, an estimated workforce size of 108,390 FTE. It was estimated that to achieve a fully EHR with shared data, a total of 149,174 IT FTE would be needed—or an increase in the supply of 40,784 HIT personnel at that time [88]. An additional study, looking at the estimated workforce for the deployment of the nationwide health information network (NHIN) and implementation of electronic records for the 400,000 practicing physicians who did not have them, estimated the need for another 7600 FTEs. For the 4000 hospitals that still needed EHRs, another 28,600 specialists and about 420 other professionals were needed to build the infrastructure in communities to interconnect all these systems [89]. After the rollout of EHRs afforded by HITECH incentive funding these authors revisited the data and found their original figures vastly underestimated the actual and needed HI professionals [22]. Using 2014 hospital data through the HIMSS analytic database they found the HI workforce to be 161,160—a figure substantially above the calculated need of 149,174. And an additional 19,852 (or 11% higher) would be needed for further growth and an additional 153,114 FTE if hospitals were to reach the advanced use functions sought through the meaningful use program (i.e., equivalent to HIMSS EMRAM (Electronic Medical Record Adoption Model) Stage 7, a fully integrated EHR).

The only environmental scan on HIE/HIO human resources to date, the white paper issued by HIMSS and AHIMA based on the results of a 2012 survey on "Trends in Health Information Exchange Organizational Staffing" reiterated the need to pay attention to the staffing needs of HIEs [90], p. 5].

> Many initiatives are underway at the federal, state and local levels, and in the private sector, to foster and enable interoperable electronic health information exchange, most of which is facilitated through Health Information Exchange Organizations or Networks (HIO). Significant focus is placed on the governance, business models, policies, standards and technical infrastructure required for long-term sustainability; however, *little attention is focused on the staffing of HIOs. This is an unfortunate oversight—even the most well-designed HIO cannot operate in a silo. It is therefore essential to consider current and future staffing needs of these organizations.* (Italics added)

The HIMSS and AHIMA workgroup noted three roles as particularly important to HIEs:

- Health information management and exchange specialists,
- Health information privacy and security specialists, and
- Programmers and software engineers.

Roles within the technology category included: security, data integration, data integrity, connectivity, data quality/compliance, payment processing, technical project management, software application support, business intelligence, specification/design/coding or testing, and help desk/support [90], p. 17]. The most prevalent technical roles were software applications support, help desk support, and data integration. Operations roles were dominated by marketing/sales/PR (note—related to a source of income and sustainability for the HIE), executive management roles, project management, and administrative assistant roles. Fewer positions were filled for privacy and security (but likely to be on-site rather than outsourced) and HIM [90], p. 20]. Organizations used a variety of staffing mixes including full-time and part-time employees, job sharing, on-site contractors, and outsourcing.

Over half (58%) of organizations were hiring positions at the bachelor's level with areas of specialization in finance, accounting, HIM, HIT, business, provider relations, computer science, or IT; and the predominant credential sought was that of project management professional followed by CPHIMS and RHIA. Even while stating that the most common staffing challenge was a lack of available qualified candidates, few respondents at that time were involved with the federally funded HITECH Workforce Development Program either through partnerships with one of the educational development consortia (usually a community college) or use of interns in the training programs or hiring of HITECH graduates.

In a follow-up survey of C-suite executives in 16 HIEs, a growth within these organizations just within the elapsed two-year time span was noted, with a shift in staffing numbers of participating organizations from 50 or less in 2012 to greater than 400 (in more than half) in 2014 and a broader range of participants beyond hospital and physician practice (payers, emergency medical services (EMS), long-term care, nursing homes, behavioral health centers, state public health) [90]. IT still represented over half of the staff, and within this category three problem areas identified in the first survey—data integrity, connectivity, data integration—were further explored.

Participants in the survey reported the following experiences in hiring and recruiting for these positions:

- difficulty finding Project Management experience specific to HIEs,
- extended periods needed to find qualified candidates that had both a cultural and technical fit to the organization, and
- lack of a system for networking with peers to identify qualified candidates [90,91].

Globally although there has been considerable interest in mapping strategies to achieve digital technologies and integrated HIE systems and more than 120 WHO member states have developed such strategies and policies [32] there is considerable variation in LMICs depending on the state of the available infrastructure, finances, healthcare professional human resources, government backing, and governance structures [31]. WHO has also addressed health human resources globally with an emphasis on education and training of care providers [92], but in achieving the vision of integrated HIEs no mention is made of the necessary HI, HIM, or HIT personnel.

2.4 Skills and training of digital health professionals

Outside of the long-standing accredited programs and credentialing in HIM through the colleges of the professional associations AHIMA and CHIMA in the United States and Canada, respectively [44,50,51], training programs for digital health and/or HI professionals are relatively new and, at best, producing well under the number of graduates needed to address the projected demand [84,85,87–89,93]. Each year about 3000 new graduates enter the HIM profession in the United States. In Canada, roughly 100 students graduate every year from HI programs, and only 250–300 graduates from HIM programs from a variety of college, degree, and certificate programs [94]. These numbers are not enough to provide the thousands needed for EHR and HIE implementation in the short-term and are increasingly insufficient to meet long-term demands for the development, operation, and management of the health information infrastructure in nations around the world and the ongoing work with EHRs and HIEs and meaningful use of health data and information.

2.4.1 Current credentials offered

Several certifications in eHealth/digital health information fields are available and often sponsored through a recognized professional college or commission (e.g., CCHIM, Commission on Certification for Health Informatics and Information Management) or professional association (e.g., AHIMA, AMIA, HIMSS) or state certifying body (see Table 2.1). Certification distinguishes an individual as competent and knowledgeable in a specific area, adds credibility to the profession, and offers some assurance to employers that these individuals have demonstrated proficiency and possess a broad base of knowledge by undertaking studies in an accredited educational program and/or passing a rigorous national examination. Certification demonstrates a commitment to ongoing professional development and maintenance of certification.

In some instances, the criterion for eligibility to write the credentialing examination requires graduation from an accredited program. Accreditation is a voluntary process that educational programs participate in as a means to demonstrate to the public and potential students that a program meets or exceeds stated standards of educational quality. AHIMA developed an accreditation program for medical record programs in 1943, and currently, CAHIIM is recognized by the Council for Higher Education Accreditation. Program accreditation by CAHIIM is necessary for eligibility for the AHIMA/CCHIIM professional HIM Certification Exams and CAHIIM accredits programs in HIM at the associate, baccalaureate, and master's level and in HI at the master's level [44,50,51,93]. Required curriculum in these programs has been established by subject matter experts in the field, industry leaders, and educators for HIM and HI [61,79,80,95].

Distinctions in HIE versus the longer-standing HIM and HI professionals are still being identified and clarified. HITComp, or health IT competencies, were a key component of the EU-US eHealth Work Project [96], a European Commission-funded project to advance digital skills development for the healthcare workforce. The project had a four-fold mission: to measure, inform, educate, and advance eHealth skills, education, and knowledge throughout the European Union, United States, and globally. HITComp hosts a repository of tools and resources for educators, health professionals, engineers, students, or others in learning about eHealth/digital health. A look through HITComp's competency listings (of 1025 total) provides resources for 26 specific competency areas related to "HIE/ Interoperability/Interfaces/Integration" in the domains of Direct Patient Care, Administration, Informatics, Engineering/Information Systems/ ICT, Research/Biomedicine (see Table 2.2). Twenty-one learning modules are available in the Foundational Curriculum available on the HITComp website (http://ehealthwork.eu/).

Within HIM, CCHIIM administers two certifications: RHIA and RHIT (see Table 2.1). Individuals who hold the **RHIA** credential are experts in managing patient health information and medical records, administering computer information systems, collecting and analyzing patient data, and using classification systems and medical terminologies. They have comprehensive knowledge of medical, administrative, ethical, and legal requirements, and standards related to healthcare delivery and the privacy of protected patient information.

Professionals holding the **RHIT** credential ensure the quality of medical records by verifying their completeness, accuracy, and proper entry into computer systems. RHITs use computer applications to assemble and analyze patient data. They often specialize in coding diagnoses and procedures in patient records for reimbursement and research.

Several specializations and advanced coding certifications are also offered by AHIMA including Coding Associate (**CCA**), Coding Specialist (**CCS**), and a physician-based coding specialist (**CS-P**). Specialty certifications and training programs are offered in health data analysis (**CHDA**), clinical documentation improvement (**CDIP**), healthcare privacy and security specialist (**CHPS**), and healthcare technology specialist (**CHTS**). The advanced and specialized certifications offered by AHIMA require (1) prior training through an HIM program at the college, baccalaureate, or Masters level; (2) prior certification in HIM at RHIT or RHIA levels; (3) certification in a variety of health professions (e.g., RN, MD, PhD, DO) plus related work experience; or (4) an associate-level degree and various years of related experience (see Table 2.1).

Within the field of HI there are currently two credentials, Certified Professional in Healthcare Information and Management Systems (**CPHIMS**) and Certified Associate in Healthcare Information and Management Systems (**CAHIMS**), offered in the United States, with a Canadian extension, **CPHIMS-CA**, offered in Canada through HIMSS (see Table 2.1). CAHIMS certification is designed for emerging professionals within the industry (five years or less of experience) who demonstrate knowledge of health IT and management systems. CPHIMS professionals demonstrate mastery of knowledge considered important for competent practice in the healthcare

TABLE 2.2 Online ONC-HIT learning modules (Workforce Development Program) and digital health information exchange learning modules (US*EU eHealth Work Project).

ONC-HIT Workforce Development Program[a]	HITComp[b]
	HIE/interoperability/interfaces/integration
1. Introduction to Healthcare and Public Health in the United States	Assess risks in relation to health information exchanges (HIEs) between different healthcare systems
2. The Culture of Healthcare	Compare how administrative, legal, financial, and management HIT/eHealth systems interface with other systems
3. Terminology in Healthcare and Public Health Settings	Compare how your organizational health information systems interface with external health information systems (e.g., EHR to community pharmacy systems, etc.) from a process and workflow perspective, and maximize interoperability between systems, per your role in patient care
4. Introduction to Information and Computer Sciences	Improve interoperability among health IT/eHealth and related information systems, applications, programs, devices, and tools
5. History of Health Information Technology in the United States	Integrate health IT/eHealth systems with other systems where appropriate such as departmental, radiology, laboratory systems, etc., and lead the development and approval processes for the methods for transferring data and messages between systems
6. Health Management Information Systems	Participate in the evaluation and selection of portable and mobile devices to facilitate data input and management of health IT/eHealth systems
7. Working with Health IT Systems	Recognize that for successful interoperability or integration to be achieved systems must either adhere to certain informatics standards or rely on middleware to supplement any technology or data transformation resulting from lack of standardization
8. Installation & Maintenance of Health IT Systems	Convey the importance of interfaces between systems, how systems are interdependent upon each other, and how the health record can be impacted by systems interfacing out of and into the EHR, including the flow of data inputs and outputs in the EHR
9. Networking and HIE	Describe basic interface design standards and design principles
10. Healthcare Workflow Process Improvement	Explain the difference between semantic and syntactic interoperability and the role each plays in overall interoperability
11. Configuring EHRs	Identify information systems that support HIE, and describe some basic features
12. Quality Improvement	Understand the concepts of and technologies used in mobile, telehealth, and system interoperability and how these relate to HIE
13. Public Health IT	Understand what is meant by system integration and interfacing and the challenges of integrating disparate but similar systems
14. Special Topics Course in Vendor-Specific Systems	Formulate processes and structures that support multidirectional flow of information and data (such as HIE, patient portals, remote access, and teleworking)
15. Usability and Human Factors	Implement HIE solutions to facilitate team-based patient care

(*Continued*)

TABLE 2.2 (Continued)

ONC-HIT Workforce Development Program[a]	HITComp[b]
	HIE/interoperability/interfaces/integration
16. Professionalism/Customer Service in the Health Environment	Manage the process leading to an environment that supports interoperability, interfacing and integration of components of health information technology applications
17. Working in Teams	Define HIE, interoperability, interfaces and integration in health IT/eHealth
18. Planning, Management, and Leadership for Health IT	Understand how HIEs and telehealth can improve communication between providers
19. Introduction to Project Management	Apply knowledge of different standards and enterprise models to facilitate the interoperability and assimilation of data and information from multiple sources
20. Training and Instructional Design	Consider the opportunities and constraints predicated by standards and consciously apply these to healthcare systems and interface design
21. Population Health	Demonstrate how HIEHIE enhances patient care, and use appropriate procedures for submitting and accessing medical information through an HIE
22. Care Coordination and Interoperable Health IT Systems	Assess risks in relation to HIEs between different healthcare systems
23. Value-Based Care	Compare how administrative, legal, financial and management HIT/eHealth systems interface with other systems
24. Healthcare Data Analytics	Compare how your organizational health information systems interface with external health information systems (e.g., EHR to community pharmacy systems, etc.) from a process and workflow perspective, and maximize interoperability between systems, per your role in patient care
25. Patient-Centered Care	Improve interoperability among health IT/eHealth and related information systems, applications, programs, devices, and tools
	Integrate health IT/eHealth systems with other systems where appropriate such as departmental, radiology, laboratory systems, etc., and lead the development and approval processes for the methods for transferring data and messages between systems

[a]*HealthIT.gov. (last reviewed on Feb 21, 2020). Health IT Curriculum Resources for Educators. The workforce components include an updated and expanded set of health IT instructional materials to help healthcare workers and others stay current in the changing digital healthcare environment and deliver care more effectively. Links to learning modules available at: https://www.healthit.gov/topic/health-it-resources/health-it-curriculum-resources-educators.*

[b]*HITComp (2021). Health Information Technology Competencies. HITComp is a searchable database designed for educators, workforce developers, current and future workforce members, students, eHealth managers, staffing experts and others interested in healthcare information technology/eHealth. HITComp is a part of the EU*US eHealth Work Project, a European-Commission funded project with a goal of mapping skills and competencies, providing access to knowledge tools and platforms, and strengthening, disseminating, and sharing success outcomes for a skilled transatlantic eHealth workforce. See* ***HIE/Interoperability/Interfaces/Integration*** *under Area of Competency. Available at: http://hitcomp.org/competencies/.*

EHR, Electronic health record; *HIT*, health information technology.

information and management systems field. The certification covers general healthcare and technology areas as well as in-depth knowledge of health IT systems, including analysis, design, selection, implementation, support, maintenance, testing, evaluation, privacy, and security with a focus on the administration and management of IT systems used in healthcare environments.

Additional certification for those with advanced degrees in health informatics (minimum Master's level) and HI work experience (minimum 4–6 years depending on prior training) has been developed by AMIA (see Table 2.1) and the inaugural certification examination will be offered in the late fall of 2021 (the examination testing window is open from October 1, 2021, to January 16, 2022) [AMIA Health Informatics Certification (AHIC)] [49].

2.5 Defining and executing a future strategy for health informaticians and health information exchange professionals

2.5.1 Health information workforce development

The US government, through the American Recovery and Reinvestment Act (ARRA), released millions of dollars to universities and colleges to train 50,000 health IT professionals as part of its $2 billion strategy to achieve widespread meaningful use of healthcare IT and provide for the use of an EHR for each person in the United States—the number of trainees needed based largely on the NHIN Workforce Study [21,89]. Funds were administered in the *Information Technology Professional in Health Care Program* (the "Workforce Program") developed through the Office of the National Coordinator for Health Information Technology (ONC) and in 2010 four programs were initiated. Training programs at the college and university level were funded as well as several Curriculum Development Centers (at five universities) for the development of modules and curriculum content that could be shared across educational institutions. A short-lived Competency Examination—the HIT Pro examination—was awarded to North Virginia Community College to fund the design and initial competency exams in health IT for individuals who completed one of the college consortium programs [21].

An evaluation of all four workforce development programs conducted by the nonpartisan and objective research organization NORC at the University of Chicago [97] indicated that the program was at least partially successful in that it trained 1704 students through the university programs, 19,733 students through the college programs, and administered 9500 HIT Pro exams (as of the end of December 2013 at the time of the survey). Among the university and college-trained students, about two-thirds were employed in health IT or health IT-related positions six months after program completion [97]. Curricular materials developed for the program were generally found to be useful by schools, and programs were able to choose which elements they wanted to include in their courses. Some concerns were noted about the quality of the materials, but these have been improved with the revised and expanded versions of the material funded through the ONC-HIT [98]. Five additional modules were added in areas relevant to improved care delivery: population health, care coordination and interoperable health IT systems, value-based care, healthcare data analytics, and patient-centered care. All material and instructional modules are available online (available at https://www.healthit.gov/topic/onc-hitech-programs/workforce-development-programs).

Many employers were either unaware of the ONC workforce program or skeptical that a six-month training period alone could provide the skills needed for employability. Within the workforce program, schools that established relationships with employers for student placements and hands-on experience were better able to support students in finding employment after graduation [97].

Additional research into workforce development programs through ONC and more broadly across the globe is still needed to identify and define the "skills and experience required to meet the demands and advance the profession of both current and future HIOs" [36,93,97]. Talent is critical to leveraging opportunities and advantages afforded by electronic records and the exchange of health information in improving healthcare delivery and integration of care, health outcomes, cost savings, and patient satisfaction. A national human resources strategy is needed to address the current shortage of skilled workers and to develop a long-term strategy for education and training of digital health and health information personnel necessary to ensure the continued quality of health data collected, its security and confidentiality, and to manage and maintain the systems and data in the future. The majority of work to date has been concentrated in a few countries (i.e., United States, Canada, Australia, and the United Kingdom) and only within a few health information professions (i.e., HIM, HI, health IT).

Labor statistics and expanded national occupational codes beyond the categories currently available are needed—and this is true not only of the US statistics (the Standard Occupational Classification system used in the collection of the Bureau of Labor Statistics data) but is also seen in Canada in their National Occupation Codes and internationally in the International Standard Classification of Occupations (ISCO) [99]. In the latter, they are limited to only three classifications: Health Information Technicians, Filing and Copying Clerks, and Librarians and Related Information Professionals. A classification or multiple classifications of digital health workers and/or health information workers needs to be generated, applied, monitored, and tracked. Ideally, these classifications should be consistent across countries as well as implemented within the ISCO standards. In addition, the ONC Health IT Workforce Development Program needs to continue to support HIOs and HIEs in addressing their skilled workforce needs. In many instances, existing health professionals in the domains of informatics and/or information management can transition into roles supporting HIE. All healthcare workers, no matter what their role, will need to be familiar with the digital environment and have basic information literacy skills that include knowledge of IT, informatics, information management, information governance, cybersecurity, and digital professionalism.

2.6 Emerging trends

One of the defining characteristics of the national HIE landscape is variability; both technically and operationally, every state and region has a unique solution to facilitating the exchange of medical information securely, and this is even more so when one looks globally at the introduction of HIEs. It follows that human resource needs will also be variable across HIEs and the best that can be done is broadly define the types of roles and functions needed and the competencies required to carry those out. Current certifications in HI and HIM cover the core content of information technology (hardware and software), legal and regulatory requirements (federal and state, but these may vary state to state), workflow processes and change and project management, network architecture, data stewardship (including data and information governance), data analysis, and telehealth (see Tables 2.1 and 2.2).

The advantages of credentialed employees versus noncredentialed employees are still debated and still to be determined. In many instances, employers are looking for individuals who can fulfill multiple roles so that narrowly defined certifications or credentials may not be desirable. The proliferation of certifications, subtle differences in their curriculum and competencies are confusing to potential employers and students alike. Many of these programs are short-term and offered online with limited opportunities for a hands-on experience that develops true expertise and competency in a given task or skill; the same is true for the training materials offered through the ONC-HIT educational modules.

2.6.1 Education

We have previously argued that within the fields of HI and HIM there is a convergence of knowledge, skills, and roles that will shape the training of future health information professionals and shape the programs being offered [44]. There are now several "merged" or "balanced" programs in health informatics and information management (HIIM), such as Conestoga College's Bachelor of Applied Health Information Science program and the University of Regina's newly accredited Masters in Health Informatics and Information Management (MHIIM) that provide education in both HI and HIM [100,101] and whose graduates are eligible to sit the Canadian HIM credentialing exam; Louisiana Tech University has an HIIM department that offers an HIIM Bachelor of Science degree and a Master of Health Informatics [102]. The University of Tennessee Health Science Center offers an entry-level and Postgraduate HIIM program entirely online [103]. Both programs are accredited by CAHIIM. The University of Mississippi's online MHIIM program also accredited through CAHIIM may be completed on a part-time basis. The program "prepares healthcare professionals for leadership roles in a healthcare system that increasingly relies on information technology" [104].

The "HIDDIN" workforce concept spearheaded by Australian and New Zealand researchers[9] takes "convergence" a step further to define health information professionals as "anyone who self-identifies as part of the health information workforce ... You are part of the workforce if you work (including volunteer or actively seeking) in a role where the primary function is related to developing, maintaining, or governing the systems for the management of health data, health information, or health knowledge"—a holistic approach in defining and quantifying this workforce [105]. Within their 2018 Australian health information workforce census of 1597 survey participants, 37% identified as Health Information Managers, 22% as Health Informaticisits, 16% in Clinical coding and classification, 14% as Health Librarians, 9% working in data analytics, and 2% in costing [106,107]. Preparation for these roles was primarily a bachelor's degree (43.5%) followed by Masters degrees (21.7%) or graduate diploma (15.3%) [107].

Parallel data collected from a scoping review of the international literature (between 1946[10] and 2018) on health information work disclosed a variety of roles, job titles, and skills [105,106]. The health information occupation identities reported in the publications were grouped into nine broad categories; HITs, health information managers and medical or health librarians, medical informaticians, appear in the earliest years (from the 1970s on) with health informaticians and health information professionals emerging as roles/titles in the mid-1990s, and in more recent years (since 2005) the clinical informaticians and clinical subgroups (e.g., nursing, pharmacy, pathology, public health, bioinformaticians). Consumer health informatician and

[9] See the text "The Health Information Workforce: Current and Future Developments" edited by KerrynButler-Henderson, KarenDay, and KathleenGray. Springer Nature, Switzerland AG, 2021. https://link.springer.com/book/10.1007/978-3-030-81850-0

[10] Explicit publications about the health information workforce first appeared in 1973, remained low (at 9) for the first two decades (1973–1990), and from 1991 the number of publications steadily increased to 56 between 2016 and 2018.

consumer health librarian appear as terms/roles in the mid-90s [105, p. 31].

Although most people currently working within HIEs are entering at the baccalaureate level, professional associations are moving toward master's level preparation as the new level of entry for these highly skilled professionals who are dealing with greater complexity in the workplace [54–56]. Professional associations in the United States, Canada, Australia, and globally have repeatedly outlined the need for positions requiring new skills and experience with EHR technology, project management, team leadership, data analytics, or strategic planning and recommended the transition to "a stage where HIM professionals at an advanced level of practice are master's degree-prepared upon entry into the work force" [36,52,54–56,61,108].

Many universities and educational institutions, often in partnership with relevant businesses or industry, are investigating the practicality and advantages/disadvantages of delivering micro-credentials. Micro-credentials are short, concentrated groups of courses that are flexible, innovative, timely, and are based on industry needs. They are designed to be high quality, competency-based, and meaningful credentials; many are offered online or in a hybrid format. In some institutions, micro-credentials may be stackable and can be combined to form a part of a larger credential. Micro-credential requirements vary significantly from credential to credential since anyone can grant them and there are no official requirements [43].

Short-term certification programs (e.g., in Privacy and Security, Decision Support or Data Analytics, Data and Information Standards) may have their greatest value in providing more in-depth information and knowledge to post-baccalaureate trainees who already have a rudimentary foundational knowledge of informatics and information management. We are seeing this trend in some HIIM programs and departments, including the University of Illinois-Chicago [109] and the Indiana University School of Informatics and Computing [110], which offer undergraduate degrees in HIM and graduate degrees that focus on HI. Many of these existing programs are accredited through CAHIIM so that their graduates can sit the national RHIA examination. It may not be necessary, or desirable, to accredit all health information certificate programs but, at the very least, the curriculum should follow some generally agreed upon and necessary curricular competencies.

2.6.2 Continued ONC-HIT Workforce Development—public health informatics

The most recent component of the ONC-HIT Workforce Development program specifically targets building up the public health IT workforce [111,112]. During the COVID-19 epidemic, deficiencies in the current training and supply of individuals with necessary skills in epidemiology, informatics, health information management, and data analysis as well as data quality and information exchange were highlighted and evident. Also, disparities in health outcomes in different racial and ethnic groups, many based on the social determinants of health (SDOH), were exposed. The 10 awardees, comprising Historically Black Colleges and Universities, Hispanic Serving Institutions, Asian American and Native American Pacific Islander-Serving Institutions, and other collaborating institutions, received $73 million to form consortia to train 4000 individuals over four years through an interdisciplinary approach in public HI and technology. Similar to the earlier workforce training programs the consortia will develop curricula, recruit and train participants, secure paid internship opportunities, and assist in career placement, in this instance, at public health agencies, public health-focused nonprofits, or other public health-focused organizations [112].

The development of new curricular modules is expected to build upon the previous ONC workforce training program components and may include new subject areas such as health equity; data science, data privacy/security; data aspects of outbreak investigation; epidemiology; public health analytics; lab-based and remote diagnostics; public health reporting (e.g., immunizations, syndromic surveillance, electronic lab reporting and electronic case reporting); public health emergency preparedness and response; HL7 FHIR basics, vocabularies and terminologies; public policy and combining multiple data streams (e.g., clinical data from EHR, lab results, immunizations, demographic data, utilization metrics, and claims data, and data from other nonhealthcare sources such as SDOH, waste-water, etc.) for analytical and HIE purposes.

2.7 Summary

Although great progress has been made over the past decade in introducing the EHR in healthcare facilities and physicians' offices, many systems remain siloed and movement toward a fully integrated electronic network and HIE has been slow. Hampering the implementation of the technical infrastructure is the lack (in numbers and skills) of digital health professionals who can not only assist in the deployment of systems but who can also work with the data and information that they contain, and who can be instrumental in the establishment of standards for capture, transmission, sharing, and governance of health data. The previous workforce development program from ARRA/HITECH provided an initial impetus to develop and define the needed competencies to educate a portion of the estimated 50,000 digital health workers (in the United States), but further work is needed on the definition of HI and HIE competencies and skills, and the continued provision of digital health information professionals. Development of training programs for individuals interested in building HIE skills can be stand-alone (e.g., certification/micro-credential in HIE) or as additional postgraduate training for other health professionals (e.g., HIMs, HIs, HITs). There is a continued need for additional training for clinical health professionals (e.g., physicians, nurses, pharmacists) in informatics and information management skills who will be working with electronic records as well as HIE. The newly introduced subspecialty in CI will provide specialized training to physicians. The latest workforce development initiative through the ONC-HIT and HHS has targeted public health and the recruitment and development of a more diverse and inclusive workforce among blacks, Hispanics, and Asian communities.

Given the state of the workforce and training options for HI and HIE professionals, a national human resources strategy for digital health information professionals is needed in every country for monitoring both supply and demand for these crucial healthcare workers. We need to be able to better track and even identify those individuals who work in digital health and health information, above and beyond the current labor statistics monitoring health records technicians, health administrators and managers, and computer technologists alone, and in monitoring the supply of individuals through current training and/or educational programs. We need to identify the various professionals working on and within the health information systems to not only fully realize their potential in securely providing quality data for decision-making but also to ensure that the data collected are complete, equitable, timely, and correct.

It is hard to imagine any other group of specialists in the health workforce that is accountable for such crucial outcomes as health data, information and knowledge are expected to deliver in the twenty-first century, and yet is so diffuse and disjointed. In the era of digital health, an apparently mission-critical part of the health workforce is ill-defined and fragmented... ([105, p. 39]

Questions for discussion

1. In which roles within a hospital, clinical or health system would knowledge and/or expertise in HIE be useful?
2. Describe how HIE specialists might interact with or support operations within a national health system. How about within an individual hospital or clinic or within a family physician(s)'s practice?
3. What knowledge and skills might be important for HIE specialists to develop over time to complement the larger digital health workforce?
4. What kind of ongoing professional certification or development might be necessary for HIE specialists to seek as they mature in their careers?

References

[1] Schoen C, Osborn R, Doty MM, Squires D, Peugh J, Applebaum SA. Survey of primary care physicians in 11 countries: perspectives on care, costs, and experience. Health Aff 2009;28(6):w1171–83.

[2] Schoen C, Osborn R, Squires D, Doty M, Rasmussen P, Pierson R, et al. Survey of primary care doctors in ten countries shows progress in use of health information technology, less in other areas. Health Aff 2012;31 (12):2805–16.

[3] Hsiao CJ, Hing E. Use and characteristics of electronic health record systems among office-based physician practices: United States, 2001–2012. NCHS Data Brief 2012;111:1–8. Available from: http://www.cdc.gov/nchs/data/databriefs/db111.pdf.

[4] Collier R. National physician survey: EMR use at 75%. CMAJ 2015;187:E17–18. Available from: https://doi.org/10.1503/cmaj.109-4957, https://www.cmaj.ca/content/cmaj/187/1/E17.full.pdf.

[5] Myrick KL, Ogburn DF. Table. Percentage of office-based physicians using any electronic health record (EHR)/electronic medical record (EMR) system and physicians that have a certified EHR/EMR system, by specialty: National Electronic Health Records Survey, 2017. National Center for Health Statistics. Available from: https://www.cdc.gov/nchs/data/nehrs/2017_NEHRS_Web_Table_EHR_Specialty.pdf; January 2019.

[6] Office of the National Coordinator for Health Information Technology (ONC-HIT). Office-based physician electronic health record adoption. Health IT Quick-Stat #50. Available from: https://www.healthit.gov/data/quickstats/office-based-physician-electronic-health-record-adoption; January 2019.

[7] Charles D, Gabriel M, Furukawa MF. Adoption of electronic health record systems among U.S. non-federal acute care hospitals: 2008–2013. ONC Data Brief, No. 16. Washington, DC: Office of the National Coordinator for Health Information Technology; May 2014.

[8] Gabriel M, Jones EB, Samy L, King J. Among critical-access hospitals progress and challenges: implementation and use of health information technology. Health Aff 2014;33(7):1262–70. Available from: https://doi.org/10.1377/hlthaff.2014.0279.

[9] Furukawa MF, Patel V, Charles D, Swain M, Mostashari F. Hospital electronic health information exchange grew substantially in 2008-12. Health Aff (Millwood) 2013;32(8):1346–54 Epub 2013/08/07.

[10] Henry J, Pylypchuk Y, Searcy T, Patel V. Adoption of electronic health record systems among U.S. non-federal acute care hospitals: 2008–2015. ONC Data Brief, No. 35. Washington, DC: Office of the National Coordinator for Health Information Technology. Available from: https://www.healthit.gov/sites/default/files/briefs/2015_hospital_adoption_db_v17.pdf; May 2016.

[11] Apathy NC, Holmgren AJ, Adler-Milstein J. A decade post-HITECH: critical access hospitals have electronic health records but struggle to keep up with other advanced functions. J Am Med Inform Assoc 2021. PMID: 34198342. Available from: https://doi.org/10.1093/jamia/ocab102.

[12] CDC National Center for Health Statistics (NCHS). National Electronic Health Records Survey (NEHRS). 2019 National Electronic Health Records Survey public use file national weighted estimates. Available from: https://www.cdc.gov/nchs/data/nehrs/2019NEHRS-PUF-weighted-estimates-508.pdf; August 2021.

[13] DesRoches CM, Campbell EG, Rao SR, Donelan K, Ferris TG, Jha A, et al. Electronic health records in ambulatory care — A national survey of physicians. N Engl J Med 2008;359:50–60.

[14] Audet A-M, Squires D, Doty MM. Where are we on the diffusion curve? Trends and drivers of primary care physicians' use of health information technology. Health Serv Res 2014;49(1 Pt 2):347–60. Available from:

https://doi.org/10.1111/1475-6773.12139; Published online 2013 Dec 21.

[15] Office of the National Coordinator for Health Information Technology. Office-based physician electronic patient engagement capabilities. Health IT Quick-Stat #54. Available from: https://www.healthit.gov/data/quickstats/office-based-physician-electronic-patient-engagement-capabilities; December 2016.

[16] Johnson C, Pylypchuk Y. Use of certified health IT and methods to enable interoperability by U.S. non-federal acute care hospitals, 2019. ONC Data Brief, No.54. Office of the National Coordinator for Health Information Technology: Washington DC; February 2021.

[17] Adler-Milstein J, Holmgren AJ, Kralovec P, Worzala C, Searcy T, Patel V. Electronic health record adoption in US hospitals: the emergence of a digital "advanced use" divide. JAMIA 2017;24(6):1142–8. Available from: https://doi.org/10.1093/jamia/ocx080.

[18] Adler-Milstein J, Jha AK. HITECH Act drove large gains in hospital electronic health record adoption. Health Aff 2017;36(8):1416–22. Available from: https://doi.org/10.1377/hlthaff.2016.1651.

[19] Hersh W. Health information technology workforce: identifying the gaps [Internet]. Available from: https://www.ruralcenter.org/sites/default/files/Rural%20HIT%20Workforce.pdf; no date - a.

[20] Hersh W. Finding the future workforce to support data-driven healthcare. AAMC Workforce PowerPoint Slides [Internet]. Available from: https://dmice.ohsu.edu/hersh/aamc-workforce.pdf; no date - b.

[21] Hersh W. A retrospective on the HITECH Workforce Development Program. Available from: https://www.healthit.gov/buzz-blog/community-college-consortia/retrospective-workforce-development-program; March 10, 2014.

[22] Hersh WR, Boone KW, Totten AM. Characteristics of the healthcare information technology workforce in the HITECH era: underestimated in size, still growing, and adapting to advanced uses. JAMIA Open 2018;1(2):188–94. Available from: https://doi.org/10.1093/jamiaopen/ooy029.

[23] Centers for Medicare and Medicaid Services (CMS.gov.). Promoting Interoperability Programs [Internet]. Available from: https://www.cms.gov/regulations-and-guidance/legislation/ehrincentiveprograms; last modified December 1, 2021.

[24] Agency for Healthcare Research and Quality (AHRQ). Practice facilitation handbook. Module 17. Electronic Health Records and Meaningful Use [Internet]. Rockville, MD: Agency for Healthcare Research and Quality. Available from: https://www.ahrq.gov/ncepcr/tools/pf-handbook/mod17.html; content last reviewed May 2013.

[25] Furukawa MF, Vibbert D, Swain M. ONC Data Brief. HITECH and health IT jobs: evidence from online job postings. Available from: https://www.healthit.gov/sites/default/files/pdf/0512_ONCDataBrief2_JobPostings.pdf; May 2012.

[26] HealthIT.gov. ONC Cures Act Final Rule. 21st Century Cures Act: Interoperability, Information Blocking, and the ONC Health IT Certification Program [Internet]. Office of the National Coordinator for Health Information Technology. Available from: https://www.healthit.gov/curesrule/; no date.

[27] Oderkirk J. Readiness of electronic health record systems to contribute to national health information and research. OECD Health Working Papers, No. 99. Paris: OECD Publishing; 2017. Available from: https://doi.org/10.1787/9e296bf3-en.

[28] OECD/European Union. Adoption and use of electronic medical records and ePrescribing. In: Health at a glance: Europe 2018: state of health in the EU cycle [Internet]. Paris: OECD Publishing /Brussels: European Union. Available from: https://doi.org/10.1787/health_glance_eur-2018-56-en; 2018 [Access the Excel file – OECD (2012 and 2016) OECD HCQI Questionnaire on Secondary Use of Health Data: Electronic Health Records at https://doi.org/10.1787/888934259788].

[29] Zelmer J, Ronchi E, Hypponen H, Lupianez-Villanueva F, Codagnone C, Nøhr C, et al.On behalf of the OECD Health ICT Benchmarking Pilot Group International health IT benchmarking: learning from cross-country comparisons. JAMIA 2017;24(2):371–9.

[30] Payne TH, Lovis C, Gutteridge C, Pagliari C, Natarajan S, Yong C, et al. Status of health information exchange: a comparison of six countries. J Glob Health 2019;9(2):1–16. Available from: https://doi.org/10.7189/jogh.09.020427.

[31] Akhlaq A, McKinstry B, Bin Muhammad K, Sheikh A. Barriers and facilitators to health information exchange in low- and middle-income country settings: a systematic review. Health Policy Plan 2016;31(9):1310–25. Available from: https://doi.org/10.1093/heapol/czw056.

[32] World Health Organization (WHO). Global strategy on digital health 2020–2025. Licence: CC BY-NC-SA 3.0 IGO. Geneva: World Health Organization. Available from: https://www.who.int/publications/i/item/9789240020924; August 18, 2021.

[33] World Health Organization (WHO). Health data: a critical element to meet the SDGs [Internet]. Available from: https://www.who.int/data/stories/health-data-a-critical-element-to-meet-the-sdgs; May 13, 2020.

[34] World Health Organization (WHO). The triple billion targets [Internet]. Available from: https://www.who.

int/news-room/questions-and-answers/item/the-triple-billion-targets; April 18, 2020.

[35] Gibson CJ, Covvey HD. Chapter 13: Demystifying E-health human resources Medical information science reference In: Kabene SM, editor. Human resources in healthcare, health informatics and healthcare systems. Hershey, PA: IGI Global; 2010.

[36] Butler-Henderson K, Day K, Gray K. Chapter 1: The specialized data, information, and knowledge workforce in health: present and future. In: Butler-Henderson K, Day K, Gray K, editors. The health information workforce: current and future developments. Cham: Springer Nature; 2021. p. 3–20. Available from: https://link.springer.com/book/10.1007/978-3-030-81850-0.

[37] Koonin LM, Hoots B, Tsang CA, Leroy Z, Farris K, Tilman Jolly B, et al. Trends in the use of telehealth during the emergence of the COVID-19 pandemic – United States, January–March 2020. MMWR 2020; 69 (43):1595–99. Available from: https://doi.org/10.15585/mmwr.mm6943a3.

[38] Demeke HB, Pao LZ, Clark H, Romero L, Neri A, Shah R, et al. Telehealth practice among health centers during the COVID-19 pandemic—United States, July 11–17, 2020 MMWR 2020;69(50):1902–5PMID:33332297. Available from: https://doi.org/10.15585/mmwr.mm6950a4.

[39] Demeke HB, Merali S, Marks S, Zilversmit Pao L, Romero L, Sandhu P, et al. Trends in use of telehealth among health centers during the COVID-19 pandemic—United States, June 26–November 6, 2020. MMWR 2021;70(7):240–4. Available from: https://doi.org/10.15585/mmwr.mm7007a3.

[40] Mehrotra A, Chernew ME, Linetsky D, Hatch H, Cutler DA, Schneider EC. The impact of the COVID-19 pandemic on outpatient visits: changing patterns of care in the newest COVID-19 hot spots. New York: Commonwealth Fund. Available from: https://www.commonwealthfund.org/publications/2020/aug/impact-covid-19-pandemic-outpatient-visits-changing-patterns-care-newest; August 2020.

[41] Eysenbach G. What is e-health? J Med Internet Res 2001;3(2):e20. Available from: https://doi.org/10.2196/jmir.3.2.e20.

[42] World Health Organization (WHO). Digital health [Internet]. Available from: https://www.euro.who.int/en/health-topics/Health-systems/digital-health; 2019.

[43] Saskatchewan. Saskatchewan's guide to micro-credentials. Available from: https://www.saskatchewan.ca/residents/education-and-learning/microcredentials-in-saskatchewan; 2021.

[44] Gibson CJ, Dixon B, Abrams K. Convergent evolution of health information management and health informatics – a perspective on the future of information professionals in health care. Appl Clin Inf 2015;6. Available from: https://doi.org/10.4338/ACI-2014-09-RA-0077.

[45] Gardner RM, Overhage JM, Steen EB, Munger BS, Holmes JH, Williamson JJ, et al.AMIA Board of Directors Core content for the subspecialty of clinical informatics. JAMIA 2009;16(2):153–7. Available from: https://doi.org/10.1197/jamia.M3045.

[46] Safran C, Shabot MM, Munger BS, Holmes JH, Steen EB, Lumpkin JR, et al. Program requirements for fellowship education in the subspecialty of clinical informatics. JAMIA 2009;16(2):158–66. Available from: https://doi.org/10.1197/jamia.M3046.

[47] Lehmann CU, Gundlapalli AV, Williamson JJ, Fridsma DB, Hersh WR, Krousel-Wood M, et al. Five years of Clinical Informatics Board Certification for Physicians in the United States of America. Yearb Med Inf 2018;27:237–42. Available from: https://doi.org/10.1055/s-0038-1641198.

[48] Desai S, Mostaghimi A, Nambudiri VE. Clinical informatics subspecialists: characterizing a novel evolving workforce. JAMIA 2020;27(11):1711–15. Available from: https://doi.org/10.1093/jamia/ocaa173.

[49] AMIA. AMIA Health Informatics Certification (AHIC) [Internet]. Available from: https://amia.org/careers-certifications/amia-health-informatics-certification-ahic; 2021 [and AMIA AHIC Certification Guide (April, 2021): https://amia.org/careers-certifications/amia-health-informatics-certification-ahic/ahic-certification-guide].

[50] Crook G, Abrams K, Arnold GB. Chapter 2: The health information management profession. In: Abrams K, Gibson C, editors. Fundamentals of health information management. 2nd ed. Ottawa, ON: CHIMA, CHA Press; 2013.

[51] Brodnick MS. Chapter 2: the health informatics and information management professional. In: Abdelhak M, Hanken MA, editors. Health information: management of a strategic resource. 5th ed. St. Louis: Elsevier Saunders; 2016.

[52] Gibson CJ, Abrams K, Crook G. Health information management workforce transformation: new roles, new skills and experiences in Canada. Perspectives in health information management (International issue); May 2015.

[53] Marc DT, Robertson J, Gordon L, Green-Lawson ZD, Gibbs D, Dover K, et al. What the data say about HIM professional trends. J AHIMA 2017;88(5):24–31.

[54] AHIMA. Vision 2016: a Blueprint for Quality Education in HIM. Chicago, IL: American Health Information Management Association. Available from: http://library.ahima.org/xpedio/groups/public/documents/ahima/bok1_035517.pdf; September 24, 2007.

[55] Calhoun M, Rudman WJ, Watzlaf VJM. Vision 2016 to reality 2016: building a profession. J AHIMA 2012;83 (8):18–23.

[56] Abrams K, Carlon S, Haugen MB, Mancilla D, McElroy K, Millen M, et al. HIM reimagined outlines bold new future for HIM profession. J AHIMA 2017;88(6):22–5.
[57] AHIMA. 2018 AHIMA Health Information Management Curricula Competencies. Available from: https://www.ahima.org/education-events/academic-center/resource-pages/academic-curricula/; 2021.
[58] Bureau of Labor Statistics, U.S. Department of Labor. Occupational outlook handbook, computer and information technology occupations. Available from: https://www.bls.gov/ooh/computer-and-information-technology/home.htm; last modified September 8, 2021 [accessed 05.10.21].
[59] Bureau of Labor Statistics, U.S. Department of Labor. Occupational outlook handbook, computer and information research scientists. Available from: https://www.bls.gov/ooh/computer-and-information-technology/computer-and-information-research-scientists.htm; last modified January 3, 2022.
[60] Bureau of Labor Statistics, U.S. Department of Labor. Occupational outlook handbook, software developers, quality assurance analysts, and testers. Available from: https://www.bls.gov/ooh/computer-and-information-technology/software-developers.htm; 2021 [accessed 28.10.21].
[61] Global Health Workforce Council (GHWC). Global academic curricula competencies for health information professionals. Collaboration of AHIMA, AHIMA Foundation and IFHIMA. Available from: https://ifhimasitemedia.s3.us-east-2.amazonaws.com/wp-content/uploads/2018/01/20033722/AHIMA-GlobalCurricula_Final_6-30-15.pdf; June 30, 2015.
[62] IBM Security & the Ponemon Institute. Cost of a data breach report 2021. Available from: https://www.ibm.com/security/data-breach; 2021.
[63] Abelson R, Goldstein M. Anthem hacking points to security vulnerability of health care industry. The New York Times. Retrieved from: https://www.nytimes.com/2015/02/06/business/experts-suspect-lax-security-leftanthem-vulnerable-to-hackers.html; February 5, 2015.
[64] National Audit Office, Department of Health. Investigation: WannaCry cyber attack and the NHS. Report by the Comptroller and Auditor General. Retrieved from: https://www.nao.org.uk/wp-content/uploads/2017/10/Investigation-WannaCry-cyber-attack-and-the-NHS.pdf; April 2018.
[65] Collier R. NHS ransomware attack spreads worldwide. CMAJ 2017;189:E786–7. Available from: https://doi.org/10.1503/cmaj.1095434.
[66] Bureau of Labor Statistics, U.S. Department of Labor. Occupational outlook handbook, information security analysts. Available from: https://www.bls.gov/ooh/computer-and-information-technology/information-security-analysts.htm; 2021 [accessed 09.01.22].
[67] Deyan G. 25 + alarming healthcare data breaches statistics 2021 [and the largest healthcare data breaches]. Techinjury [blog] (last updated on Dec 6, 2021). Available from: https://techjury.net/blog/healthcare-data-breaches-statistics/.
[68] AHIMA. Certifications and careers. Certifications: Certified Health Data Analyst (CHDA®). Available from: https://www.ahima.org/certification-careers/certification-exams/chda/; 2021.
[69] Torpey E. Math at work: using numbers on the job. Occup Outlook Q Fall 2012;56(3):2–13. Available from: https://files.eric.ed.gov/fulltext/EJ990990.pdf.
[70] Bureau of Labor Statistics, U.S. Department of Labor. Occupational outlook handbook, mathematicians and statisticians. Available from: https://www.bls.gov/ooh/math/mathematicians-and-statisticians.htm; last modified September 8, 2021 [accessed 17.01.22].
[71] Bureau of Labor Statistics, U.S. Department of Labor. Occupational outlook handbook, epidemiologists. Available from: https://www.bls.gov/ooh/life-physical-and-social-science/epidemiologists.htm; last modified September 8, 2021 [accessed 04.01.22].
[72] Health IT Certification. CPHIT, CPEHR, CPHIE and CPORA overview. Available from: http://www.healthitcertification.com/overview.html; n.d.
[73] Bhyat R, Gibson C, Hayward R, Shachak A, Borycki EM, Condon A, et al. Implementing informatics competencies in undergraduate medical education: a national-level "train the trainer" initiative. In: Shachak A, Borycki EM, Reis SP, editors. Health professionals' education in the age of clinical information systems, mobile computing and social networks. London, UK: Elsevier; 2017. p. 347–70. Available from: https://www.sciencedirect.com/book/9780128053621/health-professionals-education-inthe-age-of-clinical-information-systems-mobile-computing-and-social-networks.
[74] CASN/Infoway. Nursing informatics: entry to practice competencies for registered nurses. Available from: https://www.casn.ca/wp-content/uploads/2014/12/Nursing-Informatics-Entry-to-Practice-Competencies-for-RNs_updated-June-4-2015.pdf; 2014, updated June 2015.
[75] AFMC-Infoway. eHealth competencies for undergraduate medical education. Available from: https://afmc.ca/en/priorities/projects-resources;https://www.ehealthresources.ca; 2014.
[76] AFPC-Infoway. e-Learning for health care professionals: e-medication reconciliation and e-prescribing. Available from: https://www.afpc.info/system/files/public/AFPC%20IPE%20Informatics_Digital%20Health%20FACTS_project%20overview_19Dec18.pdf; 2018 [and see e-learning resource at https://elearnhcp.ca/].

[77] Baker C, Charlebois M, Lopatka H, Moineau G, Zelmer J. Influencing change: preparing the next generation of clinicians to practice in the digital age. J Healthc Q 2016;18:5–7.

[78] AMIA. AMIA joins CAHIIM to lead informatics program accreditation. Available from: https://www.amia.org/news-and-publications/press-release/amia-joins-cahiim-lead-informatics-program-accreditation; 2014.

[79] CAHIIM. HI curriculum requirements. 2017 health informatics Master's degree curriculum requirements. Available from: https://www.cahiim.org/accreditation/health-informatics/curriculum-requirements.

[80] CAHIIM. HIM curriculum requirements. 2018 AHIMA curriculum requirements. Available from: https://www.cahiim.org/accreditation/health-information-management/curriculum-requirements.

[81] Mantas J, Ammenwerth E, Demiris G, Hasman A, Haux R, Hersh W, et al. IMIA recommendations on education task force. Recommendations of the International Medical Informatics Association (IMIA) on education in biomedical and health informatics. First Revision. Methods Inf Med 2010;49(2):105–20. Available from: https://doi.org/10.3414/ME5119.

[82] Bureau of Labor Statistics, U.S. Department of Labor. Occupational outlook handbook, medical records and health information specialists. Available from: https://www.bls.gov/ooh/healthcare/medical-records-and-health-information-technicians.htm; [accessed 05.10.21].

[83] Bureau of Labor Statistics, U.S. Department of Labor. Occupational outlook handbook, medical and health services managers. Available from: https://www.bls.gov/ooh/management/medical-and-health-services-managers.htm; [accessed 05.10.21].

[84] Prism Economics and Analysis. Health informatics and health information management: human resources outlook 2014–2019. Toronto, ON: Prism Economics and Analysis; 2014.

[85] O'Grady J. Health informatics and health information management: human resources report [Internet]. Toronto, ON: Prism Economics and Analysis;; 2009. Available from: http://www.ictc-ctic.ca/uploadedFiles/Labour_Market_Intelligence/E-Health/HIHIM_report_E.

[86] Hersh W. Who are the informaticians? What we know and should know. JAMIA 2006;13:166–70. Available from: https://doi.org/10.1197/jamia.M1912.

[87] Hersh W, Wright A. What workforce is needed to implement the health information technology agenda? Analysis from the HIMSS Analytics™ Database. AMIA Annu Symp Proc 2008;2008:303–7.

[88] Hersh W. The health information technology workforce: estimations of demands and a framework for requirements. Appl Clin Inf 2010;1:197–212. Available from: https://doi.org/10.4338/ACI-2009-11-R-0011.

[89] Altarum Institute. Nationwide Health Information Network (NHIN) workforce study: final report. Submitted to the Department of Health and Human Services (DHHS): Assistant Secretary for Planning and Evaluation. Available from: http://aspe.hhs.gov/sp/reports/2007/NHIN/NHINReport.shtml; 2007.

[90] AHIMA/HIMSS HIE Technology Staffing Workgroup. Trends in health information exchange organizational staffing: Part 2: a deeper look at staffing challenges. Available from: https://library.ahima.org/PdfView?oid = 300624; October 2014.

[91] AHIMA/HIMSS HIE Technology Staffing Workgroup. Trends in health information exchange organizational staffing, AHIMA/HIMSS HIE staffing model environmental scan. Available from: https://library.ahima.org/PdfView?oid = 106103; December 2012.

[92] World Health Organization (WHO). Global strategy on human resources for health: workforce 2030. Geneva: World Health Organization; 2016.

[93] Ritchie A, Siemensma G, Fenton SH, Butler-Henderson K. Chapter 5: Competencies, education, and accreditation of the health information workforce. In: Butler-Henderson K, Day K, Gray K, editors. The health information workforce: current and future developments. Cham: Springer Nature; 2021. p. 79–95. Available from: https://doi.org/10.1007/978-3-030-81850-0_5.

[94] Covvey HD, Fenton SL., Ovenden M. Survey of Health Informatics Programs and Health Information Management Programs in Canada 2020 [Internet]. Searchable database Available from: http://www.nihi.ca/listings.php?ListType = HIMProgram; 2021.

[95] CHIMA. Learning outcomes for health information management, Version 3.0; 2015. ISBN: 978-0-9783332-1-8.

[96] Health Information Technology Competencies (HITComp). See hitcomp.org and hitcomp.org/education. http://ehealthwork.eu/FC/overview0.html; 2021.

[97] Lowell K. Final report. Evaluation of the information technology professionals in health care ("Workforce") program – summative report. NORC at University of Chicago; 2014.

[98] HealthIT.gov. Workforce development programs: health IT curriculum resources for educators. Available from: https://www.healthit.gov/topic/onc-hitech-programs/workforce-development-programs; last reviewed November 11, 2021.

[99] Marc DT, Dua P, Fenton SH, Lalani K, Butler-Henderson K. Chapter 4: Occupational classifications in the health information disciplines. In: Butler-Henderson K, Day K, Gray K, editors. The health information

workforce: current and future developments. Cham: Springer Nature; 2021. p. 71–8. Available from: https://doi.org/10.1007/978-3-030-81850-0_5.
[100] Conestoga College. Applied health information science (Bachelor of) (Co-op). Program details. Available from: https://www.conestogac.on.ca/fulltime/bachelor-of-applied-health-information-science-honours.
[101] University of Regina, Johnson-Shoyoma Graduate School of Public Policy. Health informatics and Information Management (HIIM) within the MHA program. Program details. Available from: https://www.uregina.ca/gradstudies/future-students/programs/jsgs.html.
[102] Louisiana Tech University, Department of Health Informatics & Information Management. Available from: https://ans.latech.edu/health-informatics-information-management/.
[103] The University of Tennessee Health Science Center. Health informatics & information management. Available from: http://www.uthsc.edu/health-professions/him/index.php.
[104] The University of Mississippi Medical Center. Health informatics and information management. Available from: https://www.umc.edu/shrp/Health%20Informatics%20and%20Information%20Management/Health-Informatics-and-Information-Management.html.
[105] Gilbert C, Gray K, Pritchard S. Chapter 2: Health Information work: a scoping review. In: Butler-Henderson K, Day K, Gray K, editors. The health information workforce: current and future developments. Cham: Springer Nature; 2021. p. 23–54. Available from: https://doi.org/10.1007/978-3-030-81850-0_5.
[106] Gray K, Gilbert C, Butler-Henderson K, Day K, Pritchard S. Ghosts in the machine: identifying the digital health information workforce. In: Lau F, et al., editors. Improving usability, safety and patient outcomes with health information technology. Amsterdam: IOS Press; 2019. Available from: https://doi.org/10.3233/978-1-61499-951-5-146.
[107] Butler-Henderson K, Gray K. Australia's health information workforce: census summary report 2018. Launceston: University of Tasmania. Available from: http://www.utas.edu.au/__data/assets/pdf_file/0003/1163487/Australias-HIW-Census-SummaryReport-2018.pdf; 2018.
[108] IFHIMA. Module 9 – Emerging trends in health information management [Internet]. Contributors: M Hocking, M Taylor, R Osatohanmwen. Available from: https://ifhima.org/wp-content/uploads/2019/07/Learning-Module-NUMBER-9-Emerging-Trends-in-Health-Information-Management.pdf; 2019.
[109] University of Illinois at Chicago. Masters in Health Informatics & Health Information Management degrees. Available from: http://healthinformatics.uic.edu/.
[110] Indiana University-Purdue University Indianapolis, School of Computing and Informatics, Department of BioHealth Informatics. Available from: http://soic.iupui.edu/departments/biohealth/.
[111] ONC-HIT. Notice of funding opportunity. Public health informatics & technology workforce development program (The PHIT workforce development program). Available from: https://www.healthit.gov/sites/default/files/page/2021-06/PHIT-Workforce-ARP-NOFO-508.pdf; June 2021.
[112] Department of Health and Human Services (DHHS). DHHS announces funding for public health IT workforce development program news release. Available from: https://www.hhs.gov/about/news/2021/09/22/hhs-announces-funding-for-public-health-it-workforce-development-program.html; September 22, 2021.

CHAPTER

3

Policies and incentives for adoption: toward broader use

Saurabh Rahurkar[1,2], *Pallavi Jonnalagadda*[1], *Japjit Kaur Tutt*[3], *Brian E. Dixon*[2,3] *and Nir Menachemi*[4]

[1]The Center for the Advancement of Team Science, Analytics, and Systems Thinking in Health Services and Implementation Science Research (CATALYST), The Ohio State University College of Medicine, Columbus, OH, USA [2]Department of Epidemiology, Richard M. Fairbanks School of Public Health, Indiana University, Indianapolis, IN, USA [3]Center for Biomedical Informatics, Regenstrief Institute, Inc., Indianapolis, IN, USA [4]Health Policy and Management, Richard M. Fairbanks School of Public Health, Indiana University, Indianapolis, IN, USA

LEARNING OBJECTIVES

By the end of this chapter the reader should:

1. Identify and list major initiatives as well as stakeholders that play a role in the adoption of health information exchange (HIE).
2. Report the current levels of HIE adoption in the United States as well as globally.
3. Understand the salient barriers to HIE adoption.
4. Describe historic and current efforts taken to address barriers to HIE adoption and generally promote adoption and implementation.
5. Discuss the usage of HIE by providers.
6. Discuss the role of policy in shaping HIE adoption and utilization.
7. Discuss HIE policy at state and national levels.
8. List and describe emerging trends influencing the adoption and use of HIE.

3.1 Introduction

A consistent thread in health policy over the past two decades internationally has been a focus on the need to adopt health information technology (HIT) and connect HIT systems through health information exchange (HIE).

Health Information Exchange
DOI: https://doi.org/10.1016/B978-0-323-90802-3.00010-1

The primary motivation or reason for this focus is a global belief that HIT and HIE systems can improve efficiencies in the delivery of care as well as the quality and safety of health care [1]. Therefore it is worthwhile to briefly discuss two seminal reports by the Institute of Medicine (IOM) that played a pivotal role in stimulating the advent of HIT in the United States. The first report—*To Err is Human*, was released in 1999, and reported that up to 98,000 people died each year due to medical errors which included medication errors, surgical errors, and other errors such as incorrect diagnoses [2]. The report emphasized the role played by poorly designed care delivery systems that created an environment that was conducive to committing errors by otherwise competent clinicians.

In 2001 the IOM released a second report which played an instrumental role in the shift toward HIT [3]. Entitled *Crossing the Quality Chasm*, this report marks a major milestone in the national quality movement. Specifically, the report provided a formal definition of quality of care as consisting of six main components (see Fig. 3.1). First, high-quality care is focused on *patient safety*, that is, it is free from harmful effects such as those associated with medical errors. High-quality care is both *effective* and *efficient*, that is, it is evidence-based and does not result in wasteful use of resources. Additionally, to be of high quality, care needs to be *timely*, *patient-centered*, and *equitable* to address extant disparities. Most importantly, the report argued that HIT addresses all six components of quality of care, and the report called for the adoption of HIT to improve health care quality in the United States.

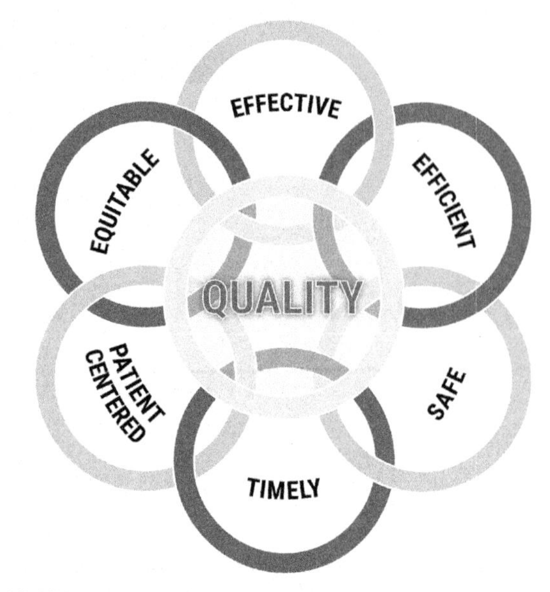

FIGURE 3.1 The six dimensions of high-quality care. Source: *Adapted from the Institute of Medicine. To err is human: building a safer health system (Kohn LT, Corrigan JM, Donaldson MS, editors). The National Academies Press; 1999.*

Following the IOM reports, health policy discussions, including the State of the Union address by President George W. Bush in 2004 calling for all Americans to have electronic health records (EHRs) by 2014, shifted to include HIT adoption. Furthermore, reports by the Center for IT Leadership emphasize that the maximum benefit from HIT adoption could only be achieved through the widespread exchange of data [4]. This expanded the policy discussions to include HIE as a critical component of the American roadmap toward the Triple Aim of improving the quality of and satisfaction with patient care while improving the health of populations and reducing the per capita cost of health care [5,6].

The push to adopt HIE was further bolstered by research that identified specific instances in medical decision-making or clinical workflow where HIT or HIE could help avoid errors. For example, researchers at Brigham and Women's Hospital suggested that HIE could eliminate up to 18% of patient safety errors generally; and as much as 70% of adverse drug events by delivering appropriate information to providers during decision-making processes [7]. Additional research on HIE and its potential impact on quality, safety, as well as costs continues to emerge [8]. A 2013 re-evaluation of IOM estimates of medical error indicates that between

210,000 and 400,000 Americans die each year due to preventable medical errors [9]. Continued lapses in quality of care and estimates that medical errors cost the US health system approximately $980 billion only bolster the argument in the favor of HIE adoption [10].

A similar pattern is observed globally. In New Zealand, adoption of EHR systems dominated policy and research during the first decade of the 21st century. Once EHR systems were established, researchers and policy advocates pushed for HIE [1]. The same pattern can be found in Denmark (see Chapter 28), Taiwan (the Republic of China, see Chapter 30), and Israel (see Chapter 31). Over time, as adoption of EHR systems expanded, nations updated their policy efforts to focus on HIE. International efforts to strengthen quality and safety were bolstered in 2018 when researchers found that development of HIT in Organisation for Economic Co-operation and Development (OECD) countries had a "significant positive impact" on outcomes [11]. National eHealth strategies, or as they are now referred to as Digital Health strategies, have evolved over time from the adoption of HIT toward adoption and use of HIE.

This chapter begins by orienting the reader to the HIE marketplace and examining the landscape of information sharing and interoperability adoption in the United States as well as globally. Next, we present factors that have been linked as impediments to adoption and use of HIE, followed by an overview of efforts directed at addressing these barriers. In the final section, we briefly examine emerging trends in HIE adoption and use.

3.2 Landscape of the health information exchange marketplace

In this section, we first examine the state of HIE adoption and use in the United States and globally. First, we look at HIE as a verb (refer to Chapter 1) by examining the prevalence of HIE across various sectors of the health care ecosystem. Next, we look at HIE as a noun (also defined in Chapter 1) and focus on the growth of HIE organizations. Evaluating HIE trends from the perspective of general availability and use as well as the organizations that are facilitating HIE presents a deeper understanding of the multifaceted nature of HIE.

Here we note that organizational ability to participate in HIE (e.g., organizational adoption) need not represent actual use of HIE. Much of the existing literature focuses on *organizational adoption* of HIE, which implies that hospitals or health facilities have the ability to exchange information. For example, an EHR system vendor may implement functionality in which clinicians or other authorized users at a hospital can press a button to export data or send data to another facility. Yet, utilization of such technological functions or HIE interfaces is often not measured or described in past studies. In other words, we know little about the actual *use of HIE* by health facilities and clinicians. Most of the literature we describe instead uses surveys of health care administrators in which they are asked about whether their facility has adopted a specific type of standard (syntactic or semantic), possesses the ability to interface with an HIE network, or sent at least one clinical document to another health facility. Details about the volume or depth of HIE in a city, state, or nation are often challenging to find when reviewing the existing literature [12].

3.2.1 Adoption of health information exchange functionalities

At the time of President Bush's 2004 State of the Union address calling for EHR adoption, no information on the electronic exchange of data between hospitals and other health care providers was routinely captured. However, given estimates in 2003 regarding the adoption of EHR systems at 27% of providers, it is likely that HIE adoption was significantly less than 25% [13]. Over time, national surveys began to ask questions annually about the adoption of both EHR systems, EHR functionality, and HIE between various health system actors.

By 2015 96% of all nonfederal acute care hospitals (referred to as hospitals henceforth in alignment with the source publications) in the United States had a certified EHR [14]. Eighty-two percent of hospitals participated[1] in HIE, representing a 100% increase from 2008 before the passage of the Health Information Technology for Economic and Clinical Health (HITECH) Act [15–17]. These hospitals, therefore, can exchange laboratory results, radiology reports, clinical care summaries, and medication histories with outside system providers [15,16]. These data and other recent studies consistently demonstrate upward trends in the adoption of both EHR systems and HIE among hospitals. Yet, hospitals prioritize HIE with providers within a health system (e.g., enterprise HIE networks) than HIE with providers outside a health system due to challenges arising from a decline in state-led efforts for HIE along with a rise in EHR-vendor-mediated HIE (see Chapter 1 for definitions) [18,19].

HIE trends among office-based physicians differ from those of hospitals. In 2014 4-in-10 office-based physicians exchanged health information electronically with any providers—within or outside their system [20]. Twenty-six percent of all physicians electronically exchanged health information with ambulatory providers outside their system. Whereas, fewer than 1-in-10 physicians electronically exchanged information with hospitals with which they are not affiliated [20]. Considerable variation was found among physicians regarding the various HIE related capabilities. For example, in 2013, while almost 83% of physicians had the capability to order prescriptions electronically, only 39.1% had the capability to electronically report to immunization registries [21]. These rates, however, only represent capabilities and not actual exchange of health information.

Although adoption of HIE has been slower for providers in office-based settings than in hospitals, steady increases in the adoption of EHR systems and HIE (verb form) have been reported in recent years. In 2004 about 21% of physicians utilized an EHR system. Per the National Electronic Health Records Survey, this percentage has increased to about 86% as of 2017 [22]. Also consider electronic prescriptions (eRx), which involves electronically transmitting a prescription from a clinic to a pharmacy. In 2020 84% of prescribers used eRx, which increased since 2018 (73%) and 2014 (70%) and represents a more than a 14-fold increase since 2008 [15,23].

Surveillance of communicable diseases, a cornerstone of public health [24], is in the spotlight in the wake of the COVID-19 pandemic. The pandemic highlighted that many reports of the novel SARS-CoV-2 virus were submitted to public health agencies in the United States using fax machines [25,26], delaying downstream action by epidemiologists and policymakers to mitigate disease spread. Over the past two decades, a dramatic progress in electronic HIE between laboratories and public health authorities has been made. In 2005 only eight state health departments could receive electronic laboratory reports. By 2021, according to the US Centers for Disease Control and Prevention, 80% of laboratory reports were received electronically [27]. However, there remain challenges to electronic laboratory reporting. In 2018 and 2019 7-in-10 hospitals experienced one or more challenges related to public health reporting with 50% of hospitals reporting

[1] HIE participation was defined as electronically exchanging laboratory results, radiology reports, clinical care summaries, or medication lists with ambulatory care providers or hospitals outside their organization

capacity-related challenges like staffing and technical expertise [28]. Furthermore, six states still do not have any capacity to receive reports electronically [27].

3.2.2 Evolution of health information exchange organizations

In 2004 there were just nine operational HIE organizations in the United States [29], then referred to as Regional Health Information Organizations (RHIOs) (see Chapter 1). Like HIE functionalities, significant growth in the number of HIE organizations has occurred in the two decades since. In 2014 the eHealth Initiative identified 125 HIE organizations, which consisted of 74 community-based HIEs, 26 private HIEs, and 25 government-facilitated HIEs [30]. However, evidence suggests that the number of HIEs is declining with the end of the HITECH Cooperative Agreement Program and competition from HIE offerings from EHR vendors. As of 2022, there were a total of 77 HIE organizations in the United States [31].

Some HIE organizations merged with neighboring HIOs to form larger HIE networks that create economies of scale to improve sustainability, which might explain part of the drop in the number of HIE organizations in recent years. Yet many barriers remain including but are not limited to, sustainability, integration into provider workflow, lack of funding, resources to implement interface standards, and competition from EHR vendors [19]. Below is a select list of HIE organizations that expanded and other large HIE initiatives in the United States:

1. The Indiana Network for Patient Care (INPC), managed by the Indiana HIE in partnership with the Regenstrief Institute, is one of the largest and the oldest community-based HIEs in the United States [32]. The INPC grew from just a handful of hospitals in the early 2000s to more than 53,004 health care providers, 123 hospitals representing 38 hospital systems, 18,738 practices, public health departments, and other health care organizations representing over 18 million patients and over 15 billion clinical data elements [33,34]. The INPC is discussed in more detail in Chapter 22.
2. Kaiser Permanente (KP)—the largest not-for-profit integrated health care delivery system in the United States—operates and maintains an EHR system called *KP HealthConnect* and facilitates enterprise HIE across its network. Overall, participation consists of over 600 medical offices and 37 hospitals, and connects providers across eight states [35].
3. Vendor-facilitated HIE—like Care Everywhere by Epic Systems and Cerner HIE by the Cerner Corporation are HIE platforms embedded within the EHR system. Epic and Cerner are the leading EHR vendors in the United States and have established large HIE networks. For example, over 1700 hospitals and 34,000 clinics are live on Care Everywhere as of 2017. Further, 99% of these hospitals and clinics are connected to over 70,000 provider sites using other EHRs and HIEs.
4. The eHealth Exchange, originally established by the US Office of the National Coordinator for HIT (ONC) in 2004 through a program called the Nationwide Health Information Exchange or NwHIN [36], established operations with two entities in 2009. As of 2015, the eHealth Exchange included participants from all 50 states, including 30% of all US hospitals, 10,000 medical groups, 8200 pharmacies, and over 900 dialysis centers [37,38]. Additionally, the eHealth Exchange also connects 101 state HIEs and four federal agencies—the Veterans Health Administration, US Department of Defense, US Social Services Administration, and the US Centers for Medicare and Medicaid Services (CMS) [39].

3.2.3 International growth in the adoption of health information exchange

Adoption of HIE internationally is more difficult to assess due to the varying descriptions of HIE functions and availability across various countries. A study from Adler-Milstein and colleagues [40] found that many developed nations, especially in Europe, have some level of HIE adoption. Efforts to exchange data in developed countries appear to be like those in the United States—transmission of data between hospitals and general practitioners as well as specialists—albeit with a distinct set of drivers and barriers, with many nations aligning HIE efforts to universal health coverage (see Chapters 15 and 32).

HIE outside Europe is more difficult to assess. In the Middle East and North Africa region, infrastructure for HIE varies dramatically. For example, the literature suggests that Iran is developing the capacity to advance HIE in support of public health, specifically in the exchange of immunization registry data nationwide [41]. In this book, Chapter 31 describes the development and evolution of HIE in Israel, which currently hosts a robust nationwide HIE network among hospitals and clinics. Elsewhere in the book, Chapter 32 describes the more recent fast-expanding HIE activity in the United Arab Emirates.

Low-to middle-income countries (LMICs) have also made progress on HIE adoption. Efforts, however, in many LMICs have focused on laying the foundation for a robust eHealth infrastructure that will eventually support HIE. Yet there do exist working implementations of HIE in the following nations: South Africa, Rwanda, Sierra Leone, Tanzania, Bangladesh, and the Philippines [42]. Other initiatives in the Thai-Cambodian region, Pakistan, South Africa, and Kenya have largely been pilot-based interventions [43]. Several chapters in the book examine the successes and challenges faced in LMICs, which equally recognize the importance of HIE as a component of their digital health/eHealth national strategies.

3.2.4 Health information exchange usage by providers

HIE usage by providers has continued to increase as research advances, incentive programs are offered, and positive outcomes associated with HIE are highlighted. In 2016, as a result of the Medicare and Medicaid (CMS) EHR incentive programs (now called the Promoting Interoperability programs), around 60% of providers (office-based) utilized health IT to better patient outcomes [44,45]. Findings from a project funded by the Agency for Healthcare Research and Quality (AHRQ) presented results on the characterization of HIE use. The report indicates substantial increases in usage over time in the outpatient, inpatient, and emergency department settings. The data showcases differences in usage among different settings. Usage of HIE in inpatient was 17.6% and 3.7% in the outpatient setting. The emergency department usage was higher than outpatient (4.4%) but still substantially lower than inpatient [46].

Trends in HIE usage analyzed from 2011 to 2017 suggest an increase of 29% in inpatient settings [46]. An important variable to consider in usage is a patient's need for HIE, as perceived by the provider. Patients with low complexity medical history records or frequent patient encounters may not require as extensive use of HIE compared to patients with high-complexity medical history records. This correlates to lower HIE usage by providers in the outpatient and emergency department, as indicated by the data presented earlier [47].

3.2.5 Barriers to adoption

Although there is great potential for HIE to improve health care delivery and outcomes, there has been resistance to its adoption among nations, organizations, and individual providers. Research on the implementation and adoption of HIE among providers has identified several challenges that warrant discussion. The following factors have consistent evidence in the literature for being barriers to the adoption and implementation of HIE:

1. *Costs*: Adoption and implementation of HIE often require a large upfront investment of time and money by a provider or health system [48–51]. These costs include those related to hardware, software, labor, and technical assistance costs, as well as the indirect costs associated with loss of productivity in the initial phase following implementation. In addition to start-up costs, providers must account for recurrent costs associated with HIE. These ongoing costs include those related to maintenance expenses, as well as those related to connectivity such as membership or subscription fees and transaction fees. Further, the commonly theorized benefits from HIE such as reduction in medical errors, reduced diagnostic and imaging tests are accrued primarily by payers (e.g., insurance carriers), and providers may potentially lose revenue generated by extraneous services utilization. Overall, these factors present an uncertainty from the perspective of gaining a positive return on investment for the decision to participate in HIE (see Chapter 5 for a full discussion of HIE value).
2. *Resources*: HIE implementation is dependent on the availability of numerous resources in addition to funding sources. These include technical or human resources, infrastructure, and availability of time. Providers routinely indicate their facilities lack the hardware, software, or network connectivity required for HIE. Even when infrastructure is present, providers suggest it is insufficient for efficient (e.g., fast) exchange of data. Furthermore, a lack of sufficiently trained human resources knowledgeable in HIE presents a bottleneck to adoption of HIE. In addition, providers often resist adoption due to a perception that HIE leads to increases in physician and administrative workload.
3. *Privacy*: Stakeholders consistently express concern regarding the privacy and confidentiality of data captured, stored, and shared via HIE [48–52]. While federal law in the United States provides a core set of regulations that govern confidentiality, privacy, and security of data in HIT and HIE systems, laws in the 50 states vary and can be more restrictive making HIE complex and challenging. For example, some states require patients to give consent before their data can be exchanged by an HIE while other states only require the ability for patients, who so desire, to remove themselves from the HIE. In addition to varying and complex regulations, up to 75% of patients report in surveys being "somewhat" to "very concerned" regarding the privacy of their health data [52]. Patients' concerns are legitimate and need to be addressed by health care providers as well as HIEs because unauthorized breaches of health information are reported every week in addition to breaches of databases that contain financial data. Chapter 6 contains a detailed discussion of the privacy, security, and confidentiality of data in the context of HIE.
4. *Interoperability*: EHR systems have historically been silos unto themselves, thus lacking interoperability [5,48,51–53]. Therefore providers and health care organizations consistently ask the federal government as well as international authorities to create and/or dictate the use of technical standards by EHR vendors to facilitate interoperability. Complaints by

providers about the absence of standards, as well as the complexity of available standards, have been an excuse, by some, to avoid adoption of HIE. While limited, adoption of available standards has grown over time. Yet interoperability is still limited, which makes it an important issue for HIEs to address. An assessment of available and emerging technical standards, as well as their adoption, is presented in Chapter 8.

5. *Competition*: Competition has traditionally been a salient barrier to adoption of HIE with vendors and providers in highly competitive markets refusing to share data with competitors [48,51–53]. Even when they shared data, stakeholders limited the type and amount of data shared [51]. Given that the financial benefits of data exchange are principally accrued by payers, sharing data with competitors, especially as new models of care such as accountable care organizations emerge in the marketplace, could put a hospital or physician practice at financial risk.

3.2.6 Drivers of adoption

Although there are barriers, there also exist two significant forces that drive the market to adopt and use HIE. First, there is a natural force in the market that seeks to exchange data electronically now that many organizations have transitioned from paper charts to EHR systems. Recall from Chapter 1 that data are fragmented in the health care system and providers have an inherent need to access patient information, no matter where it might be stored when making clinical decisions. The rise of EHR systems naturally breeds a desire to access other institutions' HIT systems.

Yet a much larger force is driving adoption of HIE in most nations. Federal governments in both the United States and globally are directly tackling the aforementioned barriers through policy, which is having a direct effect on adoption of HIE. As previously mentioned, then-President George W. Bush challenged America to adopt EHR systems by the year 2014. As of 2015, 96% of hospitals have adopted EHR systems. The President followed his State of the Union address with several policies that stimulated adoption of EHR systems as well as HIE among hospitals.

President Bush, via executive order, established the Office of the National Coordinator for HIT (ONC) as a division within the US Department of Health and Human Services (HHS) following his address to Congress. He then charged ONC with coordinating the adoption of HIT across the federal government and private sector through public–private partnerships. While the initial focus of ONC was on EHR, eRx, computerized provider order entry, and clinical decision support (CDS) systems, ONC quickly advanced the agenda for HIE. This was due, in part, to reports and urging from private sector actors. For example, the Markle Foundation, which established a public–private collaborative in 2002 called *Connecting for Health* [54], created a *Common Framework* in 2006 that identified barriers to widespread sharing of health information and prioritized key policy and technical aspects that needed to be addressed to promote interoperability [50].

Leaders at HHS, ONC, Markle, and the eHealth Initiative along with several academic medical centers and private IT consulting firms then launched the formation of a Nationwide Health Information Network (now referred to as the eHealth Exchange) to connect enterprise HIEs, community-based HIEs, and federal agencies to bring HIE to scale in the United States [55,56]. Over several years, national HIE efforts culminated in a set of policies, technical specifications, and implementation guides that provided a foundation for nationwide HIE. In parallel, AHRQ, also part of HHS, funded several statewide initiatives aimed at cultivating HIE at that level [57,58]. While successful, these efforts by HHS were not enough to create a tipping point in which providers overwhelmingly sought to create and adopt HIE.

Arguably the tipping point came following the passage of HITECH in 2009 and the Patient Protection and Affordable Care Act (PPACA) in 2010. While the earlier efforts by HHS created a pathway for others to follow, these policies create sufficient incentives to overcome the aforementioned barriers while leading others down the path. These policies specifically address barriers of cost, resources, privacy, and competition.

HITECH principally promoted adoption of HIT by creating incentives for the *meaningful use* (MU) of EHR systems by eligible hospitals and providers. Through CMS, HITECH provisioned financial incentives to certain eligible hospitals and providers, specified in the law, which could demonstrate criteria established through administrative rule-making processes part of the MU program. CMS also outlined criteria for three stages with incentives offered through 2019 followed by penalties for providers who did not adopt certified EHR technology or meet MU criteria. Each successive stage of the program, informed by experts and comments from the industry, added increasingly advanced capabilities to both the EHR technology and the use of that technology by eligible hospitals and providers. By the first quarter of 2015, CMS had distributed $28.1 billion through the MU program [59]. These dollars mediated the cost of adopting EHR systems and connecting those systems together via HIE technologies.

Criteria relevant to HIE, defined in Stage 2 of the MU program are summarized in Table 3.1. These criteria create a *floor* or minimum level of adoption. While many providers may only be able to achieve the floor, other providers will operate at a higher level or possess more advanced EHR and/or HIE functionality. For example, Stage 2 requires eligible hospitals to electronically deliver "more than 55% of all clinical lab test results ordered by an authorized provider ... for patients admitted to its inpatient or emergency department." Many hospitals that have fully implemented interfaces between their lab information systems and their EHR systems will likely exchange upward of 80%–90% of lab results. Yet the regulations set a bar for others to work toward. These criteria focus resources within health systems to implement HIE technologies that are necessary to meet the MU criteria.

3.2.7 Health information exchange policy at the state and national level

Over the years, there have been many changes in HIE policy, both at the state and national levels. Fig. 3.2 visualizes the evolution of HIE policy over the years. One of the most major updates to HIE policy at the national level was the establishment of Stage 3, Promoting Interoperability, of the Meaningful Use Program. Stage 3 was released in 2015 and was effective through the years 2016–17 and 2018–beyond. It outlined eight new objectives, summarized in Table 3.1, that eligible professionals and hospitals must abide by in order to participate in the Promoting Interoperability Programs. A major component of this new addition to the program was flexibility in certain objectives. This provided an opportunity for qualifying professionals/hospitals to better align the objectives with the needs of the populations they serve [61].

An update to HIE policy came in the form of the Medicare Access and CHIP Reauthorization Act (MACRA) of 2015. MACRA required CMS to shift from volume-based to value-based healthcare business models, collectively referred to as the Quality Payment Program (QPP). Under the QPP, two participation tracks were

TABLE 3.1 Summary of core health information exchange (HIE)-related criteria in Stages 1, 2, and 3 of the meaningful use program [60].

Health outcomes policy priority	Meaningful use objective	Meaningful use measure	HIE implication
Stage 1			
Improving quality, safety, efficiency, and reducing health disparities	EPs only: Generate and transmit permissible discharge prescriptions electronically (eRx).	Requires EPs to transmit 40% of all permissible prescriptions to be transmitted using a certified electronic health record (EHR).	Explicit HIE implication
	Defined CQMs under meaningful use definition: reporting of clinical quality measures to the Centers for Medicare & Medicaid Services (CMS) or the states.	Requires EHR to import, export, and submit CQMs electronically.	Explicit HIE implication
	Incorporate clinical lab-test results into the EHR.	Requires more than 55% of all clinical lab tests to be incorporated into the EHR structured data.	Explicit HIE implication
Engage patients and families in their health care	EPs only: Provide patients the ability to view online, download, and transmit their health information within the EHR reporting period (4 business days of the information being available to the EP).	Requires provision of online access to 50% of all unique patients seen by the EP to health information during the EHR reporting period subject to EP's discretion to withhold certain information.	Potential HIE implication
	Provide patients the ability to view online, download, and transmit their health information within 4 business days of the information being available to the EP.	More than 50% of all unique patients seen by the EP during the EHR reporting period are provided timely (within 4 business days after the information is available to the EP) online access to their health information subject to the EP's discretion to withhold certain information.	Potential HIE implication
	Provide patients the ability to view online, download, and transmit information about a hospital admission.	More than 50% of all patients who are discharged from the inpatient or emergency department of an eligible hospital or CAH have their information available online within 36 h of discharge.	Potential HIE implication
Improve care coordination	Capability to exchange key clinical information (ex: problem list, medication list, medication allergies, diagnostic test results), among providers of care and patient authorized entities electronically.	Performed at least one test of the Certified EHR Technology's capacity to electronically exchange key clinical information.	Explicit HIE implication

Stage 2

Improving quality, safety, efficiency, and reducing health disparities	Generate and transmit permissible prescriptions electronically (eRx).	More than • 50% of all Rx, or • All Rx written by the EP and queried for drug formulary and transmitted electronically using certified EHR.	Explicit HIE implication
	Incorporate clinical lab-test results into Certified EHR Technology as structured data.	More than 55% of all clinical lab tests results ordered by the EP or by authorized providers of the eligible hospital or CAH for patients admitted to its inpatient or ED during the EHR reporting period whose results are either in a positive/negative affirmation or numerical format are incorporated in Certified EHR Technology as structured data.	Potential HIE implication
	EP only: Use clinically relevant information to identify patients who should receive reminders for preventive/follow-up care and send these patients the reminder, per patient preference.	More than 10% of all unique patients who have had two or more office visits with the EP within the 24 months before the beginning of the EHR reporting period were sent a reminder, per patient preference when available.	Potential HIE implication
Engage patients and families in their health care	EP only: Provide patients the ability to view online, download, and transmit their health information within 4 business days of the information being available to the EP.	**1.** More than 50% of all unique patients seen by the EP during the EHR reporting period are provided timely (within 4 business days after the information is available to the EP) online access to their health information subject to the EP's discretion to withhold certain information. **2.** More than 5% of all unique patients seen by the EP during the EHR reporting period (or their authorized representatives) view, download, or transmit to a third party their health information.	Potential HIE implication

(*Continued*)

TABLE 3.1 (Continued)

Health outcomes policy priority	Meaningful use objective	Meaningful use measure	HIE implication
	EH/CAH only: Provide patients the ability to view online, download, and transmit information about a hospital admission.	**1.** More than 50% of all patients who are discharged from the inpatient or emergency department of an EH or CAH have their information available online within 36 h of discharge.	Potential HIE implication
		2. More than 5% of all patients (or their authorized representatives) who are discharged from the inpatient or emergency department of an EH or CAH view, download or transmit to a third party their information during the reporting period.	
	EP only: Provide clinical summaries for patients for each office visit.	Clinical summaries provided to patients or patient-authorized representatives within 1 business day for more than 50% of office visits.	Potential HIE implication
	Use Certified EHR Technology to identify patient-specific education resources and provide those resources to the patient.	Patient-specific education resources identified by CEHRT are provided to patients for more than 10% of all unique patients with office visits seen by the EP during the EHR reporting period. More than 10% of all unique patients admitted to the eligible hospitals or CAH's inpatient or emergency department are provided patient-specific education resources identified by Certified EHR Technology.	Potential HIE implication
	EP only: Use secure electronic messaging to communicate with patients on relevant health information.	A secure message was sent using the electronic messaging function of Certified EHR Technology by more than 5% of unique patients (or their authorized representatives) seen by the EP during the EHR reporting period.	Potential HIE implication
Improve care coordination	The EP, EH, or CAH who transitions their patient to another setting of care or provider of care or refers their patient to another provider of care provides a summary of care record for each transition of care or referral.	**1.** The EP, EH, or CAH that transitions or refers their patient to another setting of care or provider of care provides a summary of care record for more than 50% of transitions of care and referrals.	Explicit HIE implication

		2. The EP, EH, or CAH that transitions or refers their patient to another setting of care or provider of care provides a summary of care record for more than 10% of such transitions and referrals either (1) electronically transmitted using CEHRT to a recipient or (2) where the recipient receives the summary of care record via exchange facilitated by an organization that is a eHealth Exchange participant or in a manner that is consistent with the governance mechanism ONC establishes for the Nationwide Health Information Network. **3.** An EP, EH, or CAH must satisfy one of the two following criteria: (A) Conducts one or more successful electronic exchanges of a summary of care document with a recipient who has EHR technology that was developed designed by a different EHR technology developer than the sender's EHR technology. (B) Conducts one or more successful tests with the CMS designated test EHR during the EHR reporting period.	
Improve population and public health	Capability to submit electronic data to immunization registries or immunization information systems (IIS) except where prohibited, and in accordance with applicable law and practice.	Successful ongoing submission of electronic immunization data from Certified EHR Technology to an immunization registry or IIS for the entire EHR reporting period.	Explicit HIE implication
	EH/CAH only: Capability to submit electronic reportable laboratory results to public health agencies, except where prohibited, and in accordance with applicable law and practice.	Successful ongoing submission of electronic reportable laboratory results from Certified EHR Technology to public health agencies for the entire EHR reporting period.	Explicit HIE implication
	Capability to submit electronic syndromic surveillance data to public health agencies, except where prohibited, and in accordance with applicable law and practice.	Successful ongoing submission of electronic syndromic surveillance data from Certified EHR Technology to a public health agency for the entire EHR reporting period.	Explicit HIE implication
	Ensure adequate privacy and security protections for personal health information.	Protect electronic health information created or maintained by the Certified EHR Technology through the implementation of appropriate technical capabilities.	Explicit HIE implication

(*Continued*)

TABLE 3.1 (Continued)

Health outcomes policy priority	Meaningful use objective	Meaningful use measure	HIE implication
Stage 3			
Improve patient's access to health information	Patient Electronic Access—The EP provides patients (or patient-authorized representative) with timely electronic access to their health information and patient specific education.	EPs must satisfy both measures in order to meet this objective: • Measure 1: For more than 80% of all unique patients seen by the EP: (1) The patient (or the patient-authorized representative) is provided timely access to view online, download, and transmit his or her health information; and (2) The provider ensures the patient's health information is available for the patient (or patient-authorized representative) to access using any application of their choice that is configured to meet the technical specifications of the application programming interface (API) in the provider's CEHRT. • Measure 2: The EP must use clinically relevant information from CEHRT to identify patient-specific educational resources and provide electronic access to those materials to more than 35% of unique patients seen by the EP during the EHR reporting period.	Explicit HIE implication
	Coordination of Care—Use CEHRT to engage with patients or their authorized representatives about the patient's care.	Providers must attest to all three measures and must meet the thresholds for at least two measures to meet the objective: • Measure 1: For an EHR reporting period in 2017 and 2018, more than 5% of all unique patients (or their authorized representatives) seen by the EP actively engage with the EHR made accessible by the provider and either—(1) View, download, or transmit to a third party their health information; or (2) access their health information through the use of an API that can be used by applications chosen by the patient and configured to the API in the provider's CEHRT; or (3) a combination of (1) and (2). Threshold for 2019 and Subsequent Years: The resulting percentage must be more than 10%.	Explicit HIE implementation

		• Measure 2: For an EHR reporting period in 2017 and 2018, more than 5% of all unique patients seen by the EP during the EHR reporting period, a secure message was sent using the electronic messaging function of CEHRT to the patient (or the patient authorized representative), or in response to a secure message sent by the patient or their authorized representative. Threshold in 2018 and Subsequent Years: The resulting percentage must be more than 25% in order for an EP to meet this measure. • Measure 3: Patient-generated health data or data from a nonclinical setting is incorporated into the CEHRT for more than 5% of all unique patients seen by the EP during the EHR reporting period.	
Use CEHRT to improve health outcomes	Protect electronic protected health information created or maintained by the CEHRT through the implementation of appropriate technical, administrative, and physical safeguards.	Conduct or review a security risk analysis in accordance with the requirements under 45 CFR 164.308(a)(1), including addressing the security (including encryption) of data created or maintained by CEHRT in accordance with requirements under 45 CFR 164.312(a)(2)(iv) and 45 CFR 164.306(d)(3), implement security updates as necessary, and correct identified security deficiencies as part of the provider's risk management process.	Potential HIE as data received need to be protected
	Generate and transmit permissible prescriptions electronically (eRx).	More than 60% of all permissible prescriptions written by the EP are queried for a drug formulary and transmitted electronically using CEHRT.	Explicit—Requires electronic transmission of Rx data
	Health Information Exchange—The EP provides a summary of care record when transitioning or referring their patient to another setting of care, receives or retrieves a summary of care record upon the receipt of a transition or referral or upon the first patient encounter with a new patient, and incorporates summary of care information from other providers into their EHR using the functions of CEHRT.	• Measure 1: For more than 50% of transitions of care and referrals, the EP that transitions or refers their patient to another setting of care or provider of care: (1) Creates a summary of care record using CEHRT, and (2) electronically exchanges the summary of care record. • Measure 2: For more than 40% of transitions or referrals received and patient encounters in which the provider has never before encountered the patient, the EP incorporates into the patient's EHR an electronic summary of care document.	Explicit—Requires EP to exchange data electronically with another provider

(*Continued*)

TABLE 3.1 (Continued)

Health outcomes policy priority	Meaningful use objective	Meaningful use measure	HIE implication
		• Measure 3: For more than 80%of transitions or referrals received and patient encounters in which the provider has never before encountered the patient, the EP performs a clinical information reconciliation. The provider must implement clinical information reconciliation for the following three clinical information sets: (1) Medication: Review of the patient's medication, including the name, dosage, frequency, and route of each medication. (2) Medication allergy: Review of the patient's known medication allergies. (3) Current Problem list: Review of the patient's current and active diagnoses.	
	Public Health Reporting—the EP is in active engagement with a public health agency or clinical data registry to submit electronic public health data in a meaningful way using Certified EHR Technology, except where prohibited, and in accordance with applicable law and practice.	• Measure 1—Immunization Registry Reporting: The EP is in active engagement with a public health agency to submit immunization data and receive immunization forecasts and histories from the public health immunization registry/IIS. • Measure 2—Syndromic Surveillance Reporting: The EP is in active engagement with a public health agency to submit syndromic surveillance data from an urgent care setting. • Measure 3—Electronic Case Reporting: The EP is in active engagement with a public health agency to submit case reporting of reportable conditions. • Measure 4—Public Health Registry Reporting: The EP is in active engagement with a public health agency to submit data to public health registries.	Explicit—All of these require electronic exchange of data with public health agencies

		• Measure 5—Clinical Data Registry Reporting: The EP is in active engagement to submit data to a clinical data registry.	
Reduce cost associated with meeting program requirements	An important component of Stage 3 is the ease of requirements for certain objectives.	The three objectives with flexibility are Coordination of Care through Patient Engagement, Health Information Exchange, and Public Health Reporting.	Potential HIE implication

CAH, Critical access hospitals; *CEHRT*, certified electronic health record technology; *CMS*, Centers for Medicare and Medicaid Services; *CQM*, clinical quality measure; *EH*, eligible hospital; *ED*, emergency department; *EP*, eligible professionals.

Adapted from regulations published by the US Department of Health and Human Services.

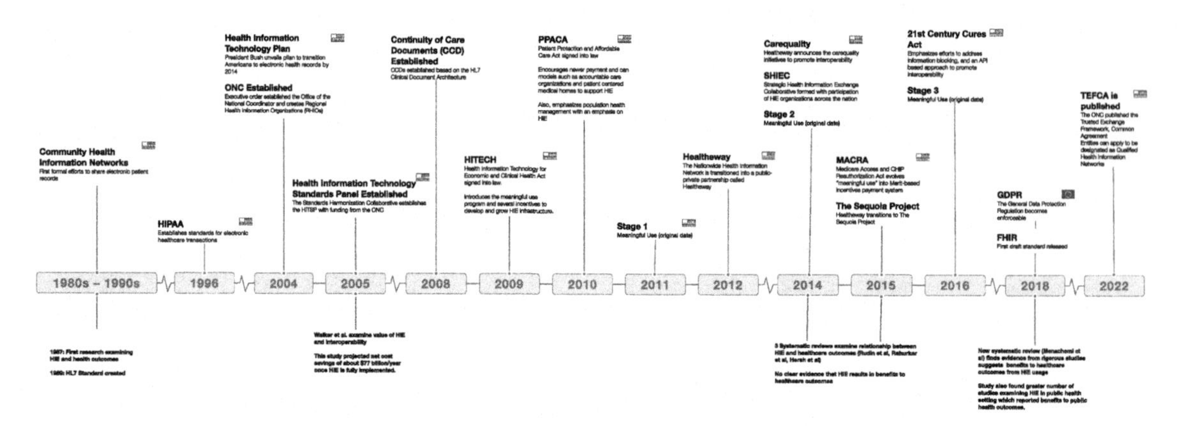

FIGURE 3.2 Timeline of major policies and governmental programs that impacted HIE adoption and use within the United States.

available to eligible providers: the Merit-based Incentive Payment System (MIPS) and Alternative Payment Models. In addition to rewarding providers for value over volume, MACRA also replaced the Medicare EHR Incentive Program, also known as MU, with MIPS [62]. Promoting Interoperability is one of the four performance categories tracked by MIPS, requiring the meaningful use of EHRs. In addition to the use of certified EHR technology for the secure exchange of health information, other requirements include reporting measures under each of the following HIE objectives: Provider to Patient Exchange, Public Health and Clinical Data Exchange, ePrescribing, and Query of Prescription Drug Monitoring Program [63].

Another major advancement in HIE policy came with the passage of the 21st Century Cures Act in 2016. Alongside Stage 3 of the Meaningful Use Program, advancing interoperability and EHR adoption are two of the emphasized components of the Cures Act. The ONC serves as the administrator of monitoring and promoting the development of HIE standards [64,65], which is discussed further in Chapter 10.

The ONC is responsible for implementing provisions of the 21st Century Cures Act that advance interoperability; support access, exchange, and use of electronic health information; and address information blocking. The 21st Century Cures Act also establishes requirements for application programming interfaces (APIs) that include requirements for patients' access to their health information. The API approach in turn offers health care providers the independence to choose "provider-facing" third-party services to interact with their certified API technology. In addition to calling for the development and support of a trusted exchange framework, the 21st Century Cures Act also supports a common agreement among health information networks (HINs) across the country. To this effect, the Trusted Exchange Framework and Common Agreement (TEFCA) describes a common set of nonbinding, foundational principles for trust policies and practices that can facilitate HIE. In addition, TEFCA also supports the ability of patients, their health care providers, and other authorized health care stakeholders to electronically access health information anytime and anywhere to improve care coordination and health care quality. In line with the seven principles of the trusted exchange framework (Table 3.2), HINs should prioritize industry-recognized standards, policies, best practices, and procedures; conduct

TABLE 3.2 Principles for trusted exchange.

Principle	
Principle 1—Standardization: HINs should prioritize federally recognized and industry recognized technical standards, policies, best practices, and procedures.	**A.** HINs should prioritize health information technology standards for interoperability that the US Department of Health & Human Services (HHS) has adopted in regulations, ONC has identified in the Interoperability Standards Advisory (ISA), or a standards developing organization (SDO) accredited by the American National Standards Institute (ANSI) has published. **B.** HINs should prioritize health information technology standards for interoperability that the US Department of Health & Human Services (HHS) has adopted in regulations, ONC has identified in the Interoperability Standards Advisory (ISA), or a standards developing organization (SDO) accredited by the American National Standards Institute (ANSI) has published.
Principle 2—Openness and Transparency: HINs should conduct activities openly and transparently, wherever possible.	**A.** HINs should make terms, conditions, and contractual agreements that govern the exchange of digital health information easily and publicly available. **B.** HINs should make terms, conditions, and contractual agreements that govern the exchange of digital health information easily and publicly available. **C.** HINs should make terms, conditions, and contractual agreements that govern the exchange of digital health information easily and publicly available. **D.** HINs should establish and, where applicable, conduct any dispute resolution processes in an equitable and transparent manner.
Principle 3—Cooperation and Non-Discrimination: HINs should collaborate with stakeholders across the continuum of care to electronically exchange digital health information, even when a stakeholder may be a business competitor.	**A.** HINs should not seek to gain competitive advantage or discriminate against competitors by limiting access to individuals' digital health information, and HINs should not treat digital health information as an asset that can be restricted in order to obtain or maintain a competitive advantage. **B.** HINs should practice data reciprocity. **C.** HINs should not use contract provisions or proprietary technology implementations to unduly limit connectivity with other HINs.
Principle 4—Privacy, Security, and Safety: HINs should exchange digital health information in a manner that supports privacy; ensures data confidentiality, integrity, and availability; and promotes patient safety.	**A.** HINs should ensure that digital health information is exchanged and used in a manner that promotes safe care and wellness, including consistently and accurately matching digital health information to an individual. **B.** Within the context of applicable law, HINs should enforce policies concerning individuals' ability to consent to the access, exchange, or use of their digital health information.

(*Continued*)

TABLE 3.2 (Continued)

Principle	Strategies
Principle 5—Access: HINs should ensure that individuals and their authorized caregivers have easy access to their digital health information and understand how it has been used or disclosed and HINs should comply with civil rights obligations on accessibility.	**A.** HINs should not impede or impose any unnecessary barriers to the ability of individuals or their legal representatives to access or direct their digital health information to designated third parties, or to learn how information about them has been accessed or disclosed. **B.** HINs should not impede or impose any unnecessary barriers to the ability of individuals, or their legal representatives, to learn how their health data have been accessed or disclosed.
Principle 6—Equity: HINs should consider the impacts of interoperability on different populations and throughout the lifecycle of the activity.	**A.** HINs should employ a health equity by design approach and should consider the health equity consequences of policy and technology choices up front. **B.** HINs should evaluate interoperability efforts, ensure health equity is being achieved, and adjust when it is not.
Principle 7—Public Health: HINs should support public health authorities and population-level use cases to enable the development of a learning health system that improves the health of the population and lowers the cost of care.	**A.** HINs should enable use cases that advance the mission of public health authorities. **B.** HINs should advance population-level use cases, including quality improvement and research.

HIN, Health Information Network, aka HIE Network.

Adapted from The Office of the National Coordinator for Health Information Technology (ONC). Trusted Exchange Framework and Common Agreement (TEFCA). Available from: https://www.healthit.gov/topic/interoperability/trusted-exchange-framework-and-common-agreement-tefca.

activities openly and transparently; collaborate with stakeholders across the continuum of care even when the stakeholder might be a competitor; exchange health information in a manner that supports privacy, security, and safety; consider the impacts of interoperability on different populations; and support public health and population health. The goal of the Common Agreement is to establish a universal floor of interoperability across the United States by establishing the infrastructure model and governing approach for users in different HINs to securely share health information under commonly agreed-to expectations and rules [66]. More information on TEFCA can be found in Chapter 21.

Although many states in the United States have HIE legislature that aligns with the national measures and recommendations offered, there are a few states that deviate. Minnesota, for example, has a unique HIE system and policies. A study conducted and presented in a report showcased many barriers in efficient statewide HIE for the state. There is a lack of uniformity in reporting of HIE and lack of communication between various organizations involved. The state would benefit from policy provisions that would establish a uniform HIE infrastructure and connected networks model. States with gaps and room for improvement in execution of HIE should consider the recommendations provided at the national level [67].

On the other end of the spectrum, the state of New York has a state-wide health information system and extensive funding for advancements in HIE. Statewide Health Information Network—New York (SHIN-NY) is a tool available state-wide for professionals and hospitals to utilize in exchanging health information, in accordance with HIPAA. The HIE in New York is distinct from the one in Minnesota in that it is a "Network of Networks" [68]. The SHIN-NY connects Qualified Entities (QEs) thereby creating secure access to patient information. Each QE is a regional network that enrolls participants in its community from hospitals, clinics, FQHCs, home care agencies, payers, ambulatory practices, and other entities so they can exchange electronic health information with other participants in their region [68]. In 2020 Version 3.8 of the SHIN-NY Privacy and Security Policies for QEs and their Participants was released with modifications. The modifications include various improvements that further quality information exchange initiatives. Continuous improvement is at the forefront of New York's HIE legislature. States looking to expand their HIE networks and modify legislature around the topic can look to larger states like New York to develop a similar framework [69]. More information on New York's approach to HIE at the state level can be found in Chapter 24.

In addition to addressing the cost and resource barriers by providing financial incentives for adoption of activities involving HIE, HITECH further addressed interoperability and privacy barriers. Beyond funds for CMS incentives, HITECH allocated funds for the advancement of technical standards. For example, ONC received funding for what it calls the Standards & Interoperability framework, which aims to create best practices for interoperability [70]. More than half a billion US dollars were also allocated to state government-designated entities to create HIE infrastructure in all 50 states and territories. Moreover, HITECH supported the creation of Regional Extension Centers as well as Beacon communities to provide technical assistance and model the possibilities for what a connected, interoperable health information infrastructure might do for quality and safety of care. Under the Workforce Development Program, HITECH created a highly skilled HIT workforce to support providers in the adoption and implementation as well as in achieving meaningful use of an EHR system. Finally, HITECH modified prior federal law referred to as the Health Insurance Portability and Accountability Act (HIPAA) of 1996. These changes are discussed at length in Chapter 6, but essentially, they expanded protections for the privacy and security of health information as it is captured, stored, managed, and shared by both health care providers and HIE organizations.

Finally, we examine the impact thus far of the PPACA. The PPACA is helping to align provider, patient, and payer interests by making major changes to reimbursement policies. Whereas existing fee-for-service payment models reward providers for the "volume" of care they provide (e.g., ordering unnecessary or redundant tests could result in higher fees collected for these services), the PPACA focuses more on "value" by rewarding providers for higher quality care that is more patient-centric and less costly. This shift from volume to value forces providers to identify ways to prevent costly hospitalizations and direct patients toward the most cost-effective care settings as a way to earn higher reimbursement rates. Moreover, the new payment models now utilized routinely collect patient satisfaction data to help determine providers' reimbursement amounts. Thus providers can earn higher fees when their patients are more satisfied. Ultimately, under the new models of care, providers are required to take on more financial risk for the prevention of costly health services utilization, assuring adequate patient satisfaction, and clinical management of patients appropriately such that they are routed to the most efficient use of resources. Being able to coordinate patient care under this new payment model requires HIE to be successful. Chapter 25 illustrates how the HIE in the State of Maryland is supporting a range of population health management services to support providers' transition to new models of care delivery.

Internationally, countries are moving towards the adoption of HIE as a component of their eHealth Strategy. As discussed in Chapter 1, the World Health Organization encourages member states to develop and implement integrated eHealth strategies to advance care delivery and public health. Many nations are seeking to formulate their national strategies, yet it will likely be a decade or more before some of them can achieve broad-scale HIE.

It is noteworthy that in countries that successfully adopted HIE, the impetus came from the government in the form of economic incentives and policies [71]. In some European countries like Switzerland and Germany, government-led initiatives to develop HIE infrastructure have been relatively recent. For instance, in Switzerland, a federal law has enforced a shared patient record since 2017. Incentives in the form of financial support are available to inpatient facilities to become interoperable. Acute care facilities had until 2020 and long-term care facilities have until 2022 to be interoperable or be subject to penalties on reimbursement claims from the universal coverage health insurance system [71]. In Germany a combination of legislative and public policy initiatives in the form of the 2019 Digital Healthcare Act, the 2020 Hospital Future Act, and the 2021 Digital Healthcare and Nursing Care Modernization Act have been launched to drive digital transformation in health care [72].

In other countries like the United Kingdom, the National Programme for IT (NPfIT) was created in 2002 with the aim to computerize the National Health Services over the span of a decade. While the NPfIT was dismantled due to the unpopularity of its top-down approach, it did lay down the foundation for HIE [71]. HIE for primary care is incentivized through the Quality and Outcomes Framework [73], a voluntary annual reward and incentive program for general practitioners introduced in 2004. On the other hand, provider resistance and variations in systems and data practices have hindered implementation of HIE in secondary care [71]. Government-led HIE is also seen in China, where the government has established programs to improve secure sharing of health care data to support the basic insurance schemes covering over 1.3 billion population. Barriers to HIE in China mostly arise from differing standards and infrastructures to develop EHR systems [71].

Although financial constraints are an important barrier to HIE adoption, the chief barrier to HIE adoption especially in LMICs arises from a lack of political will [43]. In India HIE remains virtually nonexistent, despite the push from the central government encouraging the adoption of health IT through various programs [71,74,75]. Notwithstanding the potential of standard and secure HIE in strengthening public health systems and supporting the growing healthcare tourism industry in India, fierce market competition precludes the development of infrastructure or standards to exchange clinical information across providers [71].

Apart from the barriers arising from cost, privacy, interoperability, competition, and availability of resources as in the United States, LMICs face additional barriers. These barriers, identified through a systematic review of the published literature [43], included cultures giving low importance to using data for making clinical decisions; health care workers who perform duties in unsafe environments; shortage of electricity, and lack of infrastructure like supplies, computers, office space, etc.; a dearth of software developed in languages other than English; lack of awareness of technology, applications, or processes; and a lack of data analysis tools and data quality issues.

Throughout the book, we present examples of efforts in several LMICs. While these efforts may appear to be small steps towards HIE, they are important nonetheless, because they (1) align with the nation's overall eHealth strategy and (2) they establish a foundation upon which the nation can build in the future. Some experts believe that a few of these nations might eventually leapfrog the United States in HIE in the same way many adopted cellular infrastructures and mobile phones long before Americans.

While policies have been instrumental in the adoption and use of HIE across organizations, trust and perception play a substantial role in provider utilization of HIE. Physician attitudes and perceptions of HIE must be considered in determining susceptibility to adoption of HIE methods. Results from a survey administered to physicians in 2009 indicate that a majority (89%) of providers believe HIE correlates with communication improvement amongst health care professionals. A majority (70%) of respondents also responded favorably to HIE financial incentives in an effort to increase use and purchasing of health IT equipment. Provider attitudes toward HIE are justifiably positive; however, barriers to adoption are still prevalent [76].

3.3 Emerging trends

In this section, we briefly discuss five emerging trends that are likely to have an impact on HIE adoption in the coming years. First, we discuss the transition at the policy as well as practice level, from adoption of EHRs to engaging in health HIE to using and integrating the shared information at the point of care. To this end, we discuss the potential implications of TEFCA under the 21st Century Cures Act. Second, we examine the fervor in health care around *Big Data* and how it is likely to drive adoption of HIE. Third, we discuss the potential role of blockchain technology in secure data exchange. Fourth, we briefly discuss the potential impact of the General Data Protection Regulation (GDPR) legislation in the European Union (EU). Finally, we discuss an important challenge of *information blocking* and the proposed action by the US federal government to curtail it.

3.3.1 New policies to advance health information exchange adoption and use

An emerging trend in HIE has been promotion of interoperability to further quality outcomes but also increase patient access and engagement with their health information. As the benefits are showcased, we can expect further development on the matter in the coming years [77].

In January 2022 the ONC and The Sequoia Project announced the publication of TEFCA so that entities can apply to be designated Qualified Health Information Networks. TEFCA is expected to increase secure and appropriate access to data; ensure that a core set of data is available among networks connected through the Common Agreement; decrease costs and improve efficiency by eliminating or reducing the need to join multiple HINs, and provide HINs and HIT developers with a common set of privacy and security requirements for protecting patient data [78].

While Stage 3 MU and MIPS under MACRA focused on adoption of the ability to engage in an exchange of information, TEFCA strongly emphasizes actual use of shared information. The ONC's 21st Century Cures Act provides new and updated criteria that increase protection of patient health information in addition to easier patient accessibility and HIE among various stakeholders. TEFCA also emphasizes standardization, encouraging HINs to use standards adopted by the HHS in regulations, those identified by the ONC in the Interoperability Standards Advisory, or those published by standards developing organization accredited by the American National Standards Institute [66]. The Health Level Seven Fast Interoperability Healthcare Resource (FHIR) has gained popularity for its potential to facilitate EHR-agnostic HIE. To accelerate the adoption of FHIR APIs for general use on all ONC-certified EHRs, The Sequoia Project has released a three-year FHIR RoadMap [79].

3.3.2 Blockchain may advance security of health information exchange

A major component of the 21st Century Cures Act is the privacy and security of information. As technology advances and usage of HIE increases, the need for heightened privacy and security measures can be expected to increase. Blockchain technology has drawn attention for its potential applications in the secure exchange of electronic health information [80–82]. Characteristics such as decentralization of data, data integrity verification, and data auditability make blockchain technologies appealing in HIE. In an acknowledgment of its potential, the ONC organized an ideation challenge soliciting white papers on the potential uses of blockchain in health care in 2016 [82]. However, health care implementations of blockchain remain at the concept stage [81,83,84]. Barriers to large-scale deployments of blockchain technology include scalability, security, and cost-effectiveness [82].

3.3.3 Driving health information exchange adoption through Big Data initiatives

In the past couple of years, two major initiatives have begun to unfold in the United States. First, the IOM issued a series of reports on what it calls the *Learning Health System*. Second, the White House and Congress launched a campaign for *precision medicine*. Both initiatives require collection, management, and use of extremely large-scale data sets, otherwise known as Big Data. To date, Big Data have demonstrated utility in monitoring seasonal outbreaks as well as predicting their spread [85–88]. They have further shown promise in predicting health care utilization and monitoring drug safety [89,90]. Data-driven health care is the cornerstone for both the IOM and White House initiatives. Yet to effectively capture, store, manage, and make use of Big Data, the nation will require a robust HIE infrastructure to move data and transform it into information and knowledge. The drive to deliver CDS at scale through these initiatives could add additional fuel to push adoption of HIE.

As of 2015, 96% of hospitals had adopted EHRs. This near-ubiquitous adoption of EHR has resulted in vast amounts of data that can be harnessed for improving health care quality, reducing health care costs, carrying out public health activities, and research [91]. The use of FHIR APIs can potentially address the challenge of curating this data. The dynamic structure of the FHIR standard confers advantages over other standards in that it minimizes implementation complexity while preserving data integrity. Further, these characteristics also facilitate the use of predictive modeling algorithms at the point of care. As current policy efforts through TEFCA are aligned to support the adoption of the FHIR standard [66,79], the potential for deploying real-time CDS tools in clinical practice [92] could facilitate HIE adoption.

3.3.4 Impact of General Data Protection Regulation on health information exchange adoption

As HIE entails the exchange of sensitive information, the security of health data poses a challenge. In response the EU has implemented the GDPR, where the patients are "joint-controllers" of their health data. Under the GDPR, patients have to provide explicit consent for use of their health data and can withdraw this consent at any time. Further, failure to comply with the GDPR can result in fines as high as 2% of the annual revenue to 4% of global annual revenue for healthcare organizations. Evaluations of the GDPR policy indicate that it is effective in health data protection as evidenced by the increased financial input on the part of healthcare organizations to comply with it [93]. As the GDPR regulates the collection, use, disclosure, or other processing of health data, its reach is extraterritorial. Controllers and processors of health data of individuals located in the EU may be US entities. Therefore the GDPR has implications for health care operations in the United States and medical tourism in the United States and elsewhere [94]. In providing heightened health data protections and significant penalties, the GDPR could affect the importance attached to HIE potentially impacting its adoption.

3.3.5 Information blocking policies

In the early period of HIE implementation, it was observed that numerous entities sought to control electronic health information and limit its availability and use. This was evidenced in the form of numerous complaints received by the ONC [95]. The ONC termed this behavior on the part of the stakeholders, *information blocking*. According to the ONC, "Information blocking occurs when persons or entities knowingly and unreasonably interfere with the exchange or use of electronic health information." [95]

Three definitive criteria must be met to identify information blocking: **Interference** in the form of an act or course of conduct that impedes authorized persons or entities from accessing health information, the decision to engage in this practice must be *willful* [1], and with the stakeholder's *knowledge* [2], and this conduct should be such that there is *no reasonable justification* [3] to interfere with the access to authorized personnel.

It is vital to differentiate information blocking from interference with access for legitimate reasons such as patient safety, privacy, and security concerns, or the potential to improve patient health care. Reasons for interference should be thoroughly scrutinized to differentiate them from any of the barriers discussed in the previous sections before such behavior is categorized as information blocking. Based on a national survey of HIE organizations, 55% reported that EHR vendors sometimes engaged in information blocking, while 30% reported that health systems also engaged in information blocking [96]. Information blocking is a complex issue and while some of the precipitating factors are well understood, efforts are ongoing to identify and understand others.

When present, however, information blocking presents a serious problem. In addition to interfering with effective HIE, it adversely affects aspects of health care such as clinical decision making, and the safety, quality, and effectiveness of care provided to patients. It also presents an impediment to patient engagement by preventing access to health care that may be used by consumers to make informed decisions about their health and health care [95]. Finally, information blocking presents a barrier to advances in biomedical and public health resources which depends on the ability to analyze information from numerous sources to enable data-driven health care. By defining information blocking, the 21st Century Cures Act facilitates the identification of actions that constitute information blocking and when they have occurred so these actions may be identified and investigated [97]. The investigations then enable HHS to either impose civil monetary penalties or refer the party engaging in information blocking to the appropriate agency to impose civil penalties. Congress has granted the Office of the Inspector General (OIG) the authority to investigate allegations of information blocking. The Act also enables the OIG to levy civil monetary penalties of up to $1 million per violation [97]. Thus the 21st Century Cures Act established a legal framework to prevent information blocking, address the use and exchange of health data through HIT, and strengthen interoperability.

3.4 Summary

HIE has been linked to benefits in health care utilization, health care costs, and coordination of care. Moreover, major changes to how hospitals and other providers are reimbursed are increasing the need for seamless exchange of clinical data. HIE is now considered an important prerequisite for a modern health care system. However, many HIE networks are still in their early developmental stage. In fact, as an organization type, HIE networks need further maturation which will involve innovations and technology that are expected to continue to evolve. As more and more providers adopt HIE, and more data are exchanged leading to the creation of ever-larger datasets, opportunities open up to truly unleash the potential of improving the quality and cost of care. Benefits accrued from these developments may eventually address shortcomings that have plagued the health care system in the United States. Globally, HIEs have the potential to strengthen and transform health systems that are similarly facing challenges.

Questions for discussion

1. What is the historic role of government in the adoption of health information technologies including health information exchange? What should it be?
2. Which policy-driven incentives within the United States are most likely to influence health systems to adopt HIE? How about providers? Is there is a difference between these two groups?
3. What is the adoption of HIE like outside the United States? What are some reasons for greater or lesser levels of adoption?
4. Which emerging trend will have the greatest impact on HIE adoption? Why?
5. What additional activities should governments, including ministries of health,

be doing to encourage the adoption and use of HIE?

6. Which barriers to adoption of HIE are unlikely to be solved by governmental health policy? How might these barriers be addressed?

References

[1] Bowden T, Coiera E. Comparing New Zealand's 'Middle Out' health information technology strategy with other OECD nations. Int J Med Inform 2013;82(5): e87–95 PMID: 23287413, Epub 2013/01/05.

[2] Institute of Medicine. To err is human: building a safer health system (Kohn LT, Corrigan JM, Donaldson MS, editors). The National Academies Press; 1999.

[3] Institute of Medicine. Crossing the quality chasm: a new health system for the 21st century. National Academies Press; 2001.

[4] Walker J, Pan E, Johnston D, Adler-Milstein J, Bates DW, Middleton B. The value of health care information exchange and interoperability. Health Aff (Millwood) 2005;Suppl Web Exclusives:W5-10–W5-18. PMID: 15659453.

[5] Dixon BE. A roadmap for the adoption of e-Health. e-Service J 2007;5(3):3–13.

[6] Berwick DM, Nolan TW, Whittington J. The triple aim: care, health, and cost. Health Aff (Millwood) 2008;27(3):759–69.

[7] Kaelber DC, Bates DW. Health information exchange and patient safety. J Biomed Inform 2007;40(6 Suppl): S40–5 PMID: 17950041.

[8] Rahurkar S, Vest JR, Menachemi N. Despite the spread of health information exchange, there is little evidence of its impact on cost, use, and quality of care. Health Aff (Millwood) 2015;34(3):477–83.

[9] James JT. A new, evidence-based estimate of patient harms associated with hospital care. J. Patient Saf 2013;9(3):122–8.

[10] Andel C, Davidow SL, Hollander M, Moreno DA. The economics of health care quality and medical errors. J Health Care Finance Fall 2012;39(1):39–50 PMID. 1095371694, 23155743.

[11] Rana RH, Alam K, Gow J. Development of a richer measure of health outcomes incorporating the impacts of income inequality, ethnic diversity, and ICT development on health. Glob Health 2018;14(1):72 PMCID: PMC6054722. Epub 2018/07/22.

[12] Apathy NC, Vest JR, Adler-Milstein J, Blackburn J, Dixon BE, Harle CA. Practice and market factors associated with provider volume of health information exchange. J Am Med Inform Assoc 2021;28(7):1451–60 PMCID: PMC8279783. Epub 2021/03/07.

[13] Bates DW. Physicians and ambulatory electronic health records. Health Aff (Millwood) 2005;24 (5):1180–9 PMID; 16162561.

[14] Henry J, Pylypchuk Y, Searcy T, Patel V. Adoption of electronic health record systems among U.S. non-federal acute care hospitals: 2008–2015. Washington, DC: Office of the National Coordinator for Health Information Technology; 2016.

[15] Office of the National Coordinator for Health Information Technology. Update on the adoption of health information technology and related efforts to facilitate the electronic use and exchange of health information. The Office of the National Coordinator for Health Information Technology, Office of the Secretary, United States Department of Health and Human Services, Services (USDoHaH); 2014.

[16] Swain M, Charles D, Patel V, Searcy T. Health information exchange among U.S. non-federal acute care hospitals: 2008–2014. ONC Data Brief 2015;24:1–12.

[17] Patel V, Henry J, Pylypchuk Y, Searcy T. Interoperability among U.S. non-federal acute care hospitals in 2015. Washington, DC: Office of the National Coordinator for Health Information Technology; 2016.

[18] Vest JR, Simon K. Hospitals' adoption of intra-system information exchange is negatively associated with inter-system information exchange. J Am Med Inform Assoc 2018;25(9):1189–96.

[19] Adler-Milstein J, Lin SC, Jha AK. The number of health information exchange efforts is declining, leaving the viability of broad clinical data exchange uncertain. Health Aff 2016;35(7):1278–85.

[20] Heisey-Grove D, Patel V, Searcy T. Physician electronic exchange of patient health information, 2014. Washington, DC: Office of the National Coordinator for Health Information Technology; 2015.

[21] Furukawa MF, King J, Patel V, Hsiao CJ, Adler-Milstein J, Jha AK. Despite substantial progress in EHR adoption, health information exchange and patient engagement remain low in office settings. Health Aff (Millwood) 2014;33(9):1672–9.

[22] Office of the National Coordinator for Health Information Technology. 'Office-based Physician Electronic Health Record Adoption,' Health IT Quick- Stat#50. healthit.gov. Office of the National Coordinator for Health Information Technology, Department of Health and Human Services; 2019.

[23] Gabriel MH, Swain M. E-prescribing trends in the United States. Washington, DC: Office of the National Coordinator of Health Information Technology; 2014.

[24] Thacker SB, Qualters JR, Lee LM. Centers for Disease Control and Prevention. Public health surveillance in

the United States: evolution and challenges. MMWR Suppl 2012;61(3):3–9.
[25] Dixon BE, Caine VA, Halverson PK. Deficient response to COVID-19 makes the case for evolving the public health system. Am J Prev Med 2020;59 (6):887–91 PMCID: PMC7448961. Epub 2020/09/27.
[26] Kliff S, Sanger-Katz M. Bottleneck for U.S. coronavirus response: The fax machine. The New York Times; Jul 13, 2020; Sect. Upshot.
[27] Office of Public Health Scientific Services. Public health surveillance: preparing for the Future. Atlanta, GA: Centers for Disease Control and Prevention; 2018.
[28] Richwine C, Marshall C, Johnson C, Patel V. Challenges to public health reporting experienced by non-federal acute care hospitals, 2019. Washington, DC: Office of the National Coordinator for Health Information Technology; 2021.
[29] Overhage JM, Evans L, Marchibroda J. Communities' readiness for health information exchange: the National Landscape in 2004. J Am Med Inform Assoc 2005;12(2):107–12 PMCID: 551542.
[30] Snell E. eHealth Initiative Survey: HIEs lacking in interoperability [Online]. Available from: http://healthitsecurity.com/news/ehealth-initiative-survey-hies-lacking-in-interoperability; 2014.
[31] Strategic Health Information Exchange Collaborative (SHIEC). HIE Members List 2022. Available from: https://strategichie.com/membership/hie-members-list/.
[32] McDonald CJ, Overhage JM, Barnes M, Schadow G, Blevins L, Dexter PR, et al. The Indiana network for patient care: a working local health information infrastructure. An example of a working infrastructure collaboration that links data from five health systems and hundreds of millions of entries. Health Aff (Millwood) 2005;24(5):1214–20.
[33] Schleyer TKL, editor. Big data in healthcare: The Indiana network for patient care. Informatics: "Big Data" uses and challenges in the life sciences. Indiana Government Center; 2014.
[34] Indiana Health Information Exchange. Indiana network of patient care 2022. Available from: https://www.ihie.org.
[35] Kaiser Permenente. Kaiser Permanente share: connectivity. kaiserpermanente.org. Kaiser Permenente. Available from: http://share.kaiserpermanente.org/total-health/connectivity/; 2013.
[36] Office of the National Coordinator for Health Information Technology. What is the NHIN? [Office of the National Coordinator for Health Information Technology, Department of Health and Human Services, editors]. Office of the National Coordinator for Health Information Technology. Available from: healthit.gov.; 2009.
[37] Slabodkin G. eHealth exchange claims title of largest U.S. HIE network. In: Goedert J, editor, HealthData management; 2015.
[38] The Sequoia Project. About the Sequoia Project. sequoiaproject.org. Available from: http://sequoiaproject.org/ehealth-exchange/about/; 2015.
[39] The Sequoia Project. The Sequoia Project – Participants. sequoiaproject.org. Available from: http://sequoiaproject.org/ehealth-exchange/participants/; 2015.
[40] Adler-Milstein J, Ronchi E, Cohen GR, Winn LA, Jha AK. Benchmarking health IT among OECD countries: better data for better policy. J Am Med Inform Assoc 2014;21(1):111–16 PMCID: 3912720.
[41] Hosseini M, Ahmadi M, Dixon BE. A service oriented architecture approach to achieve interoperability between immunization information systems in Iran. AMIA Annu Symp Proc. 2014;2014:1797–805. PMID: PMC4419958.
[42] OpenHIE. Our work online. Ohie.org. Available from: https://ohie.org/#ourwork; 2013.
[43] Akhlaq A, McKinstry B, Muhammad KB, Sheikh A. Barriers and facilitators to health information exchange in low- and middle-income country settings: a systematic review. Health Policy Plan 2016;31 (9):1310–25.
[44] Dixon BE, Vest JR, Finnell JT, Rahurkar S, Wiensch A, Miller M, et al. Exploring utilization of and outcomes from health information exchange in emergency settings. Indiana University Richard M. Fairbanks School of Public Health; 2020.
[45] Office of the National Coordinator for Health Information Technology. 'Office-based Health Care Professionals Participating in the CMS EHR Incentive Programs' Health IT Quick-Stat #44. 2017.
[46] Rahurkar S, Vest JR, Finnell JT, Dixon BE. Trends in user-initiated health information exchange in the inpatient, outpatient, and emergency settings. J Am Med Inform Assoc 2020;28(3):622–7.
[47] Flaks-Manov N, Shadmi E, Hoshen M, Balicer RD. Health information exchange systems and length of stay in readmissions to a different hospital. J Hosp Med 2016;11(6):401–6.
[48] Adler-Milstein J, Bates DW, Jha AK. U.S. regional health information organizations: progress and challenges. Health Aff (Millwood) 2009;28(2):483–92 PMID: 19276008. Epub 2009/03/12.
[49] Dixon B, Miller T, Overhage M. Barriers to achieving the last mile in health information exchange: a survey of small hospitals and physician practices. J Healthc Inf Manag 2013;27(4):55–8.

[50] Markle Foundation. The common framework: overview and principles. Markle Foundation; 2006.
[51] Vest JR, Gamm LD. Health information exchange: persistent challenges and new strategies. J Am Med Inform Assoc 2010;17(3):288–94 PMCID: Pmc2995716. Epub 2010/05/06.
[52] Fontaine P, Ross SE, Zink T, Schilling LM. Systematic review of health information exchange in primary care practices. J Am Board Fam Med 2010;23(5): 655–70.
[53] Vest JR. More than just a question of technology: factors related to hospitals' adoption and implementation of health information exchange. Int J Med Inform 2010;79(12):797–806 Epub 2010/10/05.
[54] Markle Foundation. Health 2002. Available from: http://www.markle.org/health.
[55] Rishel W, Rielhl V, Blanton C. Summary of the NHIN prototype architecture contracts. Washington, DC: U. S. Department of Health and Human Services; 2007.
[56] Gravely SD, Whaley ES. The next step in health data exchanges: trust and privacy in exchange networks. J Healthc Inf Manag 2009;23(2):33–7 Spring.
[57] Agency for Healthcare Research and Quality. State and regional demonstration projects. Rockville, MD: Agency for Healthcare Research and Quality. ahrq.gov. Available from: http://healthit.ahrq.gov/ahrq-funded-projects/state-and-regional-demonstration-projects; 2009.
[58] Banger AK, Dullabh P, Eichner J, Kissam S. Lessons learned from AHRQ's state and regional demonstrations in health information technology (Prepared by RTI International, under Contract No. HHSA2902009000027i). Rockville, MD: AHRQ. AHRQ Publication No. 10-0075-EF.
[59] Centers for Medicare and Medicaid Services. Medicare & Medicaid EHR Incentive Programs; 2015.
[60] American Academy of Pediatrics. Meaningful use overview. American Academy of Pediatrics; 2021. Available from: https://www.aap.org/en/practice-management/health-information-technology/meaningful-use-overview/.
[61] Centers for Medicare & Medicaid Services. Stage 3 program requirements for providers attesting to their state's medicaid promoting interoperability (PI) programs. Available from: https://www.cms.gov/Regulations-and-Guidance/Legislation/EHRIncentivePrograms/Stage3Medicaid_Require.
[62] AAPC. What is MACRA and MIPS? Available from: https://www.aapc.com/macra/macra.aspx#WhatIsMacra.
[63] AAPC. MIPS – What is MIPS (merit-based incentive payment system). Available from: https://www.aapc.com/macra/mips.aspx#promotingInteroperability.
[64] HIMSS. 21st Century Cures Act—a summary 2017. Available from: https://www.himss.org/resources/21st-century-cures-act-summary.
[65] Dieker L. State connection: state-level efforts in health information exchange. J. AHIMA 2008;79(5):40–3.
[66] The Office of the National Coordinator for Health Information Technology (ONC). Trusted Exchange Framework and Common Agreement (TEFCA). Available from: https://www.healthit.gov/topic/interoperability/trusted-exchange-framework-and-common-agreement-tefca.
[67] Minnesota Department of Health. Health information exchange legislative study; 2018.
[68] New York eHealth Collaborative. What is the SHIN-NY. Available from: https://www.nyehealth.org/shin-ny/what-is-the-shin-ny/.
[69] New York eHealth Collaborative. 2020 SHIN-NY policy changes reflected in SHIN-NY privacy and security policies and procedures for QEs and their participants V3.8: summary chart 2021. Available from: http://www.nyehealth.org/nyec16/wp-content/uploads/2021/02/2020-SHINNY-PP-Policy-Changes-Chart.pdf.
[70] Office of the National Coordinator for Health Information Technology. Standards & interoperability (S&I) framework. www.siframework.org. Available from: http://wiki.siframework.org/Frequently + Asked + Questions + %28FAQs%29; 2010.
[71] Payne TH, Lovis C, Gutteridge C, Pagliari C, Natarajan S, Yong C, et al. Status of health information exchange: a comparison of six countries. J Glob Health 2019;9(2):0204279 PMID: 31673351.
[72] Goldwasser Y, Gordon WJ, Brönneke JB, Stern AD. Health Affairs Blog [Internet]; 2021.
[73] Roland M. Linking physicians' pay to the quality of care—a major experiment in the United Kingdom. N Engl J Med. 2004;351(14):1448–54.
[74] Government of India Ministry of Health & Family Welfare. e-Health & telemedicine. Available from: https://main.mohfw.gov.in/Organisation/departments-health-and-family-welfare/e-Health-Telemedicine.
[75] NHP India. National Identification Number to Health Facility in India (NIN-TO-HFI). Available from: https://nin.nhp.gov.in/about_nin2hfi.php.
[76] Patel V, Abramson EL, Edwards A, Malhotra S, Kaushal R. Physicians' potential use and preferences related to health information exchange. Int J Med Inform 2011;80(3):171–80.
[77] The Office of the National Coordinator for Health Information Technology (ONC). ONC's Cures Act Final Rule. Available from: https://www.healthit.gov/curesrule/final-rule-policy/2015-edition-cures-update.

[78] ONC TEFCA RCE. What is the ONC Trusted Exchange Framework and Common Agreement? Available from: https://rce.sequoiaproject.org/tefca/.
[79] ONC TEFCA RCE. FHIR roadmap for TEFCA exchange; 2022.
[80] Kuo T-T, Zavaleta Rojas H, Ohno-Machado L. Comparison of blockchain platforms: a systematic review and healthcare examples. J Am Med Inform Assoc 2019;26(5):462–78.
[81] Spanakis EG, Sfakianakis S, Bonomi S, Ciccotelli C, Magalini S, Sakkalis V. Emerging and established trends to support secure health information exchange. Front Digit Health 2021;3:636082.
[82] Angraal S, Krumholz HM, Schulz WL. Blockchain technology: applications in health care. Circ Cardiovasc Qual Outcomes 2017;10(9):e003800.
[83] Azaria A, Ekblaw A, Vieira T, Lippman A, editors. MedRec: using blockchain for medical data access and permission management. In: 2016 2nd international conference on open and Big Data (OBD); 22–24 August 2016.
[84] Mettler M, editor. Blockchain technology in healthcare: the revolution starts here. In: 2016 IEEE 18th international conference on e-Health networking, applications and services (Healthcom); 14–16 September 2016.
[85] Carneiro HA, Mylonakis E. Google trends: a web-based tool for real-time surveillance of disease outbreaks. Clin Infect Dis 2009;49(10):1557–64.
[86] Cho S, Sohn CH, Jo MW, Shin SY, Lee JH, Ryoo SM, et al. Correlation between national influenza surveillance data and Google trends in South Korea. PLoS One 2013;8(12):e81422 PMCID: 3855287.
[87] Cook S, Conrad C, Fowlkes AL, Mohebbi MH. Assessing Google flu trends performance in the United States during the 2009 influenza virus A (H1N1) pandemic. PLoS One 2011;6(8):e23610 PMCID: 3158788.
[88] Hulth A, Rydevik G, Linde A. Web queries as a source for syndromic surveillance. PLoS One 2009;4(2):e4378 PMCID: 2634970.
[89] White RW, Horvitz E. From health search to healthcare: explorations of intention and utilization via query logs and user surveys. J Am Med Inform Assoc 2014;21(1):49–55 PMCID: 3912725.
[90] White RW, Tatonetti NP, Shah NH, Altman RB, Horvitz E. Web-scale pharmacovigilance: listening to signals from the crowd. J Am Med Inform Assoc 2013;20(3):404–8 PMCID: 3628066.
[91] Menachemi N, Rahurkar S, Harle CA, Vest JR. The benefits of health information exchange: an updated systematic review. J Am Med Inform Assoc 2018;25(9):1259–65.
[92] Khalilia M, Choi M, Henderson A, Iyengar S, Braunstein M, Sun J. Clinical predictive modeling development and deployment through FHIR web services. AMIA Annu Symp Proc 2015;2015:717–26. PMID: 26958207.
[93] Yuan B, Li J. The Policy Effect of the General Data Protection Regulation (GDPR) on the Digital Public Health Sector in the European Union: an Empirical Investigation. Int J Environ Res Public Health 2019;16(6):1070.
[94] Broccolo BM, Gottlieb DF. Does GDPR regulate clinical care delivery by US health care providers. Natl Law Rev 2018;VIII(57).
[95] Office of the National Coordinator for Health Information Technology. Report on health information blocking. Washington, DC: The Office of the National Coordinatior for Health Information Technology, Department of Health and Human Services; 2015.
[96] Everson J, Patel V, Adler-Milstein J. Information blocking remains prevalent at the start of 21st Century Cures Act: results from a survey of health information exchange organizations. J Am Med Inform Assoc 2021;28(4):727–32.
[97] Black JR, Hulkower RL, Ramanathan T. Health information blocking: responses under the 21st Century Cures Act. Public Health Reports 2018;133(5):610–13.

SECTION 2

Organizational aspects of managing health information exchange

CHAPTER

4

Engaging and sustaining stakeholders: toward governance

Brian E. Dixon[1,2] *and Sue S. Feldman*[3,4]

[1]Department of Epidemiology, Richard M. Fairbanks School of Public Health, Indiana University, Indianapolis, IN, USA [2]Center for Biomedical Informatics, Regenstrief Institute, Inc., Indianapolis, IN, USA [3]Department of Health Services Administration, School of Health Professions, University of Alabama at Birmingham, Birmingham, AL, USA [4]Informatics Institute, Keersink School of Medicine, University of Alabama at Birmingham, Birmingham, AL, USA

4.1 Introduction

Governance, in the context of health information exchange (HIE), refers to the establishment and oversight of a common set of behaviors, policies, and standards that enable trusted, electronic HIE among a set of participants [1]. Before data can be shared, the parties involved in an HIE network must establish a governing body with a set of broad and representative stakeholders. The *governing body* defines what data will be shared, how it will be shared, and under what circumstances it will be shared. The governing body establishes and maintains a *governance framework* for the HIE network to ensure compliance with legal, technical, and operational requirements related to the protection, use, and disclosure of protected health information. This includes the establishment of *participation agreements* or *charters* and *data sharing agreements* that codify the policies and procedures established by the governing body. All of these elements are essential for health system actors (e.g., hospitals, clinics, governmental agencies) to develop a strong foundation of mutual trust and operational processes within which HIE can occur within a community, state, or nation.

Governance for HIE is complex and often multilayered as depicted in Fig. 4.1. There are three essential layers of governance found in HIE networks around the world:

1. *Organizational governance*—This layer of governance pertains to the legal corporation or entity that manages the HIE network. In many cases this will be a health information organization (HIO, defined in Chapter 1) or a governmental agency such as a Ministry of Health (MOH). The entity requires a Board of Directors or other governing body that holds the HIO leadership accountable for its operational performance and financial

Health Information Exchange
DOI: https://doi.org/10.1016/B978-0-323-90802-3.00028-9

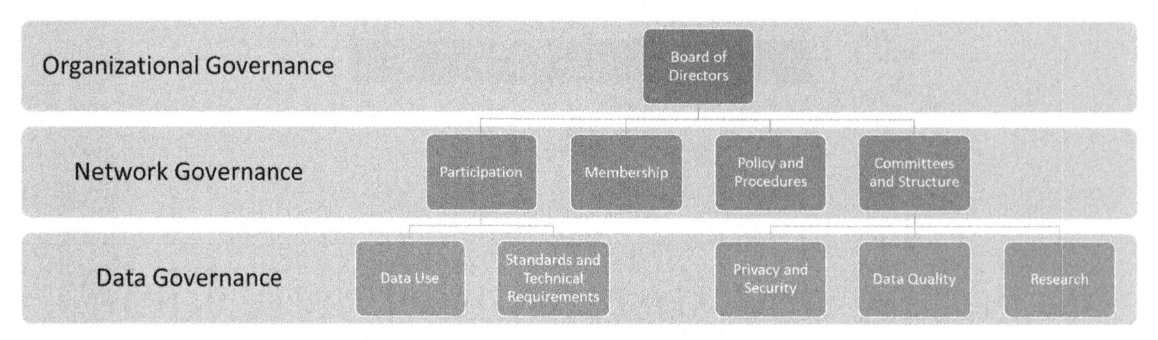

FIGURE 4.1 A governance framework for health information exchange.

sustainability. In the case of a MOH, this will likely be a directorate or office that focuses on digital health or data services.

2. *Network governance*—This layer of governance pertains to the HIE network, providing oversight of the network. The governing body for this layer will establish rules and regulations for participating in data exchange activities, including membership in the HIE network. This layer may or may not directly report to the managing entity. In the United States, the governing body is likely to be a public–private collaborative board, independent from the HIO. In many nations, the governing body is likely to be a committee formed by the MOH.
3. *Data governance*—This layer of governance pertains to the use of data exchanged in the HIE network. Governance might consist of multiple committees that report up to the HIE network governing body, each of which focuses on an aspect of HIE (e.g., technical standards, legal requirements). The Network governing body will define these committees and their purpose. Some HIE networks will manage this governance layer through the network governing body, although as HIE efforts expand it may be more prudent to have multiple working groups.

It is important to note that these layers are not orthogonal. Naturally these layers will overlap, and collaboration between them is essential. For example, there must be a shared understanding of policies and procedures between organizational and network governance, especially as network organizations begin to increase in size and reach. One area where this is very apparent is in consent structures that govern data exchange among the participants and between the participants and the organization that manages the HIE network.

Governance layers and their roles and responsibilities are discussed throughout this chapter.

As the volume and type of data exchanged expands, the importance of governance grows. The governance framework must be flexible enough to scale and evolve over time. Policies and procedures should be defined for how the framework can be changed by the governing body. A governance framework requires active engagement with participating organizations and the populations they serve to establish transparency and achieve consensus. Governance is important for all types of HIOs, but it is more critical as membership diversity, approved use cases, and the geographic footprint of the HIE network expands. Due to the complexities associated with large exchanges consisting of several competing and diverse organizations, this chapter will focus on regional, state, and nationwide HIOs.

4.2 Governing bodies

Governing bodies serve several key functions. They:

1. Embody the governance principles of the HIO for all those who are involved in exchanging information using the HIO's technology infrastructure;
2. Provide a forum for ideas to be discussed, questions to be asked, and policy to be debated;
3. Demonstrate the ongoing commitment of the key stakeholders to the HIO through their continued participation on the governing body;
4. Present an externally facing entity, which is important as governments consider the correct level of oversight and the public decides whether to trust electronic data exchange;
5. Offer an opportunity for the HIO to demonstrate representativeness, by including diverse stakeholders from the area served by the HIO; and
6. Reinforce the message that the policies of the HIO need to be followed because they will be enforced if necessary.

4.2.1 Governing body types

As illustrated in Fig. 4.1, there are three types of governing bodies found in HIE networks, each one corresponding to a distinct layer of governance. Each of these governing body types is discussed next.

4.2.1.1 Board of directors

An HIO Board of Directors holds the HIO leadership accountable for its operational performance and financial sustainability. It provides oversight to ensure proper management controls are in place, including human resources and financial accounting. This entity does not typically provide direct oversight of the HIE network but the organization that manages the technical and operational aspects of the network.

This body is typically found in the United States and other nations in which the HIO is a legal corporation distinct from the MOH. The governing body for the HIO provides separation of powers from the network governing body, enabling the Board of Directors, for example, to approve a pricing structure for HIE services without influence from the membership of the network. This body can also approve mergers with other HIE networks and establish strategies for HIE network growth.

4.2.1.2 Network governing committee

This governing body is responsible for managing governance for the HIE network. It is distinct from the managing entity in that it consists of representation from stakeholder groups participating in the exchange. A governing body establishes and maintains policies and procedures regarding data management and use. These are the "rules of the road" for HIE networks, including the rules for which health system entities can join the network, which data or clinical document types are required to be shared with other network members, and the process for removing a participant (e.g., data breach, illegal use of data).

The governing body serves as a trusted agent on behalf of all stakeholders to achieve consensus regarding data use and data access. The decisions must strike an effective balance between making data available and proper security controls. For example, consider the following data access request that occurred at a regional HIE.

> *A group of primary care physicians and specialists would like approval to access a care summary from the exchange without a patient registration transaction, which is the approved use case. Instead, they would like to self-attest to a patient relationship to access a care summary. They would only do this for their patients, and they understand they*

could be subject to audit to ensure that they weren't accessing patients who did not belong to them. This request was brought to the governing body three years ago, and it was declined. However, the physicians feel strongly that approval will improve patient care.

This governing body is the primary HIE network decision-making body and influences the day-to-day activities of the network. This body could influence strategy of the HIO, although it principally focuses on ensuring the data are captured, stored, exchanged, and used within the law and the permitted purposes adopted by the network.

4.2.1.3 Data governance committees

Many HIE networks, especially as they expand in scope, employ the use of data governance committees. These governing bodies are subcommittees that usually report up to the main HIE network governing body. They can be standing committees outlined in the network's governance charter, or they could be ad hoc committees created to focus on a specific task, such as examining data quality or providing oversight for a temporary initiative (e.g., COVID-19 pandemic task force).

A common standing committee in many HIE networks focuses on data use. This committee meets outside of the governing body meetings to review, propose, discuss, and debate the merits of various data use cases. For example, the network may consider expanding to support a new HIE service that would allow nursing homes to share Do Not Resuscitate (DNR) orders with emergency departments and hospitals. The committee would discuss how the exchange would function, which entities could author DNR orders, which systems would need to synchronize to ensure DNR orders are up-to-date and authorized, and how a DNR order would be deleted or sunset if the patient signed a new DNR. The committee would debate the details of the proposal and then make recommendations to the full HIE network governing body for adoption. More established, complex HIE networks might divide some of these discussions across multiple committees, such that a separate committee would discuss the technical aspects of the exchange. A data use committee would also discuss and make recommendations with respect to new HIE data uses, such as providing chronic disease data to public health authorities or substance use disorder information at the point of care. As the use of data to manage chronic diseases intensifies, population health divisions of public health authorities could accelerate the specificity of programs offered to certain populations. The relaxation of 42 CFR part 2 (August 14, 2020 and March 27, 2021), Confidentiality of Substance Use Disorder Patient Records, now allows transmission of certain substance use disorder data, previously unsharable, to an organization as opposed to a particular provider, under a general consent instead of a specific consent, called authorization.

4.2.2 Participants

Who should be a part of a governing body or committee? Any governing body or committee should be representative of the stakeholders engaged in data exchange and the population(s) served by the HIO. Yet while each participant should have a voice in HIE governance, not every participant needs to have a formal vote or seat on every governing body. For example, Carequality (a national HIE network defined in Section 4.3) uses an Advisory Council that has 24–30 members to discuss and provide input and guidance to its Steering Committee, which is a smaller (18 members) governing body that makes decisions for the network [2].

Several HIOs use governance models in which participants (e.g., each organization engaged in the HIE network) elect representatives to the network governing body. The governing bodies then represent various classes or types of participants. For example, there may be 70 hospitals in a network, yet the governing body has four hospital representatives elected for 1–2 year terms from the larger pool of hospital executives, much like members of the US House of Representatives represent large constituencies.

Common participant types include the following:

1. Health systems, such as integrated delivery networks (IDNs) or accountable care organizations;
2. Hospitals, including community, critical access and for-profit;
3. Physician practices of all sizes;
4. Behavioral health providers, including independent psychiatrists and mental health centers;
5. Long-term postacute care organizations, such as nursing homes;
6. Laboratories, including hospital-based or independent labs;
7. Radiology centers;
8. Public health agencies;
9. Insurance companies;
10. Quality improvement organizations;
11. Patients or patient advocates;
12. Community health workers; and
13. Nongovernmental organizations that address health and well-being (e.g., Red Cross).

The Board of Directors for the HIO might have nonhealth system participants, such as representatives from legal firms or major businesses in the region served by the HIO. Governing bodies for network governance are more traditionally composed of representatives from the groups above.

Committees are often composed of individuals drawn from the network governing body. However, some HIE networks do have committee members who are not members of the network governing body. For example, a Chief Medical Informatics Officer at a hospital might serve on an Architecture and Standards Committee for the HIE network, but they would not attend the larger governing body meetings except when their committee is making a recommendation on changes to the standards required for network participants (e.g., moving from clinical document architecture to fast healthcare interoperability resources [FHIR] standards as discussed in Chapter 9). Rules about who can serve on committees would be decided by the network governing body.

4.2.3 Representativeness

When the HIO identifies the stakeholders who will make up the governing body, it is important to have a body that is large and diverse enough to be representative of the stakeholders engaged in HIE, but not so large that efficiency and effectiveness are compromised. More importantly, this governing body must be responsive to stakeholder, environmental, state, and federal changes. Once these members are identified, they will establish bylaws or organizational policies, such as how often to meet, what establishes a quorum, and who are the officers. They will also need to be apprised of federal, state and, sometimes, local laws that govern health data use so that they can develop policies and procedures that are in accordance with those laws.

Given a strong focus on equity following the COVID-19 pandemic and Black Lives Matter protests, it is increasingly important for HIOs to ensure their governance bodies reflect the racial and ethnic diversity in their community or nation. Representativeness means balancing organizational stakeholder involvement (e.g., hospital, pharmacy, general practitioners), but it also requires representation from the populations for which the HIO seeks to improve individual and population health through data exchange. HIOs should consider inviting community members, community health workers, and minority group leaders to be members of their governing bodies so that issues such as health equity, inclusiveness, and access to care are part of the consideration for HIO priorities and HIE services. Furthermore, nonmedical voices can help ground the HIO in its community and create opportunities for collaboration across sectors to address the breadth of health and well-being issues that are critical to achieving the goals of the World Health Organization Global Action Plan [3].

Note: Although the Board of Directors for a HIO is important, the remainder of the chapter focuses on the activities of the network governing body and those of the data governance committees, provided the network elects to use one or more committees to govern aspects of the network. This is because most HIE networks outside the United States will not have a separate Board of Directors for the HIO. Moreover, the main responsibilities of a Board of Directors are better described in Chapter 5 which focuses on sustainability of HIE networks.

4.3 Policies and procedures

Once the network governing body is established, policies and procedures for operationalizing health data exchange are developed. A contracting structure is implemented to make these policies and procedures are legally enforceable and to ensure accountability, sustainability, and scalability. This document is often referred to as a *charter* or *participation agreement*. Common elements included in a charter include setting definitions, establishing permitted purposes of the data, subsequent data use, participation, consent, and data protection (e.g., security, privacy).

Table 4.1 provides a high-level outline of what the policies and procedures should address. Each area is defined, and the table further provides examples of policies and procedures.

Some HIE networks make their governance charters publicly available, including the following:

TABLE 4.1 Policies and procedures by area of governance.

Area of governance	
Policy	**Procedure**
Permitted purposes	
Use for the purposes of payment, treatment, operations, public heath reporting, meaningful use, care coordination, disability determination, research, system audits, accountable care management, etc.	• Each participant is responsible for ensuring that data requested are for a permitted purpose. • Each participant organization is responsible for auditing and monitoring usage.
Permitted users	
Types of participants as well as the types of users and the type of access (based on the permitted purposes) each user has, what actions the user can perform with that access. Participants include hospitals, physician offices, laboratories, free-standing same-day surgery centers, public health clinics, payors, long-term postacute care facilities, etc. Users include physicians, nurses, nurse practitioners, clinical researchers, billing personnel, etc. Access types include payment, treatment, operations, public health reporting, etc. User actions include sending information, obtaining information, reading information, etc.	• To enforce roles-based access, each participant can assign each user a role consistent with a standardized role code (e.g., SNOMED). • Each participant is responsible for ensuring that permitted users are appropriate and that unauthorized users are not requesting data. • Each participant organization is responsible for auditing and monitoring each permitted user.

(Continued)

TABLE 4.1 (Continued)

Area of governance	
Policy	**Procedure**
Subsequent use of information received through the HIE network	
Policies around reuse promote trust. Common subsequent use policies establish if the information is: read-only without reuse, retained without reuse unless patient authorization is received, retained, and reused for only the original purpose, or retained with reused governed by applicable law.	• Participants are responsible for ensuring that record retention policies and procedures are followed. • If applicable law requires that Participant obtain a patient consent or authorization before it reuses or re-discloses information, then it is the responsibility of Participant to obtain this consent or Authorization prior to such use or re-disclosure.
Minimum requirements for participation	
Minimum participation levels mitigate participation for the purpose of receiving information without equally providing information and ensure data exchange will ensue. Examples of minimum participation levels include: exchanging only with each other, exchanging for like purposes (e.g., treatment only), a minimum number of transactions, laboratory results routing, etc.	• Participants are responsible for monitoring compliance related to the agreed-upon minimum requirements. Monitoring can be accomplished through central auditing, reports of noncompliance from requesting participants, or self-reporting
Consent and authorization expectations	
Consent and authorization are different in that consent is a general form allowing use and disclosure of health information, whereas authorization is a specific form allowing use and disclosure of specific health information for specific purposes. Consent policies are around establishing opt-in or out-out policies and can have varying degrees of granularity, whereas authorization policies are around what information will be provided to an organization, such as the US Social Security Administration who uses clinical data from medical records for disability determination.	• Depending on the granularity of the consent, the participant is responsible for ensuring that only consented to data are exchanged.
Privacy and security requirements	
Privacy and security requirements are well established by Health Insurance Portability and Accountability Act (HIPAA). However, stakeholders frequently use privacy and security policies as a mechanism to bring these requirements to the forefront. These include areas such as virus protection, password complexity and security, establishing stakeholder privacy and security requirements, etc. Additional information on privacy and security can be found in Chapter 6.	• The participant is responsible for monitoring compliance and mitigating and managing breaches. • The participant is responsible to adhere to breach response and reporting requirements by applicable law. • The participant is responsible for ensuring risk management, auditing and incident procedures, password management, data back up, and disaster recovery plan are current at all times.

HIE, health information exchange.

1. *Carequality*—This vendor-facilitated network in the United States (self-described as a "network to network trust framework") has a Governance Charter that defines the network's governance principles as well as the multiple governing bodies and their

hierarchy in making decisions about data use, participation, etc. The charter does not, however, specify details about policies and procedures [2].

2. *Multistate EHR-based Network for Disease Surveillance (MENDS)*—This multiple state effort in the United States created an HIE governing body even though the network is not managed by an HIO. The network is facilitated by a public–private partnership involving the US Centers for Disease Control and Prevention (CDC) and the Public Health Informatics Institute, a nongovernmental organization. The charter includes many details on the network's policies and procedures, including the software selected for managing the information in the network as well as data quality and the process for requesting data from the network [4].

4.4 Data sharing "Trust" agreements

In addition to participation agreements, HIE networks also create *data sharing agreements* to constrain the use of shared data between participating organizations and the network (typically the HIO entity). These documents further facilitate the development of *trust* among network participants, because each participant is held accountable to the same standards as the other participants. More details on these agreements, which are contractual structures, are described in Chapter 6.

These agreements must be specific enough to constrain the use of shared data to specific use cases. However, such agreements also need to be flexible enough to incorporate new use cases as they are approved or modified by the governance body. Creating these agreements is not easy in the early stages of establishing HIE. For this reason, formal governance may be deferred as the exchange develops and the use cases are being defined and approved. Once policies and procedures are established, then data sharing agreements can be drafted, finalized, and executed by the parties involved in the HIE network.

Governance describes how data are handled, shared, used, and secured. It creates a mechanism for monitoring compliance with the policies and procedures of the exchange. The HIO must be trusted to provide information to improve the safety, efficiency, and effectiveness of patient care. For this reason, data sharing agreements are critical to successful governance programs.

Table 4.2 provides several types of trust agreements commonly used by HIOs [5]. The table outlines the components of each agreement type and provides definitions.

TABLE 4.2 Types, definitions, and components of data sharing agreements.

Type of agreement	Definition	Components
Data Use Agreement	Data Use Agreement (DUA): A covered entity may use or disclose a limited data set if that entity obtains a data use agreement from the potential recipient. This information can only be used for: Research, Public Health, or Health Care Operations.A limited data set is protected health information that excludes direct identifiers of the individual or of relatives, employers, or household members of the individual [3].	• Establishes what the data will be used for, as permitted above. The DUA must not violate this principle. • Establishes who is permitted to use or receive the limited data set. • Provides that the limited data set recipient will: ◦ Not use the information in a matter inconsistent with the DUA or other laws. ◦ Employ safeguards to ensure that this does not happen.

(*Continued*)

TABLE 4.2 (Continued)

Type of agreement	Definition	Components
		◦ Report to the covered entity any use of the information that was not stipulated in the DUA. ◦ Ensure that any other parties, including subcontractors, agree to the same conditions as the limited data set recipient in the DUA. ◦ Not identify the information or contact the individuals themselves.
Business Associate Agreement	A business associate is a person or entity that performs certain functions or activities involving the use or disclosure of protected health information on behalf of, or provides services to, a covered entity. A covered entity's contract or other written arrangement with its business associate must contain the elements specified at 45 CFR 164.504(e) [4].	• Describes the permitted and required uses of protected health information by the business associate. • Provides that the business associate will not use or further disclose the protected health information other than as permitted or required by the contract or as required by law. • Requires the business associate to use appropriate safeguards to prevent a use or disclosure of the protected health information other than as provided for by the contract.
Data Use and Reciprocal Support Agreement (DURSA)	The DURSA is the legal, multiparty trust agreement that is entered into voluntarily by all entities, organizations, and federal agencies that desire to engage in electronic health information exchange with each other using an agreed upon set of national standards, services, and policies developed in coordination with the office of the National Coordinator for Health IT (ONC) in the US Department of Health and Human Services [6].	Multiparty agreement that specifies: • Participants actively engaged in health information exchange • Privacy and security obligations • Requests for information based on a permitted purpose • Duty to respond • Future use of data received from another participant • Respective duties of submitting and receiving participants • Autonomy principle for access • Use of authorizations to support requests for data • Participant breach notification • Mandatory nonbinding dispute resolution • Allocation of liability risk
Participation Agreement	Designed to ensure that participants comply with the data sharing policies and procedures, Participation Agreements spell out the terms of the relationship, including the roles, rights, and responsibility of each party as they pertain to the initiative [7].	May include or reference one or more of the above-named agreements.

Adapted from Allen C, Des Jardins TR, Heider A, Lyman KA, McWilliams L, Rein AL, et al. Data governance and data sharing agreements for community-wide health information exchange: lessons from the beacon communities. EGEMS (Wash DC). 2014;2(1):1057.

4.5 Governance key success factors

Governance builds trust, scales to accommodate new stakeholders, and adapts to change. Steady and important progress can be achieved by HIE networks as they incorporate the key elements.

4.5.1 Trust

It is said that it takes years to build trust and seconds to lose it. This saying holds true for HIE. Health care organizations must have a high confidence of trust that the HIE network will be good stewards of their data. This is becoming more critical as the frequency and size of data breaches continue to grow. Some forming HIE networks identify a tipping point when health care organizations acknowledge they should not compete on the data; rather, they should compete on *what they do with* the data. By agreeing to share their data, they are also agreeing to trust the network to manage it effectively. Effective governance builds trust among participants, and it must always be a top priority.

4.5.2 Scale

The success of an HIE network hinges on its ability to securely send and receive clinical data to a variety of stakeholders to support payment, treatment, and operations. Data governance becomes more complex as more organizations participate, especially among diverse stakeholders. For example, a governance framework may need to account for the needs of health plans, which are different than a health care provider. The HIE network may also adopt new use cases, including public health, population health, and research. The governance framework should be able to expand to support a variety of use cases.

While data governance exists in single health care organizations and IDNs, the governance requirements are more complex for HIE networks. As the exchange grows beyond state lines and incorporates new types of health care organizations, the governance structure must scale to meet these new demands. For example, as the Indiana Health Information Exchange (IHIE) grew from a central Indiana focus to a statewide focus, its governance needs evolved. The representation expanded to include health care leaders throughout the state. Consensus-based decisions needed to account for the needs of small rural facilities in addition to large urban-based hospital systems.

4.5.3 Flexibility

Sharing information has become more common due to federal legislation and health care reform. HIE improves care coordination, creates efficiencies to reduce medical errors and improve clinical outcomes, and provides support for accountable care organizations. As new uses of HIE are identified, the data governance model must be flexible to adapt to these changes. The contracting structure must also be flexible to accommodate changes through the governance mechanism.

The governance model must be prepared to respond to environmental changes. For example, when the HIPAA Omnibus Rule was finalized, many HIEs needed to make governance adjustments. A change in the administrative rule prohibits information from being shared with a health plan at the patient's request if the patient self-pays. If an HIE network's governance model had previously allowed sharing data with health plans, the data use policy must be revised to adhere to the HIPAA final rule. Likewise, when 42 CFR Part 2 was relaxed, many HIEs and organizations had to make adjustments in terms of consent versus authorization allowing substance use disorder information exchange.

4.6 Governance challenges

Enterprise, regional, state, and nationwide HIE networks have some common governance challenges. For example, all exchanges must convince stakeholders to place the network needs for data sharing above the needs of the individual participating organizations. However, some governance challenges are unique. Only a nationwide exchange organization must address the "one size fits all" challenge of establishing governance that works equitably across all stakeholders in the country. Thus it is difficult to develop a single governance structure for all types of exchanges. Fig. 4.2 illustrates four governance challenges and each type of HIE to which they apply.

4.7 Enterprise exchange challenges

Enterprise HIE networks (see definition in Chapter 1) have basic governance needs. Since participating organizations belong to the same enterprise (e.g., IDN) or are closely affiliated (e.g., an independent practice association), they generally agree on data governance. The primary challenge is to place the network needs of the exchange above the interests of each participating organization (e.g., hospital, clinic).

4.8 Regional exchange challenges

Regional HIOs, referred to as community-based HIEs (see definition in Chapter 1), typically include competing health care organizations, which adds a level of complexity to governance. Because the participating organizations compete, they will likely have different opinions about data management and use by the HIE network. They might also have different interpretations of legal requirements and how much risk is acceptable.

In addition to placing network needs above the interests of each organization, regional HIE networks have the difficult task of building consensus among participants. Achieving consensus can be difficult between large, urban and small, rural organizations. It can also be challenging between health care providers and commercial health plans. Large regional HIE networks have sophisticated governance needs, especially if they cross state lines or include diverse health care organization types. Most large regional HIE networks establish formal governance structures to serve the needs of its stakeholders. Mature HIEs have evolved these structures over many years and there is variability in their governance models. This is to be expected because there is variability in the business models of HIOs.

Many regional exchanges struggle to establish a robust governance structure. If the

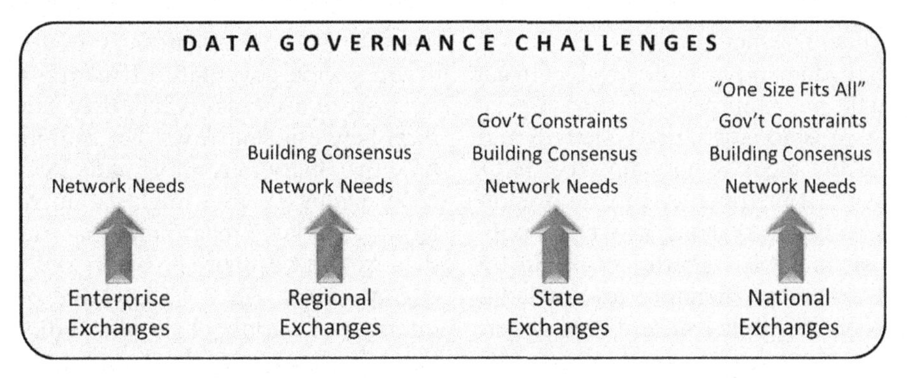

FIGURE 4.2 Data governance challenges at various levels of health information exchange.

network extends across state lines, there may be conflicting state laws. For example, patient consent laws may be different between neighboring states. Differences in state laws must be identified and addressed in a way that participating state laws can support. One approach to address this is through legislative changes. Some regional exchanges have successfully convinced state government to update certain legislation to enable new use cases. However, this can be time consuming and is not always successful. Another challenge is managing conflicts between nationwide governance structures and regional governance structures. These conflicts are only beginning to surface, but it is anticipated that more conflicts will arise.

4.9 State health information organization challenges

State HIOs, or Government-facilitated HIE (see definition in Chapter 1) because they are sponsored by or part of state government, have similar governance needs of Regional HIE networks with an important difference. Because it is associated with state government, a new layer of complexity associated with state government regulations and laws is introduced. The network needs of the exchange may be constrained by state government policies or processes, and it may be difficult to achieve consensus among stakeholders when the exchange is directed by a state government agency.

Stakeholders demand a high level of trust that there will be reciprocal stewardship of patient data that is accessed, used, shared, and reused. When the focus is on state level HIO, consideration must be given to private organizations, such as health systems, as well as public agencies, such as the Department of Health or Medicaid agencies. Therefore acknowledging that there are multiple levels of data governance to be addressed when trust agreements are developed, this is accomplished under the goal of simultaneously sending and receiving clinical data to multiple disparate entities.

4.10 Nationwide exchange challenges

Like the other types of exchanges, Nationwide HIE networks, like the eHealth Exchange, have governance challenges related to network needs, consensus building, and government influence. Nationwide exchanges have the most complexity because they must deal with the differences of all state laws, the diversity of all health care organizations, and a desire to have a single governance structure that works for the entire nation. Gaining support for a "one size fits all" governance solution is arduous when much of health care is managed locally and regionally. If important decisions about sharing health data are made nationally, there may be unintended consequences that create problems in parts of the country. For example, in Indiana there is a robust clinical and claims repository that has been standardized and normalized. It is a unique asset that does not exist in much of the country. How would a nationwide governance structure make decisions regarding this unique asset?

Each state can create laws regarding the sharing of health data. For example, most states have created patient consent laws that are not consistent across the country [8]. Until differences in state laws regarding HIE are addressed, a nationwide governance structure will be constrained to use cases where they can avoid conflicts between state laws. For example, consider how the ability to conduct nationwide reporting of infectious diseases might be impacted by differing state laws regarding what kind of health data can and cannot be shared and under what circumstances. Fig. 4.3 shows the public health information supply chain, illustrating how data flow up from local health departments, state

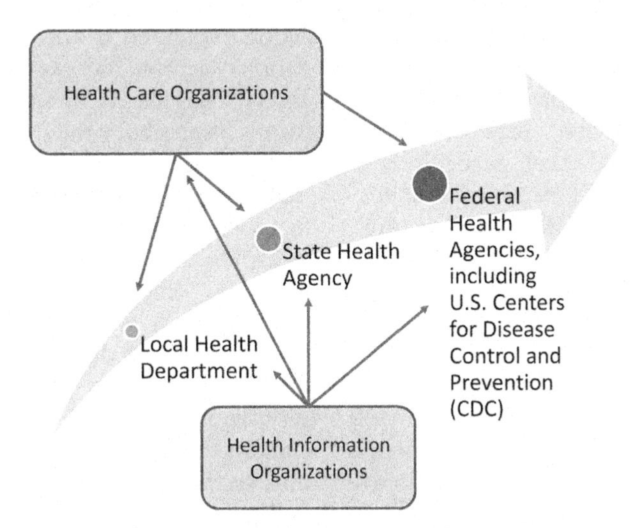

FIGURE 4.3 Flow of public health information in the United States across multiple stakeholders who all have independent relationships with one another.

health agencies and the national Centers for Disease Control and Prevention (CDC). The figure also illustrates that individual health care organizations and HIOs have relationships at all levels of the public health system. The ability of CDC to act in the best interest of the public with comprehensive surveillance and alerts becomes incomplete when just one state has laws limiting data sharing or restricting data use.

This scenario played out during the COVID-19 pandemic causing confusion on the part of citizens as well as government officials who were unfamiliar with the public health system in the United States. Each state established its own website and/or dashboard where it presented data on cases and deaths related to COVID-19. Some states, like Ohio, Indiana, and New York posted a lot of details about cases, hospitalizations, and deaths. Other states never posted public information or posted only very limited data. Individuals living in states with no dashboards accused their states of hiding information. Yet it is plausible that the states that limited information simply did not have a culture of collecting such information or did not know how to collect the information, especially at the start of the pandemic.

In order for CDC to capture data from states, the agency had to provide guidance to state health agencies on which data should be captured from hospitals and clinics. These data evolved over time and states had to update their guidance to hospitals. Furthermore, many states had to implement methods to capture the data CDC requested, but they were not data they normally collect on individuals with influenza, diabetes, or other conditions. Bed capacity and availability are two examples. Several HIE networks assisted their states in capturing these data, although not all of the HIEs were capturing those data before the start of the pandemic.

In the chaos of the pandemic, especially with increasing hospitalizations and workload on health systems, it became frustrating for hospitals to change their workflows and interfaces to keep up with evolving requests from local, state, and federal public health agencies. Even more frustrating was the fact that those three groups did not always agree on what were the most important data for hospitals to report. This example illustrates the complexity of defining consistent, common "one size fits all" approaches at the national level, particularly in the United States. It should be noted that several nations with national HIE infrastructures, including Denmark (Chapter 28) and Israel (Chapter 31), were able to quickly deploy common metrics and approaches for public health reporting during COVID-19.

Postpandemic, there is a push to reengineer this system and establish common data and pathways for public health reporting. Although many HIOs and the CDC seek to harmonize data sharing efforts, national guidelines will be subject to applicable state law and practices, meaning that health data exchange could differ from state to state without stronger national law. Furthermore, because health care organizations and HIOs have independent relationships with the various levels of public health, clear and consistent pathways for data sharing are challenging given the technical capacity and HIE engagement among the various public health agencies in a given state or region. Therefore solving this challenge will require not only stronger governance through policy, but also human and fiscal resources to support enhanced technical capabilities not currently existing in most public health jurisdictions.

4.11 Community-based health information exchange network governance example: Indiana Network for Patient Care

In the mid-1990s, the Regenstrief Institute created one of the first HIE governance bodies, called the Indiana Network for Patient Care (INPC), which is now facilitated by the IHIE. The governance structure was originally created to serve the Indianapolis market and a few use cases. Over the past three decades, the scope expanded to include health care organizations across the state and dozens of use cases. Chapter 22 in this book has additional information about the INPC and IHIE.

The governance framework in Indiana is multilayered. IHIE has a Board of Directors that focuses on the management and strategy of IHIE as an HIO. In addition, the INPC has a governing body known as the INPC Management Committee. It is this committee that provides governance and direction for the HIE network that IHIE manages. While IHIE develops HIE services it can offer to customers (e.g., hospitals, clinics), the INPC focuses on network participation, security, data use, and data quality.

The composition of the INPC Management Committee is as follows:

1. Founding hospital systems (5)
2. Regenstrief Institute (2)
3. Indiana Health Information Exchange (1)
4. Indiana Department of Health (1)
5. Indiana State Family and Social Services Agency (1)
6. Health plans or third-party payers (2)
7. Acute care hospitals, but which are not part of a Founding Member (2)
8. Physician practice groups (must be physician), but which are not part of a Founding Member (2)
9. Independent clinical laboratory (1)
10. Patient and consumer representative (1)
11. EMT, radiology, and long-term care (2)

4.12 Government-facilitated health information exchange network example: Virginia Health Information

In 2019 ConnectVirginia, the statewide HIE, merged with Virginia Health Information (VHI) to form a statewide, government-facilitated HIE network that includes an all-payer claims database (APCD). That same year, the Department of Health in the

Commonwealth of Virginia mandated providers use the APCD, providing strong incentives for exchange of data with VHI.

Although VHI and ConnectVirginia are government-facilitated, they are managed by a nonprofit organization and public funds are only a part of VHI's overall budget. The HIO has a primary governing body, the Board of Directors for VHI. From the Board, VHI creates task forces and subcommittees to perform focused governance work for the HIE network.

The Board of Directors includes the following classes of membership:

1. Business community leaders (5)
2. State representatives (4)
3. Consumer representatives (3)
4. Physician representatives (2)
5. Nursing facility representatives (2)
6. Health insurance representatives (2)
7. Hospital representatives (2)
8. HIE representatives (1)

The network has a transparent budget, which is published as part of its annual report [6], likely due to the fact it is a government (public)-sponsored entity. Previously, ConnectVirginia operated using a very transparent governance process that involved almost exclusively public governing body meetings. This transparency may be reflected in the openness of the merged HIO.

4.13 National health information exchange network governance example: eHealth Exchange

The vision of fully interoperable, nationwide electronic health records was first articulated as early as the 1980s.[1] The eHealth Exchange (formerly known as the Nationwide Health Information Network or NwHIN) was designed as a "network of networks" to enable HIE between a diverse range of stakeholders including HIOs, IDNs, federal and state government agencies, and health plans. eHealth Exchange was founded on the principal that "point-to-point" data sharing agreements, in which two data sharing organizations negotiate a specific data sharing agreement to support the sharing of specific types of data, are not scalable on a national level.

The eHealth Exchange model of a network of networks, where a wide variety of organizations can share health information safely and securely using a common trust framework, is preferred over the point-to-point model. The common trust framework includes both technical requirements to enable data sharing and policy requirements that govern the use and disclosure of data sharing. Initially, developing a common trust framework for the NwHIN was very challenging from both a technical and policy perspective. It became clear during the NwHIN Trial Implementation, sponsored by the Office of the National Coordinator for Health Information Technology (ONC), that a common trust framework would have to be created. ONC established national work groups charged with developing specific components of the trust framework. The effort of these work groups resulted in a universal trust framework, depicted in Fig. 4.4, which was ultimately endorsed by the Health Information Technology Policy Committee in 2010.

Technical specifications, while essential for electronic health systems to communicate, are not sufficient to support widespread interoperability. There are many reasons why this is true. Some organizations consider health data to be proprietary information, some health care provider organizations fear losing a

[1] The Workgroup for Electronic Data Interchange was formed in 1991 by the Secretary of Health and Human Services to promote the use of Health IT to improve the quality, cost, and efficiency of health care delivery. There were years of discussion at the national level leading up to the formation of Workgroup for Electronic Data Interchange (WEDI).

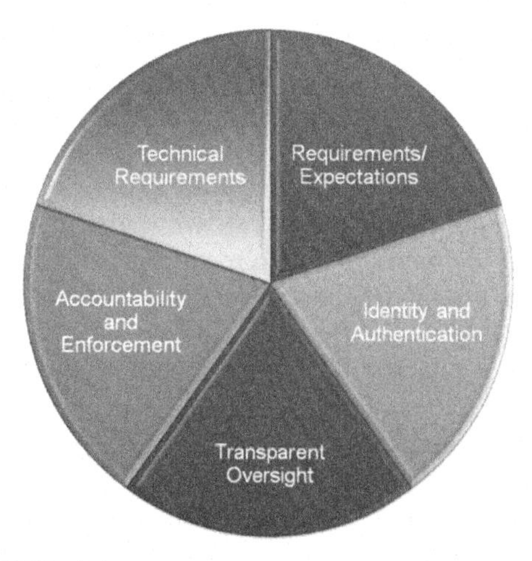

FIGURE 4.4 Universal trust framework developed by the eHealth Exchange.

competitive advantage by sharing health data, and others are simply too fearful of liability for data breach. It became clear that widespread interoperability would not happen unless there was a set of data use policies that governed the use of the HIE technology, that all participants in the network agreed to comply with the policies, and that there was a means to enforce those policies in the event of noncompliance. The conundrum was how to create a common trust framework that would be legally binding in the absence of a comprehensive federal legislative or regulatory scheme. This was complicated by the fact that the legal framework which did exist consisted primarily of data privacy laws, such as HIPAA and state laws, which were often contradictory.

ONC recognized this challenge and created a national workgroup to develop a data sharing trust agreement that would support the NwHIN's model of network-to-network data sharing. ONC named this trust agreement the Data Use and Reciprocal Support Agreement (DURSA).[2] The DURSA has since become the foundational legal document of the eHealth Exchange and a model for HIE data sharing networks generally. The DURSA is a multiparty, legally binding agreement that identifies key requirements that every organization participating in eHealth Exchange agrees to follow. However, it is more than that; it also embodies the policy framework that undergirds the eHealth Exchange.

The DURSA memorializes the set of core data sharing principles on which all eHealth Exchange participants agreed. These principles address how the eHealth Exchange can be used (Permitted Purposes), by whom it can be used (Participants and Permitted Users), the level of use that is required of each Participant to maintain a healthy data sharing community (minimum level of participation), respect for the rights of Participants (autonomy principle), requirements for reporting data security incidents, the allocation of risk, a method for dispute resolution, and details on how eHealth Exchange is governed. Each eHealth Exchange Participant knows what the requirements are and that every other Participant is required to comply with the same requirements. Failure to comply will result in penalties including suspension of data exchange privileges or, in extreme cases, expulsion from eHealth Exchange. Knowing that common rules exist and must be followed is a key component of any trust community. In the case of eHealth Exchange, it has created a foundation for governance of the multiparty network of very diverse stakeholders.

While a section-by-section analysis of the DURSA is beyond the scope of this book, some of the key provisions of the DURSA are:

1. *Permitted purposes*: Use of eHealth Exchange is limited to specific permitted purposes. Participants may not request information for

[2] The current version of the DURSA is available online at http://sequoiaproject.org/ehealth-exchange/onboarding/dursa/.

reasons that fall outside the scope of these enumerated permitted purposes.

2. *Permitted users*: Every Participant is responsible for deciding which individuals within its organization or network are allowed to access eHealth Exchange. Each Participant must have a process to authenticate its Users and to monitor their use of eHealth Exchange.
3. *Minimum level of participation*: This requires that any eHealth Exchange Participant that submits a request related to treatment is required to respond to requests from other Participants when the permitted purpose of those requests is also treatment.
4. *Autonomy principle*: Participants in eHealth Exchange are diverse and include health plans, IDNs, HIEs, federal government agencies, and other governmental organizations. It is important to respect the business rules that these Participants have in place.
5. *Notification of security incidents*: Participants are required to notify the eHealth Exchange Coordinating Committee within 1 h of determining that a security incident may have occurred involving the transmission of information using eHealth Exchange. A Participant must submit a detailed report which includes specific information set out in the DURSA within 24 h of the suspected incident. This is an extremely aggressive notification standard that meets the strictest federal requirements.
6. *Allocation of risk*: Governmental agencies cannot agree to indemnify nongovernmental parties so the DURSA does not include traditional indemnification provisions by design. However, Participants do agree to be responsible for their own actions when using eHealth Exchange that cause damage or injury to another Participant. In this way, risk is allocated to the party that is most able to control it.
7. *Data privacy*: The DURSA establishes the requirements of HIPAA as a contractual standard even if a Participant is not otherwise subject to HIPAA as a covered entity or a business associate.
8. *Mandatory "Flow Downs"*: Participants are required to flow down to every organization or individual in their network the DURSA requirements related to Security Incident notification and other critical provisions. This assures that everyone using eHealth Exchange is following the same set of rules.

Having a common set of rules that are known by all participants and are mandatory for participation in eHealth Exchange helped to create a trust framework that is both durable and flexible. However, there must be oversight of the community so that participants know the requirements are being followed and there are consequences for not following them.

eHealth Exchange is not a legal entity, so traditional governance models, like a boards of director, were not available to it. Additionally, there was no federal legislation that granted authority to a governance body over eHealth Exchange. Careful thought was given to determining the key characteristics of an effective governance model for data exchange. The following key principles of governance were developed by NeHC[3] under contract to ONC:

1. *Distributed governance*: Governance should not be solely vested in any single organization or group. The complexity of the governance functions and the diversity of core competencies required to execute these functions make it very clear that effective governance will require the active participation of multiple organizations,

[3] The National eHealth Collaborative (NeHC) was a public–private partnership established through an ONC grant. NeHC's efforts focused on enabling secure and interoperable health information exchange through education and stakeholder engagement. NeHC merged with The HIMSS Foundation in December 2013.

individuals, and groups, including consumers. Governance of the "network of networks" is and will continue to be inherently complex and requires a diverse range of competencies and perspectives, thus making it very clear that effective governance requires active participation by and distribution among public and private organizations.

2. *Representative governance*: One of the hallmarks of eHealth Exchange is its diversity in terms of those who participate in the exchange of health information. The ONC Strategic Plan affirms that this diversity is purposeful and should be encouraged. The governance model should be designed to balance the collective needs of eHealth Exchange with the unique needs of individual stakeholders, thus promoting stakeholders' continued use of and participation in eHealth Exchange. Many stakeholders including, but not limited to governmental stakeholders, are subject to specific legal requirements that govern their participation in eHealth Exchange. Any governance structures should take these requirements into consideration.
3. *Transparency and openness*: The foremost basis for establishing trust is engaging in governance activities that are transparent and open to stakeholders. The degree, type, and mechanism for openness and transparency will vary in accordance with the specific functions or activities.
4. *Responsive*: Governance exists for the benefit of the governed. This concept has many implications and challenges for governance but among the most significant is that the governance process be responsive to the needs and concerns of both governmental and nongovernmental stakeholders. This responsiveness includes giving timely attention to governing issues and remaining flexible enough to accommodate multiple demands on the governing body.
5. *Accountability*: Those charged with eHealth Exchange governance occupy a position of public trust. eHealth Exchange is a vital component of the national infrastructure as part of both the health care system and the electronic HIE infrastructure. Individuals and organizations who participate in the governance process must recognize that they, as well as the actual governing authority(ies), are accountable to the stakeholders, and the public more broadly, in the discharge of their duties. To the extent that multiple groups are involved in governance, their individual interests may at times be in conflict with the interests of eHealth Exchange. There will need to be processes to address such conflicts.

Using the principles of governance, the eHealth Exchange decided that the best approach to governance of the network of networks was a self-governance model that was driven by the eHealth Exchange participants themselves. The result is a Coordinating Committee composed of representatives of the participants. eHealth Exchange was not created by a legislative or regulatory action, and it was not originally a legal corporation. Therefore the legal basis for the Coordinating Committee had to be created. The DURSA created the Coordinating Committee by agreement of all signatories and identifies the scope of the Coordinating Committee's authority. Each eHealth Exchange Participant, by signing the DURSA, agrees contractually to submit to the authority of the Coordinating Committee to oversee eHealth Exchange. The authority of the Coordinating Committee is specifically set out in the DURSA. While broad, it is not unlimited. Following the principle of distributed governance, each eHealth Exchange participant is responsible for governing itself and those who exchange information via eHealth Exchange using that participant's digital credentials.

Section 4.03 Grant of authority.

The Participants hereby grant to the Coordinating Committee the right to provide oversight, facilitation and support for the Participants who Transact Message Content with other Participants by conducting activities including, but not limited to, the following:

1. Determining whether to admit a New Participant;
2. Maintaining a definitive list of all Transaction Patterns supported by each of the Participants;
3. Evaluating requests for and approving new Use Cases;
4. Developing and amending Operating Policies and Procedures in accordance with Section 4.11 of this Agreement;
5. Receiving reports of Adverse Security Events and acting upon such reports in accordance with Section 14.04 of this Agreement (Adverse Security Event Notification);
6. Suspending or terminating Participants in accordance with Section 19 of this Agreement (Suspension and Termination);
7. Resolving Disputes between Participants in accordance with Section 21 of this Agreement (Dispute Resolution);
8. Managing the amendment of this Agreement in accordance with Section 23.02 of this Agreement;
9. Approving the adoption of Network Utilities;
10. Evaluating, prioritizing and adopting new Performance and Service Specification, changes to existing Performance and Service Specifications and the artifacts required by the Validation Plan in accordance with Section 10 of this Agreement;
11. Maintaining a process for managing versions of the Performance and Service Specifications, including migration planning;
12. Coordinating with ONC to help ensure the interoperability of the Performance and Service Specifications with other health information exchange initiatives including, but not limited to, providing input into the broader ONC specifications activities;
13. Entering into agreements to broaden access to data to enhance connectivity across platforms and networks as provided in accordance with Operating Policies and Procedures which shall include an express opt-out right for every Participant; and
14. Fulfilling all other responsibilities delegated by the Participants to the Coordinating Committee as set forth in this Agreement.

The composition of the Coordinating Committee is a critical issue. The governance principles developed as part of creating eHealth Exchange require that a governing body be representative in order to be effective. The eHealth Exchange has evolved since it was formed in 2007 and the composition of the Coordinating Committee has evolved as well in order to remain representative of the stakeholders. Initially, the Coordinating Committee was composed of representatives from the first governmental and nongovernmental signatories to the DURSA (the "charter Participants"). This approach was taken to assure that the Coordinating Committee reflected the input of those with the most at stake in the success of eHealth Exchange.

This was a transitional model, however, and the DURSA required this approach to sunset after a period of years in favor of a more representative model in which nongovernmental

Participants elected a specific number of Coordinating Committee members and each federal agency that participated in eHealth Exchange appointed individuals. Over time, the role of various federal agencies changed such that it seemed more prudent to have the federal agencies, as a group, select up to four individuals to serve on the Coordinating Committee as voting members. This approach assures that the perspective of the federal agencies involved in eHealth Exchange is retained with the Coordinating Committee, which is critical, while not imposing an undue burden on each agency to designate a representative. The remaining nine voting members of the Coordinating Committee are selected by the nonfederal Participants across three classes of membership: (1) HIOs; (2) Health system, academic institution, provider collaboratives; and (3) Other. There is also an *ex officio* seat (nonvoting) reserved for ONC to assure that the Coordinating Committee and ONC continue to communicate effectively.

This Coordinating Committee governance model has proven to be effective in leading eHealth Exchange through its initial years as major policy issues were debated and resolved. The business and legal environment for HIE has changed dramatically since eHealth Exchange was created in 2007 and the Coordinating Committee has been responsible for keeping eHealth Exchange current and relevant in a rapidly changing landscape. This has been very challenging and yet, because the Coordinating Committee was built on solid governance principles, it has been able to adapt and remain effective. Governance must be flexible and responsive to be effective and we expect the Coordinating Committee will continue to evolve as the environment changes.

Another evolution since the start of the eHealth Exchange, the network formed a legal entity to serve as the HIO for managing the HIE network. In 2011 Healtheway, Inc. was incorporated as a nonprofit organization in the Commonwealth of Virginia as the HIO for the eHealth Exchange. The creation of Healtheway, Inc. led to the creation of a Board of Directors to oversee Healtheway the HIO the nongovernmental organization. The Coordinating Committee remains the governing body for the eHealth Exchange. Thus the eHealth Exchange looks similar now to regional, community-based HIE structures.

4.14 Emerging trends

With respect to governance, the largest emerging trend is TEFCA, the Trusted Exchange Framework and Common Agreement. The 21st Century Cures Act of 2016 [6] directed ONC to "develop or support a trusted exchange framework and common agreement" that would establish common rules for trusted exchange, including organizational and operational policies and methods to authenticate participants in exchange. TEFCA is the result of listening to health system stakeholders and completion of a multistep rulemaking process.

TEFCA does not create a new HIE network. Rather, it creates a governance and legal structure to allow existing, and possibly new, HIE networks and organizations to exchange information and sets common expectations, obligations, and technical approaches for those that choose to join. By setting a single set of rules that are embedded in legal contracts, TEFCA allows those participating in TEFCA exchange to share information across networks without having to develop one-off agreements. It also creates a single set of technical requirements to support TEFCA exchange. The vision is to allow participants such as health care providers, payers, public health agencies, and individuals to be able to share and gather information nationwide through a single connection of their choosing. In many ways, TEFCA builds on the legacy of the DURSA created by the eHealth Exchange, yet it scales those efforts and introduces a new structure and framework to facilitate nationwide HIE in the United States

To date, ONC established a Recognized Coordinating Entity (RCE), the Sequoia Project, to develop and operationalize TEFCA through a public–private collaborative funded under a Cooperative Agreement with the federal government. The RCE is tasked with operationalizing the TEFCA, including providing governance, oversight, and creating a sustainability plan.

In January 2022 ONC and the RCE released two foundational governance documents:

1. The Trusted Exchange Framework, which sets forth principles that embody the federal approach to guide nationwide exchange [8].
2. The Common Agreement, Version 1, which is the legal agreement outlining the expectations and requirements for participation in TEFCA exchange, key elements of which will also flow down to other entities participating in exchange [9].

A key feature is that HIE at the national level will focus on connecting multiple Qualified Health Information Networks (QHINs), or qualified health information networks, together for interoperable data exchange. Each QHIN can be a community-based HIE network, government-facilitated HIE network, enterprise HIE for an IDN, or a vendor-facilitated HIE network. New types of networks might also choose to participate in the future. Regardless of the structure of the QHIN in terms of its membership, the QHIN would follow the technical and governance rules of TEFCA, enabling exchange across the nationwide network.

The governance structure for the Common Agreement is depicted in Fig. 4.5. Under the Common Agreement, QHINs, Participants, and Subparticipants have the opportunity to engage in governance of TEFCA. The overarching Governing Council is composed of

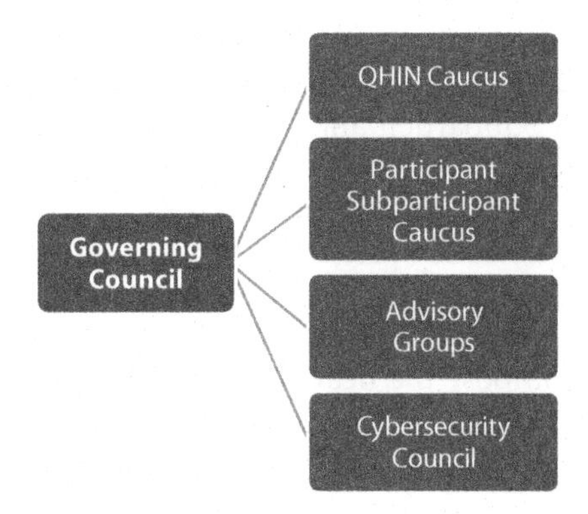

FIGURE 4.5 Governance structure for the Common Agreement, the common set of terms and conditions that facilitate HIE in the United States. Each caucus, council, or group provides recommendations to the overarching Governing Council of the Common Agreement.

representatives from the QHIN and Participant/Subparticipant Caucuses. Among other things, its responsibilities include reviewing amendments to the Common Agreement, QHIN Technical Framework (QTF), and Standard Operating Procedures; serving as a resource to the RCE and a forum for discussion; and providing oversight for resolution of disputes. The two caucuses and various advisory groups/councils may also make recommendations to the Governing Council for consideration on specific issues, like cybersecurity.

The Governing Council is composed of 21 members, as follows:

1. The QHIN Caucus, a community-of-practice involving all certified QHINs, elects 10 individuals affiliated with a QHIN.
2. The Participant/Subparticipant Caucus, a group composed of all Participants and Subparticipants, elects 10 individuals affiliated with either a Participant or Subparticipant.
   a. A Participant is an individual or organization (entity) that enters into a contract to participate in a QHIN. This could be a community-based HIE, a

health system, a physician practice, a solo practitioner, or a federal agency.
   - **b.** A Subparticipant is person or entity that uses the services of a Participant to send and receive electronic health information. If a health system is a Participant, then a Subparticipant would consist of the hospitals, clinics, and providers that compose the health system.
3. The RCE elects one representative.

The RCE further released technical documents that are outside the scope of this chapter, including a FHIR Roadmap. It should be noted that the first version of the QTF [10], released in July 2021, does outline data governance requirements that QHINs must follow. Comments from health system stakeholders were solicited in late 2021. At the time of writing, a second version had not yet been published. The RCE intends to vet HIE networks that wish to apply to become QHINs by the end of 2022.

Given its newness, TEFCA is likely to evolve and the details of its governance framework and governing body are likely to change over the coming years. The success of TEFCA is not known. However, TEFCA is a focal point for nationwide HIE in the United States, and it will likely influence HIE governance at regional and local levels beyond its role at the national level. All stakeholders in HIE should become familiar with its goals, framework, and governance principles.

4.15 Summary

Governance is an essential requirement of HIE. Yet governance is a voluntary activity, which must be embraced by all stakeholders. Stakeholder engagement is vital as an HIO seeks to gain consensus regarding data access and data use policies. A governing body needs to be representative of the diversity in an HIE network and establish data sharing agreements to enforce the policies and practices. Governance defines what data will be shared, how it will be shared, to whom it will be shared, and when it will be shared. An effective governance framework engenders trust, scales to accommodate additional stakeholders and approved use cases, and adapts to market and regulatory changes.

Successful HIOs will persuade participants to place HIE needs above the needs of their individual organizations. They will also facilitate trusted exchange of data and information that impacts care delivery as well as population health outcomes. Current efforts in the United States are focused on a new model for nationwide HIE, known as TEFCA. This national governance framework will take time to become established and evolve. The process will present challenges to existing HIOs and new organizations alike that seek to participate in nationwide HIE efforts. Regardless of its fate, TEFCA seeks to evolve governance of HIE at the national level, and only time will reveal whether it succeeds. Similarly, other nations will likely evolve their HIE governance as a result of TEFCA and the COVID-19 pandemic.

Questions for discussion

1. As detailed in the Governing Body section, a group of primary care physicians and specialists request approval to access a care summary from the exchange without a patient registration transaction, which is the approved use case. Why do you think the governing body denied the request? Should it have been approved?
2. An established regional HIO is considering joining the eHealth Exchange at the request of a nationwide health care organization (e.g., retail pharmacy chain) operating in its market. However, the policies and data sharing agreements of the regional HIO conflict with the policies and DURSA supported by the eHealth Exchange.

The HIO does not want to change its policies and data sharing agreements, but it wants to share data with the nationwide health care organization. What recommendation would you make to the parties involved?

3. How can HIE networks ensure their governing bodies are representative of the populations they serve? How would you convince a governing body to diversify its membership?
4. What impact do you believe TEFCA will have on HIE governance? Why?

Acknowledgments

The authors thank Keith W. Kelley, MBA and Steven D. Gravely, MHA, JD for their contributions to the first edition of this chapter. Their ideas and materials provided a strong foundation upon which this revision builds. We further acknowledge the Sequoia Project, specifically Dawn Van Dyke and Zoe Barber, who provided feedback and support for the descriptions of the eHealth Exchange and TEFCA.

References

[1] Office of the National Coordinator for Health Information Technology. Health information exchange governance. Washington, DC: U.S. Department of Health and Human Services. Available from: <http://www.healthit.gov/policy-researchers-implementers/health-information-exchange-governance>; 2015 [cited 2015, August 20].

[2] Carequality Steering Committee. Operating policy and procedure. Available from: <https://carequality.org/wp-content/uploads/2022/03/Carequality-Steering-Committee-OPP-Updated-7-1-2021.pdf>; 2014 [updated July 2021; cited 2022, March 2].

[3] World Health Organization. Stronger collaboration, better health: the global action plan for healthy lives and well-being for all. Available from: <https://www.who.int/initiatives/sdg3-global-action-plan>; 2021 [cited 2022, March 2].

[4] Public Health Informatics Institute. Multi-State EHR-based Network for Disease Surveillance (MENDS) governance principles, policies, and processes. Available from: <https://chronicdisease.org/wp-content/uploads/2021/07/MENDS_Governance_Document_V2_approved.pdf>; 2021 [cited 2022, March 2].

[5] Allen C, Des Jardins TR, Heider A, Lyman KA, McWilliams L, Rein AL, et al. Data governance and data sharing agreements for community-wide health information exchange: lessons from the beacon communities. EGEMS (Wash DC) 2014;2(1):1057.

[6] Virginia Health Information. Uniting to Support Care: Annual report & strategic plan update (32 p.). Richmond, VI: Virginia Health Information. Available from: <https://www.vhi.org/About/annual_report.pdf>; 2020 [cited 2022, March 3].

[7] Text - H.R.34 - 114th Congress (2015–2016): 21st Century Cures Act. (2016, December 13). <https://www.congress.gov/bill/114th-congress/house-bill/34/text>.

[8] Office of the National Coordinator for Health Information Technology. The Trusted Exchange Framework (TEF): principles for trusted exchange. Washington, DC: U.S. Department of Health and Human Services. Available from: <https://www.healthit.gov/sites/default/files/page/2022-01/Trusted_Exchange_Framework_0122.pdf>; January 2022 [cited 2022, March 3].

[9] Office of the National Coordinator for Health Information Technology. Common Agreement for Nationwide Health Information Interoperability. Version 1. Washington, DC: U.S. Department of Health and Human Services. Available from: <https://rce.sequoiaproject.org/wp-content/uploads/2022/01/Common-Agreement-for-Nationwide-Health-Information-Interoperability-Version-1.pdf>; January 2022 [cited 2022, March 3].

[10] ONC TEFCA Recognized Coordinating Entity. QHIN technical framework: public stakeholder feedback opportunity. Washington, DC: Sequoia Project. Available from: <https://rce.sequoiaproject.org/qhin-technical-framework-feedback/>; 2021 [cited 2022, April 10].

CHAPTER

5

Managing the business of health information exchange: moving towards sustainability

Saira N. Haque[1], *John P. Kansky*[2] *and Brian E. Dixon*[3,4]

[1]Pfizer Medical Outcomes and Analytics, New York, NY, USA [2]Indiana Health Information Exchange, Indianapolis, IN, USA [3]Department of Epidemiology, Richard M. Fairbanks School of Public Health, Indiana University, Indianapolis, IN, USA [4]Center for Biomedical Informatics, Regenstrief Institute Inc., Indianapolis, IN, USA

LEARNING OBJECTIVES

At the end of the chapter, the reader should be able to:

- Define sustainability and explain how applies to health information exchange (HIE).
- Explain how sustainability varies based on the organizational arrangements of the HIE network.
- Describe, in financial terms, the ways in which an unsustainable HIE organization can move to a sustainable financial position.
- Describe the importance of the alignment of mission, organizational structure, and business model and examples of how misalignment can undermine an HIE network's sustainability.
- Identify and understand challenges to HIE sustainability resulting from factors outside the network itself.
- Describe the concept of a statewide health data utility. Compare and contrast this concept with that of an HIE network.
- Discuss the role and importance of relationships with governmental agencies to the sustainability of an HIE network.

5.1 Introduction

Much has been written, presented, and debated about the sustainability of health information exchange (HIE). In fact, the healthcare industry in the United States and, more

Health Information Exchange
DOI: https://doi.org/10.1016/B978-0-323-90802-3.00009-5

recently, government seem to have a mild obsession with how to achieve and sustain HIE. Whether for-profit or not-for-profit, organizations that are created to perform HIE (the verb) are businesses (HIE, the noun). Recall from Chapter 1 that these organizations are most often referred to as Health Information Organizations (HIOs). The obsession with the sustainability of HIE networks and HIOs can be attributed, in part, to the fact that most HIE networks were founded in the last 10–15 years; and, as with many young businesses, many HIOs operate using temporary funding sources and generate more expenses than revenue.

At the base of the debate is usually the question of whether HIE networks can be run sustainably. This is the wrong question. HIEs can certainly be run sustainably. Therefore a much better set of questions, explored in this chapter, are related to how to operate a sustainable HIE network. Although this chapter is written from a US perspective, the principles of how to sustain HIE can be applied globally even though the context for HIE and market actors vary by region and nation.

5.2 Sustainability for the various forms of health information exchange is different

An exploration of sustainability in the context of HIE must begin with a working definition. The following is John Kansky's proposed definition of sustainability based on experience in the field of health information technology and, specifically, the work of growing and managing a large HIE:

> Sustainability: The ability to continuously operate a company or organization that fulfills a defined mission while remaining financially viable. In the context of HIE this means delivering HIE services in some useful way without going broke – indefinitely. [1]

Sustainability in this context refers to *financial* sustainability. For an HIE network to achieve the above definition, it must be performing HIE (the verb) in some useful way (i.e., HIE services) and generating enough money to keep operating. As covered in Chapter 1, there are several forms of HIEs: *Enterprise HIE, Government-facilitated HIE, Vendor-facilitated HIE, Health Record Banking, and Community-basedHIE*. The sustainability considerations for each type can be quite different, and each situation is explained briefly below. However, when people in the healthcare industry debate or question HIE sustainability, they are focusing on a specific challenge: the challenge of creating value through HIE and monetizing this value (i.e., getting someone to pay) with enough success to financially sustain the HIE network. This chapter is dedicated to an exploration of that sustainability challenge. As you will see, this specific challenge of sustainability is most typically characteristic of independent, community-based HIE businesses that are not part of a larger company or government.

5.2.1 Sustaining enterprise health information exchange networks

The sustainability of private, enterprise HIE networks is at the will of the central organization that operates and controls the HIE. That organization created the HIE network to serve some business purpose and as long as the HIE is perceived to be fulfilling that purpose, the central organization will sustain its operation—financially and otherwise. For example, if a large health system decided to create an enterprise HIE to share information across its affiliated hospitals and with selected business partners, it creates and sustains that HIE "function" with revenue generated through patient care. If the health system ever decided the enterprise HIE was no longer providing value in excess of the cost of its operation, the health system would simply stop operating the HIE. This scenario is not a very interesting or controversial sustainability challenge, so it will not be further explored in this chapter.

5.2.2 Sustaining government-facilitated health information exchange networks

The sustainability of HIE networks facilitated by governments are often similar to that of enterprise HIEs. The source of funding of the HIE network is identified or created by the government. This could be from tax revenues, through a levy (e.g., a fee charged on all health insurance claims), or covered within the budget of the agency in which it operates (often the public health department or Medicaid agency). If the government perceives value in continuing to operate the HIE network, it will continue to identify and provide the funds to do so. However, in some US states with government-facilitated HIEs, state leaders believe the HIE should be able to provide value to stakeholders, independent of the government, and that the value of HIE should be monetized to cover the cost of its operation. Therefore the government may also expect the leaders of the HIE to figure out how to operate sustainably without relying upon any (or limited) government funds. This sustainability challenge is similar or identical to the challenge faced by independent, community-based HIE networks, which is the focus of this chapter.

5.2.3 Sustaining vendor-facilitated health information exchange networks

Health IT vendors, especially electronic health record (EHR) vendors, operate and sustain HIE network for two primary reasons: (1) to meet requirements of government regulations and (2) in response to customer demand. With respect to regulations, as long as governmental agencies either require EHR vendors to provide HIE functionalities or incentivize HIE function usage by their customers, vendor-facilitated HIE networks will exist. Policy in the United States, specifically "meaningful use," HITECH, and the 21st Century Cures Act (all discussed in Chapter 3), required EHR systems to meet specific criteria that included interoperability and HIE functions. Many vendors now go beyond those minimums to provide HIE networks to which customers can subscribe, enabling customers to share data with other healthcare organizations. These networks were developed based on EHR strategies, policy considerations, and customer demands. Costs are sometimes included in annual subscription fees, or the vendor charges an additional fee for access to outside records. These costs are generally coupled with existing agreements that are difficult to change. Regardless of the fee structure, creating value is similar or identical to the challenge faced by independent, community-based HIE networks as described further in the chapter.

5.2.4 Sustaining Health Record Banks

Health Record Banks (HRBs) are the least common form of HIE. The sustainability of HRBs is similar to that of community-based HIE networks yet also distinct. On the one hand, HRBs are organized as grassroots, community-based organizations. They rely upon voluntary membership into the HIE network, and they work hard to directly recruit patients to use the network for gathering and curating health data. Yet, unlike other forms of HIE, HRBs start off with a very limited number of patients for whom data are available. A community-based HIE network might recruit a large health system which can prepopulate the network with records for thousands of patients. Meanwhile, an HRB might start off with records for 20–50 initial volunteers.

This number can grow substantially, yet the amount of data in the network may be limited at first. This can make it challenging for HRBs to create value for the individuals and organizations HRBs rely upon to financially sustain the network. This sustainability challenge is similar or identical to the challenge faced by independent, community-based HIE networks as described further in the chapter.

5.2.5 Sustaining community-based health information exchange networks

While the name "community HIE" might sound quaint or parochial, the largest and most robust HIE networks in the United States are of this form. A community-based HIE is typically a free-standing, not-for-profit business whose mission and purpose are to improve the quality, safety, and efficiency of health and/or healthcare through HIE. The organization (often called a HIO per Chapter 1) fulfills that mission by providing HIE services to customers throughout the healthcare supply chain (e.g., hospitals, health insurance companies, physician groups, state government agencies). These services produce value for customers, and in return, customers are willing to pay fees to the HIO, as long as the fees charged by the HIO are less than the customers' perceived value of the service. If the cost of operating a given HIE service is at or below the fees customers are willing to pay, the service is sustainable. If not, it is not. Community HIE networks that operate sustainably create a profile of sustainable services (i.e., more than one or two) which together generate enough revenue to exceed the total cost of operating the HIE. Simple, right?

The explanation above is an accurate description of the basis of sustainable HIE, but it glosses over details and nuance that we will now explore. Much of what comes next is more about business than HIE.

5.3 *Business 101* for Health Information Organizations

HIOs, dry cleaners, oil refineries, and health clubs are all businesses, and all have certain basic characteristics in common. Whether for-profit or not-for-profit, to be sustainable they all must produce revenue in excess of expenses. They all have fixed and variable costs as well as overhead. At the beginning of the chapter, we asserted simply that if an HIO delivers a profile of sustainable services, and if the total revenue from all services exceeds the cost of operating the HIE network, then it is sustainable. While true, it is important to explore a few key business and microeconomics concepts embedded in that simple explanation.

5.3.1 Key business definitions

- Total revenue—The sum of all income produced and earned by the HIO—presumably from fees charged to customers through the delivery of services.
- Total expense—The sum of all costs of operating the HIO including all fixed and variable costs.
- Variable costs—The costs that grow as the provision of services grows. New customers or growing transaction volumes cause variable costs to rise. Typical variable costs for an HIE network include data storage and any vendor fees that vary with volume. (If we operated a hot dog cart, buying more hot dogs would be a variable cost.)
- Fixed costs—The costs that the HIO incurs regardless of transaction volumes or the addition of new customers. Typical fixed costs for an HIO include rent, insurance, depreciation, and salaries. (If we operated a hot dog cart, the rental of the cart would be a fixed cost.) Some fixed costs can be directly attributed to the cost of delivering services while the rest are sometimes referred to as overhead.

TABLE 5.1 Facts describing the hypothetical case study HyHIE.

HyHIE's portfolio of sustainable services:	Service 1 (S1), Service 2 (S2), Service 3 (S3), and Service 4 (S4)	• Each service generates $1 million per year in revenue. • Each service costs $700k to deliver (but only $200k of the cost of each service is variable cost). • Therefore each service generates a "gross margin" of $1M − $700k = $300k
Total revenue	= S1 revenue + S2 revenue + S3 revenue + S4 revenue	= $4M/year
HyHIE's fixed costs	For example rent, insurance, and salaries	= $3 M/year (this would include the $2M fixed-cost component of S1, S2, S3, and S4 plus other costs like rent)
HyHIE's variable costs	For example, the variable cost component of delivering S1, S2, S3, and S4	= $200k + $200k + $200k + $200k = $800k/year
Total expense	= Fixed costs + variable costs	= $3.8 M/year
Excess revenue over expense	= Total revenue − total expense	= $4M − $3.8 = $200k/year

- Overhead—The portion of fixed costs that an HIO incurs that are not directly related to the delivery of its products or services, but rather, support the overall business operations. Overhead[1] includes rent, selling and marketing costs, and management salaries.
- Gross margin—The amount of revenue each service generates in excess of its own costs.
- Excess revenues (over expenses)—As the name suggests, when the HIO's total revenue is greater than its total expenses, it generates *excess revenue over expenses*. In for-profit businesses, this is called *profit* or *net income*.

5.4 Hypothetical case study to illustrate sustainability

So, for a given HIO to be sustainable, total revenue must be greater than total expenses over the long-term. Let us explore that more deeply through the example of a hypothetical HIO we will call *HyHIE* (Table 5.1).

In the simple example above, HyHIE is sustainable and can add $200k a year to its "rainy-day and reinvestment fund." However, what if circumstances were subtly different? What if HyHIE had 7% fewer customers? Or one fewer service? Or had to charge 8% lower prices? Or had an increase of 9% in fixed costs? In all these scenarios, HyHIE is no longer sustainable.

What we learn from the HyHIE example is that moving an HIO business from an unsustainable to a sustainable financial position means some combination of the following:

- Increasing revenue by:
  - Adding more customers
  - Adding more services
- Increasing the gross margin per service by:
  - Raising prices
  - Reducing service delivery costs
- Reducing overhead costs

[1] To be clear, some fixed costs are part of overhead and some are not. For example, rent and management salaries are not considered directly related to the delivery of its products or services—and therefore overhead. The salary of a database administrator or helpdesk associate would not be overhead since their effort is directly part of service delivery. This nuance is relevant to good accounting, but not important to the concepts of HIE sustainability in this chapter.

5.5 Increasing health information exchange revenue

HIE networks can increase their revenue in three ways[2]: by adding customers, by adding services, or by increasing service prices to their customers. A closer examination of each reveals some important microeconomic and business principles that are important to HIOs. Since price increases are directly related to gross margin, a means of increasing revenue that will be discussed as part of increasing the gross margin per service.

5.5.1 Increasing revenue by adding customers

Since an HIO sells services that yield revenue it uses to cover its cost of operations, each additional customer provides a little more revenue. And since we are assuming we cannot offer services that cost more to deliver than they generate in revenue, we know that some of the revenue from each additional customer helps us cover our fixed costs and gets us closer to sustainability. Let us suppose we are an HIE network with a service we offer to hospitals. If only half the hospitals in our market currently buy the service, we can add more customers simply by convincing more hospitals of the value of participating in the service. Alternatively, the same service could be used by independent labs or imaging centers. We could therefore add customers by selling the service to them.

But what if we operate in one specific healthcare market and all (or nearly all) the potential customers already buy the service? Can we expand into a new market (e.g., a nearby city that has some referral traffic with our market)? Or can we expand our definition of customers (e.g., a community services organization with referral traffic with healthcare providers in our organization)? If we continue extrapolating this a bit, it allows us to see how an important microeconomic principle applies to HIE sustainability. Since we see that each additional customer makes it easier to be sustainable, does not having more potential customers also make sustainability easier? If we sell services to hospitals, it is easier to sell services to more hospitals if there are 100 hospitals in our market than if there are 10. In addition, having more customers providing information adds to the value of information the HIE can offer [2,3]. Similarly, if we expand the definition of a customer, they will see more value if we already sell to the majority of hospitals in the area [4]. Therefore it is easier to sustain an HIE business in a large market than in a small one. This leads to a question that cannot be answered precisely here (we leave it to the economists). The question is "What is the optimal size market for sustainable health information exchange?" Given that many community-based HIE networks historically operated in markets smaller than an entire state (or in small states[3]), experience tells us the answer is bigger.

Since the first edition of this book was published, multiple HIOs have consolidated into bigger networks that cover larger markets (and geographic areas). For example, Indiana used to possess three independent, community-based HIOs. From 2019 to 2020, the three HIOs merged into the Indiana HIE, the largest of the three networks. The larger, statewide HIE network now has more customers as well as the opportunity to add even more customers among those facilities that do not belong to any network.

[2] HIEs often have temporary sources of revenue, such as one-time government grants. These temporary sources, while they are revenue, are almost always specifically intended to financially support the HIE while it builds itself into a truly sustainable organization.

[3] For example, the state of Delaware includes about a dozen hospitals.

5.5.2 Increasing revenue by adding services

Community-based HIE networks that operate sustainably create a profile of sustainable services which together generate enough revenue to exceed the total cost of operating the HIE. More specifically, financial sustainability is achieved when the portfolio of services is generating enough gross margin to cover the HIO's overhead costs. Since we know that each sustainable HIE service provides additional revenue and gross margin, each new service helps get the HIE closer to sustainability. Sharing information in and of itself does not demonstrate value; HIE networks must demonstrate that they can support organizational objectives through using the data they have [5–7], which may support sustainability. Therefore successful HIE businesses keep adding services to diversify revenue streams that (1) advance their mission and purpose and (2) generate additional revenue and gross margin.

But how does one identify HIE services that are sustainable? By no means specific to HIE, there is an entire field of study around the identification, development, and management of products and services known as product management.[4] In general, HIE services, like services in any industry or market, produce value for customers by making something in their world better or easier. A good service enables the customer to do something useful that they either cannot do on their own or cannot do as efficiently or effectively on their own. In practice, there are four main sources of new service ideas or concepts as summarized in Table 5.2.

Regardless of the source, identifying the concept for a HIE network's next potential sustainable service is the easy part. Concepts must be vetted for technical, economic, and legal/cultural feasibility; prioritized; developed; launched; marketed; and managed.

TABLE 5.2 Sources of new health information exchange (HIE) revenue streams through additional services.

Sources of new HIE service ideas	Explanation/examples
The service portfolios of other successful HIE networks	If another HIE network is successfully sustaining, for example, an electronic results delivery service, your HIO may be able to offer a similar or identical service.
Business challenges (pain points) brought to the HIE by customers (or potential customers)	A customer, knowing the data and capabilities of the HIE, may present a business problem to the HIE. For example, they might ask if the HIE can improve a specific population health management initiative by providing additional data.
Self-generated service concepts (through formal or informal idea generation)	Whether through formal product development ideation or concepts that come up opportunistically, members of the HIE's product management team will occasionally recognize new opportunities to create value for customers.
Opportunities created by federal or state regulations	Government regulations, such as promoting interoperability as well as information blocking, create opportunities for HIE networks to produce valuable services for customers.

[4] Readers can learn more about best practices in the identification and development of services—not specifically HIE services—by researching Product Management and New Product Development.

To yield one sustainable service offering, HIE networks should expect to pursue 3–5 service concepts. Abandoning concepts that prove to be unfruitful at the earliest possible stage of development is healthy as it keeps product development costs to a minimum. This is where learning from the experience of other HIE networks can be useful. One adage of entrepreneurship and innovation also applies to product development—*fail early, fail often*. That is to say, do not be afraid to pursue new ideas but also do not be afraid to *pull the plug* if an idea does not work out.

As an HIE network seeks to grow its profile of sustainable services, the importance of the HIO's mission and the economic realities of sustainability must be considered simultaneously and balanced. It helps to think of potential HIE services in two groups illustrated in Fig. 5.1.

There are many services that an HIE could deliver that are consistent with its mission (the left side of the Venn diagram in Fig. 5.1). Some of these services will have ready customers who are willing to pay for value they perceive, but some services will not. Consider an example of a service that could improve the quality of healthcare. An HIE could combine and analyze large and complex healthcare data sets from multiple payors and provider organizations and identify specific gaps in best practice clinical care for specific patient populations. These identified gaps could be communicated to healthcare providers who are treating these patients—even in real-time as the patients present in different settings across the healthcare system. However, it could be difficult to identify the customer segment(s) who would be willing to cover the significant cost of such a service given its complexity and the volume of data needed to provide it at scale.

Alternatively, there are services an HIE could deliver that have ready, paying customers (the right side of the Venn diagram in Fig. 5.1). Some of these services will be consistent with a given HIO's mission, but some services will not. For example, an HIE network might have access to data that a for-profit marketing research firm would value to support product planning for its customers. However, most community-based HIEs would view this use of the data as outside their mission.

Having access to a large number of healthcare organizations in a given region offers the possibility for partnering for group purchasing. Approximately one-third of the nation's independent HIE networks offer some form of group purchasing [2]. The organizations that participate in the HIE network have greater

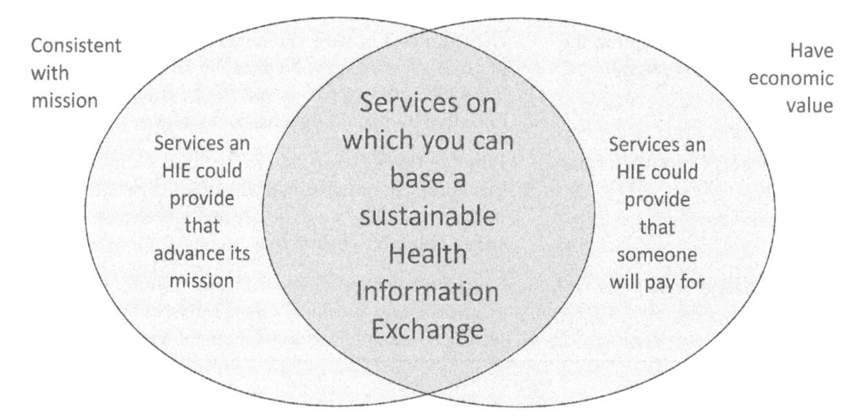

FIGURE 5.1 There are services that a health information exchange (HIE) could theoretically provide for which there is no apparent business model. There are also services that have business models that are outside the mission of a typical HIE.

negotiation power for products and services together than they would alone. The HIE can support supplier rebate programs where each member receives a rebate. The HIE benefits financially from receiving a small portion of the rebate, operationally but having more information about providers and their needs that they can use for other efforts, and can better a more stable membership. The participating organizations benefit from not having to spend time in negotiations to save time and in better pricing or rebates on products and services [6]. These savings can help offset the costs of participating in an HIE network and support ongoing membership.

As more organizations move to value-based arrangements, HIE networks can offer services to support that. Reductions in duplicate services such as laboratory or radiology tests and improved care coordination are often-cited benefits of HIE networks. If information about a patient can be displayed in an easy to access way or tied to quality measures, that might be a service that customers would appreciate. In addition, if customers or potential customers see the value in using the HIE to provide missing information and that is easy to visualize [4], the visualization and tie to existing programs might be another service HIE networks can provide. Related to this, HIEs could use information from its members to support streamlining workflows which involve using the HIE to demonstrate value to its members [2]. In addition, HIE networks can analyze information they already have, such as for alerts, and provide insights to participating organizations based on that [8]. Additional services can help with the perception of value, but also use resources.

Therefore services on which a sustainable HIE can be based are at the intersection of these two groups (the overlapping portion of the Venn diagram in Fig. 5.1). An HIE service portfolio should be composed of services that are both consistent with the mission of the organization and have intrinsic economic value to existing or new customers.

Imbedded in the above explanation is the concept of an unsustainable HIE service. An unsustainable service may serve the mission of the HIE and be technically achievable and viable in every other way, but not generate enough revenue to cover the cost of providing the service. Raise the price and customers will not buy it. Lower the price and the HIE is selling at a loss. Unsustainable. Reasons a given service might be unsustainable:

- Produces too little value (Not a good service—abandon it)
- Produces good value but costs too much to deliver

For the case in which a service produces value but costs too much, an unsustainable service could be turned into a sustainable service by sufficiently reducing the cost of delivering the service. This could occur through reduction in overhead, leveraging previously developed solutions or advancements in technology. For example, if the service is too costly because the HIE is delivering it in a cost-inefficient way, it could be rendered sustainable by finding a way to deliver it more efficiently. Alternatively, the service may be too expensive to deliver only because the scale of the customer base is too small. That service could be rendered sustainable by selling it to more customers and/or broadening the market of potential customers. In practice, it can be difficult to recognize, especially early in its life cycle, whether a service is unsustainable or whether it just needs more sales effort or more focus on cost reduction.

Before leaving the discussion of building a portfolio of sustainable HIE services, it is important to note that identifying and developing HIE services costs money. Every hour spent investigating the feasibility of a potential service offering, designing it, developing it, and selling it is 100% cost and 0% revenue until the first customer signs a contract and

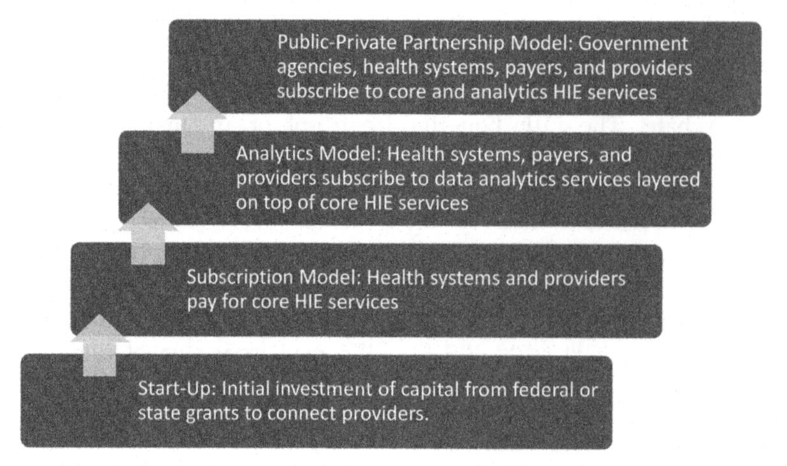

FIGURE 5.2 Strategic plan for a hypothetical health information exchange (HIE) network. The network initially received start-up funding from federal and state grants. Ultimately the HIE seeks to serve all stakeholders in the state or region.

begins paying. This is where sharing experiences across HIE networks (see Fig. 5.2) can be useful. And many more customers must be signed and implemented before the service is making a positive contribution to the organization's bottom line. The money to fund the development typically comes from one of two sources: excess revenue generated by other services or (more commonly) one-time sources of funding (e.g., a grant). Grants, while increasingly scarce, can be excellent sources of funding for the development of sustainable services as long as there is a disciplined and clearly understood goal that what the grant funds will result in a sustainable service. HIE networks cannot be operationally sustained on grant funds, which are inherently temporary.

5.6 Increasing the gross margin per service

Increasing gross margin means making slightly more *profit* from a service you already offer and deliver to customers. For a given service, an HIE can increase a service's gross margin in two ways: raise prices or reduce the cost of delivering the service.

5.6.1 Setting prices

Of these two choices, it is tempting to assume that raising prices is easier, but a customer's perspective would be different. In microeconomic terms, raising prices forces customers to seek alternatives. For community HIE networks, the most common alternatives for customers are to either stop participating in the HIE or to create an enterprise HIE that can serve the same or similar purpose (from their perspective). Both of these outcomes are harmful to the HIE network's quest of sustainability and undermines the overall value delivered by the HIE in support of its mission. Setting prices that maximize both revenue and customer participation is a theoretical goal, and there is no practical way of knowing if you have ever achieved it. Since it is important to the mission and value proposition of an HIE to have as much participation from healthcare stakeholders in the markets they serve, any price that is greater than the HIEs total cost of delivering the service that does not drive customers away is a financial victory.

Setting prices is much easier in theory than it is in practice. Establishing a price and explaining that price to potential customers is straightforward, in theory, if an HIO knows two numbers: (1) the total cost (including overhead[5]) of delivering the service to that customer and (2) the total economic benefit of the service that the customer will receive from the service. Some HIE networks are experimenting with different pricing models based on service, which adds another dimension to setting prices [5,8].

Any price that is above the first number but below the second means that both the HIE and the customer come out ahead. The problem is that in reality, an HIO is not likely to precisely know what it will cost to implement and deliver a service to a specific customer and even more unsure of the economic benefit to the customer.

What typically happens in the real world is that the HIE pleads its case for how its service will provide value, economic or otherwise, and the skeptical customer asks for empirical evidence. While there are a few research studies that support the economic value of HIE (more are needed; see Chapters 16 and 17), these studies inevitably do not fit the specific circumstances and therefore are not helpful in convincing skeptical potential HIE participants. In the end, some organizations are convinced of the value and participate while others do not. Increasingly HIE is becoming an assumed part of the healthcare supply chain, and markets are moving toward strengthening HIEs in terms of function and value as opposed to deciding whether or not to participate.

5.6.2 Reducing the cost of service delivery

Remember that financial sustainability is reached when the gross margin from all services exceeds the organization's overhead. If price is held steady and the costs associated with the delivery of services are reduced, the gross margin from that service increases. Given how difficult it can be to raise prices, reducing the cost of service delivery is extremely helpful.

Accountants refer to an organization's total cost of service (or product) delivery as *cost of goods sold* or *COGS*. For an HIE, COGS is chiefly made up of the costs associated with the people needed to deliver the HIE's services and a whole bunch of things related to data, computers, and software. Sometimes the people are employees and sometimes they are contractors. Sometimes the computers and software belong to the HIE and sometimes they are licensed or delivered as a service (e.g., cloud computing or software as a service). In either case, lowering COGS is about figuring out how to deliver the service with the lowest cost combination of people and computing. This might mean outsourcing your data center operation, or it might mean insourcing your data center operation. It might mean reducing your workforce by X people to lower payroll expenses, or it might mean hiring X people to perform a function at a lower cost than a third party was charging.

In most cases, the per-customer cost of delivering a service will drop as the customer base grows. Therefore growing the scale of your HIE helps to reduce costs and increase margin. Thus lowering service delivery cost might be achieved by merging with a neighboring HIE, for example. Significant HIE consolidation is happening as evidenced by recent mergers in New York, Michigan, and Texas.[6]

Yet there is no magical formula. Reducing service delivery costs in the pursuit of

[5]Accountants have methods of attributing the organization's overhead fairly to its various revenue-generating services. You must include a fair amount of overhead in the total cost of a service to know its gross margin at a given price.

[6]Since December 2013, at least three significant HIE mergers have been announced: Healthix and Brooklyn Health Information Exchange in New York, Michigan Health Connect and the Great Lakes HIE in Michigan, and the exchanges in Dallas and San Antonio in Texas.

sustainability is about deeply understanding your costs and working hard at exploring alternatives approaches, negotiating hard with suppliers, and sometimes making difficult business decisions.

5.7 Reducing overhead costs of an health information exchange business

HIOs tend to be high fixed-cost businesses, like an oil refinery or steel mill as opposed to a high variable cost business such as a consulting firm. Some fixed costs can be directly attributed to the cost of delivering HIE services, such as leasing a data center, while the rest, generally speaking, are overhead. Since the biggest financial challenge to sustainability for a given HIE is to generate enough gross margin from services to cover its overhead, overhead is viewed as a necessary evil. Minimizing overhead is an important mantra for the leadership of any HIE or any other high fixed-cost business.

Minimizing overhead is characterized by having a small leadership team, fair but not overly generous compensation levels, and adequate but not extravagant office space. One author (J.K.) once worked for a company that issued business cards to employees in five different colors and had an open bar at company parties, and that company soon went bankrupt.

While managing for minimal overhead might seem as simple as being fiscally conservative, there are conundrums. For example, consider sales expenses. Costs associated with sales are overhead. But stop selling, and your HIE will not grow. If an HIE network's strategy to reach sustainability hinges on increasing the number of customers, and therefore the scale of the HIE, doubling the size of the sales force may well be the key to sustainability. This, however, will double the sales component of overhead. Thus the focus should not be on simply reducing overhead but on making strategic decisions about spending [5] to support areas of focus for the HIE network. Once again, there is no magic formula.

Earlier we discussed increasing revenue by adding customers. While technically not reducing overhead, it is worth noting that as an HIE's customer base grows, overhead costs are *diluted*. That is to say that if the HIE's scale increases and overhead stays the same, the overhead per customer is reduced. Anheuser-Busch InBev produces more beer than your local micro-brewery but both businesses are sustainable. However, take note that their prices per pint are not the same. Anheuser-Busch has much lower overhead per pint and therefore can charge much lower prices. The smaller the scale of the company, the higher the prices it must charge to cover overhead. Customers are price sensitive because they have alternatives, which is usually to not participate in the HIE network.

5.8 Planning for sustainability

No different than any other businesses, HIE networks should have and follow a plan for their business which spells out their goals and strategies for achieving them.[7] This involves shifting focus from standing up the HIE network and implementation to planning for long-term sustainability [9], illustrated in Fig. 5.2. The hypothetical HIE network in this illustration seeks to move from a start-up to a statewide public–private partnership model in which the HIE network provides a range of services for providers as well as other stakeholders.

[7] Readers can learn more about best practices in planning for any business by researching Strategic Planning.

When setting goals and strategies, the mission of the organization and how best to achieve it should be the first concern. For an HIE that is not currently generating revenue over expenses, sustainability should be a close second. Just like the restaurateur who has opened a new location, obsessing over sustainability is absolutely appropriate until profitability is achieved. However, sustainability need not be a permanent preoccupation. While your HIE is moving toward sustainability (i.e., losing money), it is important to make decisions about every aspect of the HIE business with long-term sustainability in mind. However, once the HIE is sustainable, prudent management and fiscal discipline should enable the leadership team to focus on new ways of delivering value to customers and innovative means of achieving the mission. This may inform decision-making, such as what additional services to offer [6]. Sustainability, at that point, should be an ongoing reward for good, careful management.

5.8.1 Start with sustainability in mind

For a cross-country driving trip to be successful and efficient, one needs a plan for the route, places to stay along the way, and enough money to cover the expenses of the journey. But even with all these things, choosing the wrong vehicle or not packing the right accouterments can doom the journey before it begins. So it is with HIEs. Certain key characteristics of the organization, if not well chosen and correctly aligned, can make long-term sustainability difficult or impossible to achieve. These include mission, organizational structure (including corporate governance), and business model.

5.8.2 Mission

The mission of the HIE, as with any company, should be the bedrock of planning and decision-making. An HIE's mission statement might say that the organization exists to "enable the highest quality healthcare" or "raise the health status of citizens." The mission statement might say "in central Indiana" or "in the Midwest." It might say "support patient engagement" or "advance health IT research." In each case, following the mission will lead the organization in different directions. For example, a difference as subtle as "enable the highest quality healthcare" versus "raise the health status of citizens" can make a big difference. Focusing on health*care* suggests finding ways to help healthcare providers, whereas raising the health status of citizens suggests promoting or advancing public health, disease prevention, nutrition, and exercise.

5.8.3 Organizational structure

The term organizational structure, in this context, refers to whether an HIE is for-profit or not-for-profit, how its board governs it, who makes up the board, and how the bylaws of the corporation are written. While there is no one right organizational structure, a sustainable HIE is more likely to result if careful consideration is given to these most basic aspects of organizational design. In addition, Heath and Porter found that having physician involvement can help support HIE sustainability since physicians are a major contributor and end-user of information in the HIE network [10]. For example, if the mission of the organization is heavily focused on research, a board of business leaders from for-profit businesses may be a misalignment. If the organization is for-profit, a board made up of academicians or government leaders could lead to problems.

As HIEs face business challenges related to sustainability, the individuals in leadership roles and on the board of the organization will make the most important decisions. Imagine explaining to your board that the best strategy to attain sustainability is to increase the margin of services by raising prices if the board is made up of leaders from your customer organizations. The structure of the HIE should match the long-term strategy and purpose of the organization, and the governing board of the HIE must understand and support that alignment. Be prepared to make difficult changes when those changes are necessary to remove barriers and move toward sustainability.

5.8.4 Business model

In the most general terms, an HIE network's business model is a cohesive idea about how the organization will do something useful (i.e., produce value) and how the organization will generate revenue so it can do so sustainably. More specifically, the business model answers questions like:

- What kind of services the HIE will deliver?
- To which types of organizations will those services be delivered?
- What is the value proposition of the services to those organizations?
- How will the HIE generate revenue to cover its cost?

These decisions must be in line with the organization's mission, and the leadership and board of the HIE must understand and believe in the business model. For a given HIE, many possible versions of a business model could ultimately be successful, but there are many potential pitfalls. Getting the details right is important. The answer to a question as simple as "who pays the HIE" can sink an otherwise sound service concept.

As we saw in the HyHIE case study, loss of revenue from one service can render an HIE unsustainable. An example will help. Suppose the business model of the HIE is based on services that give hospital-based clinicians better information. A part of the value proposition of these services is that the additional information will prevent unnecessary procedures, thereby improving the quality of the care delivered to the patient (e.g., faster care with less trauma, less radiation) while reducing the cost of care. Does the HIE business model presume that it will charge the hospital based on the improvement in quality, or does it plan to charge the payor (e.g., insurance carrier) based on the reduction in cost? There is no "right answer."

If the leadership and board understand and believe in the business model, they will act in concert to find an answer that leads to sustainability. Together, they can make the necessary decisions around the HIE's business model and help gain support for it among healthcare and business stakeholders in the market. This alignment and understanding are necessary for a successful and sustainable HIE business. One example of a sustainable HIE business model can be found in Chapter 22.

5.8.5 Dissemination of the value of the health information exchange network

Sales, marketing, and sharing the value proposition of the HIE network to stakeholders may seem secondary to the HIE network's mission and vision. However, HIE networks are dependent on recruiting and maintaining a large network of stakeholders in a given region to contribute information, use the HIE, and pay subscription fees. Thus dissemination of the value of the HIE network, services offered by the network, and how the services integrate with stakeholders' operations should be a key part of sustainability planning [5]. More information on dissemination of value can be found in Chapter 17.

5.9 Challenges to sustainability

As we have explored in this chapter, there are many financial aspects of an HIE network that must be well managed to achieve sustainability. But outside the HIE, in the wider ecosystem of healthcare and governmental policy, there are other challenges to sustainable HIE that go beyond managerial accounting. While not an exhaustive list, Table 5.3 provides some examples of the challenges facing HIE networks.

5.10 Health data utilities, an emerging model for health information exchange networks

One way to leverage the power of HIE networks, promote efficiency, and serve communities is to consider the HIE as a public good [15]. If we consider exchange to be a public good like broadband or water, then HIE organizations would be considered health data utilities (HDUs). This is an emerging concept that serves the health data curation and analysis needs of the government (e.g., Medicaid, public health) and the private sector (e.g., hospitals, clinics) in a given state [16]. The services offered by HDUs go beyond the typical data exchange services offered by most HIE networks today.

HIE networks are regionally based, which allows them to evolve to serve the needs of the community. However, there is an opportunity to share infrastructure and take advantage of economies of scale through coordination and consolidation of HIE services. Consider Medicaid programs as an example. Today many are working to establish enterprise master person indexes to resolve patient identity as well as link clinical with claims data. These are core services of an HIE network (see Chapters 8, 11, and 12). Performing these services for governmental agencies, rather than in parallel, is a primary distinction between an HDU and an HIE network. In addition, HIEs facilitate important public health activities by being a conduit for mandatory public health reporting, helping identify hospital capacity (especially during major events like COVID-19), and supporting a broad range of population health needs (e.g., disease surveillance, multidrug resistant organisms surveillance).

HIEs can support mandatory reporting, promote broader connectivity, support value-based care, and provide information about health resources [15] in the community (e.g., facilities, providers). In some states, HIE networks already administer the prescription drug monitoring program and All-payer claims database [17,18], which are governmental functions. Conceiving the HIE as a HDU would help reduce duplicate patient records across HIE networks, promote patient safety [15,19], and reduce data fragmentation [20]. For example, during the COVID-19 pandemic, CyncHealth, the HIE in Nebraska, provided information about bed capacity and critical care availability throughout the state to promote patient transfers and manage capacity [17].

By taking advantage of economies of scale and serving the population as a whole, HIEs can perform more functions and serve larger populations. Examples of this include having more data to provide analytics by region (see Chapter 18), identifying and analyzing trends for populations of interest, and strengthening contact tracing while serving as a unified source of lab data and reviewing trends for comorbidities [20]. At the individual level, having the HIE as a HDU can help support longitudinal views of patients, alerts and notifications to providers, and facilitate care coordination [17,20] (see Chapter 27). In addition, HDUs can help support health policy decision-making through streamlined analysis of statewide data [16]. However, some states with robust regional networks may not wish to make changes to what they have already done or may perceive that they would lose functionality with the HDU approach. In addition, only a few states have statewide HIE mandates, so moving the United States toward the HDU

TABLE 5.3 Sustainability challenges that face health information exchange (HIE) networks.

Challenge	Explanation
The region does not know how to do HIE yet	HIE is in its early stages of maturity in many regions of the United States. Look at several HIE networks and observe the many differences in even the most basic aspects of their approaches. Look further at how many new standards and new government regulations have been created in the last 5–10 years. Most states and regions are still figuring out what approaches and business models will be the most effective and efficient.
Alternative to HIE is the Status Quo	Because healthcare providers and public health officials have been operating for decades in the absence of HIE, the natural tendency is to continue with the status quo. HIE leaders must not only have a compelling value proposition; they must also be able to communicate an understanding of that value to others. HIE can be a difficult concept to understand and explain, so many organizations are not participating [11,12]. The COVID-19 pandemic has shifted thinking among some healthcare and public health leaders, although there remains a natural tendency to envision modernization efforts are siloed within individual organizations rather than as a community (or public–private) effort.
Need to demonstrate value of HIE networks and services	Skeptical or confused decision-makers want evidence of the economic value of HIE. Studies demonstrating which HIE services deliver value (and which do not) are few, and value is different across stakeholders. See Chapter 16 for an assessment of the current evidence on HIE.
Adoption requires change	HIE networks cannot produce value unless the customers adopt and use their services. Just as healthcare providers are having to adapt their workflows to reap the benefits of EHRs, adoption of HIE services sometimes requires adaptation. This is of particular import for physician leaders, as physicians generate and use much of the information in the HIE network [10]. Many HIE services fail to produce improvements in health and healthcare only because they are not used or adopted by health workers (see Chapter 16).
Need to increase or maintain membership [4]	HIEs are subscription-based and rely on fees from users to be financially viable. Some healthcare organizations, such as laboratories, are underrepresented in HIE networks nationally [6]. In the absence of a clear value proposition and change management processes to support HIEs, membership sustainability is in question. In addition, several EHR vendors offer their own information exchange services, which may reduce the value proposition for new members [7].
Challenging and confusing government direction	In the last several years, the federal government has begun trying to use policy to advance and promote the interoperability of health data. The resulting regulations have elevated the level of activity and interest in HIE, but also created significant confusion and, in some cases, have forced prescriptive standards and actions that stifle innovation [13].
Understand the role of additional services	Many HIE networks are starting to offer additional services to demonstrate value. These services require time and money, and it is unclear if they result in additional, ongoing revenue through increased subscription fees, member retention, or additional members. More information is needed to prioritize additional services and share information about how best to implement them.
Patient information located in multiple HIE networks	Patient information may be located across HIE networks in multiple regions due to having providers in different areas, moving, or regularly scheduled seasonal moves. This points to the need to share information across HIEs and a need for focus on patient matching across HIE networks [5,7,14]. Although interstate exchange is occurring through efforts like the Patient Centered Data Home (see Chapter 20) and efforts like the Trusted Exchange Framework and Common Agreement (TEFCA, see Chapter 21), these efforts are nascent and will evolve in the future.

approach would involve national policy changes [2].

States and regions vary with HIE population coverage, current funding levels, and coordination with other HIEs. Considering HIE networks as HDUs could help unify HIEs throughout the country in support of public health functions, state government functions, and private-sector needs more evenly across jurisdictions.

Some HIE networks like CyncHealth and CRISP (Chapter 25) meet the definition of an HDU reasonably well. A trend toward this model may reshape HIE in the United States, enabling sustainability of HIE while more evenly distributing HIE capabilities across the nation benefiting all citizens. More on this topic is in Chapter 21 where the authors discuss future directions of HIE in the United States and globally.

5.11 Summary

HIE on any real scale has existed less than 20 years. During that period, the advancement of technology and standards, and the government's involvement in HIT policy-making, has been extraordinary [21]. The pace of change in the American healthcare system has been equally dramatic. In that context, HIE businesses have emerged, and their growth and evolution has accelerated. The keen interest in HIE sustainability is an understandable byproduct of those environmental circumstances. HIE businesses can be run sustainably. There is ample opportunity in our fragmented and inefficient healthcare system to create value—especially when technology and information are your tools. Any business that can create value can figure out the combination of mission, organizational, structure, business model, services, and disciplined financial management that are required to succeed.

Questions for discussion

1. Using concepts in this chapter, what arguments would you make to support the basic tenet that HIE businesses can be run sustainably?
2. What examples of sustainable HIE services are you aware of? Do you understand the business model behind these services?
3. For any HIE service that you are aware of, discuss ways an HIE could try to increase the gross margin from that service.
4. For any existing HIE you are aware of, discuss ways that HIE could try to increase its revenue.
5. What ideas do you have for HIE services that you feel could produce value and be sustainable?
6. What is needed in terms of government policy to make sustainable HIE a natural and indispensable element of delivering healthcare and maintaining health in our country?
7. What can the leaders of individual HIEs do to make HIE a natural and indispensable element of delivering healthcare and maintaining health in their market?
8. What progress has been made to evolve HIE networks into health data utilities? Will this concept make HIE networks sustainable in the United States?
9. Compare the concept of a Health Data Utility to the HIE models used in Denmark (Chapter 28), Israel (Chapter 31), and the United Arab Emirates (Chapter 32). What are the similarities and differences between the various approaches?

Acknowledgments

Although not an author on this chapter, many of the ideas in the Health Data Utility section were heavily influenced by David Horrocks, the President of CRISP (featured in Chapter 25). We acknowledge his thought leadership on this topic.

References

[1] Kansky JP. Managing the business of health information exchange: towards sustainability. In: Dixon BE, editor. Health information exchange: navigating and managing a network of health information systems. London: Academic Press; 2016. p. 77–90.

[2] Rajapakshe T, Kumar S, Sen A, Sriskandarajah C. Sustainability planning for healthcare information exchanges with supplier rebate program. Oper Res 2020;68(3):793–817.

[3] Langabeer 2nd JR, Champagne T. Exploring business strategy in health information exchange organizations. J Healthc Manag 2016;61(1):15–26.

[4] Ahmed A, Shen W, Khasawneh MT. Sustainability modelling of health information exchanges in dynamic environments. Int J Ind Syst Eng 2019;33(4):413–34.

[5] Feldman SS. An early model for value and sustainability in health information exchanges: qualitative study. JMIR Med Inform 2018;6(2):e29.

[6] Demirezen EM, Kumar S, Sen A. Sustainability of healthcare information exchanges: a game-theoretic approach. Inf Syst Res 2016;27(2):240–58.

[7] Adler-Milstein J, Garg A, Zhao W, Patel V. A survey of health information exchange organizations in advance of a nationwide connectivity framework. Health Aff 2021;40(5):736–44.

[8] Khuntia J, Mithas S, Agarwal R. How service offerings and operational maturity influence the viability of health information exchanges. Prod Oper Manag 2017;26(11):1989–2005.

[9] Adler-Milstein J, Lin SC, Jha AK. The number of health information exchange efforts is declining, leaving the viability of broad clinical data exchange uncertain. Health Aff 2016;35(7):1278–85.

[10] Heath ML, Porter TH. Physician leadership and health information exchange: literature review. BMJ Health Care Inform 2019;26(1):e100080.

[11] Dixon BE, Miller T, Overhage JM. Barriers to achieving the last mile in health information exchange: a survey of small hospitals and physician practices. J Healthc Inf Manag 2013;27(4):55–60.

[12] Dixon BE, Miller T, Overhage JM. Assessing HIE stakeholder readiness for consumer access: lessons learned from the NHIN trial implementations. J Healthc Inf Manag 2009;23(3):20–5.

[13] Basch P, McClellan M, Botts C, Katikaneni P. High value health IT: policy reforms for better care and lower costs. Washington: The Brookings Institution; 2015 [cited 2022 Mar 29]. Available from: <http://www.brookings.edu/~/media/research/files/papers/2015/03/16-health-it-policy-brief/16-high-value-health-it-policy-reforms-mcclellan.pdf>.

[14] Winkler TJ, Brown CV, Öztürk P, editors. The interplay of top-down and bottom-up: approaches for achieving sustainable health information exchange. ECIS; 2014.

[15] Raths D. Should HIEs Become More Like Public Utilities?: Healthcare Innovation; 2020 [cited 2022 Apr 12]. Available from: <https://www.hcinnovationgroup.com/interoperability-hie/health-information-exchange-hie/article/21151905/should-hies-become-more-like-public-utilities>.

[16] Kansky JP, editor. The importance of health data utilities in supporting public health. In: Spring rural summit; 2022; Indianapolis, IN.

[17] Bennett D. Transforming an HIE into a "Population Health Utility" is helping Nebraska fight COVID-19: NextGate; [cited 2022 Apr 12]. Available from: <https://nextgate.com/uk/2021/02/transforming-an-hie-into-a-population-health-utility-is-helping-nebraska-fight-covid-19-3/>.

[18] Tepper N. Momentum returns for health information exchanges. Mod Healthc 2021;51(15):28.

[19] Kansky JP. The Tallest Kindergartner [Internet]: anchor.fm; 2021 [cited 2022 Apr 12]. Podcast. Available from: <https://anchor.fm/indianahie/episodes/Season-2-Episode-1-From-HIE-to-Statewide-Health-Data-Utility-A-Conversation-with-David-Horrocks-epk4mj>.

[20] Horrocks D, Kansky J. HIEs are vital to public health, but need reshaping: Healthcare Information Management Systems Society; 2020 [cited 2022 Apr 12]. Available from: <https://www.himss.org/resources/hies-are-vital-public-health-need-reshaping>.

[21] Hersh WR, Totten AM, Eden K, Devine B, Gorman P, Kassakian SZ, et al. The evidence base for health information exchange. In: Dixon BE, editor. Health information exchange: navigating and managing a network of health information systems. 1st ed. Waltham, MA: Academic Press; 2016. p. 213–29.

CHAPTER

6

Managing privacy, confidentiality, and risk: towards trust

Ammon R. Fillmore[1], *Carl D. McKinley*[2] *and Eileen F. Tallman*[3]

[1]Indiana Health Information Exchange, Indianapolis, IN, USA [2]Regenstrief Institute, Inc., Indianapolis, IN, USA [3]Department of Epidemiology, Richard M. Fairbanks School of Public Health, Indiana University, Indianapolis, IN, USA

LEARNING OBJECTIVES

At the end of this chapter, the reader should be able to:

- Define trust, privacy, confidentiality, and security.
- Define an HIPAA covered entity and business associate.
- Describe how HIPAA interacts with state laws.
- Define protected health information (PHI) and electronic health information (EHI).
- Describe permissible uses and disclosures of PHI under the HIPAA Privacy Rule.
- List and describe the required and addressable security controls under the HIPAA Security Rule.
- Discuss what is considered a breach of unsecured PHI under the HIPAA Breach Notification Rule.
- Describe how the NIST Privacy Framework enables privacy protection activities in an organization.
- Discuss how the Information Blocking Regulations interact with HIPAA regulations.
- List and describe three primary contracting models for HIE network participation.

6.1 Introduction

Trust is having confidence in how another party will behave in a given situation.[1] If you

[1]This chapter will define several terms, such as trust, privacy, confidentiality, and security. The definitions are the author's description of what these terms mean in the context of health information exchange, rather than definitions from third party sources. Different parties may have different definitions; the ones provided in this chapter are used in the context of health information exchange.

Health Information Exchange
DOI: https://doi.org/10.1016/B978-0-323-90802-3.00030-7

have a high degree of confidence in how another party will behave in a given situation, then you have a high degree of trust in that other party. If the behavior of another party is unknown in a given situation, then the degree of trust in that party is low.

Laws, rules, regulations, and contracts exist to foster trust. They define how parties should behave in given situations. In a contract, one party might promise to do A in situation Z and B in situation X. The contract establishes expected behaviors in given situations and acts as a mechanism to enforce behaviors or apply penalties if a party does not behave as required by the contract. As parties behave according to the contract over time, more trust is established.

Laws, administrative rules, and regulations work in much the same way. A law might say if Z occurs, then all regulated parties must do A. The law or regulation will carry with it enforcement penalties to which regulated parties will be subject if they do not comply with the law. These penalties create accountability for HIPAA-protected entities and, as parties comply with the law or regulation over time, more trust is established across society.

These concepts of trust, built over time through contract, laws, and regulations, are paramount in developing a successful health information exchange (HIE). Healthcare providers and health plans are trusted by their patients and members to safeguard health information. In order for these entities to share health information, a sufficient fabric of trust must be created by the HIE through contracts and practices, as well as laws and regulations at both state and federal levels. Compliance with HIE contracts as well as applicable laws and regulations is demonstrated through strong HIE governance (as described in Chapter 4), which breeds further trust. As HIE participants work together over time, they develop a higher degree of certainty in how each other will act in a given situation, which translates into a higher degree of trust.

The concepts of privacy, security, confidentiality, and risk are established though contracts, laws, and regulations. They represent situations in which parties must develop a high degree of certainty around how other parties will act (i.e., trust) in order for an HIE initiative to be successful. It is the combination of contracts, laws, and regulations that define expected behaviors around privacy, security, confidentiality, and risk that establish the trust necessary for successful HIE.

6.1.1 Privacy

Privacy is the freedom to choose what information is shared or not shared with other parties. For example, privacy is an individual's right to not disclose information about themselves to others, such as not disclosing an individual's genetic predisposition to cancer on an employment application. Legislatures may choose to enact laws that prohibit the compelled disclosure of information in order to protect an individual's privacy.

6.1.2 Confidentiality

Confidentiality is the obligation to keep secret information with which one is entrusted. For example, confidentially obligations are imposed under the Health Insurance Portability and Accountability Act (HIPAA) by prohibiting covered entity healthcare providers from disclosing protected health information (PHI) to the media without a patient's authorization. Confidentiality obligations are often mislabeled as privacy obligations. For Example, the HIPAA Privacy Rule would be more appropriately labeled as the Confidentiality Rule since it imposes obligations upon covered entities not to make certain disclosures of information (i.e., to maintain confidentiality).

6.1.3 Security

Security is the combination of administrative, technical, and physical safeguards that ensure confidentiality and promote privacy. Security comprises the safeguards that prevent inappropriate uses and disclosures of information. For example, strong passwords, encryption, and door locks all represent security safeguards that exist to keep information in the right hands.

6.1.4 Accountability

Accountability refers to the norms, processes, and structures that make the population legally responsible for their actions and imposes penalties when laws are broken [1]. It is a key privacy principle that is implemented throughout HIE to varying degrees and in different ways. For example, accountability can be a cultural value of an HIE or implemented as a series of governance policies and procedures within an HIE [2].

6.1.5 Privacy risk

A privacy risk is the likelihood that individuals will experience problems as a result of data processing. Privacy risks can lead to breaches that impact individuals, such as an authorized electronic health records (EHRs) user accessing PHI for someone who is not their patient. Privacy risks can also impact a society. For example, a pharmacy experiences a cyberattack on their EHR system and PHI from medication records is exposed. Privacy risks, when exposed, reduce trust. Accountable health information organizations (HIOs) should work to identify gaps in privacy and security in order to mitigate risk.

This chapter explores how contractual and legal mechanisms exist to promote privacy, confidentiality, security, and risk reduction in fostering trust among HIE participants.

6.2 Federal and state laws pertaining to health information exchange

The "rules of the road" for HIE are defined by a combination of laws and regulations at both state and federal levels as well as contracts among HIE participants. Federal and state laws establish a baseline, and then HIE participants may create additional rules through contracts among HIE participants. Contracts among HIE participants cannot override or conflict with federal or state laws and regulations, but they may detail obligations above and beyond federal or state laws and regulations.

The interaction between state and federal law in the HIE space can be complex and confusing. Generally, federal laws preempt state laws when the two are in conflict. In many cases, Congress will "occupy the field" and create laws or regulations that preempt all state laws and regulations. For example, Congress regulates medical devices through a structure that preempts all state laws and regulations. In other cases, Congress will establish a national minimum in an area and allow states to enact more stringent laws or regulations. This is the case with HIPAA as well as regulation of uses and disclosures of health information. When in conflict, HIPAA preempts state laws except to the extent state law are more stringent than HIPAA [3]. For example, HIPAA allows healthcare providers to disclose PHI for treatment purposes without patient consent or authorization. This creates a federal "floor" or minimum standards. States are free to enact laws that require healthcare providers to obtain patient consent prior to disclosing PHI for treatment purposes, because imposing a consent requirement is more stringent than the HIPAA federal floor. Therefore an HIE initiative must analyze its state laws to determine if they are more stringent than HIPAA. If they are, then the HIE network and its participants must comply with the more stringent state law requirements, keeping in mind that if a state law is silent on an issue, then the federal floor of HIPAA must be followed.

6.2.1 Sensitive data

Many states have enacted laws that are more stringent than HIPAA with respect to several categories of "sensitive data." Data considered sensitive under state laws are often mental and behavioral health data, communicable disease data, genetic information, and sexually transmitted disease data. State laws will generally impose more stringent patient consent requirements on the disclosure of these types of data. HIPAA and federal law generally do not provide additional protections or consent requirements upon communicable or sexually transmitted diseases. HIPAA and federal law do provide specific protections for psychotherapy notes (under HIPAA) [4], which require specific patient consent each time they are disclosed unless they are needed for treatment, payment, or healthcare operations.

It is important for any HIE initiative to research state and federal laws relating to sensitive data and determine how such data will be handled by the HIE. Many HIEs take the approach of prohibiting their participants from sending HIPAA psychotherapy notes and Part II drug and alcohol addiction treatment information. They will also take the same approach with respect to state-regulated sensitive data. This way the HIE never handles data that have special consent requirements attached to it. Rather than outright prohibiting such types of data, some HIEs require that their participants specifically represent and warrant that consent for disclosure has been obtained for any data that is shared with the HIE. This allows sensitive data types to be shared via the HIE, but it imposes additional administrative burdens upon HIE participants.

6.2.2 HIPAA and the HITECH Act

The primary US federal laws applicable to HIE initiatives is the Health Insurance Portability and Accountability Act of 1996 (HIPAA) and the Health Information Technology for Economic and Clinical Health Act (HITECH Act). HIPAA was passed in 1996 and allowed for the US Department of Health and Human Services (HHS) to issue privacy and security regulations. HHS implemented these regulations in what are known as the Privacy Rule (finalized in December of 2000) and the Security Rule (finalized in February of 2003). In 2009, as part of the American Recovery and Reinvestment Act (ARRA or the Stimulus Package), the HITECH Act was passed and, among other things, made a number of changes to HIPAA, which were implemented through regulations issued by HHS. Most of these changes were finalized in January of 2013, although some of them are still forthcoming. These two laws (HIPAA and HITECH) and their implementing regulations (the Privacy Rule and the Security Rule) create the federal floor of laws and regulations that impact use and disclosure of PHI across an HIE network.

6.2.3 What is regulated?

HIPAA, by virtue of the Privacy Rule, the Security Rule, and the HITECH Act, applies to "covered entities" and their "business associates." A *covered entity* is (1) a healthcare provider that engages in certain electronic transactions (essentially any healthcare provider that accepts insurance of any kind will engage in covered electronic transactions), (2) a health plan, or (3) a healthcare clearinghouse (an entity that converts health information into standard formats required by HIPAA) [5].

A *business associate* is a person or entity (other than a member of a covered entity's workforce) that creates, receives, maintains, or transmits PHI for or on behalf of a covered entity; essentially a person or entity that performs services for a covered entity that involve PHI [5]. Examples of business associates include billing companies, practice management companies, hosted EHR vendors, and lawyers. Under the HITECH Act, an HIO or an HIE network is specifically named as a business associate [5].

HIPAA requires that all covered entities have contracts with their business associates (called business associate agreements or BAAs) [6]. BAAs must contain a number of specific provisions regarding confidentiality and security [7]. Prior to the HITECH Act, business associates were not directly subject to HIPAA; they were merely obligated to comply with the terms of their BAAs with covered entities. This left the federal government in a difficult position when a business associate suffered a breach of PHI. The federal government had no direct recourse against the business associate; it was left to the covered entity to pursue contractual remedies against the business associate under its BAA. In order to avoid this lack of recourse, the HITECH Act provided that business associates must comply with all aspects of the Security Rule and virtually all of the aspects of the Privacy Rule [8]. This means that the federal government now has a direct cause of action against a business associate in the event of a breach [9].

Having established that covered entities and business associates are the entities regulated by HIPAA, the next question is: What type of information is subject to HIPAA? HIPAA regulates *PHI*, which is individually identifiable health information transmitted or maintained in any form or medium (excluding certain education records and student medical records) [5]. *Individually identifiable health information* is health information, including demographic information, created or received by a covered entity that relates to the past, present, or future physical or mental health or condition of an individual that identifies the individual or could reasonably be used to identify the individual [5].

The Privacy Rule lists 18 specific identifiers that, when paired with some type of health information, results in PHI. Those identifiers are:

1. Names;
2. All geographic subdivisions smaller than a state, including street address, city, county, precinct, zip code, and their equivalent geocodes, except for the initial three digits of a zip code if certain population requirements are met;
3. All elements of dates (except year) for dates directly related to an individual, including birth date, admission date, discharge date, date of death; and all ages over 89 and all elements of dates (including year) indicative of such age, except that such ages and elements may be aggregated into a single category of age 90 or older;
4. Telephone numbers;
5. Fax numbers;
6. Electronic mail addresses;
7. Social security numbers;
8. Medical record numbers;
9. Health plan beneficiary numbers;
10. Account numbers;
11. Certificate/license numbers;
12. Vehicle identifiers and serial numbers, including license plate numbers;
13. Device identifiers and serial numbers;
14. Web universal resource locators (URLs);
15. Internet protocol (IP) address numbers;
16. Biometric identifiers, including finger and voice prints;
17. Full face photographic images and any comparable images; and
18. Any other unique identifying number, characteristic, or code, except for certain coding systems that allow for reidentification of data [10].

These identifiers are broad and show that HHS takes an expansive view in determining what might reasonably be used to identify an individual. Many individuals hold the false believe that if they simply remove a name, they have de-identified PHI. The truth is that only once these 18 identifiers are removed from PHI, will the PHI be considered "de-identified" under HIPAA and no longer subject to regulation under HIPAA [11–13].

Covered entities (and their business associates with permission from their covered entity) may de-identify PHI and use de-identified information for any purpose [14]. This is an important term to consider in any covered entity–business associate relationship: Will the covered entity permit the business associate to de-identify PHI and use the de-identified information for other purposes? Many vendors seek to de-identify information and monetize it through sales or licensing arrangements. Some HIE networks could benefit and increase their sustainability if they are permitted to de-identify PHI and use the de-identified data for other purposes.

De-identification can raise privacy concerns as individuals may feel that a third party should not profit from the use of their de-identified data. De-identified data can also be used for many public goods by researchers looking to promote public health or analyze the efficacy of various treatments. The issue of de-identification is an important one to discuss with HIE stakeholders and reach agreement upon how the issue will be addressed by a specific HIO or HIE network.

6.2.4 The Privacy Rule and the Security Rule

Knowing who (covered entities and business associates) and what (PHI) is regulated by HIPAA, the next question is: What is required under HIPAA? The Privacy Rule establishes permissible uses and disclosures of PHI and the Security Rule establishes a set of required and addressable security controls.

6.2.5 The Privacy Rule

Under the Privacy Rule, covered entities and business associates may only use or disclose PHI if the Privacy Rule permits the particular use or disclosure or if the person who is the subject of the PHI authorizes the use or disclosure [15]. It is important to note the distinction between "use" and "disclosure." A use of PHI is the sharing, employment, application, utilization, examination, or analysis of such information within an entity that maintains such information [5]. A disclosure of PHI is the release, transfer, provision of, access to, or divulging in any other manner of information outside the entity holding the information [5].

Under the Privacy Rule, the following are the primary uses and disclosures of PHI that are permitted without a patient's authorization:

- To the individual to whom the PHI relates;
- For treatment, payment or healthcare operations;
- For public health activities;
- As required by law;
- For certain research activities where a privacy board or an institutional review board has waived the authorization requirement [16].

Except in the case of treatment, the Privacy Rule requires that covered entities and business associates make reasonable efforts to limit uses and disclosures of PHI to the minimum amount necessary to accomplish the intended use or disclosure [17].

For the purposes of an HIE network, most uses and disclosures will be for treatment, healthcare operations, or public health activities. Just because the Privacy Rule permits a particular use or disclosures does not mean that a business associate (or an HIE network) may automatically make such use or disclosure; the business associate (or HIE network) must obtain permission from its covered entity (ies) in order to make a particular use or disclosure [18]. It is critical that an HIE network establish the types of uses and disclosures that will be made of data shared with the HIO and obtain appropriate permissions for such uses and disclosures in its agreement (including a BAA) with the HIE participants.

HIE use cases for treatment purposes are fairly straightforward and self-explanatory. For example, providing data at the point of care or delivering a clinical laboratory result is a treatment disclosure [19].

Public health use cases encompass, for example, delivering immunization reports to public health authorities or providing data for public health syndromic surveillance [19].

Healthcare operations use cases are emerging as the next frontier of HIE use cases. Healthcare operations includes, among other things, conducting quality assessment and improvement activities, including outcomes evaluation and development of clinical guidelines, provided that the obtaining of generalizable knowledge is not the primary purpose of any studies resulting from such activities; patient safety activities; population-based activities relating to improving health or reducing healthcare costs, protocol development, case management and care coordination, contacting of healthcare providers and patients with information about treatment alternatives; and related functions that do not include treatment [19]. These uses and disclosures, sometimes called "secondary use," are some of the higher-value services that an HIE can offer. Since these are permitted under the Privacy Rule without patient authorization [20], it is important for an HIE to secure permission from its covered entity participants for the HIE to make these uses of PHI if these services are part of the HIE network's plans.

An important change that the HITECH Act made to the Privacy Rule is in the area of requests by patients for their information not to be shared in certain circumstances. The Privacy Rule provides that patients may request that covered entities not make certain uses or disclosures of their information [21]. The Privacy Rule goes on to state that covered entities are not obligated to grant such requests except in one situation [22]. That situation is when a patient pays out-of-pocket in full for healthcare and requests that their healthcare provider not share information relating to such healthcare with the patient's health plan [23]. In this situation the provider must honor the request and refrain from sharing the information with the patient's health plan [23]. This can create unique challenges for HIE networks that share data with health plans, as many do and as more will to increase their sustainability. HIE networks must have in place a mechanism for their healthcare provider participants to either (1) not send information that is subject to a restriction request or (2) notify the HIO that certain data are subject to a restriction request so that the HIO can take steps to ensure that the data are not shared with the patient's health plan. This right is rarely exercised by patients, but it is nonetheless something for which HIE networks must be prepared if they are going to share data with health plans.

The Privacy Rule establishes the situations in which covered entities and business associates may use and disclose PHI. The Privacy Rule is sometimes used as an excuse for providers and health plans to not share data with each other. This is called information blocking, which will be discussed later in this chapter. The truth is that the Privacy Rule is designed to allow sharing of health data among healthcare providers and health plans in the interest of patient treatment, improving quality, and population health management. If an entity is declining to share data because "HIPAA does not allow it," it is important to do a deep analysis to determine what provision of HIPAA does not allow the particular data sharing. The truth is that if the sharing would enhance patient care or public health, then it is probably allowed under HIPAA. HIPAA does a good job of protecting confidentiality by limiting uses and disclosures to covered entities and business associates and then ensuring confidentiality by imposing security control requirements upon covered entities and business associates under the Security Rule.

6.2.6 The Security Rule

The Privacy Rule establishes permissible uses and disclosures of PHI. The Security Rule is equally as important in establishing the baseline security controls that are required or addressable by covered entities and business associates [24]. The Security Rule establishes a number of general requirements that apply to all covered entities and business associates and then describes a number of implementation specifications that are either "required" or "addressable" by covered entities and business associates [24]. This framework provides a great deal of flexibility and allows covered entities and business associates to consider their size, complexity, capabilities, technical infrastructure, cost, and probability and criticality of potential risks when implementing security controls [25]. If a particular control is required (shown as (R) in Table 6.1), then it must be implemented by a covered entity or business associate [26]. If a particular control is addressable (shown as (A) in Table 6.1), then the covered entity or business associate must assess whether each control is a reasonable and appropriate safeguard in its environment, when analyzed with reference to the likely contribution to protecting PHI and either implement the control or document its decision to

TABLE 6.1 HIPAA Security Rule controls.

Administrative procedures [28]	Physical safeguards [29]	Technical security measures [30]
Security Management Process—Policies and procedures to prevent, detect, contain, and correct security violations, including:	*Facility Access Controls*—Policies and procedures to limit physical access to PHI, including:	*Access Control*—Policies and procedures to allow PHI access only to those persons or programs that have been granted access rights, including:
• Risk assessment (R) • Reduce risk to an appropriate level (R) • Workforce sanctions (R) • Review system activities (R)	• Contingency operations plans (A) • Facility security plan (A) • Access control and validation procedures (A) • Maintenance records (A)	• Unique user identification (R) • Emergency access (R) • Automatic logoff (A) • Encryption (A)
Security Responsibility—Identify a security official (R)	*Workstation Use*—Policies and procedures that specify functions and physical attributes of workstations and the surrounding areas (R)	*Audit Controls*—Hardware, software, or mechanisms that record and examine activity in systems (R)
Work Force Security—Limit PHI access to appropriate members of the workforce, including:	*Workstation Security*—Physical safeguards for all workstations that access PHI (R)	*Integrity*—Policies and procedures to protect PHI from improper alteration or destruction, including:
• Authorization and supervision of employees (A) • Clearance of workforce members (A) • Procedures for terminating access to PHI as necessary (A)		• Mechanism to authenticate PHI to ensure it has not been altered or destroyed (A)

(*Continued*)

TABLE 6.1 (Continued)

Administrative procedures [28]	Physical safeguards [29]	Technical security measures [30]
Information Access Management—Access to PHI is limited as required by the Security Rule, including: • Isolating healthcare clearinghouse functions (R) • Access authorization policies (A) • •Access modification policies (A)	*Device and Media Control*—Policies and procedures that govern the receipt and removal of hardware and media that contain PHI, including: • Disposal of media (R) • Media reuse (R) • Accountability for movement (A) • Data backup and storage (A)	*Person or Entity Authentication*—Procedures to verify that a person or entity seeking access to PHI is the one claimed (R)
Security Awareness and Training—A security and awareness training program for all workforce members, including: • Security reminders (A) • Protection from malicious software (A) • Log-in monitoring (A) • Password management (A)		*Transmission Security*—Technical security measures to guard against unauthorized access to PHI while in transit, including: • Integrity controls (A) • Encryption (A)
Security Incident Procedures—Policies and procedures to address security incidents through response and reporting (R)		
Contingency Plan—Policies and procedures for responding to emergencies and system failures, including: • Data backup (R) • Disaster recovery plan (R) • Emergency operation plan (R) • Testing and revision of plans (A) • Application and data criticality analysis (A)		
Evaluation—Preform periodic technical and nontechnical evaluations of security controls (R)		
Business Associates—Covered entities and business associates must obtain written business associate agreements from their business associates and subcontractors, respectively (R)		

not implement the control [27]. The controls are divided into three categories: administrative, physical, and technical, as shown and described in Table 6.1.

6.2.7 Managing privacy risks

An HIE may have privacy management procedures in place, but still experience difficulties identifying and communicating gaps in those procedures over time. Personal data are not limited to the health space and are maintained by many different types of organizations governed by a multitude of domestic or international regulations and laws. The variety requires a privacy framework design flexible enough to meet the needs of these different organizations. The US National Institute of Standards and Technology (NIST) developed the NIST Privacy Framework, a voluntary tool for organizations looking to improve privacy by identifying and managing cybersecurity and privacy risks. Cybersecurity will be discussed in Chapter 7, so for this section, we will only focus on privacy components.

The Privacy Framework enhances consumer trust by helping organizations to prioritize privacy and communicate existing privacy protections and outcomes to their clients [31]. It uses a set of core functions aimed to help an organization determine how they are considering privacy risks at every stage of development [2]. In doing so, organizational staff increases their knowledge and awareness, and accountability is strengthened throughout the organization.

When HIOs apply the Privacy Framework in their organization, they should consider how to manage privacy risks with both their priorities and the HIE ecosystem priorities in mind. NIST suggests using a common language for sharing privacy requirements with HIE participants [2].

6.2.8 Breach notification rule

The HITECH Act established a national requirement for individuals to be notified in the event of a breach of their PHI [32]. The HITECH breach notification rule requires that a covered entity notify an individual of a breach of the individual's "unsecured" PHI [33]. *Unsecured PHI* is PHI that has not been encrypted or destroyed in accordance with guidelines issued by the Secretary of HHS [34]. This concept of "unsecured" PHI illustrates the value and importance of encrypting PHI (i.e., a breach of encrypted PHI is not a "breach" for purposes of the breach notification rule). Even though encryption is only an "addressable" control under the Security Rule [35], the "safe harbor" that encryption provides under the breach notification rule has made encryption a de facto requirement. An HIE needs to seriously consider encryption of data both while it is at rest (e.g., when stored) and in transit (e.g., when being transferred via email or file transfer protocol). Many covered entities will require their business associates to utilize encryption to take advantage of the breach notification rule's encryption safe harbor.

Under the breach notification rule, in the event of a breach of unsecured PHI, covered entities must notify individuals and business associates must notify covered entities after performing a risk assessment [33,36]. An impermissible acquisition, access, use, or disclosure of unsecured PHI is presumed to be a breach under the rule unless the covered entity or business associate demonstrates that there is a low probability that the PHI has been compromised based on a risk assessment of at least the following factors:

- The nature and extent of the PHI involved, including the types of identifiers and the likelihood of reidentification;
- The unauthorized person who used the PHI or to whom the disclosure was made;
- Whether the PHI was actually acquired or viewed; and
- The extent to which the risk to the PHI has been mitigated [37].

The notice to individuals (or from a business associate to a covered entity) must include, to the extent possible:

- A brief description of what happened, including the date of the breach and the date of the discovery of the breach, if known;

- A description of the types of unsecured PHI that were involved in the breach (such as whether full name, social security number, date of birth, home address, account number, diagnosis, disability code, or other types of information were involved);
- Any steps individuals should take to protect themselves from potential harm resulting from the breach;
- A brief description of what the covered entity involved is doing to investigate the breach, to mitigate harm to individuals, and to protect against any further breaches; and
- Contact procedures for individuals to ask questions or learn additional information, including a toll-free telephone number, an email address, Web site, or postal address [38].

Additionally, the media must be notified of a breach that affects more than 500 individuals and HHS must be notified of all breaches (immediately if the breach is over 500 individuals and annually for breaches that affect less than 500 individuals) [39,40].

Since all HIE networks are business associates, they must be sure to have plans and procedures in place to notify their covered entities in the event of a breach. HIE participation agreements or their BAAs should address roles and responsibilities in the event of a breach. For example, who will bear the costs associated with notification? Additionally, many BAAs will require that a business associate notify a covered entity of any impermissible use or disclosure of PHI, regardless of whether a risk assessment demonstrates that there is a low probability that the PHI has been compromised [41]. This may result in situations where a business associate notifies a covered entity of an impermissible use or disclosure, but the covered entity elects to not notify individuals based on the covered entity's risk assessment.

6.2.9 HIPAA enforcement

Prior to the HITECH Act, HIPAA had a reputation for being a "paper tiger" due to its lack of enforcement and relatively low fines and penalties when enforced. The HITECH Act greatly increased the penalties for HIPAA violations (from $100 to $50,000 up to a $1.5 million cap), which can include jail time [42]. Additionally, the HITECH Act empowered State Attorneys General to bring HIPAA enforcement actions [43]. Furthermore, HITECH calls for the sharing of HIPAA violation penalties with individuals harmed by violations (although regulations implementing this provision have not yet been issued) [44]. Lastly, the HITECH Act requires that HHS conduct HIPAA audits of covered entitles and business associates [45]. The combination of these enforcement enhancements under the HITECH Act gives HIPAA the enforcement strength that has been lacking and has made HIPAA compliance a much higher priority at covered entities and business associates.

6.3 Information blocking regulations

In 2016 the United States Congress passed the 21st Century Cures Act to empower patients and put them in charge of their health records [46]. Section 4004 of the Cure Act prohibits healthcare providers, health information network/HIEs, and health information technology developers (collectively defined as "actors") [47] from *information blocking*, or otherwise improperly interfering with access, exchange, or use of electronic health information (EHI) [48]. In 2020 the Office of the National Coordinator for Health information Technology (ONC) finalized the information blocking regulations (IBRs).

The IBR represents a substantial milestone toward healthcare information interoperability that are best understood in tandem with HIPAA and other federal privacy and security laws. While HIPAA restricted how and when Covered Entities may make available health information, the IBR implements a complementary framework that effectively requires actors to make EHI available for access, exchange, or use in response to a request for EHI. Failing to respond to a request for EHI may result in regulatory enforcement, unless the actor lacked the necessary intent or a regulatory exception applies to the request.

The IBR specifies eight distinct exceptions that function similar to regulatory safe harbors; meaning, if a request for EHI is within any of these exceptions an actor does not have to fulfill the request. These exceptions are described in Table 6.2.

6.4 Contracts

Federal and state laws establish the baseline rules of the road for HIE. When HIE participants come together to form an HIE initiative, they are likely to want to agree upon additional rules that will govern their relationship and foster trust among participants. As a threshold issue, there are different contracting structures that may be used in an HIE. Generally, these contracting structures can be divided into three categories, as shown in Table 6.3.

HIE contracting has evolved a great deal in recent years. The trend is toward multiparty agreements; however, many two-party HIE participation agreements and point-to-point agreement frameworks still exist. Each model has pros and cons and various reasons why it is used.

6.4.1 Point-to-point agreements

Party-to-party or point-to-point agreements tend to be used when the number of HIE participants is low and the parties involved do not

TABLE 6.2 Information blocking regulations exceptions.

Exceptions that involve not fulfilling EHI requests	Exceptions that involve procedures for fulfilling EHI requests
A practice will not be information blocking for an actor if:	
Preventing harm [49]	*Content and manner* [50]
• Practices that are reasonable and necessary to prevent harm to a patient or another person.	• Actors may limit the content or manner in responding to a request.
Privacy [51]	*Fees* [52]
• Practices to protect the individual's privacy.	• Actors may charge fees, including a reasonable profit margin.
Security [53]	*Licensing* [54]
• Practices to protect the security of electronic health information.	• Actors may require certain conditions for the license of interoperable elements.
Infeasibility [55]	
• The request is infeasible to fulfill (e.g., uncontrollable events like natural disasters, or EHI cannot be unambiguously segmented).	
Health IT performance [56]	
• Practices reasonable and necessary to make health information temporarily unavailable, such as routine IT system maintenance.	

TABLE 6.3 HIE contracting structures.

Structure	Characteristics
Party-to-party or point-to-point agreements	• Direct agreements between individual parties exchanging data with each other • No HIE entity involved • Example: Jurisdiction by jurisdiction agreements with the CDC for biosurveillance
Two-party HIE participation agreements	• Individual agreement between an HIE entity and a participant • HIE participants do not have direct contractual privity with each other • Involvement of an HIE entity • Example: HIE X has 27 "one-off" or individualized agreements with the 27 entities that participate in its HIE network
Multiparty agreement	• A common set of terms and conditions to which an HIE entity and all participants agree • The HIE network and all participants are in direct contractual privity with each other • Involvement of an HIE entity • Example: The DURSA governing the eHealth Exchange or the INPC Terms and Conditions used in Indiana; Trust Exchange Framework & Common Agreement (TEFCA)

wish to create a sophisticated HIE governance structure. Sometimes point-to-point agreements are referred to as data use agreements, especially in the government context. Point-to-point agreement frameworks can be found in small communities where there are, for example, only two hospitals that have decided to share data with each other in certain circumstances. The two parties will enter into direct agreements with each other that will define the circumstances under which data will be exchanged. There is no HIO to mediate the exchange; the two entities share data directly with each other.

Eventually, a third party may come a long that wants to exchange data. Under the point-to-point model, the third party would sign an agreement with both the existing parties and data sharing would occur. The obvious downside to this model is that it does not scale. If a fourth and fifth party came along in this example, they would need to each contract with the first three parties as well as each other. In other words, the number of point-to-point agreements that each party must execute and maintain will always be $N - 1$, where N is the number of parties. Once this type of growth occurs, the parties probably need to look at a different model that allows for broader participation and the possible creation of an HIE entity to mediate the exchange.

6.4.2 Two-party agreements

The two-party HIE participation agreement model comes into play when an HIO exists and it needs to contract with HIE participants to facilitate exchange. Under this model, the HIO signs an agreement with each HIE participant. The HIO will want the multiple agreements it signs to be as similar as possible, but in all likelihood there will be variation in the agreements it signs. The HIE network participants have only a contractual relationship, or privity, with the HIO. They do not have contractual relationships with each other. This model has been used by numerous HIE efforts.

The challenge to this model is that variation among the agreements the HIO signs can create challenges for the HIO in administering data exchange. If the HIO has different obligations to different HIE network participants, the administrative costs of running the HIE network will increase. Furthermore, if the HIO wishes to make changes to its agreement, for example, to allow for a new data use, the HIO must go to each HIE network participant and ask for a contractual amendment. This creates additional administrative overhead and could lead to "hold out" problems if some of the HIE network participants are not willing to agree to the amendment. Furthermore, because the HIE network participants do not have direct contractual privity with each other, they will not have contractual rights against each other in the event of a breach. For example, if an employee at participant A wrongly discloses PHI that was obtained though the HIE network from participant B, participant B may have breach notification obligations, but does not have contractual recourse against the bad actor at participant A. Participant B would only have a contractual right against the HIO (which then, in turn, would have a contractual right against participant A), which could be problematic as the HIO might lack sufficient capital or insurance coverage to make participant B whole.

6.4.3 Multiparty agreements

The multiparty agreement model is the most sophisticated model of the three and has many advantages. However, this model can be challenging to implement, as all HIE network participants and the HIO must agree to the same terms. This requires significant time for negotiations and consensus building across participants. Sometimes so much so that HIE initiatives that seek to implement this model fail to get past the contract negotiation phase.

If consensus around a common set of terms and conditions can be reached, then the HIE network will have a lower contractual administration burden as all HIE network participants have the same rights and obligations. Furthermore, contractual amendment mechanisms can be built into the agreement that allow amendments and new data uses without having to obtain signatures from each HIE network participant. Under the Data Use and Reciprocal Support Agreement (DURSA) used by the eHealth Exchange [57] and the INPC Terms and Conditions used by the Indiana Health Information Exchange (see Chapter 22), amendments and new data uses can be proposed to designated committees that have the contractual authority to approve amendments and new data uses. Once approved by the designated committee, the amendment or new data use can go into effect. Lastly, under this model, all HIE network participants and the HIO have direct contractual privity with each other, which allows for direct contractual actions in the event of a contractual breach.

Multiparty agreements may also include privacy–public partnerships. In response to the 21st Century Cures Act of 2016, the ONC, in consultation with other relevant agencies convened public and private stakeholders to develop a trusted exchange framework for trust policies and practices and for a common agreement for the exchange of EHI between participants of the same network [58]. This trusted exchange framework and common agreement, or "TEFCA," is not intended to wholly replace existing multipart agreements but operate in concert and are require to take into account existing trusted exchange frameworks and agreements used by health information networks to avoid the disruption of existing exchanges [59].

Regardless of the contracting model implemented by an HIE network, contracts among or with HIE network participants serve as a mechanism to create and build trust by defining how particular parties will behave in given situations. A thorough contract will address as many situations as possible so that HIE network participants will trust in how each other will act in those situations, which breads more trust over time.

6.5 Summary

Trust among HIE network participants is paramount to any HIE initiative. The initiative will never get off the ground and actually engage in data sharing if the participants do not trust each other. Trust is confidence in knowing what another party will do in a given situation. Laws, regulations, and contacts are mechanisms that dictate how parties will behave in given situations and therefore are trust enablers.

The HIPAA Privacy and Security Rules, as enhanced by the HITECH Act, serve as the primary pieces of federal regulation that govern privacy, security, and confidentiality in the healthcare space. They are the primary regulations that establish how healthcare entities, such as HIE network participants, will act in given situations. They establish permitted uses and disclosures of PHI and set forth the baseline security controls that healthcare entities must put in place. State laws, particularly in the area of sensitive data, can be enacted to add additional requirements on the use and disclosure of health information, particularly in the area of patient consent, and must be addressed by any HIE initiative.

Finally, contractual arrangements among HIOs and their participants can establish additional rules for how parties will behave in given situations. Different contracting models lead to different levels of trust and sophistication in HIE network arrangements. An HIE initiative that understands the federal and state legal landscape and implements a contracting structure that address critical legal issues will bread trust among its participants and enable a higher level of exchange.

Questions for discussion

1. How is "trust" defined in the context of HIE?
2. Explain the difference between "privacy" and "confidentiality."
3. What are the primary federal laws the regulate privacy and security in the healthcare space?
4. What uses and disclosures of protected information are permitted under HIPAA without patient consent or authorization?
5. May states enact legislation that is more stringent than HIPAA?
6. Is encryption a required or addressable control under the HIPAA Security Rule?
7. What benefits does encryption provide under the Breach Notification Rule?
8. What are the three categories of security controls under the HIPAA Security Rule?
9. What type of contracting structure are most HIE initiatives trending toward?

Acknowledgments

The authors acknowledge Eric Thieme, JD, who authored the corresponding chapter in the first edition of the book. Since authoring the chapter, Mr. Thieme passed away. The editor and authors appreciate the strong foundation upon which the revised chapter builds.

References

[1] United States Institute of the Peace. Accountability to the law [Internet]. [cited August 10, 2021]. Available from: https://www.usip.org/guiding-principles-stabilization-and-reconstruction-the-web-version/rule-law/accountability-the-law.

[2] National Institute of Standards and Technology. NIST privacy framework: a tool for improving privacy through enterprise risk management. Version 1.0 [Internet]. Gaithersburg, MD: U.S. Department of Commerce; 2020 [cited August 10, 2021]. Available from: https://www.nist.gov/system/files/documents/2020/01/16/NIST%20Privacy%20Framework_V1.0.pdf.

[3] General rule and exceptions, 45 CFR 160.203(b); 2002.

[4] Uses and disclosures for which an authorization is required, 45 CFR 164.508(a)(2); 2013.

[5] Definitions, 45 CFR 160.103; 2013.

[6] Uses and disclosures of protected health information: General rules, 45 CFR 164.502(e)(2); 2013.

[7] Uses and disclosures: Organizational requirements, 45 CFR 164.504(e)(2); 2013.
[8] Security standards: General rules, 45 CFR 164.306; 2013.
[9] Basis for a civil money penalty, 45 CFR 160.402; 2013.
[10] Other requirements relating to uses and disclosures of protected health information, 45 CFR 164.514(b)(2); 2013.
[11] Uses and disclosures of protected health information: General rules, 45 CFR 164.502(d)(2); 2013.
[12] Other requirements relating to uses and disclosures of protected health Information, 45 CFR 164.514(a); 2013.
[13] Other requirements relating to uses and disclosures of protected health information, 45 CFR 164.514(b); 2013.
[14] Uses and disclosures of protected health information: General rules, 45 CFR 164.502(d); 2013.
[15] Uses and disclosures of protected health information: General rules, 45 CFR 164.502(a); 2013.
[16] Uses and disclosures of protected health information: General rules, 45 CFR 164.502(a)(1); 2013.
[17] Uses and disclosures of protected health information: General rules, 45 CFR 164.502(b); 2013.
[18] Uses and disclosures of protected health information: General rules, 45 CFR 164.502(a)(3); 2013.
[19] Definitions, 45 CFR 164.501; 2013.
[20] Uses and disclosures to carry out treatment, payment, or health care operations, 45 CFR 164.506(c); 2013.
[21] Rights to request privacy protection for protected health information, 45 CFR 164.522(a)(1)(i); 2013.
[22] Rights to request privacy protection for protected health information, 45 CFR 164.522(a)(1)(ii); 2013.
[23] Rights to request privacy protection for protected health information, 45 CFR 164.522(a)(1)(vi); 2013.
[24] Security Standards for the Protection of Electronic Protected Health Information, 45 CFR 164, Subpart C; 2003.
[25] Security standards: General rules, 45 CFR 164.306(b); 2013.
[26] Security standards: General rules, 45 CFR 164.306(d)(2); 2013.
[27] Security standards: General rules, 45 CFR 164.306(d)(3); 2013.
[28] Administrative safeguards, 45 CFR 164.308; 2013.
[29] Physical safeguards, 45 CFR 164.310; 2013.
[30] Technical safeguards, 45 CFR 164.312; 2013.
[31] National Institute of Standards and Technology. Privacy framework: frequently asked questions. National Institute of Standards and Technology [Internet]. 2018 [updated January 14, 2021; cited September 02, 2021]. Available from: https://www.nist.gov/privacy-framework/frequently-asked-questions.
[32] Notification in the Case of Breach of Unsecured Protected Health Information, 45 CFR 164, Subpart D; 2009.
[33] Notification to individuals, 45 CFR 164.404; 2013.
[34] Definitions, 45 CFR 164.402; 2013.
[35] Technical safeguards, 45 CFR 164.312(e); 2013.
[36] Notification by a business associate, 45 CFR 164.410; 2013.
[37] Other requirements relating to uses and disclosures of protected health Information, 45 CFR 164.514; 2013.
[38] Notification to individuals, 45 CFR 164.404(c)(E); 2013.
[39] Notification to the media, 45 CFR 164.406; 2013.
[40] Notification to the Secretary, 45 CFR 164.408; 2013.
[41] Uses and disclosures: Organizational requirements, 45 CFR 164.504(e)(2)(ii)(c); 2013.
[42] Amount of a civil money penalty, 45 CFR 160.404; 2016.
[43] Improved Enforcement, Section 13410(e) of the HITECH Act.
[44] Improved Enforcement, Section 13410(c)(3) of the HITECH Act.
[45] Audits, Section 13411 of the HITECH Act.
[46] 21st Century Cures Act, Pub. L. No. 114-255, 130 Stat. 1033 (December 13, 2016).
[47] Definitions, 45 CFR 171.102; 2020.
[48] Information blocking, 45 CFR 171.103; 2020.
[49] Preventing harm exception – When will an actor's practice that is likely to interfere with the access, exchange, or use of electronic health information in order to prevent harm not be considered information blocking? 45 CFR 171.201; 2020.
[50] Content and manner exception – When will an actor's practice of limiting the content of its response to or the manner in which it fulfills a request to access, exchange, or use electronic health information not be considered information blocking? 45 CFR 171.301; 2020.
[51] Privacy exception – When will an actor's practice of not fulfilling a request to access, exchange, or use electronic health information in order to protect an individual's privacy not be considered information blocking? 45 CFR 171.202; 2020.
[52] Fees exception – When will an actor's practice of charging fees for accessing, exchanging, or using electronic health information not be considered information blocking? 45 CFR 171.302; 2020.
[53] Security exception – When will an actor's practice that is likely to interfere with the access, exchange, or use of electronic health information in order to protect the security of electronic health information not be considered information blocking? 45 CFR 171.203; 2020.
[54] Licensing exception – When will an actor's practice to license interoperability elements in order for electronic health information to be accessed, exchanged, or used not be considered information blocking? 45 CFR 171.303; 2020.
[55] Infeasibility exception – When will an actor's practice of not fulfilling a request to access, exchange, or use

electronic health information due to the infeasibility of the request not be considered information blocking? 45 CFR 171.204; 2020.

[56] Health IT performance exception – When will an actor's practice that is implemented to maintain or improve health IT performance and that is likely to interfere with the access, exchange, or use of electronic health information not be considered information blocking? 171.205; 2020.

[57] Reinstatement II of the Data Use and Reciprocal Support Agreement (DURSA); 2019. Available from: https://ehealthexchange.org/wp-content/uploads/2019/08/DURSA-Restatement-II-of-the-DURSA-revised-August-13-2019-EXECUTABLE-1.pdf.

[58] 21st Century Cures Act, Pub. L. No. 114-255, 130, s 4003 Stat. 1033; December 13, 2016.

[59] 21st Century Cures Act, Pub. L. No. 114-255, 130, s 4003(F)(iii) Stat. 1033; December 13, 2016.

CHAPTER

7

Managing threats to health data and information: toward security

Mitchell Parker

Indiana University Health, Indianapolis, IN, USA

LEARNING OBJECTIVES

At the end of the chapter, the reader should be able to:

- Examine the components of multiple security frameworks and discuss how they fit the needs of HIE networks.
- Describe the security requirements of the HIPAA Security Rule.
- Identify the additional requirements from the HITECH Act and Breach Notification Rule.
- Identify the additional requirements from the 21st Century Cures Act Final Rule.
    - Understand Information Blocking and Security.
    - Understand API Security.
- Define the components of a Risk Assessment.
- Define the components of a Risk Management Plan.
- Describe the requirements for addressing open risk items.
- Examine the components of the NIST Cybersecurity Framework.
- Examine how OCTAVE FORTE can be combined with multiple associated frameworks to provide an improved risk management picture for organizations.

7.1 Introduction

According to the SANS Institute, *Information Security* refers to the processes and methodologies which are designed and implemented to protect print, electronic, or any other form of confidential, private, and sensitive information or data from unauthorized access, use, misuse, disclosure, destruction, modification, or disruption [1]. *Cybersecurity*, according to Cisco, a major technology firm responsible for the development of many security technologies, is the practice of protecting systems, networks, and programs from digital attacks [2].

Health Information Exchange
DOI: https://doi.org/10.1016/B978-0-323-90802-3.00016-2

Digital systems and information protection are critically important to Health Information Exchanges (HIEs). Properly functioning computer systems are required to be able to interchange data between multiple organizations and serve as an information gathering and distributing hub. With the significant amounts of data collected by healthcare organizations, and the expected amount to be collected in 10 years, it is simply not possible to conduct this business manually in any meaningful way.

Business Partner Security Risk, which is the process by which third parties have their risks evaluated using frameworks and technologies, is a central tenet of the business of a HIE. This is because their business is the interconnection of third parties. A security risk in one organization can present multiple risks to others. Having excellent security at the hub of the HIE and spokes of each member organization is critical to all participants. This has been made especially obvious given the numerous ransomware attacks that have befallen healthcare organizations since 2016. According to the US Cybersecurity and Infrastructure Security Agency, 2084 confirmed ransomware attacks occurred between January 1 and July 31, 2021 [3]. This is a 62% increase from the same time period in 2020. The amount of losses over the same time period increased by 20%. An example of a ransomware attack is detailed in Box 7.1.

Communication is also critically important during and after ransomware attacks to protect the rest of the healthcare ecosystem. Organizations such as H-ISAC, the Health

BOX 7.1

Attack on the Erie County Medical Center.

On April 9, 2017 at 2:30 a.m., Erie County Medical Center (ECMC), a safety-net hospital and Level I Adult Trauma Center serving Buffalo, New York and surrounding areas, got the message that their computers had been held for ransom and encrypted [4]. This had the effect of shutting down 6000 computer systems, their electronic medical records (EMR) system, and communication with the outside world (Fig. 7.1).

ECMC brought in laptop computers with portable Wi-Fi hotspots that were not connected to the hospital network, and were able to connect to their local HIE, which they were active participants of. This was HEALTHeLINK, the Regional Health Information Organization, for the eight counties in Western New York State [5]. ECMC was able to strategically place these computers so clinicians could use them to access critical patient information. This enabled them to continue business under adverse conditions. They did not divert patients, and the vast majority of elective surgeries stayed on schedule [6]. ECMC did not pay the ransom. They had a two-week downtime of their EMR systems, and took approximately 45 days to recover the rest.

It was because of their active participation with their HIE that they were able to care for critical patients at the only Level I Adult Trauma Center in Western NY [7]. Critical patients that would have needed that level of care would have to have been diverted elsewhere, such as Strong Memorial Hospital in Rochester [7]. This would have had negative effects on patients that need that level of care by adding time.

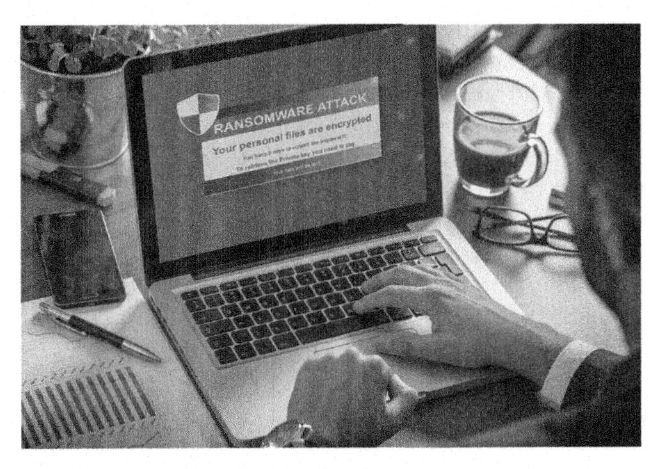

FIGURE 7.1 What a Ransomware attack looks like (simulated).

Information Sharing and Analysis Center, provide trusted communities for coordinating, collaborating, and sharing cyber threat intelligence and best practices among critical infrastructure owners and operators [8]. H-ISAC is focused on healthcare providers, payors, pharmaceutical, and medical device providers.

Their mailing lists and collaboration platforms provide means by which organizations can share specific attack details, called Indicators of Compromise. According to Trend Micro, an information security company, these serve as forensic evidence of potential intrusions. Knowing these allows other organizations to better detect if they have also been compromised, and to stop potential attacks by detecting them and improving their defenses and strategies [9].

Recently, a community hospital in the Midwest that was the main support hospital and healthcare provider for the county it is in was attacked by ransomware. This organization, instead of communicating what was happening, was difficult to reach. This impacted care because not even the state was able to reach them. Because of this, patients were diverted to other hospitals, and many appointments were rescheduled. Critical systems, such as billing and email, have been down for over two months. It took over a month for organizations to connect the local HIE to the third-party incident response team helping the organization get back online. The HIE was not able to successfully contact anyone within the organization because they did not return phone calls and did not have email available.

These examples show the importance of having a good understanding of information security and why applying it to support the business is critically important to the mission of an HIE. This chapter is not going to go over Information Security and give the same statistics that a plurality of books and training already give. Rather, it is going to focus upon what the rules and frameworks are, what they mean to HIEs, and how to use existing internationally used frameworks such as Operationally Critical Threat, Asset, and Vulnerability Evaluation Framework (OCTAVE) to meet critical business goals. HIEs must address high degrees of variety, variability, and capabilities with their member organizations and their security postures while providing critical data needs. Utilizing strict framework compliance does not address the latent security needs or flexibility, nor does it provide the resiliency needed to be that trusted business partner when members need it the most.

This chapter will start by introducing the four major sets of regulations governing Information Security in healthcare in the United States. All organizations that store or process data on behalf of healthcare providers, including HIEs, are subject to these. These are the Health Insurance Portability and Accountability Act (HIPAA) Security Rule, the Health Information Technology for Economic and Clinical Health (HITECH) Act, the 21st Century Cures Act Final Rule, and the National Institute of Standards and Technology (NIST) Cybersecurity Framework. The Ransomware and HIPAA Guidance from 2016 will also be discussed. The three primary management frameworks used to manage information security internationally, ISO/IEC 27001, the European Union (EU) General Data Protection Regulation (GDPR), and OCTAVE/OCTAVE Allegro, will then be introduced.

The chapter will next discuss the following technical/management frameworks used to identify specific technology risks and exploitation methods in the context of how they apply to HIE networks:

- Vulnerability Scanning
- The Open Web Application Security Project (OWASP) Top 10
- Health Information Trust Alliance (HITRUST) Common Security Framework (CSF)
- MITRE ATT&CK and D3FEND
- CIS Critical Security Controls

The concepts of Penetration Testing, Red Teams, Blue Teams, and Purple Teams, and their context in security for HIE networks will also be explored.

The concepts of the risk assessment, risk register, and risk management plan and how they apply in healthcare for HIEs will then be discussed. The risk management process will be explored in detail. Risk Management for HIEs using a modification of the OCTAVE For The Enterprise (FORTE) suite will be explored. This is to provide an example of how the unique organizational needs and structure of this organization type can be leveraged to provide an applicable Risk Management Framework (RMF).

Emerging trends in HIE networks, including Trusted Exchange Framework and Common Agreement (TEFCA) Security, Blockchain, and Decentralized Identifiers (DIDs) will then be discussed. Resources will then be provided for further exploration.

7.1.1 Healthcare information security regulations

7.1.1.1 HIPAA Security Rule

The HIPAA Security Rule is part of the Health Insurance Portability and Accountability Act of 1996, Administrative Simplification, 45 CFR Part 160, and Subparts A and C, 45 CFR Part 164 [10]. It establishes national standards to protect electronic protected health information (ePHI) that is created, received, used, or maintained by a covered entity [11]. It covers the interchange of ePHI between covered entities, which can be health plans, healthcare clearinghouses, or healthcare providers, and Business Associates.

Business Associates are people or organizations that are not part of the workforce of the Covered Entity and perform business functions related to the payment, treatment, or operations of it requiring the disclosure of ePHI. A Covered Entity may be a Business Associate of another Covered Entity [10]. According to the Health and Human Services (HHS) Office for Civil Rights, in their document The HIPAA Privacy Rule and Electronic Health Information Exchange in a Networked Environment, a Health Information Organization (HIO), of which an HIE is one type, is not considered a covered entity [12]. This is because the functions they typically perform do not make it a health plan, healthcare clearinghouse, or covered healthcare provider. HIOs are considered Business Associates, and cannot participate in Organized Health Care Arrangements, which involve providers and health plans, or Affiliated Covered Entities, which allow multiple legally separate covered entities to designate themselves as one for compliance purposes [12].

The Security Rule's requirements are divided into three different categories, which are Administrative, Technical, and Physical. Each specification under these three categories can be Required or Addressable [10]. If one is required, then it is marked as such. However, if one is marked as "Addressable," an covered entity or business associate is required to assess whether it is a reasonable and appropriate safeguard in its environment. Twenty-one of the Security Rule's forty-two specifications are marked as Addressable. This requires analysis as to what the contribution to protecting ePHI is. If the protection is considered reasonable and appropriate, then implement it. If not, document why it is not, and then implement an equivalent alternative measure [10,13]. Organizations are required to comply with these [11,14].

One of the many areas of confusion with the Security Rule is that its guidance has been considered vague and open to interpretation. Addressable has been interpreted as something that can be put off until another day [15]. An example of this is encryption. The final Security Rule made its use addressable [16].

However, 45 CFR 164.306 (a) [1], Security standards: General Rules, requires Covered Entities and Business Associates to ensure the confidentiality, integrity, and availability of all ePHI that they create, receive, maintain, or transmit. Encryption provides confidentiality between two or more parties that have a legitimate need to interchange data. Cryptographic Hash Functions, which are a class of mathematical functions that map bit strings of arbitrary length to fixed-length ones, are used to verify the Integrity of transmitted or stored data. These functions are one-way, meaning you cannot determine the source material from the resulting hash [17]. They are also supposed to be collision-resistant, meaning that any two given inputs cannot give the same output. However, multiple algorithms such as MD5 and secure Hash algorithm 1 (SHA-1) have been found to be vulnerable to these. The United States' National Institute of Standards and Technology, NIST, who sets the security standards for the US Federal Government and its contractors, publishes their list of approved hash algorithms in Special Publication 800-107 [18].

The Security Rule requires that organizations conduct risk analysis via risk assessments as part of their security management processes [14]. This includes evaluating the likelihood and impact of potential risks to ePHI, implementing appropriate security measures to address identified risks, documenting the chosen security measures and rationale, and maintaining continuous, reasonable, and appropriate security protections. While the Security Rule provides this guidance, it does not provide specifics on how to implement the technical methods of doing so.

The Administrative Safeguards include instituting a security management process to identify and analyze potential risks to ePHI, and the implementation of reasonable and appropriate countermeasures [14]. They also require organizations to designate a security official for developing and implementing their security policies and procedures. As part of this, Information Access Management policies and procedures that limit the use and disclosures of ePHI to the minimum necessary authorized based on user entitlements or role membership need to be implemented. Workforce Training and Management requires that the organization train the entire workforce on its security policies and procedures. They must also provide appropriate policies and procedures for management to appropriately authorize and supervise workforce members who work with ePHI. This includes Sanction Policies and Procedures for workforce members who violate the Information Access Management policies and procedures [14]. Finally, organizations must perform periodic assessments of how well their security policies and procedures meet the requirements of the Security Rule [14]. While this is not specified in the Security Rule itself, participants in the Medicare and Medicaid Electronic Health Record (EHR) incentive programs are required to complete one for each EHR reporting period [19]. In addition, many insurance companies require annual risk assessments as a condition of the policy renewal process. This was spurred on by the New York Department of Financial Services' Cybersecurity Regulations for insurance companies and financial institutions in 2017 [20].

The Physical Safeguards include Facility Access and Control, which requires organizations to limit physical facility access to only those authorized. Workstation and Device Security requires the implementation of policies and procedures to specify proper use of workstations and electronic media. It also must have policies and procedures in place that address the transfer, removal, disposal, and reuse of electronic media to protect ePHI [14]. This includes workstation timeouts, securing of workstations against theft, and use of encryption such as Microsoft BitLocker to prevent unauthorized disclosure of ePHI. Physical Safeguards can also be interpreted to mean electronic access control systems that are part of physical facility access. This includes badging systems, electronic door locks, and physical access to controlled areas such as pharmacies.

The Technical safeguards include Access Control, which requires organizations to implement policies and procedures to only allow authorized access to ePHI. Audit Controls require them to implement hardware, software, and/or procedural mechanisms to record and examine activity and access to ePHI. Integrity Controls require organizations to implement policies and procedures to protect the integrity of ePHI. This includes electronic measures such as auditing, cryptographic hashing, and encryption. Transmission Security requires organizations to implement technologies and associated policies, procedures, and processes to protect ePHI being transmitted/received over electronic networks [14]. This means the use of technologies such as Secure FTP, Secure Shell, or Transport Layer Security (TLS) 1.2 or greater (TLS 1.2 or 1.3), which use both encryption and hashing, to protect information in transit.

If a covered entity discovers that one of their business associates is undertaking activity that can be considered a data breach or a violation of their obligation, they are responsible for addressing the breach and/or ending the violation [14]. This includes failure to use reasonable and appropriate measures to protect ePHI.

Covered entities need to implement reasonable and appropriate policies, procedures, and processes to comply with Security Rule requirements. They are required to review and update them regularly in response to internal or external changes that can affect the security of ePHI [14]. They need to maintain them for six years after their creation or last effective date, whichever came last.

The Security Rule provides some excellent guidance to organizations to assist them in building out the basics for a security program focused around healthcare. However, it did not provide sufficient penalties for breaches, additional security guidance, what constitutes a certified Electronic Health Record, or when to conduct risk analysis exercises. That is what the HITECH Act clarified.

7.2 Health Information Technology for Economic and Clinical Health Act

The HITECH Act was part of the American Recovery and Reinvestment Act (ARRA) of 2009. It was part of the overall stimulus package from the beginning of the Obama administration to address the 2008 global financial crisis [21]. Three components of the Act that impact Information Security are the Medicare and Medicaid EHR Incentive Program (Meaningful Use), Enforcement Final Rule, and the Breach Notification Rule. This is because they have impacts on the use of encryption, types of encryption used, and vulnerability management. The latter is especially important, especially given ransomware and software supply chain attacks such as SolarWinds. The guidance given in the HITECH Act changed security requirements and how organizations respond to breaches. It also changed how organizations had to certify how they interchanged data with their peers.

The EHR Incentive Program, Meaningful Use, has several key objectives. It is designed to improve quality, safety, and efficiency, and reduce health disparities. It engages patients and families in their healthcare. It encourages care coordination and improves population and public health. It is intended to accomplish all of this while maintaining privacy and security [22]. It was mandated to receive incentives from the US government to implement these systems.

There were three major components of Meaningful Use in ARRA. The first was the use of a certified EHR in a meaningful way by completing 15 core usage objectives, 5 out of 10 objectives from a menu set, and 6 total clinical quality measures from a set of 38. Three of those had to be core objectives, and the other three had to come from an additional set of 38. Hospitals had to complete 14 core objectives, 5 out of 10 objectives from a menu set, and 15 Clinical Quality Measures [22].

The next component was the use of certified EHR technology for electronic exchange of health information to improve quality of care. This could be accomplished with data interchange using an HIE, or using DIRECT. Direct is a technical standard for exchanging information between healthcare entities, and was a Stage 2 Meaningful Use requirement for certified EHRs [23]. This is also where the use of NIST-approved encryption became important. Finally, organizations were required to use certified EHR technology to submit their clinical quality measures and other selected ones to the Center for Medicare and Medicaid Services (CMS).

Privacy and Security underpin the Meaningful Use requirements and the Recovery Act. It also extends out to the Enforcement Final Rule. HIPAA was limited to a maximum of $100 per violation and $25,000 for all violations of the same type within the calendar year [24]. The Enforcement Final Rule introduced four categories of violations, four corresponding penalty tiers, and maximum total Civil Monetary Penalties for violations of an identical provision in a calendar year, summarized in Table 7.1 [24].

TABLE 7.1 HIPAA Enforcement Final Rule violation categories and Civil Monetary Penalties (CMP) [24].

Violation category	Each violation	Total CMP for violations of an identical provision in a calendar year
Unknowing	$100–$50,000	$1,500,000
Reasonable Cause	$1000–$50,000	$1,500,000
Willful Neglect—Corrected	$10,000–$50,000	$1,500,000
Willful Neglect—Not Corrected	At least $50,000	$1,500,000

It also prohibits the imposition of penalties corrected within a 30-day time period, if they were not due to willful neglect. It strikes the bar on the imposition of penalties if the covered entity did not know and with the exercise of reasonable diligence would not have known of the violation. Those are now covered under the Unknowing category [25]. Also, under the Final Rule, HHS cannot impose the maximum Civil Monetary Penalties for a given violation. They need to consider [24]:

- The nature and extent of the violation, including the number of individuals affected and the time period during which the violation occurred;
- The nature and extent of the harms resulting from the violation, including whether the violation caused physical harm, whether the violation resulted in financial harm, whether there was harm to an individual's reputation and whether the violation hindered an individual's ability to obtain healthcare;
- The history of prior compliance, including previous violations; and
- The financial condition of the covered entity or business associate, including whether financial difficulties affected the ability to comply and whether the imposition of the CMP would jeopardize the ability of the covered entity to continue to provide or pay for healthcare.

On April 30, 2019, HHS exercised its discretion to apply new annual limits under a Notification of Enforcement Discretion. This limited the annual limits of Civil Monetary Penalties to the amounts summarized in Table 7.2 [26].

This has a cybersecurity impact due to several key factors:

- Even with the implementation of full cybersecurity or privacy protections on the network, a Covered Entity or Business Associate can be penalized for violations due to a data breach or other adverse event happening. An event like the SolarWinds Orion or Kaseya compromises, where compromised software was issued by the vendor to customers to address security issues that caused security and ransomware events, would still result in a penalty.
- If an organization conducts a risk assessment and indicates factors that led to a violation as an issue in it, and/or does not address these risks as per the Security Rule, the Violation Category can be indicated as Willful Neglect. If the organization participates in EHR incentive programs, they are required to conduct one of these annually.
- If an organization does not monitor and/or maintain the systems they have that store and protect ePHI, it can be considered Willful Neglect as the Security Rule requires organizations to monitor and maintain these systems for risks.
- Implementation of cybersecurity or privacy systems and not adequately staffing or

TABLE 7.2 Penalty tiers under notification of enforcement discretion (2019).

Culpability	Minimum penalty/violation	Maximum penalty/violation	Annual limit
No Knowledge	$100	$50,000	$25,000
Reasonable Cause	1000	50,000	100,000
Willful Neglect—Corrected	10,000	50,000	250,000
Willful Neglect—Not Corrected	50,000	50,000	1,500,000

maintaining them can increase the Violation Category from Unknowing or Reasonable Cause to Willful Neglect.

7.3 Breach Notification Rule

The *Breach Notification Rule* is the part of HITECH that people are most familiar with. It is an impermissible use or disclosure under the Privacy Rule that compromises the security or privacy of Protected Health Information (PHI). These are considered breaches unless the covered entity or business associate demonstrates that there is a low probability that the ePHI has been compromised based on a risk assessment of at least four key factors [27]:

1. The nature and extent of the PHI involved, including the types of identifiers and the likelihood of re-identification;
2. The unauthorized person who used the PHI or to whom the disclosure was made;
3. Whether the PHI was actually acquired or viewed; and
4. The extent to which the risk to the PHI has been mitigated.

There are three exceptions to the definition of "breach":

1. The unintentional access, acquisition, or use by someone acting under the authority of a covered entity or business associate if in good faith and within their scope of authority;
2. Inadvertent disclosure by someone authorized to someone else authorized to view the information within the same business associate, covered entity, or organized healthcare arrangement; and
3. If the covered entity or business associate believes that the unauthorized person would not have been able to retain the information.

The covered entity or business associate (if delegated) must notify individuals no later than 60 days after a breach has been discovered. The notification must include:

- A description of the breach
- A description of the types of information that were involved and data fields such as Social Security Number (SSN)
- The steps individuals need to take to protect themselves from harm
- A description of what the covered entity is doing to investigate, mitigate, and prevent further breaches
- Contact information for the covered entity, or business associate where applicable

If the breach occurs at a business associate, the covered entity is responsible for notifying; however, they can delegate the provision of individual notices to the business associate. Depending on the jurisdiction, the state Attorney General may need to be notified. The HHS Secretary needs to be notified through the HHS web site as well. If the breach has less than 500 affected individuals, then the HHS Secretary can be notified within 60 days of the end of the calendar year in which it was discovered.

If they cannot find accurate contact information for more than 10 individuals, they have to post a notice on their web site for at least 90 days. If the breach involves more than 500 individuals, the Covered Entity must notify the media, usually through a press release. The HHS Secretary also has to be notified within 60 days of discovery.

7.3.1 What's really considered Unsecured Protected Health Information

The common understanding of the word unsecured correlates to unencrypted. The Heartbleed vulnerability demonstrated that even encrypted communications can be compromised given flaws in the implementations of encryption algorithms [28]. As researchers such as the NIST continue to discover weaknesses in older encryption algorithms such as the Data Encryption Standard (DES), or hashing algorithms such as SHA-1, they cannot be considered reasonable and appropriate to sufficiently protect data, including ePHI [29,30]. In addition, the use of proprietary cryptographic functions that have not been verified by outside testing can put systems at significant risk of compromise, according to Roel Verdult, in his dissertation, the (in)security of proprietary cryptography [31].

In the Breach Notification Rule, Unsecured Protected Health Information is defined as ePHI that has not been rendered unusable, unreadable, or indecipherable to unauthorized persons through the use of a technology or methodology specified by the Secretary in guidance [27]. The guidance from Volume 74, Number 162, pages 42,742–42,743 of the Federal Register is [32]:

PHI is rendered unusable, unreadable, or indecipherable to unauthorized individuals if one or more of the following applies:

1. Electronic PHI has been encrypted as specified in the HIPAA Security Rule by "the use of an algorithmic process to transform data into a form in which there is a low probability of assigning meaning without use of a confidential process or key" and such confidential process or key that might enable decryption has not been breached. To avoid a breach of the confidential process or key, these decryption tools should be stored on a device or at a location separate from the data they are used to encrypt or decrypt. The encryption processes identified below have been tested by the NIST and judged to meet this standard.
   - **a.** Valid encryption processes for data at rest are consistent with NIST Special Publication 800-111, Guide to Storage Encryption Technologies for End User Devices.
   - **b.** Valid encryption processes for data in motion are those which comply, as appropriate, with NIST Special Publications 800-52, Guidelines for the Selection and Use of TLS Implementations; 800-77, Guide to IPsec Virtual Private Networks (VPNs); or 800-113, Guide to SSL VPNs, or others which are Federal Information Processing Standards (FIPS) 140-2 validated.
2. The media on which the PHI is stored or recorded have been destroyed in one of the following ways:
   - **a.** Paper, film, or other hard copy media have been shredded or destroyed such that the PHI cannot be read or otherwise cannot be reconstructed. Redaction is specifically excluded as a means of data destruction.
   - **b.** Electronic media have been cleared, purged, or destroyed consistent with NIST Special Publication 800-88, Guidelines for Media Sanitization, such that the PHI cannot be retrieved.

The guidance published by NIST in their special publications relies upon two programs to verify and validate the cryptographic algorithms and implementations used, which are the Cryptographic Algorithm Validation Program (CAVP), and the Cryptographic Module Validation Program. Only validated cryptographic modules utilizing validated algorithms that have been tested to conform to the appropriate federal standards, FIPS 140-2 and/or FIPS 140-3, are accepted by Federal agencies for the protection of sensitive information [33]. Algorithm validation by the CAVP program is a prerequisite to cryptographic module validation [34].

The newer FIPS 140-3 standard is based on two international standards:

- ISO/IEC 19790:2012(E), Information technology—Security techniques—Security requirements for cryptographic modules

- ISO/IEC 24759:2017(E), Information technology—Security techniques—Test requirements for cryptographic modules

What this means is the following:

- Covered Entities and Business Associates can only utilize approved encryption algorithms and implementations to protect ePHI at rest and in transport.
- NIST updates their Special Publications to address security changes, such as NIST SP 800-52, which has had two revisions since the publication of the Breach Notification Rule [35].
- Organizations need to ensure that the encryption and hashing algorithms they use are in accordance with NIST guidance.
- Transmission and/or storage of ePHI and the credentials that guard it must be done in accordance with NIST standards. Proprietary methods are not acceptable.
- Continual risk assessments to ensure that the systems used to protect data at rest and in transport are not susceptible to vulnerabilities that could compromise the Confidentiality, Integrity, or Availability of PHI is required.

7.3.2 Ransomware, HIPAA, and HITECH Act Breach Notification Rule implications

On July 11, 2016, the HHS Office for Civil Rights released the document FACT SHEET: Ransomware and HIPAA [36]. This document describes ransomware as a type of malware that attempts to deny access to a user's data using encryption until a ransom is paid, usually in cryptocurrency [36]. It also describes ransomware types that either destroy or exfiltrate data, or does so in conjunction with other malware [36]. Recent ransomware attacks, such as the one on Eskenazi Health in Indianapolis, Indiana, have resulted in the exfiltration of patient data onto a section of the Internet known as the Dark Web [37].

This document also describes how compliance with the HIPAA Security Rule, specifically its requirements of a security management process, security measures, procedures to guard against and detect malicious software, training users on malicious software protection, and implementing proper access controls can help prevent malware infections [36]. It also describes how implementation of backups, business continuity, and downtime procedures can assist organizations in recovery.

If a covered entity or business associate determines they have been infected with ransomware, they need to start with an initial analysis to [36]:

- determine the scope of the incident to identify what networks, systems, or applications are affected;
- determine the origination of the incident (who/what/where/when);
- determine whether the incident is finished, is ongoing or has propagated additional incidents throughout the environment; and
- determine how the incident occurred (e.g., tools and attack methods used, vulnerabilities exploited).

They then need to include steps such as [36]:

- containing the impact and propagation of the ransomware;
- eradicating the instances of ransomware and mitigating or remediating vulnerabilities that permitted the ransomware attack and propagation;
- recovering from the ransomware attack by restoring data lost during the attack and returning to "business as usual" operations; and
- conducting postincident activities, which could include a deeper analysis of the evidence to determine if the entity has any

regulatory, contractual, or other obligations as a result of the incident (such as providing notification of a breach of PHI), and incorporating any lessons learned into the overall security management process of the entity to improve incident response effectiveness for future security incidents.

The guidance then indicates that when ePHI is encrypted as part of a ransomware attack, it is a breach because it has been acquired by unauthorized individuals, and is a disclosure not permitted under the HIPAA Privacy Rule [36]. Only if the covered entity or business associate can demonstrate otherwise, a breach has been determined to occur, and the organization has to comply with the appropriate rules [36]. The exceptions to this are:

- If the organization can conclusively prove that the data have not been exfiltrated during the time period between initial access and ransom. According to the IBM Cost of a Data Breach Report 2020, the global average time to detect a data breach is 207 days, and 73 days to respond [38]. The HIPAA Privacy Rule requires organizations to maintain logs of ePHI access and disclosures for six years [39]. However, the requirements do not extend to the systems themselves, and logging every data conversation is an extreme undertaking with little to no benefit.
  - This type of analysis requires analyzing Internet traffic in detail to make a reasonable and appropriate determination as to whether data were exfiltrated. Ransomware attackers can use legitimate Cloud services to mask this. Unless an organization can affirmatively accomplish this, assume a breach of ransomed data.
- If the ransomware encrypts already-secured or encrypted ePHI in an encrypted state.
  - If the ransomware encrypts a PC, external storage, or flash drive with disk encryption, and they are turned on and able to access this data, then it is still considered a breach.
  - If the ransomware infects cloud-based storage, even if it is encrypted in transport and at rest, it is still considered a breach because it can be transparently encrypted or decrypted by the ransomware.
  - If the ransomware affects a hypervisor, which is a system that utilizes Virtual Machine technologies to host multiple logically separate computers on the same platform, and infects the individual virtual machines, then each virtual machine is considered breached.
  - However, if it is in a password-protected encrypted ZIP file using AES-256 encryption either locally or in the cloud, then it is not considered a breach

The summary of this fact sheet is that if a covered entity or business associate has been infected with ransomware, unless they can prove otherwise, they will need to assume that data that have been encrypted by it have been breached, including virtual machines.

7.3.3 Vulnerabilities and breaches

The effects of Ransomware bring up an interesting point. If a vulnerability can be used to provide unauthorized access to data, then that vulnerability is considered a breach. Under the Breach Notification Rule, unless one can prove otherwise, all data that could potentially be accessed have to be considered breached. A real-life example of this is with phishing attacks. If someone's credentials get compromised, and a malicious threat actor uses them to access their email, then all emails in that mailbox are considered breached unless there are log files that empirically prove otherwise. With the significant amount of cloud email providers out there, this is often a difficult task to accomplish.

With web site vulnerabilities, often those vulnerabilities allow unlogged access to the raw data. Attacks such as SQL Injection or Application Programming Interface (API) manipulation do not log access to ePHI the way an EMR would. Therefore a vulnerability on a web site that allows for unauthenticated access to ePHI could potentially lead to a breach of all of information on that site unless proven otherwise. Alissa Valentina Knight's research into vulnerabilities in Fast Health Interoperability Resources (FHIR) API implementations demonstrates exactly how vulnerable implementations can lead to data breaches [40].

Additionally, vulnerabilities such as the log4j vulnerability, which was discovered in November, 2021, demonstrate why this is the case [41]. This incredibly severe vulnerability was in a library used by multiple vendor products for logging. Log4j, according to the Apache project, is used to help programmers output log statements to a variety of targets [42]. This vulnerability allowed random code to be executed from a remote server. It had a Common Vulnerability Scoring System (CVSS) vulnerability score of 10.0, which is the highest score one can get [43]. This is an example of a common system library used as a utility by many programs with a wide reach being exploited.

Cisco, Sonicwall, and Netapp are major vendors who were affected by this [44]. Numerous others who used this library, including Oracle, were also affected [45]. Attacking the logging library itself to run code without logging actions taken demonstrates why these types of breaches are often considered breaches of all information. In addition, these vulnerabilities can be used to install and run code that takes further action, such as ransomware. That can lead to further information compromises, and potentially all data on a network that a successful threat actor has access to being considered breached.

7.4 21st Century Cures Act Final Rule

As data interchanges move from just between covered entities and business associates such as HIEs to now include consumers, interoperability and security become more paramount. This is expressed in the 21st Century Cures Act Final Rule (Cures Act). The purposes of this Act are to advance interoperability, support the access, exchange, and use of electronic health information (EHI), and address occurrences of Information Blocking [46]. Information Blocking, according to HHS, is a practice that is likely to interfere with access, exchange, or use of EHI [47]. It is also designed to allow for patients to get copies of their data using standard Application Programming Interfaces (APIs) and to put them in applications they control. Applications can be developed by anyone and voluntarily certified as long as they follow appropriate CURES Act guidelines.

The Cures Act provides for several key interoperability standards, including adopting the United States Core Data for Interoperability as a standard, FHIR 4.0.1 as a standard for healthcare data exchange with individuals, TLS 1.2 or greater as a data security standard, and OAuth 2.0 for authentication [46].

TLS 1.3 is only supported by Windows 11 and Server 2022, and is not supported by Windows 10 or previous Windows Server versions [48]. Web browsers, such as Google Chrome, Mozilla Firefox, and Microsoft Edge, however, do support it [49]. However, as 72.48% of all desktop market share is Windows, and Windows 11 was released on October 5, 2021, it would not be prudent to include a security standard that a significant portion of potential clients cannot support at the operating system level, even if it is an improvement [50,51].

From a cybersecurity perspective, the Cures Act Final Rule introduces several new risks into covered entities and business associates.

The use of FHIR 4.0.1 along with TLS 1.2 or greater and OAuth 2.0 to provide patients their information presents several new avenues of risk:

- APIs that once were only open to Covered Entities and HIEs for data interchange on closed networks such as VPNs are now open to the world.
- Any developer can develop FHIR 4.0.1-compliant applications to access EHI [52].
- Added exposure leads to additional risks from outside threat actors, such as bots, attempting to access data.
- Security issues in the FHIR API implementation can lead to potential data breaches [52].
- Programming errors in the third-party applications using the FHIR API can lead to unstable operation, denial of service through server crashes, or data breaches through malfunctioning code.
- Security issues with the exposed technology stack (web server, TLS, OAuth, etc.) can lead to data breaches through system compromise.
- Organizations may not know how to properly implement Security exceptions for Information Blocking and mistakenly think they have to let every application through to access data, even though they may cause risks.

The Security Exception, 45 CFR 171.203, discusses this [46]:

Security exception—when will an actor's practice that is likely to interfere with the access, exchange, or use of EHI in order to protect the security of EHI not be considered information blocking?

An actor's practice that is likely to interfere with the access, exchange, or use of EHI in order to protect the security of EHI will not be considered information blocking when the practice meets the conditions in paragraphs (a), (b), and (c) of this section, and in addition meets either the condition in paragraph (d) of this section or the condition in paragraph (e) of this section.

1. The practice must be directly related to safeguarding the confidentiality, integrity, and availability of EHI.
2. The practice must be tailored to the specific security risk being addressed.
3. The practice must be implemented in a consistent and non-discriminatory manner.
4. If the practice implements an organizational security policy, the policy must:
   a. Be in writing;
   b. Have been prepared on the basis of, and be directly responsive to, security risks identified and assessed by or on behalf of the actor;
   c. Align with one or more applicable consensus-based standards or best practice guidance; and
   d. Provide objective timeframes and other parameters for identifying, responding to, and addressing security incidents.
5. If the practice does not implement an organizational security policy, the actor must have made a determination in each case, based on the particularized facts and circumstances, that:
   a. The practice is necessary to mitigate the security risk to EHI; and
   b. There are no reasonable and appropriate alternatives to the practice that address the security risk that are less likely to interfere with, prevent, or materially discourage access, exchange, or use of EHI.

The methods by which Covered Entities or Business Associates can address the Security Exception and reduce the risks of implementing FHIR or other API-based security methods are:

- Implement an organizational security policy as defined by the HIPAA Security Rule that discusses assessing and addressing organizational risks by:

- Implementing the ability for organizations to deny access to resources attempting to access the network that may present a risk to the organization and/or its customers
- Documenting that the practice of addressing risks safeguards the confidentiality, integrity, and availability of EHI
- Documenting that resources that present evidence of malicious behavior as determined by the NIST Cybersecurity or MITRE ATT&CK Frameworks and people, processes, and technologies used to implement and monitor for such will be used to detect and make the determination of this behavior [53,54]
- Documenting that resources determined to be malicious by application of those third-party standard frameworks will be immediately or proactively blocked
- Providing contact information so that people or organizations that want to address nonconformance can do so easily

- Leverage people, processes, and technologies to protect FHIR APIs from:
  - Distributed Denial of Service attacks
  - Geo-blocking, that is, not allowing certain IP addresses based on reputation or propensity for attacks to access APIs
  - Bot attacks, where up to thousands of computers are used to attempt access to APIs
  - Nonconforming FHIR code
  - TLS Downgrade attacks, where an application attempts to use an older version of TLS
  - Known API security attacks
  - Web Server attacks
  - TLS Protocol attacks
  - Border Gateway Protocol hijacking attacks, where networks can be routed through malicious actors
  - Domain Name Service attacks, where malicious servers can impersonate legitimate ones
  - Spoofed Certificates, where a malicious certificate can be used to exfiltrate data to malicious third parties
- Segment the API providers to not sit directly on the corporate network so that outside attacks are less likely to penetrate the corporate network
- Leverage third-party cloud-based technologies for externally facing applications and APIs to provide adaptive protection from attacks and protect the production networks, even if already segmented
- Conduct Regular Risk Assessments of the entire environment
- Conduct regular penetration tests of the API environment, including detailed API testing
- Conduct regular vulnerability scans of the API environment

These methods are not just germane to FHIR API providers. These techniques can also be used by HIEs to protect their assets and provide better security. The Cures Act and Alissa Valentina Knight's research demonstrates areas to focus on in terms of conformance testing and security [55].

7.5 NIST Cybersecurity Framework 1.1

Organizations need to be able to organize their security activities to be able to appropriately identify, assess, and address risks. The Cybersecurity Enhancement Act of 2014 expanded the NIST's role to include identifying and developing cybersecurity risk frameworks for use by critical infrastructure owners and operators [56]. NIST, in response to the needs of organizations that required a prioritized, flexible, repeatable, performance-based, and cost-effective approach to develop their own programs, leveraged the work from version 1.0 of the framework [56]. Version 1.1 was released on April 16, 2018 after version 1.0 was released in 2014 [56].

The framework is organized into the Framework Core, Framework Implementation Tiers, and Framework Profiles. They organize into a recommended seven-step Cybersecurity program that helps organizations continually assess and address risks [56]. The use of this program helps organizations leverage the framework to improve their security.

The Framework Core is composed of five Framework Core Functions, their associated outcome Categories, their Subcategories, and Informative References. The outcome Categories represent business functions associated with needs and specific activities. Subcategories represent a further division of these into specific operational activities. Informative References provide links back to specific guidance needed to implement Categories and Subcategories within a business to appropriate standards, mainly NIST's own Special Publications [56]. The five Core Functions and associated Categories are [56]:

- Identify—Develop an organizational understanding to manage cybersecurity risk to systems, people, assets, data, and capabilities. This includes the Categories of Asset Management, Understanding the Business Environment, Governance, Risk Assessment, and Risk Management Strategy.
- Protect—Develop and implement appropriate safeguards to ensure delivery of critical services. This includes the categories of Identity Management and Access Control, Awareness and Training, Data Security, Information Protection Processes and Procedures, Maintenance, and Protective Technology.
- Detect—Develop and implement appropriate activities to identify occurrences of cybersecurity events. Categories here include Understanding Anomalies and Events, Security Continuous Monitoring, and Detection Processes
- Respond—Develop and implement appropriate activities to take action regarding a detected cybersecurity incident. These have the categories of Response Planning, Communications, Analysis, Mitigation, and Improvements.
- Recover—Develop and implement appropriate activities to maintain plans for resilience and to restore any capabilities or services that were impaired due to a cybersecurity incident. The categories of this Core Function include Recovery Planning, Improvements, and Communications.

The four organizational tiers [56] are defined as follows:

1. Partial
   a. Cybersecurity professionals (referred to as staff) and the general employee population have little to no cybersecurity-related training.
   b. The staff has a limited or nonexistent training pipeline.
   c. Security awareness is limited.
   d. Employees have little or no awareness of company security resources and escalation paths.
2. Risk Informed
   a. Staff and employees have received cybersecurity-related training.
   b. The staff has a training pipeline.
   c. There is an awareness of cybersecurity risk at the organizational level.
   d. Employees have a general awareness of security and company security resources and escalation paths.
3. Repeatable
   a. Staff possess the knowledge and skills to perform their appointed roles and responsibilities.
   b. Employees receive regular cybersecurity-related training and briefings.

c. The staff has a robust training pipeline, including internal and external security conferences or training opportunities.
d. Organization and business units have a security champion or dedicated security staff.

4. Adaptive
   a. Staff knowledge and skills are regularly reviewed for currency and applicability and new skills, and knowledge needs are identified and addressed.
   b. Employees receive regular cybersecurity-related training and briefings on relevant and emerging security topics.
   c. Staff have a robust training pipeline and routinely attend internal and external security conferences or training opportunities.

The tiers themselves are not scores. They provide context into how an organization views risk and what processes help manage it. They do describe an increase in complexity and organizational maturity as the level increases from 1 to 4. While they are not scores, organizations that rate themselves as Tier 1 are strongly encouraged to move to a higher one. The lack of awareness, training, and security response puts Tier 1 organizations at serious risk. The framework recommends that organizations move to a higher level if a cost–benefit analysis indicates that it is possible and is cost-effective.

When an organization picks the area they want to evaluate, identifies the scope, and assesses the area in scope against the Functions, Categories, and associated Subcategories/operational processes, they build what is known as a Profile of the area. These can be for an entire organization, or a specific unit or area. Large organizations will generally assess business units and areas individually. There are two types of Profile in the NIST Cybersecurity Framework:

- Current Profile: Cybersecurity outcomes currently being achieved
- Target Profile: Outcomes needed to meet targeted cybersecurity risk management goals

The recommended seven-step program that NIST illustrates to implement a Cybersecurity Program using the Framework is:

- Step 1: Prioritize and Scope. Identifies the business and mission objectives, and high-level organizational policies. This is where strategic decisions and scoping of cybersecurity are determined.
- Step 2: Orient. Associated assets and systems, federal, state, and local regulatory requirements, and the risk approach appropriate for the scope. Threats and vulnerabilities against associated systems and assets are identified.
- Step 3: Create a Current Profile. The current organizational state is evaluated against the NIST Cybersecurity Framework Core Functions, Categories, and Subcategories. The results are documented as part of the process. Intel used the Tiers as scores to evaluate each Category, and then identified outliers and differences with heat maps to identify areas to focus on [57].
- Step 4: Conduct a Risk Assessment. The area needs to conduct a risk assessment to discern the likelihood of a cybersecurity event and its impact. While the Framework itself does not specifically recommend one, NIST Special Publication 800-30 Revision 1, Guide for Conducting Risk Assessments, provides organizations with sufficient detail to conduct their own [58].
- Step 5: Create a Target Profile. Based upon the gathered evidence from creating the Current Profile, conducting a risk assessment, understanding stakeholders and their needs, and understanding the organization's desired state, the organization develops a Target Profile for the area. This identifies where the organization would like to be. The Target

Profile and target Implementation Tier need to be in alignment.

- Step 6: Determine, Analyze, and Prioritize Gaps. The Current and Target profiles and scores are compared to determine gaps. These gaps are then utilized to develop an action plan to achieve the objectives identified in the Target Profile. The organization then plans for and allocates resources to achieve them. Intel used heat maps as part of their gap analysis to identify specific areas.
- Step 7: Implement Action Plan. The action plan and associated processes and subprocesses are then executed and monitored to achieve the goals and objectives set in the Target Profile.

NIST cautions that these steps need to be repeated as needed to continuously assess and improve cybersecurity [56]. Covered Entities, due to CMS reporting requirements, are required to do so annually. Business Associates, of which HIEs are one type, are often required to follow the lead of the Covered Entities (CEs) they contract with as part of the overall risk management process.

The goal of the NIST Cybersecurity Framework is to build the skeleton that organizations can adapt to their needs for conducting risk and gap analysis. Implementations such as Intel's provide a quantitative one that can be used to provide additional weight to decision-making processes and heat maps to identify opportunities. Their method also allows them to more effectively communicate to stakeholders using a minimum increase of resources, and is aligned with their organization [57].

However, aligning with the needs of HIEs, which include analyzing application services and potential system vulnerabilities with FHIR, Health Level 7 (HL7), United States Core Data for Interoperability (USCDI), and the numerous healthcare data interchange formats means that more specific risk assessment types need to be added. Adding those types and the specific analyses they need will be part of the buildup to OCTAVE FORTE as a base by which various RMFs can be evaluated as part of a more robust overall process. The current methods, such as NIST, discuss how, and require the organizations to seek out additional guidance themselves. The rest of this chapter will discuss applicable international frameworks, and then ones specific to Application Security.

7.5.1 Global regulations and frameworks

According to the International Telecommunications Union, in their 2020 Global Cybersecurity Index 2020 Report, 133 countries have protection and privacy regulations signed into law [59]. These regulations are summarized in Fig. 7.2 by global region and policy status (e.g., passed, drafted).

Detailed information about the regulations applicable to all 133 is outside of the scope of this chapter. Interested parties will want to check with their individual nation's ministries and laws for the ones applicable for their use cases. However, this chapter will summarize the frameworks that are most prevalent by virtue of being internationally approved by standards bodies such as ISO, such as the ISO/IEC 27001 framework, used by a plurality of countries, such as GDPR, or are well-established frameworks with large adoption rates like OCTAVE and OCTAVE Allegro. Several examples of International Privacy/Security Laws and Frameworks are summarized in Table 7.3.

7.5.2 ISO/IEC 27001

Out of the numerous international frameworks and standards, the only one that helps organizations to understand the components of an Information Security Management System

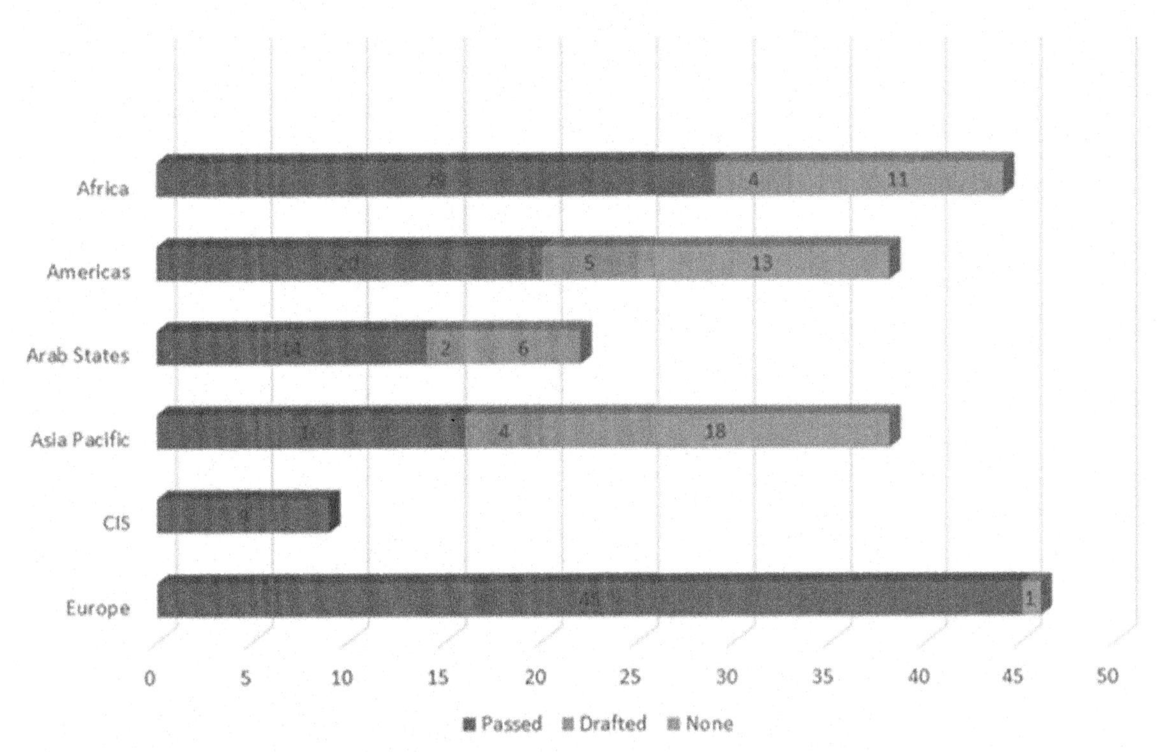

FIGURE 7.2 Global data protection legislation by region and status. Source: *Adapted from Global Cybersecurity Index 2020 [Internet]. Global Cybersecurity Index. International Telecommunications Union; [cited 2021 Dec 30]. Available from: https://www.itu.int/en/ITU-D/Cybersecurity/Pages/global-cybersecurity-index.aspx.*

(ISMS) is ISO/IEC 27001:2013 [66]. It is considered the main standard [67]. This standard has 114 security controls in 14 domains. These controls are part of the Annex A section of the standard, which provides outlines of the controls [68]. The 14 domains are:

- Information Security Policies
- Human Resource Security
- Access Control
- Physical and Environmental Security
- Operation Security
- Supplier Relationships
- Information Security Aspects of Business Continuity Management
- Organisation of Information Security
- Asset Management
- Cryptography
- Operations Security
- System acquisition, development, and maintenance
- Information Security Asset Management
- Compliance

ISO/IEC 27001 also has 10 management system clauses. These are there to provide the frameworks for implementation, management, and continual improvement [69]:

- Scope
- Normative References
- Terms and Definitions
- Context of the Organization and Stakeholders
- Leadership
- Planning, including risk assessment and risk management plan
- Support

TABLE 7.3 International Privacy/Security Laws and Frameworks.

Name	Law or framework	Description	Applies to	Date ratified	Date last amended
European Union (EU) General Data Protection Regulation	Law	Protects data subjects, their personal data, how it is processed, its movement, and how it is protected.	All applicable EU data subjects	April 27, 2016	
Canada Personal Information Protection and Electronic Documents Act	Law	Protects personal information that is collected, used, or disclosed in certain circumstances, and provides for electronic means to communicate or record information and/or transactions [60].	Canadian citizens and corporations	April 13, 2000	June 21, 2019
Brazilian General Data Protection Law	Law	Protects the processing of personal data, including electronically, with the purpose of protecting the fundamental rights of freedom and privacy of natural persons [61].	Brazilian Citizens and corporations	August 14, 2018	
Singapore Personal Data Protection Act	Law	Governs the collection, use, and disclosure of personal data by organizations. Requires organizations to develop policies and practices to meet the obligations of the Act [62].	Organizations doing business in Singapore	November 20, 2012	February 1, 2021
ISO 27001 Information technology—Security techniques—Information security management systems—Requirements	Framework	Provides the framework for an Information Security Management System and all associated components	Corporations who either elect to or are required to utilize this	October 2005	October 2013
ISO 27018—Information technology—Security techniques—Code of practice for protection of personally identifiable information (PII) in public clouds acting as PII processors	Framework	Provides commonly accepted control objectives, controls, and guidelines for implementing measures to protect PII for the cloud environment [63].	Corporations who either elect to or are required to utilize this	August 2014	January 2019
Operationally Critical Threat, Asset, and Vulnerability Evaluation Framework (OCTAVE)	Framework	The OCTAVE is a framework for identifying and managing information security risks. This was developed by the Software Engineering Institute at Carnegie Mellon University [64].	Corporations who either elect to or are required to utilize this	September 1999	

(Continued)

TABLE 7.3 (Continued)

Name	Law or framework	Description	Applies to	Date ratified	Date last amended
OCTAVE Allegro	Framework	An improved version of OCTAVE. OCTAVE Allegro is a methodology to streamline and optimize the process of assessing information security risks so that an organization can obtain sufficient results with a small investment in time, people, and other limited resources [65].	Corporations who either elect to or are required to utilize this	May 2007	

- Operation
- Performance Evaluation
- Improvement

It is structured linearly, from the establishment of the ISMS through to its review and adaption. The organization needs to start by defining the scope of the ISMS and what will fall under potential certification. Knowing the scope allows organizations to define and allocate resources to establish the ISMS project needed to complete the rest. The current 2013 version does not mandate a project-based approach or Plan-Do-Check-Act approach for performing analysis and addressing the requirements [67].

However, this is still considered an effective way to accomplish them. According to the American Society for Quality, the four steps can be summarized as such [70]:

- Plan: Recognize an opportunity and plan a change.
- Do: Test the change. Carry out a small-scale study.
- Check: Review the test, analyze the results, and identify what you've learned.
- Act: Take action based on what you learned in the study step. If the change did not work, go through the cycle again with a different plan. If you were successful, incorporate what you learned from the test into wider changes. Use what you learned to plan new improvements, beginning the cycle again.

ISO/IEC 27001 also requires a Risk Assessment to determine the security controls that the organization will need [70]. It requires organizations to do the following as part of their ISMS:

- Conduct a Risk Assessment using their methodology and quantitative rankings of choice.
- Design a set of controls to address items from the risk assessment.
- Compare the list of controls to Annex A.
- Ensure they meet necessary obligations (legal, contractual, regulatory).
- Ensure they are in place and operational.
- Ensure their effective application.

As part of the ISMS processes, organizations are also required to produce a document that details which controls have been applied due to the Risk Assessment process, and which have not. This document is called the Statement of Applicability (SoA). The ISMS scope and SoA are key to the certification audit.

Certification audits for ISO/IEC 27001 must be completed by an external reviewer or accreditation body. While there are many firms out there that offer this service, many offer consultation and certification services, which are not in line with other international standards such as ISO/IEC 17021 [71]. ISO/IEC 17021 is the standard that sets the requirements for organizations that provide audit and certification of management systems [71]. The American National Standards Institute and American Society for Quality (ANSI-ASQ) National Accreditation Board offer a directory service for accredited certification bodies that meet this standard at https://anabdirectory.remoteauditor.com/ [72]. Completing a certification from a nonaccredited firm can lead to credibility issues. This is because the firm that has completed the certification will not have met the regular performance, quality, and competence monitoring that an organization like ANSI-ASQ can provide [71]. Potential conflicts of interest on a certification for security management can lead to significant concerns with clients who will scrutinize it.

A concrete example of these is in Subsection B, Title II, Section 208 of the Sarbanes-Oxley Act, Auditor Independence. This forbids registered public accounting firms from preparing or issuing audit reports for publicly traded companies if they provide certain other services [73]. The US Securities and Exchange Commission clarified on January 22, 2003 that this included nonaudit services including expert services unrelated to the audit [74].

The ISO/IEC 27001 certification is significant. It is considered the top ISMS standard. However, it is more than just a standard. It defines a controls and management system to be used for continual management and improvement, and a certification system that emphasizes removing potential conflicts of interest in line with ISO/IEC 17021 and Sarbanes-Oxley Act. While it does not define how an organization assesses its risk, it defines the management system by which they would do so. It also provides an implementation framework compatible with laws such as the EU GDPR or HIPAA/HITECH.

7.5.3 European Union General Data Protection Regulation

GDPR, Regulation (EU) 2016/679 of the European Parliament and of the Council of 27 April 2016, is designed to protect natural persons, also known as Data Subjects, with regards to the processing of their personal data and the free movement of it. It also repeals the previous EU Directive 95/46/EC [75]. This law took effect on May 25, 2018 for EU Member States [76]. It establishes detailed requirements for companies that collect, store, and manage personal data of natural persons/data subjects within the EU. This applies if a company processes personal data and is based in the EU, even if the actual processing occurs somewhere else. It also applies if the company is based outside the EU and processes personal data in relation to goods or services to individuals in the EU, or monitors their behavior [77]. The GDPR does not apply if [77]:

- The data subject is deceased.
- The data subject is a legal person, such as a corporation.
- The processing is done by someone acting outside their scope of expertise.

GDPR identifies two main profiles that deal with the processing of Personal Data [77]:

- Data Controllers: Decide the purpose and way in which personal data is processed. This includes companies like Microsoft, Amazon, or Google.
- Data Processors: Hold and process data on behalf of Data Controllers. This can include third parties or the Controllers themselves.

The following are considered Personal Data under GDPR [77]:

- Name
- Address
- ID card/passport number
- Income
- Cultural profile
- IP address
- Personal Health Data held by a hospital or doctor

The following data are prohibited from being processed under the GDPR [77]:

- Racial or Ethnic Origin
- Sexual Orientation
- Political Opinions
- Religious or Philosophical Beliefs
- Trade Union Membership
- Genetic, Biometric, or Health Data, except when explicit consent is given or when processing is needed for legal reasons of substantial public interest
- Personal data related to criminal records unless explicitly authorized by law

Much publicity has been given to Article 17, the Right to Be Forgotten, which allows data subjects to request that data controllers erase, without undue delay, applicable personal data. There are many misconceptions about this Article, specifically that it requires total erasure of information [76]. The Article requires that controller take reasonable steps that take into account the technology available and implementation cost, to do so. They also need to inform downstream processors that the data subject has requested erasure of this data.

The cases in which information can be erased are:

- The personal data are no longer necessary for the purposes for which it was collected.
- The data subject withdraws consent and there are no other legal grounds for processing.
- The data subject objects to the processing and there are no overriding legitimate grounds to continue.
- The data subject objects to the processing due to it being for Direct Marketing processes or profiling as defined in Articles 21 and 18. This can include the use of data for training Intelligent Systems, such as Artificial Intelligence or Machine Learning.
- The personal data have been unlawfully processed.
- The personal data have to be erased for legal/compliance purposes for the EU or a Member State.
- The personal data have been collected on a data subject under the age of 16 without parental consent.
- The data subject who the personal data were collected on is age 16 or older and now objects to its collection.

The cases in which it cannot be erased are:

- When erasure would prevent the exercising the rights of freedom of expression and information;
- For compliance with legal obligations under EU or Member State law in the public interest or official authority;
- For the purposes of preventative or occupational medicine, including assessment of working capacity, medical diagnosis, provision of health or social care or treatment, or the management of health or social care systems and services under EU or Member State Law by. The data still needs to be safeguarded under strict professional and technical controls;
- For the purposes of public interest in public health, such as cross-border threats to health like COVID-19 variants;
- For healthcare quality and safety purposes; and
- For ensuring high standards for medicinal products or medical devices given

suitable and specific measures to protect the rights and freedoms of the data subject, specifically processional secrecy.

For HIEs and HIOs, the data collected, as it is collected on behalf of organizations for public health purposes such as sending immunization data and reporting quality measures, would be exempt from the Right To Be Forgotten [78]. However, GDPR does have a set of obligations and type of risk assessment that needs to be completed when organizations plan to implement new processes or technologies. This is known as a Data Protection Impact Assessment (DPIA), which is defined under Article 35 of the GDPR, Data Protection Impact Assessment [76]. The GDPR requires that organizations structure themselves to continually monitor and assess risks to Personal Data throughout the lifecycle of these products or technologies. These are supposed to be done when these present a high risk to the rights and freedoms of natural persons. As the misuse, theft, or nonprotection of personal data puts it at risk, and the data can negatively impact their rights and freedoms, DPIAs are a critical component of the product lifecycle in the EU.

Unlike other regulations and certifications, which are more organization-focused, a DPIA is focused on specific products and technologies. The closest analog to this is Failure Mode and Effects Analysis, from the Institute for Healthcare Improvement [79]. The below are the categories and items that an HIE or HIO conducting business in the EU will need to know and accomplish to be able to be in compliance with GDPR.

To provide HIEs and HIOs with a more comprehensive assessment, material from four other Articles, 13—information to be provided where personal data are collected from the data subject, 37—designation of the data protection officer, 38—position of the data protection officer, and 39—tasks of the data protection officer, will be added to the outline. The purpose of this is to provide organizations that operate under the GDPR or like laws to be able to produce the evidence of compliance they need as part of their risk assessment process [75]:

1. Article 37: The organization has Data Protection Officer(s) (DPOs) assigned. They can be either employees or contractors.
2. Article 38: The DPO will be involved in a proper and timely manner with all issues relating to the protection of personal data.
3. Article 38: The DPO will directly report to the highest management level of the controller or processor.
4. Article 38: The DPO will not be instructed on how to conduct their work or dismissed for doing it.
5. Article 38: Data subjects can contact the DPO with regards to all issues related to processing of their personal data and the exercising of their rights.
6. Article 38: The DPO will be bound by secrecy and confidentiality regarding their tasks.
7. Article 38: The DPO can do other work as long as it is not a conflict of interest.
8. Article 39: The DPOs are professional qualified to complete their duties.
9. Article 39: The DPOs have informed the Controller(s) and Processor(s) under their purview of their obligations.
10. Article 39: The DPOs need to continually monitor compliance with the GDPR and any local superseding provisions with regards to the protection of Personal Data.
    a. This includes the assignment of responsibilities, awareness, and training.
    b. They are responsible for conducting and monitoring the required audits for processes and technologies in their purview.
11. Article 35: DPIA assessment categories.

a. The intended usage of Personal Data by the Controller(s) and Processor(s)
b. The intended data elements to be used in processing operations by the products and technologies
c. A description of the processing operations used to store, process, and manipulate the data
d. A description of the responsibilities of the Controller(s) and Processor(s) in the operations.
e. A needs analysis of the reasons why the data elements used are required.
f. An assessment to the risks of rights and freedoms of Data Subjects
g. Intended countermeasures, including security measures, safeguards, and mechanisms to protect Personal Data and be in regulatory compliance. This specifically references Article 25, Data protection by design and default.
h. Intended countermeasures to protect the rights and individual interests of Data Subjects and other concerned parties
i. Consultation with the appropriate supervisory and regulatory authorities defined under Article 36, Prior Consultation. This allows them to review:
    i. The draft DPIA
    ii. Supporting processing documents
    iii. Risk assessments
    iv. Intended Countermeasures
    v. The authorities are allowed up to eight weeks for their response
    vi. They can, under Article 58, Powers:
        1. Investigate Further
        2. Issue Fines or Reprimands
        3. Withdraw Certification of the Processes and/or technologies
        4. Order the erasure of Personal Data if an organization is noncompliant

12. Article 13: Right To Data Portability. Personal Data can be copied and given to the Data Subject to be used elsewhere.
13. Article 13: Right to Rectification. Personal Data can be corrected if it has errors.

GDPR is a comprehensive framework that gives EU Data Subjects significant control of their data. The DPIA process requires specific organizational structuring reminiscent of the Chief Risk Officer's role as a board-accountable senior leader as defined by the US Office of the Comptroller of the Currency [80]. It also requires assessment and continual monitoring of all new technologies and processes that process Personal Data. These must be completed by DPOs that have been given independence to complete their tasks without interference. It is more than just framework compliance. It is a fundamental restructuring of companies mandated under EU law to ensure that they are developing and maintaining secure and private systems to protect and process Personal Data. The purpose of providing the outline was to give organizations information they need to conduct the DPIA and integrate it into other frameworks and processes such as ISO/IEC 27001 or OCTAVE.

7.5.4 Operationally Critical Threat, Asset, and Vulnerability Evaluation (OCTAVE)

OCTAVE is a framework for identifying and managing information security risks [64]. It provides for a comprehensive evaluation method that examines both technological and business assets, along with the personnel involved in these processes. This was developed in 1999 by the Networked Systems Survivability Program of the Software Engineering Institute (SEI) at Carnegie Mellon University [64]. OCTAVE is designed to allow organizations to identify critical assets of all relevant types, threats to them, and the vulnerabilities that can expose those assets to threats. It is designed to provide a more complete view of risks than the frameworks that preceded it [64]. It leverages knowledge from SEI, one of the pioneers in the fields of software engineering and cybersecurity. Since 1984, they have been one of 10 Federally Funded Research and Development Centers, a nonprofit, public–private partnership sponsored by the US Department of Defense (DoD). They are the only one authorized to work with groups outside of DoD [81]. Knowledge from their years of experience went into development of OCTAVE. It was developed to address the security challenges DoD faced in addressing the implementation of the HIPAA Privacy and Security Rules [82].

OCTAVE consists of three phases and associated subprocesses. The three phases are [64]:

- Phase 1—Build Enterprise-Wide Security Requirements
- Phase 2—Identify Infrastructure Vulnerabilities
- Phase 3—Determine Security Risk Management Strategy

Phase 1 has four associated processes. These are designed to develop requirements based on knowledge at three core levels of the organization. They are:

- Process 1—Identify Enterprise Knowledge. Senior Management is queried to discover what they perceive to be the key assets and values, the threats that may befall them, what the risk indicators are, and what the current protection strategies are. Questions include:
  - What they believe key enterprise assets are
  - Perceived threats to assets
  - Current and planned strategies for enterprise asset protection
  - Perceived gaps in current protection strategies
  - What operational areas need to be evaluated?
  - Who the key operational and support managers are?
  - Applicable Laws and Regulations
- Process 2—Identify Operational Area Knowledge. Identified Operational and Support Management is asked the same questions that Senior Management was. The expectation is that the answers will not be the same. In addition, the management is queried as to who the top staff/individual contributors are, and what projects and support functions are involved with them.
- Process 3—Identify Staff Knowledge. The staff-level personnel and individual contributors are asked the same questions that Senior-level and Operational Management were, with the same expectation of differing answers.
- Process 4—Establish Security Requirements. This phase integrates the answers and perspectives from the first three processes. The enterprise outputs are:
  - Security Requirements
  - Prioritized view of Assets/Asset Map
  - View of Threats
  - Current view of Protection Strategies
  - Operational Risk Indicators
  - Protection Strategy Blueprint

Phase 2 has two associated processes. It uses the asset and threat information collected in Phase 1 to prioritize the physical and computing infrastructure components, and evaluates them to identify vulnerabilities [64]. The processes are:

- Process 5—Map High-Priority Information Assets to Information Infrastructure. This takes the information gathered in Phase 1 to identify asset locations, access paths, and most important, data flows. These help identify what the highest priority components are.
- Process 6—Perform Infrastructure Vulnerability Evaluation. This combines the gathered Phase 1 knowledge with staff infrastructure and asset knowledge, and standard information about intrusion

scenarios and vulnerabilities such as the CIS Controls, OWASP Top 10, or MITRE's Common Vulnerabilities and Exposures (CVE) database [83]. The gap analysis performed between these identifies missing policies and practices, along with infrastructure vulnerabilities and potential ones.

Phase 3 has two processes. It takes the information gathered in the first two phases to produce a Security Risk Management Strategy. The purpose of this is to generate a prioritized list of risks based on impact and probability. The processes are:

- Process 7—Conduct a multidimensional risk analysis. This is where risks are identified and prioritized based on impact and probability. The outputs are:
  - Validated intrusion scenarios
  - Exposed assets
  - Impact of exposed assets
  - Threat probability
  - Prioritized List of Risks
- Process 8—Develop Protection Strategy. The information from the previous seven steps is integrated to select mitigation approaches to improve enterprise security. The following information sources are considered:
  - Candidate Mitigation Approaches
  - Asset Impact of Approaches
  - Number of Assets at Risk
  - Solution Cost
  - Resource and Staff Availability

  The outputs from this process are:
- Candidate mitigation approaches
- Defined protection strategy
- Security Risk Management Plan
- Risk Management Measurement Information

OCTAVE is a framework that builds upon knowledge of all levels of the organization to develop a risk management plan that addresses the highest-priority risks. It does not proscribe prioritization methods or what specific inputs to use to do so; however, it provides that basic framework to do so. It can be used in combination with ISO/IEC 27001, GDPR, or other methods that require a RMF and do not specify one to be used.

7.5.5 OCTAVE Allegro

The OCTAVE Allegro framework is a streamlined version of the OCTAVE framework based upon field experience with its usage, specifically in Clark County, Nevada [82]. It was released in May 2007, in the publication Introducing OCTAVE Allegro: Improving the Information Security Risk Assessment Process. It is designed to be an evolution of OCTAVE that allows for broad assessment of the operational risk environment without extensive risk assessment knowledge [82]. It is designed to work with less resources than a full OCTAVE evaluation. It has eight key steps, much like OCTAVE's eight processes. It also has an extensive set of worksheets and templates organizations can use to streamline processes and increase repeatability included in the publication.

These steps are:

- Step 1—Establish Risk Measurement Criteria. This establishes the organizational drivers used to evaluate risk effects to an organization's mission and business objectives. Qualitative Risk measurement criteria are created and captured as part of the initial step. These are from an organizational view.
- Step 2—Develop an Information Asset Profile for information assets. These are representations of assets describing their unique features, qualities, characteristics, and values. They are clearly and consistently described. There is an unambiguous definition of asset boundaries, and the security requirements are defined.

The publication contains single worksheets that can be used for each profile.

- Step 3—Identify Information Asset Containers. Containers are the places where information assets are stored, transported, and processed. These can be local, in the cloud, or outsourced to a third party. These third parties, in turn, can outsource to fourth or even fifth parties. This step identifies all of these containers used by organizational assets.
- Step 4—Identify Areas of Concern. This step involves brainstorming about possible conditions or situations that can threaten information assets. These are referred to as Areas Of Concern and represent threats and possible outcomes. The purpose of this step is not to be comprehensive. It is to immediately capture initial thoughts on what threats are on the minds of the team.
- Step 5—Identify Threat Scenarios. The Areas Of Concern are expanded to full scenarios to better detail threat properties. Additional threats are considered by examining threat scenarios. The structure known as a Threat Tree, brought over from the OCTAVE method, is used to extrapolate those. The identified threat scenarios are defined as branches off one of the threat tree scenarios. The four types of scenarios represented in the Threat Tree are:
  - Human actors using technical means
  - Human actors using physical access
  - Technical problems/concerns
  - Other problems such as natural disasters, critical infrastructure risks, third-party risks, and other interdependency risks
- Step 6—Identify Risks. The organizational consequences of threat realization are captured. Threats can have multiple potential impacts, and the threat tree structure helps visualize this for the organization.
- Step 7—Analyze Risks. A simple quantitative analysis of the threat impacts is computed. This is derived from the risk impact and relative asset importance. This is done to prioritize risks to address.
- Step 8—Select Mitigation Approach. This is where organizations determine which of the identified risks require mitigation and develop strategies to do so. This involves prioritizing them based on the relative risk scores identified in Step 7. Then, mitigation strategies are developed based on asset values, security requirements, containers of residence, and the organization's unique environment.

OCTAVE Allegro is the result of significant customer input. It provides standard criteria and worksheets to address the concerns of needing to have significant risk management expertise. It allows organizations to conduct risk assessments without having to spend significant amounts to get that expertise either internally or externally. It is better for resource-constrained organizations that may not be able to afford ISO/IEC 27001 certification and still need to comply with regulations such as GDPR or the HIPAA Security Rule. It can be interchanged with them. In addition, more technical risk evaluation processes such as Vulnerability Scanning, the OWASP Top 10, CIS Controls, and CVE can be integrated within Step 5 to provide a more detailed threat picture. HIEs can leverage free and low-cost items such as these to perform risk assessments with limited resources and achieve results and continual improvement from doing so.

7.6 Technical risk management analysis methods

While there are a plethora of frameworks to help organizations more efficiently manage their information security processes, these frameworks do not cover how to discover or address specific technical vulnerabilities. They also do not know how to address processes and methods by which specific groups of methodologies can be found and addressed. Vulnerability Scanning, the CIS Common Security Controls, the HITRUST CSF, MITRE ATT&CK, MITRE D3FEND, and Penetration Testing all provide those additional details, controls, and control sets to augment laws and frameworks to address specific vulnerabilities and types of vulnerabilities. They provide the depth that is one level down from high-level frameworks to help organizations understand threats to their assets.

7.6.1 Vulnerability Scanning

Vulnerability Scanning is a critical component of risk analysis. It identifies where security risks are in assets and systems. It allows organizations to programmatically discover these and prioritize them so they can be mitigated. This is a type of risk analysis that the HIPAA Security Rule requires that organizations undertake for the purpose of continually assessing and addressing risks.

According to Holm, Sommestad, Alroth, and Persson in their paper A quantitative evaluation of vulnerability scanning, Vulnerability Scanning is when a database of vulnerability signatures is compared to the information obtained from a scan of the network to produce a list of vulnerabilities that are presumably present in the network [84]. These signatures are carefully constructed queries that attempt to verify their presence without service disruption. They also can assign severity to the vulnerabilities.

The most effective type of scan, according to them, is an authenticated one. This is where administrative credentials to target systems are utilized to scan for vulnerabilities. The vulnerability detection rate, in their paper, is 80%, as opposed to 44% for unauthenticated [84].

Vulnerability scores are usually identified using the NIST National Vulnerability Database (NVD) CVSS, version 3.0 Ratings [85]. This is a common scoring system used by multiple vendors and products to communicate the characteristics and severities of software vulnerabilities. It is designed to be, and used as, a standard measurement system for them. The NVD provides CVSS scores for almost all known vulnerabilities [85]. These ratings are summarized in Table 7.4.

Vendor vulnerabilities from products are reported, along with the CVSS score, in the CVE database at https://cve.mitre.org/index.html [83]. This site is maintained by the CVE Program [83]. Their purpose is to identify, define, and catalog publicly disclosed cybersecurity vulnerabilities [86]. Published vulnerabilities are assigned CVE records and identifiers.

Multiple vendors, such as Tenable, Rapid7, and Qualys provide vulnerability scanners that organizations can use. There are also numerous consulting and service firms that can also scan as a service. These vendors, products, and services utilize the CVE Identifier and CVSS score.

When an organization performs a vulnerability scan, it is critical to address the vulnerabilities with the highest CVSS numbers first, as they have the most critical risks. It is also critical to scan using an authenticated scan to

TABLE 7.4 Common vulnerability ratings and scores, according to National Institute of Standards and Technology [85].

Severity	Base score range
None	0.0
Low	0.1–3.9
Medium	4.0–6.9
High	7.0–8.9
Critical	9.0–10.0

identify more vulnerabilities. These also need to be regularly run as researchers discover new ones daily. With the numerous software products HIEs use, the business partner vendor risk, and the HITECH Act's requiring organizations to affirmatively prove that records were not exfiltrated during an attack, it is mission-critical to scan for and address vulnerabilities in their environments.

If an HIE develops or utilizes customized software, there is also the need to address security risks in the development or customization environments. The OWASP, which is a nonprofit foundation that works to improve software security via multiple means, publishes a list of the top 10 Web Application Security Risk categories on their web site [87]. They arrive at this list through community utilization of open source tools they develop, sponsor and vendor input, community education, and community feedback [87]. The OWASP Top 10, as it is known, is a standard for improving web application security. Utilizing it and its associated tools to examine code and customizations will greatly improve product security by addressing common vulnerabilities. Again, it will also help address the need to reduce environmental vulnerabilities that can result in data exfiltration and breaches.

7.6.2 CIS Critical Security Controls

Encompassing the entire technical environment is also incredibly important. Both the OWASP Top 10 and vulnerabilities can be encompassed in a set of 18 Critical Security Controls from the Center for Internet Security known as the CIS Critical Security Controls. Unlike the other frameworks discussed earlier, this is a technically focused one specific to technical security controls [88]. This was originally developed by the SANS Institute and called the SANS Top 20. It has been shortened to 18 controls. Its purpose is to provide an inventory of security controls organizations need as a baseline to protect themselves. These controls are [88]:

- CIS Control 1: Inventory and Control of Enterprise Assets
- CIS Control 2: Inventory and Control of Software Assets
- CIS Control 3: Data Protection
- CIS Control 4: Secure Configuration of Enterprise Assets and Software
- CIS Control 5: Account Management
- CIS Control 6: Access Control Management
- CIS Control 7: Continuous Vulnerability Management
- CIS Control 8: Audit Log Management
- CIS Control 9: Email Web Browser and Protections
- CIS Control 10: Malware Defenses
- CIS Control 11: Data Recovery
- CIS Control 12: Network Infrastructure Management
- CIS Control 13: Network Monitoring and Defense
- CIS Control 14: Security Awareness and Skills Training
- CIS Control 15: Service Provider Management
- CIS Control 16: Application Software Security
- CIS Control 17: Incident Response Management
- CIS Control 18: Penetration Testing

Utilizing these controls in conjunction with a framework like ISO 27001, OCTAVE, or OCTAVE Allegro will help provide a better understanding of actual technical control sets required to reduce risk.

7.6.3 HITRUST Common Security Framework (CSF)

The HITRUST is a nonprofit organization that creates and maintains the HITRUST CSF and HITRUST Assurance Program [89]. This was developed specifically for healthcare. Its goal is to provide organizations with a combination of over 40 control sets from authoritative sources, including ISO/IEC 27001, GDPR, the NIST Cybersecurity Framework, and Payment Card Industry-Data Security Standards (PCI-DSS) in one comprehensive framework [90]. Its goal is to Assess Once, Report Many. Unlike ISO/IEC 27001, the NIST Cybersecurity Framework, or the CIS Controls, it provides low-level technical details as part of the CSF.

Organizations can download the HITRUST CSF for free and identify the controls they need to address. They can then self-assess using a two-year Readiness Assessment using the MyCSF platform. Organizations then need to use an authorized HITRUST External Assessor to help with a two-year r2 Validated Assessment. This assessment is good for a certain version of the framework for two years. The organization then undergoes an r2 Validated Assessment, which is then audited by the HITRUST Assurance team. If the assessment score is high enough, the assessment passes. HITRUST then issues a Letter of Certification that is good for 2 years. Organizations are then required to conduct an r2 Interim Assessment at the one-year mark, and then recertify the year after [90].

This is popular because numerous payors and providers accept the HITRUST CSF. This means that the onboarding time for new products and services is drastically reduced as organizations do not have to do as much due diligence to assess the security of a new vendor. However, this will require the usage of a Certified Assessor to be properly certified. Gerry Miller, in his article What is the Cost of HITRUST CSF Certification in 2022?, gives a price range of $60K–$285K for a total cost [91]. This needs to be appropriately budgeted and planned for. However, due to its high degree of acceptance in healthcare, many organizations opt to use this. It can significantly reduce the time an HIE needs to prove their security is valid to provider organizations to be certified and increases credibility with them.

7.6.4 MITRE ATT&CK

The ATT&CK framework, developed by MITRE, provides documentation of common tactical goals (tactics), such as gaining credential access, with numerous techniques that can be used to do so (techniques) [92]. ATT&CK also specifies Subtechniques, which are more specific descriptions of the techniques, and procedures, which are specific implementations used for techniques or subtechniques. This framework is available in Enterprise and Mobile versions and is constantly updated. The version available at the current time is 10.1 [93]. There are 14 Enterprise tactics [94] as summarized in Table 7.5. Table 7.6 summarizes the 14 Mobile tactics [95], which are those used by mobile attackers.

The best use of ATT&CK is to use it in conjunction with a framework like OCTAVE or NIST to examine if assets are vulnerable to these tactics, what techniques can be used to exploit them, and what protection methods are most effective. Specific defense measures are covered within the D3FEND knowledge graph.

7.6.5 Mitre D3FEND

MITRE developed the D3FEND knowledge graph framework to meet the need of providing specific cybersecurity countermeasures and capabilities. It functions as a countermeasure knowledge base [96]. It also provides mappings from specific related ATT&CK tactics and techniques to actual implementations and countermeasures [96]. The matrix also provides specific definitions, digital artifacts, and references, including implementations and patents.

TABLE 7.5 Enterprise tactics from the ATT&CK framework, developed by MITRE [94].

Tactic	Description
Reconnaissance	The adversary is trying to gather information they can use to plan future operations.
Resource Development	The adversary is trying to establish resources they can use to support operations.
Initial Access	The adversary is trying to get into your network.
Execution	The adversary is trying to run malicious code.
Persistence	The adversary is trying to maintain their foothold.
Privilege Escalation	The adversary is trying to gain higher-level permissions.
Defense Evasion	The adversary is trying to avoid being detected.
Credential Access	The adversary is trying to steal account names and passwords.
Discovery	The adversary is trying to figure out your environment.
Lateral Movement	The adversary is trying to move through your environment.
Collection	The adversary is trying to gather data of interest to their goal.
Command and Control	The adversary is trying to communicate with compromised systems to control them.
Exfiltration	The adversary is trying to steal data.
Impact	The adversary is trying to manipulate, interrupt, or destroy your systems and data.

It is best used in conjunction with ATT&CK, Vulnerability Management, the CIS Controls, or Risk Management techniques to develop countermeasures to identified attack types and risks. This can be of great benefit to organizations looking to understand countermeasures without vendor bias. It is also excellent to use in Penetration Testing exercises.

7.6.6 Penetration Testing, Red Teams, Blue Teams, and Purple Teams

Penetration Testing, according to the NIST Computer Security Resource Center (CSRC), is a method of testing where testers target individual binary components or the application as a whole to determine whether intra or intercomponent vulnerabilities can be exploited to compromise the application, its data, or its environment resources [97]. This is often conflated with vulnerability scanning, which often uses carefully constructed queries to determine the existence and/or exploitation potential of vulnerabilities. Penetration Testing does not test to see whether a vulnerability exists or not. It tests just for exploitability. Tools such as Metasploit can provide an environment where Penetration Testers can determine whether or not mitigations have been mitigated [98]. Metasploit and other custom and open-source tools allow organizations to test for and demonstrate exploitation more easily.

With the emphasis on moving to more programmatic API-based frameworks such as FHIR 4.0.1 due to the Cures Act, Penetration Testing has become significantly more important. Alissa Valentina Knight's work in demonstrating exploitable application-level vulnerabilities in FHIR implementations shows its importance in protecting data [40]. More importantly, the

TABLE 7.6 Mobile tactics from the ATT&CK framework, developed by MITRE [95].

Tactic	Description
Initial Access	The adversary is trying to get into your device.
Execution	The adversary is trying to run malicious code.
Persistence	The adversary is trying to maintain their foothold.
Privilege Escalation	The adversary is trying to gain higher-level permissions.
Defense Evasion	The adversary is trying to avoid being detected.
Credential Access	The adversary is trying to steal account names, passwords, or other secrets that enable access to resources.
Discovery	The adversary is trying to figure out your environment.
Lateral Movement	The adversary is trying to move through your environment.
Collection	The adversary is trying to gather data of interest to their goal.
Command and Control	The adversary is trying to communicate with compromised devices to control them.
Exfiltration	The adversary is trying to steal data.
Impact	The adversary is trying to manipulate, interrupt, or destroy your devices and data.
Network Effects	The adversary is trying to intercept or manipulate network traffic to or from a device.
Remote Service Effects	The adversary is trying to control or monitor the device using remote services.

HITECH Act requires affirmative proof that these vulnerabilities were not exploited to not have all application data in their purview to be considered breached. As vulnerabilities do not log accesses like applications do, it is critical to perform accurate penetration tests, not just vulnerability scans, to ensure that PHI is being protected.

Red Teams, according again to the NIST CSRC, are groups of people authorized to emulate a potential adversary's attack or exploitation capabilities against an enterprise's security posture. Their objective is to improve enterprise cybersecurity by demonstrating the impacts of successful attacks and what works for the defenders in an operational environment [99]. They leverage Penetration Testing to accomplish these tasks.

Their work directly improves that of the Blue Team, who are the group responsible for defending an enterprise's use of information systems by maintaining its security posture against a group of mock attackers such as the Red Team. They must defend against real or simulated attacks over a significant period, in a representative operational context, and according to rules of engagement [100]. In a real operational environment, they are responsibly for operational monitoring and continual improvement of defenses to protect against ever-evolving attacks.

Purple Teams are a newer concept designed to enhance information sharing between the Red and Blue teams to maximize their respective and combined effectiveness [101]. According to SCYTHE, a vendor in this space, it is an open engagement where attack activity is explained to the Blue Team as it occurs. The goal is to improve people, process, and technology in real time [102]. They emulate known Tactics, Techniques, and Procedures leveraged by real-world threat actors. Usage of the ATT&CK and D3FEND frameworks, along with other vendor platforms, can help facilitate communication here.

The use of Red, Blue, and Purple Teams as part of Penetration Testing can assist HIEs in ensuring that the services they provide customers are reasonably and appropriately secure. They can also assist with information sharing and providing current information on real-world attacks.

7.7 Risk assessments, risk management plans, and risk registers in the healthcare management process for Health Information Exchanges

While this chapter has discussed several interpretations of risk assessments in the context of various frameworks, it has not in the context of HIEs. NIST classifies a risk assessment as the process of identifying risks to organizational operations, organizational assets, individuals, other organizations, and the Nation [103]. The purpose of doing one for an HIE is to gather an understanding of the internal and external threats to the organization and to business partners. Much of the security risk assessment material out there is geared toward Covered Entities, not Business Associates.

The Office of the National Coordinator for Health Information Technology released a Security Risk Assessment tool that can be run locally. While it is designed for providers that participate in the EHR incentive program, it can also be leveraged for HIEs [104]. This was released in October 2018. This tool provides an assessment of Physical, Administrative, and Technical security requirements in line with the HIPAA Security Rule, and is enough to do a basic assessment.

For the findings, NIST recommends the NIST RMF. It integrates security, privacy, and cyber supply chain risk management into the system development lifecycle [105]. The RMF has seven key steps:

- Prepare—Identify key management roles, establish organizational strategy and risk tolerance, conduct an organization-wide risk assessment, identify common controls, and develop an organization-wide strategy for continuous monitoring.
- Categorize—Inform organizational risk management processes and tasks by determining the adverse impact to system confidentiality, integrity, and availability, and the information stored, processed, or transmitted by them.
- Select—Select, tailor, and document the controls necessary to protect the system and organization commensurate with risk.
- Implement—Implement the controls in the security and privacy plans for the system and organizations.
- Assess—Determine if the controls are implemented correctly, operating as intended, and producing the desired outcome with respect to meeting the security and privacy requirements for the system and organization.
- Authorize—Senior official makes a risk-based decision to authorize the system.
- Monitor—Continuously monitor control implementation and system risks.

The Risk Management Plan that HHS and other organizations require aligns with the NIST RMF, and the NIST Cybersecurity Framework. However, the items implemented needed to implement the controls required need to be tracked and monitored. It is just not about implementing them. The Security Rule, ISO/IEC 27001, and the NIST Cybersecurity

Framework all require controls implementation tracking, assessment, and monitoring.

The Risk Register is the document that captures that information in one central place for the purposes of communicating and tracking risks. It needs to be used consistently, iteratively, and to review and track even closed risks. It is a critical part of the risk management process to demonstrate closure.

NIST, in their NISTIR 8286 document, Integrating Cybersecurity and Enterprise Risk Management (ERM), documents their recommended Risk Register elements [106]. The purpose is to provide info on all identified risks and statuses in one place and categorize them. These elements are summarized in Table 7.7.

Risk Registers provide an important tool for following up from Risk Assessments and Risk Management Plans. They help organizations such as HIEs track outstanding and closed risks to ensure they are being worked on, addressed, and monitored for continual effectiveness. However, while NIST puts together a good framework, it does not address many of the basic functions that modern security functions that HIEs need, specifically cross-organizational governance.

7.7.1 OCTAVE FORTE for Health Information Exchange networks and modern needs

One of the major concerns with cybersecurity for HIEs is that many of the governance frameworks assume nondistributed organizations that do not depend on third-party data interchange. OCTAVE has had multiple iterations courtesy of Carnegie Mellon University's (CMU) SEI's continued evolution of the framework. OCTAVE FORTE provides a 10-step process by which organizations can manage Cyber and Enterprise Risk [107].

This evolution of the framework came out in 2020. It is designed to help organizations use ERM principles to bridge the gap between enterprise and operational risks. Like the original OCTAVE framework, it focuses on risk at the Executive, Management, and Practitioner levels [107]. CMU SEI also provides significant resources and templates at https://resources.sei.cmu.edu/library/asset-view.cfm?assetID = 644636 for implementing this [108].

This example implementation will go through the 10 steps of OCTAVE FORTE and adapt each to the unique needs of HIEs. The purpose of this is to not only explain this iteration of OCTAVE. It is to also provide a nonprovider specific version of RMFs that can also be adapted for other organizations in Business Associate capacities.

7.7.1.1 Step 1—Establish risk governance and appetite

In this step, the organization needs to establish a governance structure for its ERM program. This needs to have guidance about roles, responsibilities, policies, resources, and information flow [107]. FORTE recommends a three-tier governance structure. These levels all need to operate according to a documented and board-approved charter that establishes authority, sets direction, and sets operational procedures [107].

- Tier 1: Executive Board. This includes the roles of senior executives, an advisory board in a nonprofit, or a group of senior executives/appointees in a public organization. For HIEs, the inclusion of Chief Information Officers (CIOs), Chief Information Security Officers (CISOs), and Chief Medical Information Officers (CMIOs) from member organizations is recommended at this level so that they have a view into the organization's security and processes. This group sets the strategic direction and approves policy. They institute authority into the governance structure.

TABLE 7.7 Risk register elements from the NISTIR 8286 [106].

Register element	Description
ID (Risk Identifier)	A sequential numeric identifier for referring to a risk in the risk register
Risk Description	A brief explanation of the cybersecurity risk scenario (potentially) impacting the organization and enterprise. Risk descriptions are often written in a cause and effect format, such as "if X occurs, then Y happens"
Risk Category	An organizing construct that enables multiple risk register entries to be consolidated [e.g., using SP 800-53 Control Families: Access Control (AC), Audit and Accountability (AU)]. Consistent risk categorization is helpful for comparing risk registers during the risk aggregation step of Enterprise Risk Management
Current Assessment—Likelihood	An estimation of the probability, before any risk response, that this scenario will occur. On the first iteration of the risk cycle, this may also be considered the initial assessment
Current Assessment—Impact	Analysis of the potential benefits or consequences that might result from this scenario if no additional response is provided. On the first iteration of the risk cycle, this may also be considered the initial assessment
Current Assessment—Exposure Rating	A calculation of the probability of risk exposure based on the likelihood estimate and the determined benefits or consequences of the risk. Throughout this report, the combination of impact and likelihood is referred to as exposure. Other common frameworks use different terms for this combination, such as level of risk (e.g., ISO 31000, NIST SP 800-30 Rev. 1). On the first iteration of the risk cycle, this may also be considered the initial assessment
Risk Response Type	The risk response (sometimes referred to as the risk treatment) for handling the identified risk
Risk Response Cost	The estimated cost of applying the risk response
Risk Response Description	A brief description of the risk response. For example, "Implement software management application XYZ to ensure that software platforms and applications are inventoried," or "Develop and implement a process to ensure the timely receipt of threat intelligence from [name of specific information sharing forums and sources]"
Risk Owner	The designated party responsible and accountable for ensuring that the risk is maintained in accordance with enterprise requirements. The Risk Owner may work with a designated Risk Manager who is responsible for managing and monitoring the selected risk response
Status	A field for tracking the current condition of the risk and any next activities

- Tier 2: Risk Committee. This includes executive leaders from across the organization such as the Chief Financial Officer (CFO), CISO, and Chief Operating Officer (COO). They set policy and procedure, and partner with the audit team. They provide advocacy and resources. They also periodically review the policies and procedures.
- Tier 3: Risk Subcommittee(s). These include high-performing managers from across the organization. They enforce policy and oversee processes. They oversee risk response plans and risk management

performance. They also advise on technical aspects. These are function-based.

The purpose of these tiers is to gather input at all levels and build workable policies that can be enforced. Including HIE partners at the board level ensures the interlocks needed with partner organizations to improve security and share risks.

As part of their role, these committees help define the risk appetite as part of their work. This is the general amount and type of risk the organization is willing to take to meet its strategic objectives. The risk appetite statement describes this. It needs to align with the strategic objectives of the organization. It also needs to realize them as risks and opportunities. This needs to be periodically reviewed, especially given the legislative, technical, and procedural changes that HIEs operate under.

Risk tolerances, especially given the negative impacts of information system implementations, need to be well defined. Financial, technical, and resource risks needs to be documented.

7.7.1.2 Step 2—Scope critical services and assets

Like the original OCTAVE framework, this step involves understanding the critical services, assets, and resources a company needs. These resources need to be documented in an asset catalog. These need to include people, information, technologies, and facilities. They also need to include cloud-based resources. Based on real-life examples of ransomware attacks, people and resource information at client facilities need to be considered part of an HIE asset catalog and kept updated and maintained. The risk of not having someone to contact in case of an attack, or when suspicious traffic is seen from a machine for the first time is significant. Knowing what assets clients use to connect and interchange info and knowing who to contact when something goes wrong are critical.

7.7.1.3 Step 3—Identify resilience requirements of assets

This step is normally ambiguous about the methods used to identify and document resilience requirements. Healthcare has utilized a standardized method for years called Failure Mode and Effects Analysis (FMEA). This is a systematic method of identifying product and process problems before they occur [109]. It is aimed at the prevention of tragedy. It does not require previous bad experiences. It is also designed to make systems more robust and fault-tolerant.

It was begun in the 1940s by the US military as a process analysis tool. It is normally used for continual improvement [110]. It is designed to be used:

- When a process, product, or service is being designed or redesigned, after quality function deployment;
- When an existing process, product, or service is being applied in a new way;
- Before developing control plans for a new or modified process;
- When improvement goals are planned for an existing process, product, or service;
- When analyzing failures of an existing process, product, or service; and
- Periodically throughout the life of the process, product, or service.

Risk analysis fits into several of these categories.

The recommended process is to follow the American Society for Quality's process, which is available at https://asq.org/quality-resources/fmea, for each identified critical asset [110]. Calculate the Severity, which is how serious each effect is, from a scale of 1–10, the Occurrence, which is the probability of failure, also from 1–10, and the Detection Rating, which is how well the current controls can detect either the cause or failure more after they have happened, but before the customer is affected. That is also 1–10. Multiply the three together to get the Risk Priority Number. Identify recommended actions to reduce this number. Leverage this for each identified asset to get a prioritized list of assets by highest risks to resilience.

7.7.1.4 Step 4—Measure current capabilities and Step 5—Identify risks, threats, and vulnerabilities to assets

In these steps, there are three components. The risk manager reviews the organization's existing controls, assesses their effectiveness, and creates a prioritized list of controls. There are several options organizations can utilize to complete this review, based on previously discussed controls sets:

- Use of the Systems Readiness Assessment/ Security Risk Assessment Tool from the US Department of Health and Human Services (HHS)
- ISO/IEC 27001 Controls Assessment
- NIST Cybersecurity Framework assessment, using Intel's application of it as a model
- HITRUST CSF MyCSF Analysis
- GDPR Data Protection Impact Analysis
- OCTAVE or OCTAVE Allegro Risk Analysis
- CIS Controls Analysis

In addition to using one or more of those frameworks, complete the following analyses:

- Full testing of Endpoint Detection and Response (EDR) Software used on endpoints and servers
- Full credentialed vulnerability scan of all internal and external assets
- Full penetration tests of all externally available services, prioritizing API communications, file interchange, and communications first
  - This is to ensure that assets using FHIR, HL7, or similar APIs are assessed
- OWASP Top 10 Analysis on code and customizations
- Physical walkthroughs and penetration tests on protected physical assets
- Modeling attack types and identified vulnerabilities detected in FMEA, penetration testing, and vulnerability scanning against MITRE ATT&CK

Use the information from the completed frameworks and the identified effects from the FMEA in Step 3 to create a prioritized list of controls to address. Add the greatest risks and controls gaps identified by the FMEA, vulnerability scans, and penetration tests. Use the combined list as the prioritized list of controls.

These two steps are combined because the current technical capabilities and risks, threats, and vulnerabilities are combined when performing a technical risk analysis. One of the major gaps in security risk analysis of technical assets is a lack of penetration testing or evaluation against the OWASP Top 10. As healthcare and HIEs move toward API-based models of data interchange, the combination becomes critical to be able to assess and address risks, threats, and vulnerabilities in these systems that a vulnerability scan or risk assessment will not pick up.

7.7.1.5 Step 6—Analyze risks against capabilities

The data from Steps 4 and 5 is prioritized, categorized, and analyzed against the organization's risk appetite statement. The impacts and likelihood are determined from the risk analyses, FMEA, penetration tests, and vulnerability scans. They are plotted against current capabilities to determine where the gaps are and where improvement can occur. A Risk Register, preferably in NISTIR 8286 format, is constructed to catalog this. The risk scores from the FMEA are used to prioritize the risks. It needs to be effectively managed and updated to reflect changes.

7.7.1.6 *Step 7—Plan for response*

This step involves developing the response plans to determine what the organization will do to reduce and respond to risk. These are normally developed by the risk owners and address risks. These plans are designed to disrupt, reduce, or avoid the following [107]:

- risk triggers from taking place
- consequences from making meaningful impact
- conditions aligning that would allow risks to become a reality

Risk owners need to be educated about risk, how risk response affects the bottom line, and because some stakeholders are still reticent about spending for risk mitigation. This is despite the significant amount of ransomware attacks that have crippled healthcare organizations, and that there is still the belief among many executives that it will not happen to them.

Modeling planned responses and identified vulnerabilities and risks against MITRE D3FEND is also recommended to implement the best solutions for addressing vulnerabilities. It also provides credible methods mapped against industry standards to demonstrate that the most applicable risk mitigations are being implemented.

This makes it critical for risk owners to develop plans consistent with the risk policy, risk register, and risk appetite statements. These also need to align with a business case and the organization's strategy. For each identified risk, a response plan using one of the seven Risk Response Strategies is developed. These strategies are [107]:

- Mitigate—Take actions to limit the likelihood that the risk will occur or limit its impact if it does occur.
- Transfer—Distribute the exposure of the risk to others to minimize the risk's impact.
- Avoid—Cease activity or avoid conditions that may enable the risk to become an issue.
- Accept—Take no action to mitigate the risk while continuing activities that constitute it.
- Enhance—Take action to bolster the positive impacts of the risk when it becomes a reality (typically used for opportunistic risks).
- Exploit—Take action to raise the likelihood of a risk becoming a reality (typically used for opportunistic risks).
- Share—Partner with others to divide the impacts of a risk among amenable parties.

Most organizations have finite resources to address risks. Addressing the highest priority ones through use of the risk scores is in alignment with the principle of preserving scarce resources. Identifying interdependent risks, which can help increase support and reduce resource requirements by spreading them across multiple groups and reduce silos. It can also help gather the governance support required.

The plans to address risks need to have Specific, Measurable, Attainable, Relevant, and Timely (SMART) goals for the response plans [107]. They need project plans developed. These plans need to be maintained, updated in the risk register, and kept updated.

7.7.1.7 *Step 8—Implement the response plans*

In this step, there are three components [107]:

1. Ensure that the projects are well resourced
2. Have the following:
   a. A project plan with scope, schedule, budget, requirements, and risks
   b. Measurable success criteria
   c. Milestones toward success
   d. A project manager that leads the project and is responsible for operation and completion

3. Standardized measurement and performance reporting metrics

This step involves making sure that the risk management plans are organized into projects.

7.7.1.8 *Step 9—Define metrics*

These projects need to have [107]:

1. Metrics attached to them to define progress that are tailored to objectives, progress, and the overall ERM program.
2. Measured overall ERM program effectiveness through the following metrics:
   a. Response plan implementation progress.
   b. Risk exposure monitoring. If the exposure continues or increases, then this may become a bigger issue
3. Monitored impacts from risk exposure, and whether they are greater or lesser than expected. Postimpact analysis, such as from an actual attack, can help assess this.

7.7.1.9 *Step 10—Review, update, and repeat*

This step discusses if the risk program has controlled risks effectively through stakeholder input. These inputs are developed into an improvement plan that addresses investment, training, communication, policy changes, contingency planning, org changes, and asset procurement. The improvement plan is then implemented and monitored. This entire process is repeated.

The OCTAVE FORTE process can capture the needs of a risk management program for HIEs. It is also capable of adapting for more modern needs, such as penetration testing. The overall program developed from its 10 steps can also accommodate other required frameworks such as GDPR, HIPAA, or the NIST Cybersecurity Framework. Technical vulnerability testing as a separate part alongside these frameworks helps identify technical risks from emerging technologies such as APIs and FHIR for the purpose of better and more accurate risk mitigation. The use of FMEA for risk resilience uses a standard process to score these in line with its use in healthcare. The goal of this improved program is to leverage a popular framework in a way that it can be used internationally independent of country-dependent security frameworks such as HIPAA or GDPR. Integrating newer frameworks including MITRE ATT&CK and D3FEND to help model risks and mitigations, along with application and penetration testing, addresses gaps that these frameworks do not cover.

7.8 Emerging trends

7.8.1 Trusted Exchange Framework and Security

The TEFCA has the goals of scaling HIE nationwide and ensuring that all stakeholders have real-time access to interoperable health information [111]. A single network is not possible. However, having multiple networks that can interoperate allows EHI to follow the patient, and can scale at a national level. These need common operating procedures and technical standards. As part of these standards, FHIR is being considered as an interchange standard in this framework for patient data interoperability. The first release of this framework is scheduled for Q1 2022.

Alissa Valentina Knight's research into FHIR implementations demonstrates that there is significant implementation quality, variety, and security issues in many of them [55]. However, the security requirements in Draft 2 of the TEFCA framework only address compliance with the HIPAA Privacy and Security Rules, and the NIST Cybersecurity Framework. It does not integrate the people, processes, and technologies needed to address conformance testing as part of security, penetration testing, vulnerability management, or API security.

Further clarification, and the adoption of stronger security practices, can help address significant potential security and privacy risks in TEFCA.

7.8.2 Blockchain/Distributed Ledger Technologies

The use of Blockchain/Distributed Ledger Technologies as a potential interchange method for healthcare data exchange has been discussed by many. The HIMSS Blockchain Task Force, in their article TEFCA and Blockchain: Enabling Trusted Data Flow Between Health Networks, discusses how the technology can be used in conjunction with HL7 and FHIR APIs to provide peer to peer data exchange between organizations [112].

Blockchain is a type of Distributed Ledger Technology that distributes cryptographically signed data in a shared ledger across a network. There is no inherent central administration of the ledger [113]. Changes are made by consensus and associated algorithms. These algorithms can change depending on the implementation. Blockchain networks can be public/permissionless, where everyone has access to participate pseudonymously, or private/permissioned, where only trusted partners can operate.

The "block" in blockchain is a set of transactions that are bundled together in a block, cryptographically signed, and secured, ordered chronologically, and then appended to the previous block. It is based on the Linked List data structure developed in computer science and used as a base element of software development. Each block contains the hash of the previous block, the timestamp when added, the Merkle Root Hash for all transactions in the block, and a nonce, aka number only used once, which is the cryptographic challenge being solved for to propose a new block [113].

Blockchain data can be stored either on-chain, which has the potential of violating the HIPAA Privacy and Security Rules, or off-chain on third-party storage [113]. The Interplanetary File System was designed to allow for third-party storage while preserving privacy and security by allowing individual files to be protected [114].

Smart Contracts, which are automated programs that can run on top of Blockchain, are also prevalent. Enterprise Resource Planning systems such as SAP and Oracle already integrate it [115].

There are many projects that are still in pilot stages. There are also companies such as IBM, Deloitte, and Hashed Health providing services to companies wishing to implement these solutions [116]. Hashed Health, for example, has the ProCredEx credentials exchange already in production. While there have been many false starts, there are credible projects being used in the marketplace now and large firms providing advisory services. This technology, due to improvements in security, is going to increase in usage. As HIEs increase use of distributed technologies via technologies like TEFCA, Blockchain and Smart Contracts will likely see a corresponding increase.

7.8.3 Decentralized Identifiers

DIDs enable verifiable decentralized digital identity. These can refer to any subject, such as a person, organization, thing, data model, or abstract entity [117]. These are designed to be decoupled from central registries, providers, and Certificate Authorities. These are Universal Resource Indicators that allow interactions associated with subjects using defined APIs.

Due to the decentralized nature of newer web technologies, there will be multiple means by which subjects can prove identity. DIDs provide a general syntax for large and small systems to interoperate, and works with technologies such as Blockchain to provide systems for verifying distributed identities. This is under current development with the W3C and has been implemented by companies such as Hashed Health and Evernym. With the implementation of TEFCA and its de-emphasizing monolithic technologies, the use of DIDs to provide interchange between participants may increase.

7.9 Summary

Cybersecurity for HIEs can best be described as a gray area. Much of the guidance available for organizations that have to comply with HIPAA is aimed at providers, not business associates. There are a significant amount of frameworks that exist. However, these frameworks do not address the technical and risk assessment needs that organizations require to make decisions on scarce resource allocations. Specific explanations on risk management processes, encryption requirements, and quantitative risk analysis have not been fully explained, which is what this chapter attempts to do. Aligning security requirements internationally with the GDPR and/or other applicable international privacy laws, and OCTAVE is also important. Providing a set of controls, tests, and processes that HIEs can use in conjunction with security risk management processes adds additional details they can use to better assess and address risks.

As HIEs move into an API-based world from one driven by file-based interchange, being able to address the cybersecurity needs of protecting these systems is critical. Application Security, Vulnerability Management, use of the MITRE ATT&CK and D3FEND frameworks, and Penetration Testing are important to providing distributed security that affirmatively protects patient data.

More importantly, leveraging international standards and the latest version of OCTAVE, OCTAVE FORTE, to be able to develop an HIE-specific enterprise information security RMF that can be used worldwide while providing the means for organizations to protect themselves against emerging threats was the goal of this chapter. HIEs are a key component in providing patient care when adverse events, such as downtimes or ransomware attacks, occur. They need the best protection possible because of that and asking them to utilize frameworks meant for providers is not going to meet their needs. The material provided today hopefully provides an illustration on what regulations apply, what the real threats are, and a path forward for organizations to follow to improve their security.

Questions for discussion

1. The HITECH Act requires the use of NIST-Approved encryption. Can encryption algorithms have their approvals revoked because of age or weakness even if previously approved? Provide an example of how NIST Special Publications have evolved since the initial Breach Notification Rule
2. Does the GDPR require security by design? How does this compare and contract with the NIST Cybersecurity Framework in how they approach application of security?
3. Is it recommended, if your organization wants an ISO/IEC 27001 certification, to use an independent auditor? Why or why not? Where would there be a potential conflict of interest?
4. Does the GDPR Right To Be Forgotten applies to public health data?
5. Since the HIPAA Security Rule indicates that encryption is addressable, it means that my organization does not have to do it

and can claim it is too much effort. Why or why not is not this the case?

6. Why are data ransomed in a ransomware attack considered breached?
7. True or False? The NIST Cybersecurity Framework is a skeleton that organizations can use to build their own frameworks.
8. Does the NIST Cybersecurity Framework cover penetration testing? What category does it fall under in the framework, and why?
9. Do any current frameworks cover MITRE ATT&CK or D3FEND? If not, what frameworks would it best work in conjunction with?
10. Does GDPR mandate specific types of encryption? How is its application different than the Breach Notification Rule?
11. Is FIPS 140-3 based off of international standards? If so, which ones?
12. How do the OCTAVE frameworks handle organizational perceptions of risk at multiple levels?

References

[1] SEC401: Security essentials: network, endpoint, and cloud [Internet]. SANS Institute; [cited 2021 December 21]. Available from: https://www.sans.org/information-security/.

[2] Cisco. What is cybersecurity? [Internet]. Cisco; 2021 [cited 2021 December 21]. Available from: https://www.cisco.com/c/en/us/products/security/what-is-cybersecurity.html#:~:text=Cybersecurity%20is%20the%20practice%20of,or%20interrupting%20normal%20business%20processes.

[3] Alert (AA21-243A) [Internet]. CISA; [cited 2021 December 21]. Available from: https://www.cisa.gov/uscert/ncas/alerts/aa21-243a.

[4] Snell E. How an HIE aided in recovery from a ransomware attack [Internet]. HealthITSecurity; 2018 [cited 2021 December 21]. Available from: https://healthitsecurity.com/news/how-an-hie-aided-in-recovery-from-a-ransomware-attack.

[5] HEALTHeLINK. Who we are [Internet]. HEALTHeLINK; 2021 [cited 2021 December 29]. Available from: https://wnyhealthelink.com/who-we-are/.

[6] Snell E. How an HIE aided in recovery from a ransomware attack [Internet]. HealthITSecurity; 2018 [cited 2021 December 29]. Available from: https://healthitsecurity.com/news/how-an-hie-aided-in-recovery-from-a-ransomware-attack.

[7] Department of Health [Internet]. New York State Trauma Centers; 2021 [cited 2021 December 29]. Available from: https://www.health.ny.gov/professionals/ems/state_trauma/trauma2.htm.

[8] Home – Health Information Sharing and Analysis Center: H-ISAC [Internet]. H-ISAC. Healthcare ISAC; 2021 [cited 2021 December 29]. Available from: https://h-isac.org/.

[9] Trend Micro. Indicators of compromise [Internet]. Definition; 2021 [cited 2021 December 29]. Available from: https://www.trendmicro.com/vinfo/us/security/definition/indicators-of-compromise.

[10] HIPAA administrative simplification – HHS.gov [Internet]. HIPAA Administrative Simplification. US Department of Health and Human Services; 2013 [cited 2021 December 29]. Available from: https://www.hhs.gov/sites/default/files/ocr/privacy/hipaa/administrative/combined/hipaa-simplification-201303.pdf.

[11] (OCR) Ofor CR. The security rule [Internet]. HHS.gov.; 2021 [cited 2021 December 29]. Available from: https://www.hhs.gov/hipaa/for-professionals/security/index.html.

[12] Health Information Technology and HIPAA – HHS.gov [Internet]. The HIPAA Privacy Rule and Electronic Health Information Exchange in a Networked Environment. US Department of Health and Human Services; 2008 [cited 2021 December 29]. Available from: https://www.hhs.gov/sites/default/files/ocr/privacy/hipaa/understanding/special/healthit/introduction.pdf.

[13] Editor CSRCC. Addressable – glossary [Internet]. CSRC. National Institute of Standards and Technology; 2021 [cited 2021 December 29]. Available from: https://csrc.nist.gov/glossary/term/addressable.

[14] (OCR) Ofor CR. Summary of the HIPAA security rule [Internet]. HHS.gov. US Department of Health and Human Services; 2021 [cited 2021 December 29]. Available from: https://www.hhs.gov/hipaa/for-professionals/security/laws-regulations/index.html.

[15] HIPAA encryption requirements [Internet]. HIPAA Journal; 2020 [cited 2021 December 29]. Available from: https://www.hipaajournal.com/hipaa-encryption-requirements/.

[16] (OCR) Ofor CR. Summary of the HIPAA security rule [Internet]. HHS.gov. US Department of Health and Human Services; 2021 [cited 2021 December 29].

Available from: https://www.hhs.gov/hipaa/for-professionals/security/laws-regulations/index.html.

[17] Editor CSRCC. Cryptographic hash function – glossary [Internet]. CSRC. National Institute of Standards and Technology; 2021 [cited 2021 December 29]. Available from: https://csrc.nist.gov/glossary/term/cryptographic_hash_function.

[18] Dang Q. Recommendation for applications using approved hash algorithms [Internet]. CSRC. National Institute of Standards and Technology; 2012 [cited 2021 December 29]. Available from: https://csrc.nist.gov/publications/detail/sp/800-107/rev-1/final.

[19] Stage 3 medicaid security risk analysis tip sheet – CMS [Internet]. Stage 3 Medicaid security risk analysis tip sheet: protect patient health information. US Department of Health and Human Services; 2016 [cited 2021 December 29]. Available from: https://www.cms.gov/Regulations-and-Guidance/Legislation/EHRIncentivePrograms/Downloads/SecurityRiskAnalysis_Tipsheet_Stage3Medicaid.pdf.

[20] Karlinsky FE, Fidei RJ, Stanfield TF, Brito C. Cybersecurity and data privacy in the insurance industry: maintaining a culture of compliance with evolving standards [Internet]. The Demotech Difference; 2020 [cited 2021 December 29]. Available from: https://www.gtlaw.com/-/media/files/insights/published-articles/2020/02/cybersecurity-and-data-privacy-in-the-insurance-industry.pdf.

[21] (OCR) Ofor CR [Internet]. HITECH Act Enforcement Interim Final Rule. US Department of Health and Human Services; 2021 [cited 2021 December 29]. Available from: https://www.hhs.gov/hipaa/for-professionals/special-topics/hitech-act-enforcement-interim-final-rule/index.html.

[22] Medicare & Medicaid Ehr Incentive Program – CMS. US Department of Health and Human Services; 2010 [cited 2021 December 29]. Available from: https://www.cms.gov/Regulations-and-Guidance/Legislation/EHRIncentivePrograms/Downloads/MU_Stage1_ReqOverview.pdf.

[23] Direct basics: Q&A for providers. National Learning Consortium; 2014 [cited 2021 December 29]. Available from: https://www.healthit.gov/sites/default/files/directbasicsforprovidersqa_05092014.pdf.

[24] HIPAA omnibus final rule implements tiered penalty structure for HIPAA violations. RMcGuireWoods; 2013 [cited 2021 December 29]. Available from: https://www.mcguirewoods.com/client-resources/Alerts/2013/2/HIPAA-Omnibus-Final-Rule-Implements-Tiered-Penalty-Structure-HIPAA-Violations.

[25] (OCR) Ofor CR. HITECH Act Enforcement Interim Final Rule [Internet]. HHS.gov. US Department of Health and Human Services; 2021 [cited 2021 December 29]. Available from: https://www.hhs.gov/hipaa/for-professionals/special-topics/hitech-act-enforcement-interim-final-rule/index.html.

[26] Notification of Enforcement Discretion Regarding HIPAA Civil Money Penalties. US Department of Health and Human Services; 2019 [cited 2021 December 29]. Available from: https://www.federalregister.gov/documents/2019/04/30/2019-08530/notification-of-enforcement-discretion-regarding-hipaa-civil-money-penalties.

[27] (OCR) Ofor CR. Breach notification rule [Internet]. HHS.gov. US Department of Health and Human Services; 2021 [cited 2021 December 29]. Available from: https://www.hhs.gov/hipaa/for-professionals/breach-notification/index.html.

[28] CVE-2014-0160 detail. National Institute of Standards and Technology; 2020 [cited 2021 December 29]. Available from: https://nvd.nist.gov/vuln/detail/CVE-2014-0160.

[29] Computer Security Division ITL. Block cipher techniques: CSRC [Internet]. National Institute of Standards and Technology; 2020 [cited 2021 December 29]. Available from: https://csrc.nist.gov/projects/block-cipher-techniques.

[30] Computer Security Division ITL. NIST policy on hash functions – hash functions: CSRC [Internet]. National Institute of Standards and Technology; 2020 [cited 2021 December 29]. Available from: https://csrc.nist.gov/projects/hash-functions/nist-policy-on-hash-functions.

[31] Verdult R. The (in)security of proprietary cryptography [Internet]. KU Leuven; 2015 [cited 2021 December 29]. Available from: http://roel.verdult.xyz/publications/phd_thesis-roel_verdult.pdf.

[32] 45 CFR Parts 160 and 164 Breach Notification for Unsecured Protected Health Information; Interim Final Rule. US Department of Health and Human Services; 2009 [cited 2021 December 29]. Available from: https://www.govinfo.gov/content/pkg/FR-2009-08-24/pdf/E9-20169.pdf.

[33] Computer Security Division ITL. Cryptographic module validation program: CSRC [Internet]. National Institute of Standards and Technology; 2021 [cited 2021 December 29]. Available from: https://csrc.nist.gov/projects/cryptographic-module-validation-program.

[34] Computer Security Division ITL. Cryptographic algorithm validation program: CSRC [Internet]. National Institute of Standards and Technology; 2021 [cited 2021 December 29]. Available from: https://csrc.nist.gov/projects/cryptographic-algorithm-validation-program.

[35] Computer Security Division ITL. TLS guidelines: NIST publishes SP 800-52 Revision 2 [Internet]. National

Institute of Standards and Technology; 2019 [cited 2021 December 29]. Available from: https://csrc.nist.gov/News/2019/nist-publishes-sp-800-52-revision-2.

[36] FACT SHEET: Ransomware and HIPAA. US Department of Health and Human Services; 2016 [cited 2021 December 29]. Available from: https://www.hhs.gov/sites/default/files/RansomwareFactSheet.pdf.

[37] WTHR Indianapolis. Data stolen in Eskenazi Cyberattack leaked on Dark Web [Internet]. wthr.com. WTHR Indianapolis; 2021 [cited 2021 December 29]. Available from: https://www.wthr.com/article/news/local/eskenazi-cyberattack-personal-data-leaked-dark-web/531-6c02dacb-6ba3-48d6-b0a2-9b456f7d2226.

[38] IBM. Cost of a data breach report 2020 [Internet]. IBM; 2020 [cited 2021 December 29]. Available from: https://www.ibm.com/downloads/cas/RZAX14GX.

[39] ECFR: 45 CFR part 164 – security and privacy [Internet]. US Department of Health and Human Services; 2002 [cited 2021 December 29]. Available from: https://www.ecfr.gov/current/title-45/subtitle-A/subchapter-C/part-164.

[40] Bazzoli F. HL7 statement responds to security worries about FHIR [Internet]. Health Data Management; 2021 [cited 2021 December 29]. Available from: https://www.healthdatamanagement.com/articles/hl7-responds-to-concerns-about-security-concerns-about-fhir.

[41] Message lookups should be disabled by default [Internet]. [LOG4J2-3198] Message lookups should be disabled by default – ASF JIRA. Apache Software Foundation; 2021 [cited 2021 December 29]. Available from: https://issues.apache.org/jira/browse/LOG4J2-3198.

[42] Apache log4j 1.2 – frequently asked technical questions. Apache Software Foundation; 2012 [cited 2021 December 29]. Available from: https://logging.apache.org/log4j/1.2/faq.html.

[43] Apache Log4j security vulnerabilities [Internet]. Log4j – Apache Log4j Security Vulnerabilities. Apache Software Foundation; 2021 [cited 2021 December 29]. Available from: https://logging.apache.org/log4j/2.x/security.html.

[44] CVE-2021-44228. MITRE; 2021 [cited 2021 December 29]. Available from: https://cve.mitre.org/cgi-bin/cvename.cgi?name = CVE-2021-44228.

[45] BlueTeam cheatsheet * log4shell*: Last updated: 2021-12-20 2238 UTC [Internet]. BlueTeam CheatSheet * Log4Shell*; 2021 [cited 2021 December 29]. Available from: https://gist.github.com/SwitHak/b66db3a06c2955a9cb71a8718970c592.

[46] 21st Century Cures Act: Interoperability, Information Blocking, and the ONC Health IT Certification Program. US Department of Health and Human Services; 2020 [cited 2021 December 29]. Available from: https://www.federalregister.gov/documents/2020/05/01/2020-07419/21st-century-cures-act-interoperability-information-blocking-and-the-onc-health-it-certification.

[47] Information Blocking. US Department of Health and Human Services; 2021 [cited 2021 December 29]. Available from: https://www.healthit.gov/topic/information-blocking.

[48] Kennedy J, Krynitsky J, Shores T, Vissoultchev V, suntsu42, Sharkey K, et al. Protocols in TLS/SSL (schannel SSP) [Internet]. Win32 apps | Microsoft Docs; 2021 [cited 2021 December 29]. Available from: https://docs.microsoft.com/en-us/windows/win32/secauthn/protocols-in-tls-ssl-schannel-ssp-

[49] Silverlock M, Redner G. Bringing modern transport security to Google Cloud with TLS 1.3 [Internet]. Google; 2020 [cited 2021 December 29]. Available from: https://cloud.google.com/blog/products/networking/tls-1-3-is-now-on-by-default-for-google-cloud-services.

[50] Desktop operating system market share worldwide. Statcounter, Inc.; 2021 [cited 2021 December 29]. Available from: https://gs.statcounter.com/os-market-share/desktop/worldwide.

[51] Windows 11 – release information [Internet]. Windows 11 – release information | Microsoft Docs. Microsoft Corporation; 2021 [cited 2021 December 29]. Available from: https://docs.microsoft.com/en-us/windows/release-health/windows11-release-information.

[52] Muoio D. HHS' final interoperability rules standardize APIs for patient health data access through apps [Internet]. HIMSS Media; 2020 [cited 2021 December 29]. Available from: https://www.mobihealthnews.com/news/hhs-final-interoperability-rules-standardize-apis-patient-health-data-access-through-apps.

[53] Mitre ATT&CK® [Internet]. MITRE; [cited 2021 December 29]. Available from: https://attack.mitre.org/.

[54] Keller N. Cybersecurity framework [Internet]. National Institute of Standards and Technology; 2021 [cited 2021 December 29]. Available from: https://www.nist.gov/cyberframework.

[55] Playing with FHIR: hacking and securing FHIR API implementations. Critical Blue, Ltd; 2021 [cited 2021 December 29]. Available from: <https://kantarainitiative.org/confluence/download/attachments/151454472/AlissaKnightFullReport.pdf?version = 1&modificationDate = 1635428397948&api = v2.

[56] Framework for improving critical infrastructure cybersecurity. National Institute of Standards and Technology; 2018 [cited 2021 December 29]. Available from: https://nvlpubs.nist.gov/nistpubs/CSWP/NIST.CSWP.04162018.pdf.

[57] Casey T, Fiftal K, Landfield K, Miller J, Morgan D, Willis B. The cybersecurity framework in action an Intel use case brief [Internet]. Intel Corporation; 2015 [cited 2021 December 29]. Available from: < https://supplier.intel.com/static/governance/documents/The-cybersecurity-framework-in-action-an-intel-use-case-brief.pdf.

[58] Guide for conducting risk assessments – NIST. National Institutes of Standards and Technology; 2012 [cited 2021 December 30]. Available from: https://nvlpubs.nist.gov/nistpubs/Legacy/SP/nistspecialpublication800-30r1.pdf.

[59] Global Cybersecurity Index 2020 [Internet]. Global Cybersecurity Index. International Telecommunications Union; [cited 2021 December 30]. Available from: https://www.itu.int/en/ITU-D/Cybersecurity/Pages/global-cybersecurity-index.aspx.

[60] Branch LS. Consolidated federal laws of Canada, Personal Information Protection and Electronic Documents Act [Internet]; 2021 [cited 2021 December 30]. Available from: https://laws-lois.justice.gc.ca/eng/acts/P-8.6/page-1.html#h-416888.

[61] Brazilian General Data Protection Law (LGPD, English translation). International Association of Privacy Professionals; [cited 2021 December 29]. Available from: https://iapp.org/resources/article/brazilian-data-protection-law-lgpd-english-translation/.

[62] Personal Data Protection Act 2012; 2021 [cited 2021 December 30]. Available from: https://sso.agc.gov.sg/Act/PDPA2012.

[63] Information technology—Security techniques—Code of practice for protection of personally identifiable information (PII) in public clouds acting as PII processors. ISO; 2019 [cited 2021 December 30]. Available from: https://www.iso.org/standard/76559.html.

[64] Alberts CJ, Behrens S, Pethia RD, Wilson WR. Operationally critical threat, asset, and Vulnerability Evaluation (OCTAVE) framework, version 1.0 [Internet]. Software Engineering Institute; 1999 [cited 2021 December 30]. Available from: https://resources.sei.cmu.edu/library/asset-view.cfm?assetid = 13473.

[65] Caralli RA, Stevens JF, Young LR, Wilson WR. Introducing OCTAVE Allegro: improving the information security risk assessment process [Internet]. Software Engineering Institute; 2007 [cited 2021 December 30]. Available from: https://resources.sei.cmu.edu/library/asset-view.cfm?assetid = 8419.

[66] All about ISO 27001 global standard: ISO 27001 Advisory: EGS [Internet]. What do you know about ISO 27001? EC-Council; 2021 [cited 2021 December 30]. Available from: https://egs.eccouncil.org/what-do-you-know-about-iso-27001/.

[67] Watkins SG. An introduction to information security and ISO27001:2013: a pocket guide. Ely: IT Governance Publishing; 2013.

[68] Irwin L. ISO 27001 annex a controls explained [Internet]. ISO 27001 Annex A controls explained; 2020 [cited 2021 December 30]. Available from: https://www.itgovernance.co.uk/blog/iso-27001-the-14-control-sets-of-annex-a-explained.

[69] ISO 27001, the International Information Security Standard [Internet]. IT Governance. IT Governance USA; [cited 2021 December 30]. Available from: https://www.itgovernanceusa.com/iso27001.

[70] What is the plan-do-check-act (PDCA) cycle? [Internet]. American Society for Quality; [cited 2021 December 30]. Available from: https://asq.org/quality-resources/pdca-cycle.

[71] Woollven C. List of US accredited certification bodies for ISO 27001 [Internet]. IT Governance USA Blog; 2020 [cited 2021 December 30]. Available from: https://www.itgovernanceusa.com/blog/list-of-us-accredited-certification-bodies-for-iso-27001.

[72] CB Directory [Internet]. ANAB CB Directory. ANAB; [cited 2021 December 30]. Available from: https://anabdirectory.remoteauditor.com/.

[73] Sarbanes-Oxley Act of 2002; 2002 [cited 2021 December 29]. Available from: https://www.govinfo.gov/content/pkg/COMPS-1883/pdf/COMPS-1883.pdf.

[74] Commission Adopts Rules Strengthening Auditor Independence [Internet]. US Securities and Exchange Commission; 2003 [cited 2021 December 30]. Available from: https://www.sec.gov/news/press/2003-9.htm.

[75] Regulation (EU) 2016/679 of the European Parliament and of the Council of 27 April 2016. European Union; 2016 [cited 2021 December 30]. Available from: https://eur-lex.europa.eu/legal-content/EN/TXT/?uri = CELEX%3A32016R0679.

[76] Regulation (EU) 2016/679 of the European Parliament and of the Council of 27 April 2016 on the protection of natural persons with regard to the processing of personal data and on the free movement of such data, and repealing Directive 95/46/EC (General Data Protection Regulation) (Text with EEA relevance). European Union; 2016 [cited 2021 December 30]. Available from: https://eur-lex.europa.eu/legal-content/EN/TXT/?uri = uriserv%3AOJ.L_.2016.119.01.0001.01.ENG&toc = OJ%3AL%3A2016%3A119%3ATOC.

[77] Data protection under GDPR. European Union; [cited 2021 December 30]. Available from: https://europa.eu/youreurope/business/dealing-with-customers/data-protection/data-protection-gdpr/.

[78] What is HIE? US Department of Health and Human Services; 2020 [cited 2021 December 30]. Available

from: https://www.healthit.gov/topic/health-it-and-health-information-exchange-basics/what-hie.

[79] Failure Modes and Effects Analysis (FMEA) tool: IHI. Institute for Healthcare Improvement; [cited 2021 December 30]. Available from: http://www.ihi.org/resources/Pages/Tools/FailureModesandEffectsAnalysisTool.aspx.

[80] Comptroller's handbook: corporate and risk governance. US Department of Treasury – Office of the Comptroller of the Currency; 2019 [cited 2021 December 30]. Available from: https://www.occ.treas.gov/publications-and-resources/publications/comptrollers-handbook/files/corporate-risk-governance/index-corporate-and-risk-governance.html.

[81] About the SEI. Software Engineering Institute; [cited 2021 December 30]. Available from: https://www.sei.cmu.edu/about/index.cfm.

[82] Caralli RA, Stevens JF, Young LR, Wilson WR. Introducing OCTAVE Allegro: improving the information security risk assessment process [Internet]. Software Engineering Institute; 2015 [cited 2021 December 30]. Available from: https://resources.sei.cmu.edu/asset_files/TechnicalReport/2007_005_001_14885.pdf.

[83] CVE. The MITRE Corporation; [cited 2021 December 30]. Available from: https://cve.mitre.org/.

[84] Holm H, Sommestad T, Almroth J, Persson M. A quantitative evaluation of Vulnerability Scanning. Inf Manag Comput Secur 2011;19(4):231–47.

[85] Vulnerability metrics. National Institute of Standards and Technology; [cited 2021 December 30]. Available from: https://nvd.nist.gov/vuln-metrics/cvss.

[86] About the CVE Program. The MITRE Corporation; [cited 2021 December 30]. Available from: https://www.cve.org/About/Overview.

[87] Top 10 web application security risks [Internet]. OWASP Top Ten. The OWASP Foundation; [cited 2021 December 30]. Available from: https://owasp.org/www-project-top-ten/.

[88] The 18 CIS critical security controls. Center for Internet Security; 2021 [cited 2021 December 30]. Available from: https://www.cisecurity.org/controls/cis-controls-list/.

[89] Fitzpatrick A. HITRUST Certification FAQs [Internet]. Meditology Services; 2020 [cited 2021 December 30]. Available from: https://www.meditologyservices.com/hitrust-certification-faqs/.

[90] HITRUST C-level overview – HITRUST Alliance [Internet]. How HITRUST helps organizations manage risk. HITRUST Alliance; 2021 [cited 2021 December 30]. Available from: https://hitrustalliance.net/content/uploads/HITRUST-C-Level-Overview-2021.pdf.

[91] Miller G. What is the cost of HITRUST CSF certification in 2022? [Internet]. Cloudticity Blog. Cloudticity, LLC; 2021 [cited 2021 December 30]. Available from: https://blog.cloudticity.com/hitrust-certification-cost-2022.

[92] Frequently asked questions [Internet]. FAQ | MITRE ATT&CK®. The MITRE Corporation; [cited 2021 December 30]. Available from: https://attack.mitre.org/resources/faq/.

[93] Enterprise matrix [Internet]. Matrix – Enterprise | MITRE ATT&CK®. The MITRE Corporation; [cited 2021 December 30]. Available from: https://attack.mitre.org/versions/v10/matrices/enterprise/.

[94] Enterprise tactics [Internet]. Tactics – Enterprise | MITRE ATT&CK®. The MITRE Corporation; [cited 2021 December 30]. Available from: https://attack.mitre.org/versions/v10/tactics/enterprise/.

[95] Mobile tactics [Internet]. Tactics – Mobile | MITRE ATT&CK®. The MITRE Corporation; [cited 2021 December 30]. Available from: https://attack.mitre.org/versions/v10/tactics/mobile/.

[96] About the D3FEND knowledge graph project [Internet]. About | MITRE D3FEND™. The MITRE Corporation; [cited 2021 December 30]. Available from: https://d3fend.mitre.org/about.

[97] Editor CSRCC. Penetration testing – glossary [Internet]. National Institute of Standards and Technology; [cited 2021 December 30]. Available from: https://csrc.nist.gov/glossary/term/penetration_testing.

[98] The world's most used penetration testing framework [Internet]. Metasploit. Rapid7, Inc.; [cited 2021 December 30]. Available from: https://www.metasploit.com/.

[99] Editor CSRCC. Red Team – glossary [Internet]. CSRC. National Institute of Standards and Technology; [cited 2021 December 30]. Available from: https://csrc.nist.gov/glossary/term/red_team.

[100] Editor CSRCC. Blue Team – glossary [Internet]. CSRC. National Institute of Standards and Technology; [cited 2021 December 30]. Available from: https://csrc.nist.gov/glossary/term/blue_team.

[101] Daniel Miessler. The definition of a Purple Team [Internet]. Daniel Miessler; 2019 [cited 2021 December 30]. Available from: https://danielmiessler.com/study/purple-team/.

[102] Purple Team Exercise Framework (PTEF). SCYTHE Corporation; [cited 2021 December 30]. Available from: https://www.scythe.io/ptef.

[103] Editor CSRCC. Risk assessment – glossary [Internet]. National Institute of Standards and Technology; [cited 2021 December 30]. Available from: https://csrc.nist.gov/glossary/term/risk_assessment.

[104] Security Risk Assessment Tool. US Department of Health and Human Services; 2021 [cited 2021 December 30]. Available from: https://www.healthit.gov/topic/privacy-security-and-hipaa/security-risk-assessment-tool.

[105] Computer Security Division ITL. About the RMF – NIST risk management framework: CSRC [Internet]. About the Risk Management Framework (RMF). National Institute of Standards and Technology; [cited 2021 December 30]. Available from: https://csrc.nist.gov/projects/risk-management/about-rmf.

[106] Stine K, Quinn S, Witte G, Gardner RK. Integrating cybersecurity and enterprise risk management (ERM) [Internet]. National Institute of Standards and Technology; 2020 [cited 2021 December 30]. Available from: https://nvlpubs.nist.gov/nistpubs/ir/2020/NIST.IR.8286.pdf.

[107] Tucker BA. Advancing risk management capability using the OCTAVE FORTE process [Internet]. Software Engineering Institute; 2020 [cited 2021 December 30]. Available from: https://resources.sei.cmu.edu/asset_files/TechnicalNote/2020_004_001_644641.pdf

[108] Tucker B. Advancing risk management capability using the OCTAVE FORTE process [Internet]; 2020 [cited 2021 December 30]. Available from: https://resources.sei.cmu.edu/library/asset-view.cfm?assetID = 644636.

[109] The basics of healthcare failure mode and effect analysis. US Department of Veterans Affairs; 2006 [cited 2021 December 30]. Available from: https://www.patientsafety.va.gov/docs/hfmea/FMEA2.pdf.

[110] Failure mode and effects analysis (FMEA). American Society for Quality; [cited 2021 December 30]. Available from: https://asq.org/quality-resources/fmea.

[111] The Office of the National Coordinator for Health Information Technology. Trusted Exchange Framework and Common Agreement (TEFCA) Draft 2 [Internet]. The Office of the National Coordinator for Health Information Technology; 2019 [cited 2021 December 30]. Available from: https://www.healthit.gov/sites/default/files/page/2019-04/FINALTEFCAQTF417195-08version.pdf.

[112] Yerra K, Ekwueme O, Ingraham A, Choi W. TEFCA and blockchain: enabling trusted data flow between health networks [Internet]. HIMSS; 2019 [cited 2021 December 30]. Available from: https://www.himss.org/resources/tefca-and-blockchain-enabling-trusted-data-flow-between-health-networks.

[113] Blockchain in healthcare. HIMSS; [cited 2021 December 30]. Available from: https://www.himss.org/resources/blockchain-healthcare.

[114] IPFs powers the Distributed Web [Internet]. Protocol Labs; [cited 2021 December 30]. Available from: https://ipfs.io/.

[115] Lagasse J. Himss20: improving smart contract security in the Healthcare Supply Chain [Internet]. Healthcare Finance News. HIMSS Media; 2020 [cited 2021 December 30]. Available from: https://www.healthcarefinancenews.com/news/himss20-improving-smart-contract-security-healthcare-supply-chain.

[116] Poston A. About Hashed Health [Internet]. Hashed Health; 2021 [cited 2021 December 30]. Available from: https://hashedhealth.com/about/.

[117] Decentralized Identifiers (DIDs) v1.0 Core architecture, data model, and representations. W3C; 2021 [cited 2021 December 30]. Available from: https://www.w3.org/TR/did-core/#:~:text = Decentralized%20identifiers%20(DIDs)%20are%20a,the%20controller%20of%20the%20DID.

SECTION 3

Technical architecture and building blocks

CHAPTER

8

Architectures and approaches to manage the evolving health information infrastructure

Brian E. Dixon[1,2], *David Broyles*[3], *Ryan Crichton*[4], *Paul G. Biondich*[2,5] *and Shaun J. Grannis*[2,5]

[1]Department of Epidemiology, Richard M. Fairbanks School of Public Health, Indiana University, Indianapolis, IN, USA [2]Center for Biomedical Informatics, Regenstrief Institute, Inc., Indianapolis, IN, USA [3]Marion County Public Health Department, Indianapolis, IN, USA [4]Jembi Health Systems, Cape Town, South Africa [5]Indiana University School of Medicine, Indianapolis, IN, USA

LEARNING OBJECTIVES

By the end of the chapter, the reader should be able to:

- Define the concept of a health information infrastructure.
- List and describe three key technical aspects of a health information infrastructure.
- Explain the concept of architecture from an information science perspective and how it is used in strategic planning for a health information infrastructure.
- Explain the role of transactions in health information exchange.
- List and describe the three types of interoperability important to health information exchange.
- Describe the role and core functions of an interoperability layer in supporting health information exchange.
- List and describe the components of an interoperability layer.

8.1 Introduction

This is the first chapter in the section of the book that covers the technical aspects of health

Health Information Exchange
DOI: https://doi.org/10.1016/B978-0-323-90802-3.00001-0

information exchange (HIE). In this chapter, we define and describe the key concept of a health information infrastructure, or the ecosystem in which HIE occurs. Information infrastructures are enabled by technical architectures, so we define a model HIE architecture and the core technical aspect of the model that facilitates HIE: the interoperability layer. Additional details on interoperability and the standards that support the syntactic form of interoperability can be found in Chapter 9. Semantic interoperability and standards are covered in Chapter 10. Additional components of a model HIE architecture are further detailed in Chapters 11–15.

8.2 The health information infrastructure

The health information infrastructure for a nation, state, or community is an ecosystem composed of the people, processes, procedures, tools, facilities, and technologies, which supports the capture, storage, management, exchange, and creation of data and information to support individual patient care and population health. While individual organizations such as hospitals possess discrete people (e.g., health care workers), processes (e.g., medication administration protocols, referral patterns), information systems (e.g., electronic health records, remote monitoring, laboratory information systems), and communities are composed of a larger set of technologies, organizations, and people that create a health information infrastructure [1]. Thus an information infrastructure is a sort of network of networks, and HIE is the method by which data and information are shared among the organizations, people, and technologies that comprise the defined ecosystem.

8.2.1 The health information infrastructure is an Ultra Large-Scale system

As described by the Institute of Medicine in its report on the digital infrastructure for supporting the Learning Health System [2], a health information infrastructure is similar to the concept of an Ultra Large-Scale (ULS) system as defined in computer science. An ULS system is a set of characteristics that tend to arise as a result of the scale of the system (in this case, the complex and fragmented organization as well as delivery of health care along with the heterogeneous nature of medicine and clinical data) rather than a prescriptive set of required technical components. Previous work on the ULS concept [3] has identified the following key characteristics of ULS systems:

- *Decentralization*: The scale of ULS systems means that they will necessarily be decentralized in a variety of ways—decentralized data, development, evolution, and operational control.
- *Inherently conflicting, unknowable, and diverse requirements*: ULS systems will be developed and used by a wide variety of stakeholders with unavoidably different, conflicting, complex, and changing needs.
- *Continuous evolution and deployment*: There will be an increasing need to integrate new capabilities into an ULS system while it is operating. New and different capabilities will be deployed, and unused capabilities will be dropped; the system will be evolving not in phases, but continuously.
- *Heterogeneous, inconsistent, and changing elements*: An ULS system will not be constructed from uniform parts: there will be some misfits, especially as the system is extended and repaired.
- *Erosion of the people/system boundary*: People will not just be users of an ULS system; they will be elements of the system, affecting its overall emergent behavior.
- *Normal failures*: Software and hardware failures will be the norm rather than the exception.
- *New paradigms for acquisition and policy*: The acquisition of an ULS system will be

simultaneous with the operation of the system and requires new methods for control.

8.3 Supporting the health information infrastructure

To organize and support an integrated health information infrastructure, where the various actors in the ecosystem can effectively exchange data and information, HIE networks must facilitate three important technical aspects of an infrastructure (the organizational, political, and legal aspects are considered in earlier chapters as well as the case studies):

- An *architecture* that defines how everything "fits together" and provides a common understanding for creating and managing the components of the infrastructure;
- Methods for *transactions* between information systems or the exchange of data and information; and
- Methods for *interoperability* or the ability for receiving information systems to do something with the data or information exchanged.

The specific information systems and applications used in HIE are defined and managed by individual hospitals, physician offices, health systems, public health agencies, and payors. These include systems such as laboratory information systems, radiology information systems, emergency department information systems, etc. In HIE speak, we often refer to them as point-of-care applications. Where an HIE infrastructure that can provide the most value is in defining the big picture and providing centralized technical services that enable data exchange among the various applications and information systems across the health care ecosystem.

8.3.1 Architecture

In computer science, the term *software architecture* refers to the high-level design of a system, the methods by which components are created, and the documentation of the system structures. In other words, the *architecture* of an information infrastructure defines how its various parts "fit together." Fig. 8.1 is an example of an architecture from the nationwide HIE in South Korea [4]. The image identifies the various components used by the HIE network, such as a registry server as well as a master patient index (MPI) server. In the context of South Korea's HIE network, the registry server contains information on clinical documents that exist for patients across various electronic health record (EHR)-based repositories. This is often referred to as a record locator service or RLS. As depicted in the architecture, the clinical document repositories are populated by EHR systems. Documents are then retrieved for viewing through either the DMZ (demilitarized zone) for clinics or the "Middleware" platform for hospitals. Architecture diagrams outline the various methods and interfaces needed to connect the various information systems and HIE network components together. The South Korea diagram further outlines the security measures used to keep data protected. An architecture like this one is derived from consensus discussions among the stakeholders involved in the network (e.g., health systems, public health authorities, pharmacies) who agree upon the components for exchange as well as the methods by which data and information will be exchanged.

When stakeholders agree upon an architecture, most often they agree to use one of several types of architectural patterns or styles. An *architectural pattern* is a general, reusable approach to a commonly occurring problem in software architecture within a given context like HIE. An *architectural style* is a reusable set of design decisions and constraints that are applied to an architecture to induce chosen desirable qualities [5]. While computer scientists disagree on the exact differences between the two idioms, they both provide a common

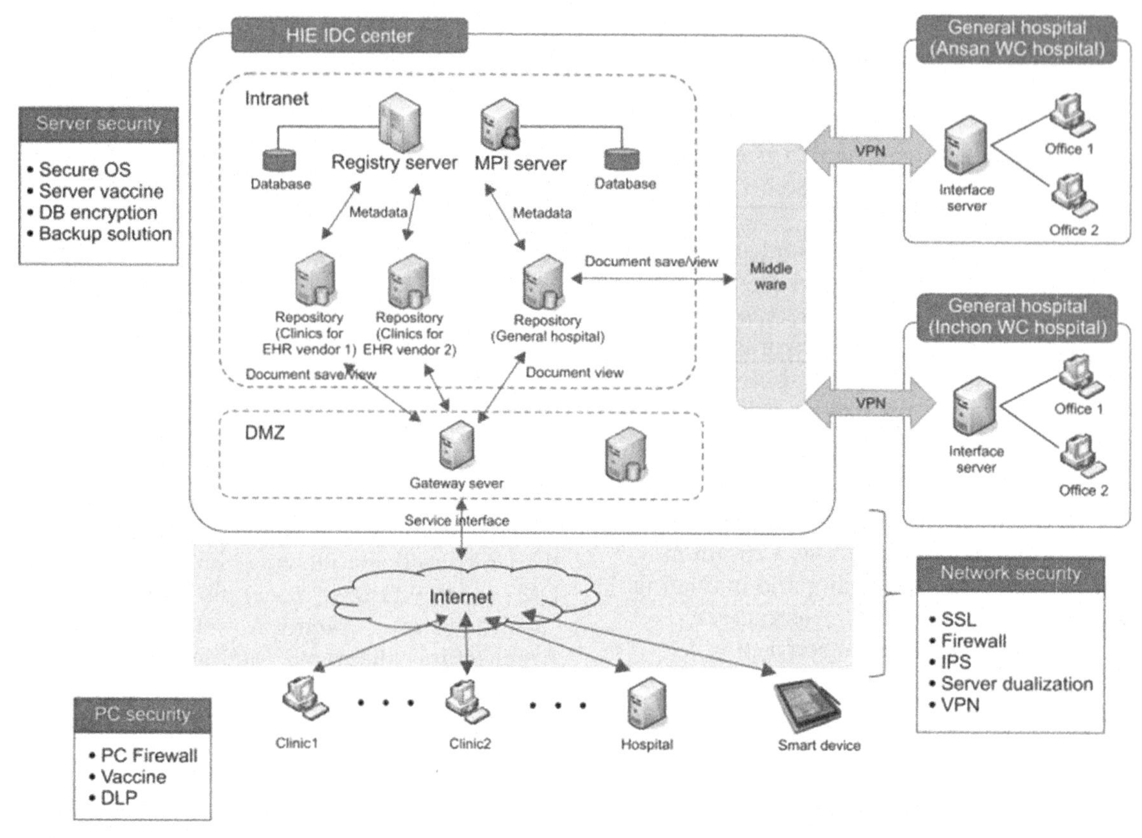

FIGURE 8.1 Example of an architecture from the nationwide HIE in South Korea. Source: *Originally published in Lee M, Heo E, Lim H, Lee JY, Weon S, Chae H, et al. Developing a common health information exchange platform to implement a nationwide health information network in South Korea. Healthc Inform Res 2015;21(1):21–9 and used with permission from the Korean Society of Medical Informatics.*

language or vocabulary with which to describe classes of systems [6]. Commonly used architectural patterns and styles include:

- Client/server—Distributed systems that involve a separate client and server system, and a connecting network. The simplest form of client/server system involves a server application that is accessed directly by multiple clients, referred to as a two-tier architectural style. Historically, the client/server style indicated a desktop application that communicated with a database server containing much of the business logic, or with a dedicated file server. This style is recommended when implementing business processes that will be used by people throughout an organization.
- Component-based architecture—Decomposes the system into reusable functional or logical components that expose well-defined communication interfaces. Essentially, the system is composed of prefabricated components that perform specific functions. A set of components function together as an application server. Aspects of a user interface are typically implemented as components. Other

common types of components are those that are resource intensive, not frequently accessed, and must be activated using the just-in-time (JIT) approach (common in distributed component scenarios); and queued components executed asynchronously using message queuing.

- Service-oriented architecture (SOA)—Application functionality is provided as a set of services that are loosely coupled because they use standards-based interfaces that can be invoked, published, and discovered. Services in SOA are focused on providing a schema and message-based interaction with an application through interfaces that are application scoped as opposed to components. SOA approaches are common for Software as a Service (SaaS) as well as cloud-based applications. The SOA style is recommended for message-based communication between segments of the application in a platform independent way, when you want to take advantage of federated services such as authentication, or you want to expose services that are discoverable through directories. Because services are independent and focus on a performing a narrow task, maintenance is easier when compared to other styles.
- Event-driven architecture (EDA) – In this paradigm, applications respond to events, which are significant changes in a state. For example, a patient is admitted to the hospital. The EDA is driven by *event notifications*, messages triggered by the event. The notifications communicate to other systems about the change in state with respect to a patient, procedure, provider, etc. Like SOA, the software components and services are loosely coupled. Systems that send notifications are referred to as *emitters* (event producers). Those that receive notifications are called *sinks* (event consumers). Sinks must react or respond to each notification, which might be to perform an action or filter, transform, and/or forward the event to another component.
- Microservices – A modern term that describes an architectural approach to a specific application rather than an enterprise (e.g., the HIE). SOA, EDA, and microservices all use a similar, loosely coupled approach and application programming interfaces (APIs), described below, to communicate between the various components within an application (e.g., medication hub) or HIE network.

Whereas client/server types are common for health information systems operating within a clinic, hospital, or health system, HIE applications typically use component-based or SOA types. Furthermore, SOA dictates that services operate in distributed environments and focus on document-centric communication [7], making this type very suitable for HIE since health information infrastructures share many aspects of an ULS system. More recent HIE initiatives have favored SOA approaches in their design and development, including the eHealth Exchange [8,9]. Some IT architects suggest that EDA and SOA models work well together, since EDAs are commonly built upon message-based frameworks and complement document-centric SOAs.

8.3.2 Transactions

A health information *transaction* can be defined as the exchange of electronic health information between two extraneous entities for a specific purpose. HIEs are designed to promote a variety of health information transactions. An example of a common transaction is the delivery of laboratory test results to the physician that ordered the test. The transaction occurs between the information system at the laboratory and the EHR system in the clinic or health system. Laboratory reports can also be

TABLE 8.1 Transaction classes commonly handled by health information infrastructures.

Transaction class	Description
Save/Update Records	Information regarding a patient encounter can be saved to the individual's electronic health record
	Demographic information about a patient can be updated in the CR
	A new patient is registered in the health system for the first time
Requests/Queries	A list of a patient's previous encounters restricted to a specific time frame can be retrieved
	Client information can be obtained by providing the client ID number
	Information about a specific health care facility can be retrieved if the point of service application calling the system provides the facility ID number
	A point of service system can request a list of a clients that match specific criteria outlined in the parameters of the query
	A point of service application can request a list of health care facilities that match specific criteria outlined in the parameters of the query
Alerts	The system can relay alert messages regarding patient care to physicians and other providers
	Public health authorities can be alerted to a new report of a disease like Ebola they may be closely monitoring in a state or nation
	Admission, discharge, and transfer messages are a special class of alert transactions commonly found in HIE environments

sent from the lab information system to other health system stakeholders such as a public health agency [10]. Thus transactions support routine business processes among health care system stakeholders. Other examples include sending medication orders to the pharmacy, retrieving a report from a specialty physician, and registering a new patient who visits the clinic for the first time.

In Table 8.1 we summarize common classes of transactions that can occur within a health system. While individual transaction types (e.g., medication order, lab result delivery) are designed around a specific process in health care, these transaction classes represent a broader set of transactions that can occur. There is a Save/Update Records class that represents the variety of transactions in which data or information about a patient is "pushed" or delivered from one system to another for either storage in the EHR or display to a clinician. Another class referred to as Requests/Queries represents transactions in which one information system asks or requests information from the EHR or another information system about a patient or population (e.g., all patients with diabetes, Veterans). A third class, Alerts, represents transactions in which a business rule is triggered by data in the system and a user is alerted about an emerging state (e.g., new blood pressure reading is high, diagnosis of a highly contagious disease).

8.3.3 Interoperability

Successful transactions between disparate information systems require multiple layers of interoperability including foundational, syntactic, and semantic [11,12]. Foundational interoperability refers to the technical infrastructure necessary to share information between systems [13]. Syntactic interoperability requires that messages sent between two information systems must be transmitted in a format that is recognized by both systems [14]. Semantic interoperability refers to the ability of one system to correctly decipher and process the information received from another information system without prior consultation [15].

8.3.3.1 Foundational interoperability

Disparate health information systems that wish to exchange information must adhere to a series of standardized communication protocols. Initially, the heterogeneous systems must be linked together to form a communication network. Many exchanges use Transmission Control Protocol/Internet (TCP/IP) connections to fulfill this requirement [11]. Information exchange also requires an application protocol such as the Hypertext Transfer Protocol (HTTP) [11,16]. Web services such as SOAP (Simple Object Access Protocol) or Representational State Transfer (REST) that define how and where to send the messages are also critical to structured information exchange [11]. Although foundational interoperability is necessary for data exchange, these requirements can be fulfilled relatively easily in relation to syntactic and semantic interoperability concerns.

8.3.3.2 Syntactic interoperability

Successful communication between systems also requires messages to be transmitted using a structure and syntax that is ascertainable to both systems [17]. Formats such as Extensible Markup Language (XML) are frequently used to satisfy this demand [11,14]. Enabling successful communication becomes increasingly complex as more heterogeneous systems with their own unique formatting are involved in the information exchange [11]. For this reason, HIEs have typically adopted messaging standards such as Health Level Seven (HL7) version 2 or 3 [4,11,18,19]. In Chapter 9, the book provides a more detailed discussion on syntactic interoperability, including HL7, and the process for developing and selecting technical standards.

8.3.3.3 Semantic interoperability

The ability to successfully receive a message does not assure that the system receiving the message will be able to interpret and complete a request. If external systems attempting to communicate with the HIE system use terminology or coding that is incompatible with the internal standards of the HIE, then the data must be translated into a standardized format before it can be interpreted. In addition, the response must be translated back into the language used by the external system. In many HIE structures, this can be a time consuming and expensive process [20–22]. In Chapter 10, the book more fully discusses syntactic interoperability as well as methods and tool for managing terminologies.

8.4 Open HIE—a model health information infrastructure

Interoperability between multiple disparate health systems presents a particularly complex challenge for HIEs to overcome [21,23,24]. The interoperability of health information systems is a prominent issue in the United States due to the fragmented makeup of the health information infrastructure [25]. Although maintaining many disassociated information systems empowers the United States to meet a diverse variety of local health care needs, this degree of flexibility also has some drawbacks [25]. Most health information systems were designed and structured to meet the unique needs of the implementing health care organization [26]. Planning for interoperability with external systems is generally a low priority in the development process [27]. Although standards for health data exist, many health care providers still identify clinical observations using locally specific terminology that is not harmonious with external systems [21]. As a result, health data are often collected in an inconsistent manner from one organization to another [28]. This often prevents the information systems of the separate organizations from corresponding with each other successfully without a uniform method of standardizing the data [28]. The lack of standardization that results from this approach makes it difficult to assemble the information from these fragmented local databases into a strong national system [25].

The *OpenHIE* framework is designed to promote the sharing of health information in countries with a diverse array of health information systems through a middle-out approach to national HIE [25]. The middle-out strategy adapts to the varying needs and capabilities of the heterogeneous entities involved in the HIE [25]. The OpenHIE framework facilitates interoperability by combining existing applications through relatively simple and inexpensive interfaces rather than implementing new systems or major re-development efforts [29]. This enables HIE efforts using the OpenHIE framework to avoid some of the financial and technical barriers experienced by many conventional HIE solutions [25,30]. As a result, OpenHIE can be implemented more quickly than other solutions and with few disruptions to any existing operational health information systems that will be participating in the HIE [18].

For numerous heterogeneous health information systems to communicate successfully, the architecture of an HIE must offer flexible processes and technologies that are capable of accommodating the constantly changing demands associated with health information. The OpenHIE model addresses this challenge through a component-based architecture. The component-based design enables multiple services to work together to provide a secure mechanism for sharing health care information while maintaining the flexibility of the system. This allows OpenHIE to meet the needs specific to the country where it is being implemented. As a result, OpenHIE has the potential to make the health care industry of an implementing nation more efficacious and boost the quality of service by enabling accurate and timely access to critical patient information [10,30–32].

The OpenHIE architecture is depicted in Fig. 8.2. Each component supports well-described, core health data management functions and interoperates with other components to ensure that health information from various point of service applications is rationalized to support person-centric and population-based health care needs. Reference implementations of each of the components exist to validate and highlight the functionality enabled within the architecture, and also are designed to support real world needs. Different compositions of these components can be used within a given environment to support myriad workflows.

The components of the OpenHIE architecture depicted in Fig. 8.2 include:

- *Interoperability layer (IL)* serves as the core method for connecting the components of the HIE with point of service applications. Detailed description of the IL is provided in the remainder of this chapter.

8.4.1 Business domain services

- *Shared health record (SHR)* that serves as a repository of person-centric records detailing visits, diagnoses, treatments, laboratory results, and other observations documented during care delivery or by public health authorities. Detailed description of the SHR is provided in Chapter 11.
- *Health management information system (HMIS)* that stores and redistributes population-level information normalized through the HIE. Detailed description of the HMIS is provided in Chapter 11.
- *Finance and insurance service (FIS)* that stores, categorizes, and facilitates the

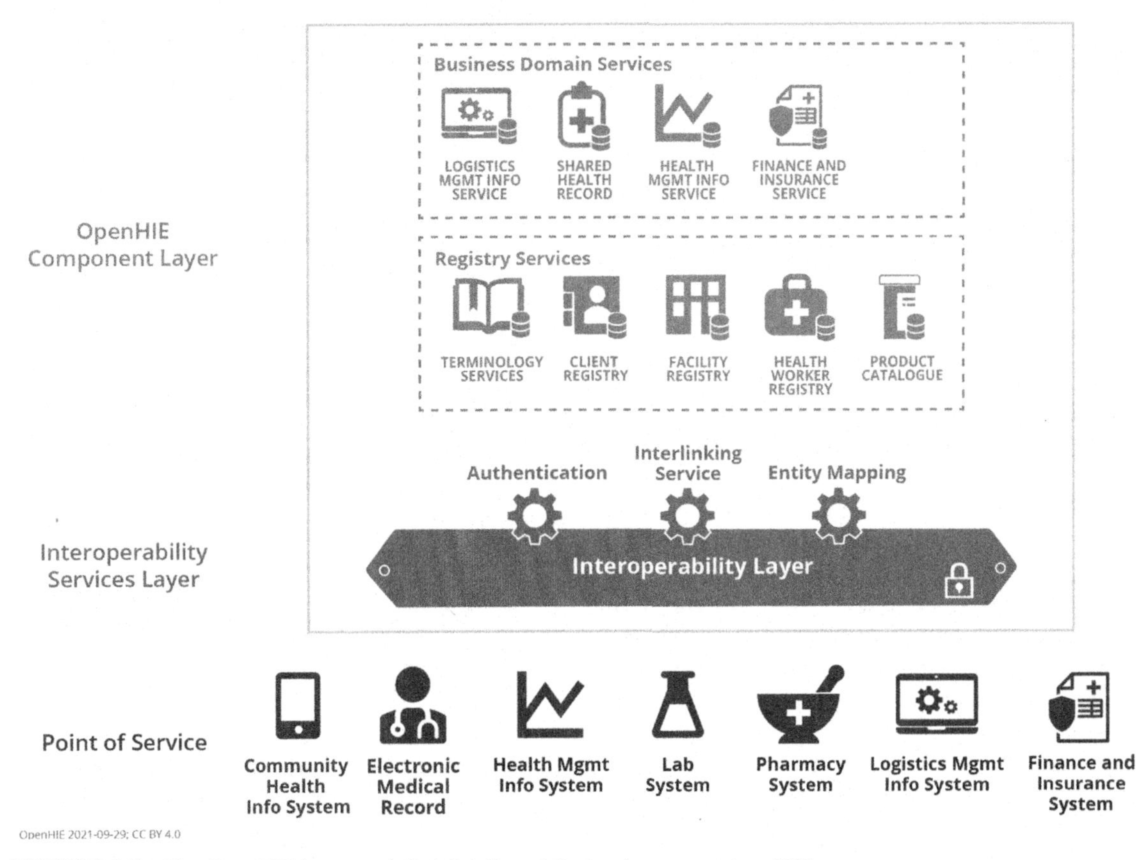

FIGURE 8.2 The OpenHIE framework that details architectural components, c.2021.

administration of centralized claims and finance-related data. The service receives claims/financial data and curates the management of them. Detailed description of the FIS is provided in Chapter 15.

8.4.2 Registry services

- *Terminology services (TS)* that manages local as well as reference terminologies, collections of unique concepts that describe diagnoses, treatments, and outcomes. Detailed description of the TS is provided in Chapter 10.
- *Client registry (CR)* that manages the unique identities of people receiving health services or who live in a community. Detailed description of the CR is provided in Chapter 12.
- *Facility registry (FR)* that manages unique health facilities located within a community, state, or nation. Detailed description of the FR is provided in Chapter 13.
- *Health worker registry (HWR)* that manages unique health workers at all levels of the health system, including doctors, nurses, pharmacists, social workers, and community health workers. Detailed description of the HWR is provided in Chapter 14.

Point of Service Applications are health information systems external to the HIE that have a need to interface with the various HIE components, which is why they are also depicted in Fig. 8.2. Mobile applications, laboratory information systems, health insurance claims systems, and home monitoring devices are examples of information systems that have a need to store data in the HIE and/or retrieve data from the HIE. These applications interact with the various HIE components via the IL.

8.4.3 Interoperability layer

In the OpenHIE model, the foundation of the flexible architecture is the *IL* [27]. The IL is a middleware system that enables easier interoperability between disparate information systems by bringing all of the infrastructure services and external applications together [33]. The OpenHIE structure includes both systems that request services and systems that provide those services. Service requestors are the external point of service applications such as a pharmacy information system or laboratory information system that are making requests of the internal OpenHIE components [27,34]. Service providers are the systems that accommodate these requests [27]. The service providers in the OpenHIE infrastructure consist of business domain services represented in Fig. 8.2 including the SHR and FIS as well as the registry services like CR, TS, and HWR. The job of the IL is to facilitate the transaction between the service requestor and the service provider.

The IL receives transaction requests from external client systems, conducts the correspondence between the internal components of the HIE, and possesses functions that can facilitate manageable interoperability between systems [35]. The IL serves several core functions that facilitate HIE for OpenHIE.

1. The IL simplifies the security for the HIE by providing a single point of access for all external systems that are attempting to communicate with the components of the HIE such as the CR, the provider registry, the FR, or the SHR.
2. The IL keeps a record of all of the transactions that take place in the OpenHIE.
3. The IL is responsible for routing messages to the appropriate service provider within the infrastructure.

In addition to the core functions provided by the IL, it also offers mediation functionality. If a point of service application sends a request in a format that is not recognizable to the service provider, the IL assists the transaction by furnishing an adapter that transforms the message into a format accepted by the internal components of the HIE. Similarly, the adapters will transform the data back into a format expected by the point of service application that initiated the transaction. When necessary, the IL orchestrates complicated transactions to remove that complexity from the consumer systems.

8.4.4 Structure of the interoperability layer

The IL was designed to address the problem of interoperability between health care systems through an architectural framework that incorporates the use of web services and progressive middleware [36]. The OpenHIE IL is composed of two components including the core component and the orchestrators and adapter services component. This architectural approach is based on the Enterprise Service Bus (ESB) model. An ESB is a middleware system that integrates messaging, web services, transformation, and routing to coordinate transactions among discordant applications [16,36]. These advanced middleware systems can be leveraged to overcome interoperability constraints between heterogeneous health information systems [16,33,37]. ESBs can accept transaction requests, and then perform mediation tasks to fulfill the transaction [16,27]. In addition, the

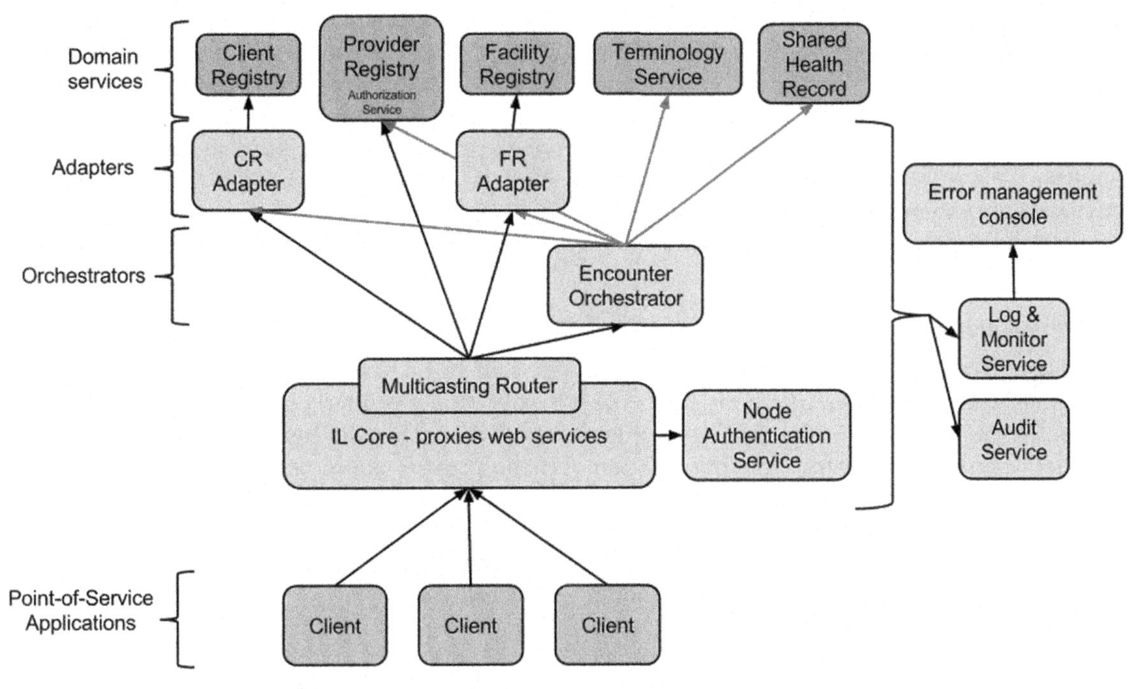

FIGURE 8.3 Architecture of the OpenHIE model illustrating the detailed components of the Interoperability Layer.

individual mechanisms of the ESB can operate independently of one another, which allows them to continue to function in the event that one component fails [27,38]. Fig. 8.3 illustrates the components of the IL and the role they serve in the OpenHIE infrastructure. The components are described in greater detail below.

8.4.5 Core component

The core component of the IL serves as the entry point into the HIE. It functions as a web service proxy and executes some supplementary tasks on the incoming requests to eliminate the need for other domain services to furnish them. It provides security for the HIE, logs transactions, identifies and displays errors that occur between services, and routes the incoming requests to the proper services. This requires an authentication and authorization service, a log service, and an audit service. When the IL receives confirmation from all of these services that the applicable information has been collected and saved, it passes the message to the router so it can be sent to the appropriate service.

Providing a single point of entry for all incoming messages serves to streamline the transaction process [39]. The IL can accommodate requests from a diverse range of systems through exposing an external PI [4,40]. The external API is publicly accessible to systems with the proper privileges and handles all transactions with point of service applications such as laboratory or pharmacy information systems. Requests from these external systems can be collected through an application protocol such as HTTP and then translated into a configuration that is recognizable to all components of the interoperability layer [27]. The use of an API enables OpenHIE services to be called in real time by external point of service systems. The point of service systems calling the IL can provide the necessary parameters for the system designated by the API, and then allow the IL to facilitate an automated response. This approach is advantageous over conventional systems that often relied on asynchronous approaches to interoperability [40].

8.4.5.1 *Security*

The core component of the IL also manages security for the entire HIE. Using the IL as the sole point of entry into the HIE mitigates potential security barriers to information exchange because the requesting systems can submit a message without ascertaining the location and security demands of the system that is providing the service [27]. The node authentication service depicted in Fig. 8.3 ensures that only authorized systems can interact with the components of the OpenHIE. Transactions that are received by the IL are acquired over a secured HTTPs connection through the external API. The IL uses the Audit Trail and Node Authentication (ATNA) profile from Integrating the Healthcare Enterprise (IHE) to authenticate transactions (see Chapter 9 for more on IHE). The ATNA profile relies on Mutual Transport Layer Security (MTLS) to ensure that transactions only take place when the digital certificate of a point-of-service application is trusted by the IL and the digital certificate of the IL is trusted by the point-of-service application.

The point of service applications that are calling the IL is responsible for authenticating users. For example, a provider may want to call the HIE to obtain a list of a patient's encounters within the last year. Once the provider has entered the correct password, they can submit a transaction request to the IL. This transaction request includes a provider ID number. When the IL receives an authenticated request, it calls the provider registry to verify the permissions associated with the provider ID number. This step verifies that the provider has the authority to make the request. This is important because some mobile point of service applications may be restricted to requesting data from specific services within the infrastructure, while other, more robust point of service applications may have unrestricted access to all of the services provided in the infrastructure. Once it is verified that the provider has the authority for the transaction, the IL will record the transaction in the SHR and notify the provider or other point of service application that the transaction was successful. If the provider does not have the authority for the transaction, an exception message would be returned to their point of service application. The results would be written to the audit log of the IL.

8.4.5.2 *Monitoring/logging*

Another function of the core component of the IL is to log and monitor the transactions that occur. The log, monitor, and audit services portrayed in Fig. 8.3 provide an audit trail for each transaction by storing every message as well as the crucial characteristics of the message including the sender's identity, details about the information that was received, the time and date the message was received, and the response to the message. This enables auditing when necessary, and provides insight into the movement of messages through HIE.

The logging mechanism of the IL also improves system performance and error-management within the OpenHIE infrastructure. Areas within the system that may be experiencing restrictions to the flow of information or inefficiencies can be identified more easily. All failed transactions are logged and can be grouped by the underlying source of the error. System administrators can use this information to correct recurring issues more efficiently [27]. Transactions that failed due to an internal system error can be re-run once the root cause of the error has been rectified without placing the burden of having to re-submit a request on the consumer.

8.4.6 Mediation component

The IL also offers a mediation component that executes the transactions that are routed from the core component. Mediators are microservices that carry out supplementary exercises on requests that are received by the IL [33]. These mediation microservices are disassociated components of the interoperability layer that each provides a distinct function. The two types of mediators that incorporated into the architecture of the IL include adapters and orchestrators. Adapters change the incoming requests into an acceptable format when necessary while orchestrators enable a business process to be carried out.

8.4.6.1 Adapters

Adapters allow the IL to transform incoming transactions into a format that the HIE recognizes [27]. Transformation ensures that the transaction will have syntactic interoperability. For example, a message that arrives in HL7 version 3 format may need to be converted into HL7 version 2 format in order to be recognized by the system because HL7 version 3 uses XML data objects to identify values while HL7 version 2 uses delimiters to separate values [19]. Adapters are also responsible for facilitating semantic interoperability for the transaction by translating the codes from the messages into the standardized language used by the IL. This requires a call to the terminology server that maps the standards used by the interoperability layer to the vocabulary used by the various participating systems [27]. The internal OpenHIE components such as the CR or FR each have a designated adapter as characterized in Fig. 8.3 to perform these services [35].

8.4.6.2 Orchestrators

The orchestration microservice enables the timely completion of transactions that require multiple tasks to be executed. The orchestrator may need to call numerous components of the HIE in order to assemble a valid response to the point of service application that initiated the transaction. For example, the completion of a request may require the verification of multiple identifiers that may be stored in separate registries within the HIE infrastructure such as the provider registry, FR, and CR. The illustration in Fig. 8.3 exemplifies how the encounter orchestrator may delegate tasks throughout the OpenHIE during a transaction.

These mediation services are summoned only when there is a requirement to translate or orchestrate a transaction. The core component will communicate directly with the domain service for transactions that do not require an adapter or orchestrator. The mediation services also log the messages that they dispatch to the domain services. The mediation components that are available in the IL are generally unique to the needs of the country that is implementing OpenHIE. Developing orchestrators and adapters as independent services within the architecture adds flexibility to the system because these subcomponents can be added or removed as needs change [35]. An alternative approach is to combine orchestration and adaptation services into a single component, referred to as an interface engine, which is described in more detail in Chapter 9.

8.5 Benefits of the OpenHIE interoperability layer

Collectively, the OpenHIE IL provides a solution to overcome many of the prominent barriers that can inhibit health information sharing. The ability to restrict access to a single entry point simplifies security, monitoring, and error management for the entire HIE infrastructure. The ability of the IL to process requests without the use of a specific message format is critical because no individual standards can exhaustively meet the demands of all prevailing and forthcoming information systems [28]. The flexibility of the IL structure enables OpenHIE to adapt as clinical guidelines, technology, and the needs of the stakeholders evolve over time [29]. Services can be added or changed as needed, and the loose component-based architecture can be leveraged to accommodate fluctuations in transaction volumes.

8.6 Emerging trends

Since the publication of the first edition, several important events triggered advancements in health information infrastructures across the globe. First, growth of the OpenHIE community amplified HIE efforts in multiple nations. Second, strong interest in nonclinical data gave rise to an evolving health information infrastructure that seeks to incorporate social, behavioral, and other data into HIE architectures. Finally, the COVID-19 pandemic triggered new investment in public health infrastructure, including HIE networks.

In 2016, the OpenHIE framework consisted of a few founding organizational partners and a handful of countries looking to implement HIE. Fast-forward to 2021, the OpenHIE community of practice now has over 10 organizational partners plus eight stories highlighting implementations of its architecture in various countries across Africa and Asia [41]. Even more impressive, the community has engaged health IT and HIE professionals from all continents working to evolve the framework and its components. Multiple nations involved in the OpenHIE community implemented standards and various architectural components during the past 5 years, and they incorporated the architecture into their nations' respective eHealth or digital health roadmaps. Their work amplifies the work of the global HIE community. The framework summarized in this chapter is an evolved form of the one first presented in the original chapter. Perhaps by the printing of the third edition, you might be part of the community and contributing to the next version of the framework.

Increasingly nations recognize the importance of the social determinants of health as well as other nonclinical factors that influence health and life expectancy. For example, access to clean water and nonpolluted air are some of the many nonclinical targets of the WHO, which seeks to promote health and well-being for citizens of all nations. Because HIE networks seek to support population health and improve health outcomes, many HIOs are working to incorporate nonclinical data into the health information infrastructure. This includes hosting data at geographic and population levels, which is quite different from the traditional patient-level focus of HIE. The trend toward supporting the capture, management, and use of nonclinical data is forcing many HIOs to re-examine their infrastructure and evolve their approaches to accommodate new data types and structures. This trend is covered in more detail in Chapter 19.

The COVID-19 pandemic exposed many flaws in the existing health information infrastructure [42]. Many public health agencies in the United States relied upon fax machines to receive laboratory confirmation of SARS-CoV-2 infections [43], and other data were captured using telephone calls from hospitals as well as manual data entry into web-based portals. Whereas HIE infrastructures were capturing patient-level characteristics and outcomes from hospitals and clinics, many public health agencies struggled to gather details on hospitalization rates as well as symptoms associated with the novel coronavirus. Given these challenges, the United States as well as other nations are investing in strategies to strengthen the health information infrastructure. For example, the American Rescue Plan Act of 2021 [44] appropriated over $50 billion to state, local, territorial, and tribal (SLTT) public health departments to, among other things, enhance their IT infrastructure and modernize their data systems. Other nations are contemplating their own digital public health strategies. All of these efforts are renewing interest in IT systems as well as HIE architectures that can help ensure during the next pandemic that patient and population health data are captured and shared electronically, and that public health authorities can readily use them to guide decision-making processes.

8.7 Summary

The technical attributes of a health information infrastructure are paramount to the effectiveness of large-scale information exchange efforts. HIEs must have a well-developed architecture, mechanisms for transmitting data from one system to another, and processes to provide interoperability between disparate information systems. In this chapter, we have discussed the core technical components of a robust health information infrastructure and described one model for achieving HIE within a community, state, or nation. While OpenHIE offers advantages, it is not the only way to achieve HIE. Regardless of the architecture selected, stakeholders who want to engage in HIE must make design decisions about the layers of interoperability or else the various, disparate information systems that exist within a given health care ecosystem will not be able to exchange data or information.

In the rest of this section of the book, we describe other important technical components of a health information infrastructure that can facilitate HIE. In Chapter 9, we discuss syntactic interoperability and available technical standards that support HIE between information systems. Then in Chapter 10 we describe semantic interoperability and available internationally recognized data standards for consistent representation of data and information across information systems. In Chapter 11 we discuss the role of a SHR that enables longitudinal examinations of individual patients as well as populations. Linking patient records from disparate facilities and health information systems requires a client or patient registry, which we discuss in Chapter 12. Then in Chapter 13 we describe facility registries, which uniquely identify the places where patients receive care in a health system. Next, we discuss health worker registries in Chapter 14 that unique identify the various individuals who provide care in a community or health system, including physicians, nurses, medical assistants, etc. Finally, in Chapter 15, we discuss the business domain service responsible for managing information about insurance and financial claims. When used together, these various components of a health information infrastructure not only facilitate HIE between information systems but they also enable providers, and community and public health organizations to answer questions about who receives care where in the community by whom as well as the outcomes of that care. This is ultimately the goal of HIE—to facilitate better quality, more efficient care that leads to improved health for individuals and populations.

Questions for discussion

1. What characteristics of the health system support the argument that a health information infrastructure can be classified as an ULS system?
2. Compare and contrast the HIE architectural styles and patterns. Which approach might be the most effective on a national scale?
3. Which type of interoperability is most important to architectural design of an HIE?

4. Why is a flexible HIE architecture so important in a country like the United States with multiple, heterogeneous health information systems?
5. What function provided by the interoperability layer is the most important to HIE endeavors? Why?

Acknowledgments

The authors thank the OpenHIE Community of Practice for sharing its collective knowledge and wisdom for use in the book, not only in this chapter but also in this entire technical section. The authors further acknowledge Mr. Ahmed Deeb, a research assistant from Earlham College, who contributed to the updates in the chapter for the second edition of the text.

References

[1] Dixon BE, Grannis SJ. Information infrastructure to support public health. In: Magnuson JA, Dixon BE, editors. Public health informatics and information systems. Health informatics. 3rd ed. Switzerland AG: Springer Nature; 2020. p. 85–104.

[2] Institute of Medicine. Digital infrastructure for the learning health system: The Foundation for Continuous Improvement in Health and Health Care: workshop series summary. Washington, DC: The National Academies Press; 2011.

[3] Feiler P, Sullivan K, Wallnau K, Gabriel R, Goodenough J, Linger R, et al. Ultra-large-scale systems: the software challenge of the future. Pittsburg: Software Engineering Institute, Carnegie Mellon University; 2006. Available from: http://resources.sei.cmu.edu/library/asset-view.cfm?assetID = 30519.

[4] Lee M, Heo E, Lim H, Lee JY, Weon S, Chae H, et al. Developing a common health information exchange platform to implement a nationwide health information network in South Korea. Healthc Inform Res 2015;21(1):21–9.

[5] Taylor RN, Redmiles DF, van der Hoek A. Architectural styles. Irvine, CA: Institute for Software Research, University of California. Available from: http://isr.uci.edu/architecture/styles.html.

[6] Microsoft Corporation. Architectural patterns and styles. Microsoft application architecture guide. 2nd ed. Redmond, WA: Microsoft Corporation; 2009.

[7] Koskela M, Rahikainen M, Wan T. Software development methods: SOA vs. CBD, OO and AOP. Available from: http://citeseerx.ist.psu.edu/viewdoc/summary?doi = 10.1.1.111.9582.

[8] Hosseini M, Ahmadi M, Dixon BE. A service oriented architecture approach to achieve interoperability between immunization information systems in Iran. AMIA Annu Symp Proc/AMIA Symp AMIA Symp 2014;2014:1797–805.

[9] Simonaitis L, Dixon BE, Belsito A, Miller T, Overhage JM. Building a production-ready infrastructure to enhance medication management: early lessons from the nationwide health information network. AMIA Annu Symp Proc 2009;2009:609–13.

[10] Dixon BE, McGowan JJ, Grannis SJ. Electronic laboratory data quality and the value of a health information exchange to support public health reporting processes. AMIA Annu Symp Proc 2011;2011:322–30.

[11] Gliklich RE, Dreyer NA, Leavy MB. Registries for evaluating patient outcomes: a user's guide [Internet]. 3rd ed. Rockville, MD: Agency for Healthcare Research and Quality; 2014.

[12] Broyles D, Dixon BE, Crichton R, Biondich P, Grannis SJ. The evolving health information infrastructure. In: Dixon BE, editor. Health information exchange: navigating and managing a network of health information systems. 1st ed. Waltham, MA: Academic Press; 2016. p. 107–22.

[13] Healthcare Information and Management Systems Society. HIMSS interoperability & HIE community. Chicago: HIMSS. Available from: https://www.himss.org/membership-participation/himss-interoperability-hie-community.

[14] Vergara-Niedermayr C, Wang F, Pan T, Kurc T, Saltz J. Semantically interoperable XML data. Int J Semantic Comput 2013;7(3):237–55.

[15] Dolin RH, Alschuler L. Approaching semantic interoperability in Health Level Seven. J Am Med Inf Assoc 2011;18(1):99–103.

[16] Andry F, Wan L. Health information exchange network interoperability through IHE transactions orchestration. International Conference on Health Informatics, Vilamoura, Portugal 2012.

[17] Healthcare Information and Management Systems Society. What is interoperability? 2013. Available from: http://www.himss.org/library/interoperability-standards/what-is-interoperability.

[18] Barbarito F, Pinciroli F, Mason J, Marceglia S, Mazzola L, Bonacina S. Implementing standards for the interoperability among healthcare providers in the public regionalized Healthcare Information System of the Lombardy Region. J Biomed Inform 2012;45(4):736–45.

[19] Viangteeravat T, Anyanwu MN, Nagisetty VR, Kuscu E, Sakauye ME, Wu D. Clinical data integration of distributed data sources using Health Level Seven (HL7) v3-RIM mapping. J Clin Bioinforma 2011;1:32.

[20] Lin MC, Vreeman DJ, McDonald CJ, Huff SM. A characterization of local LOINC mapping for laboratory tests in three large institutions. Methods Inf Med 2011;50(2):105–14.

[21] Dixon BE, Vreeman DJ, Grannis SJ. The long road to semantic interoperability in support of public health: experiences from two states. J Biomed Inf 2014;49:3–8.

[22] Baorto DM, Cimino JJ, Parvin CA, Kahn MG. Combining laboratory data sets from multiple institutions using the logical observation identifier names and codes (LOINC). Int J Med Inf 1998;51(1):29–37.

[23] Vest JR, Gamm LD. Health information exchange: persistent challenges and new strategies. J Am Med Inform Assoc 2010;17(3):288–94.

[24] Kuperman GJ. Health-information exchange: why are we doing it, and what are we doing? J Am Med Inform Assoc 2011;18(5):678–82.

[25] Coiera E. Building a National Health IT System from the middle out. J Am Med Inform Assoc 2009;16(3):271–3.

[26] Berges I, Bermudez J, Illarramendi A. Toward semantic interoperability of electronic health records. IEEE Trans Inf Technol Biomed: Publ IEEE Eng Med Biol Soc 2012;16(3):424–31.

[27] Crichton R, Moodley D, Pillay A, Gakuba R, Seebregts C. An architecture and reference implementation of an open health information mediator: enabling interoperability in the Rwandan health information exchange. In: Weber J, Perseil I, editors. Foundations of health information engineering and systems. Lecture notes in computer science 7789. Springer Berlin Heidelberg; 2013. p. 87–104.

[28] Gold MR, McLaughlin CG, Devers KJ, Berenson RA, Bovbjerg RR. Obtaining providers' 'buy-in' and establishing effective means of information exchange will be critical to HITECH's success. Health Affairs (Project Hope) 2012;31(3):514–26.

[29] Arzt NH. Service-oriented architecture in public health. J Healthc Inf Manage 2010;24(2).

[30] Adler-Milstein J, Bates DW, Jha AK. Operational health information exchanges show substantial growth, but long-term funding remains a concern. Health Aff (Proj Hope) 2013;32(8):1486–92.

[31] Dixon BE, Zafar A, Overhage JM. A framework for evaluating the costs, effort, and value of nationwide health information exchange. J Am Med Inf Assoc 2010;17 (3):295–301.

[32] Vest JR. Health information exchange: national and international approaches. Adv Health Care Manage 2012;12:3–24.

[33] Crichton R. The open health information mediator: an architecture for enabling interoperability in low to middle income countries. Durban: University of KwaZulu-Natal; 2015.

[34] Liu S, Zhou B, Xie G, Mei J, Liu H, Liu C, et al. Beyond regional health information exchange in China: a practical and industrial-strength approach. AMIA Annu Symp Proc/AMIA Symp AMIA Symp 2011;2011:824–33.

[35] El Azami I, Cherkaoui Malki MO, Tahon C. Integrating hospital information systems in healthcare institutions: a mediation architecture. J Med Syst 2012;36(5):3123–34.

[36] Koufi V, Malamateniou F, Vassilacopoulos G. A big data-driven model for the optimization of healthcare processes. Stud Health Technol Inform 2015;210:697–701.

[37] Ryan A, Eklund P. The Health Service Bus: an architecture and case study in achieving interoperability in healthcare. Stud Health Technol Inform 2010;160(Pt 2):922–6.

[38] Van Den Bossche B, Van Hoecke S, Danneels C, Decruyenaere J, Dhoedt B, De Turck F. Design of a JAIN SLEE/ESB-based platform for routing medical data in the ICU. Comput Methods Prog Biomed 2008;91(3):265–77.

[39] Khan WA, Khattak AM, Hussain M, Amin MB, Afzal M, Nugent C, et al. An adaptive semantic based mediation system for data interoperability among Health Information Systems. J Med Syst 2014;38(8):28.

[40] Blobel B, Holena M. Comparing middleware concepts for advanced healthcare system architectures. Int J Med Inform 1997;46(2):69–85.

[41] OpenHIE. Our community is improving global health: OpenHIE; 2021. Available from: https://ohie.org/impact-stories/.

[42] Dixon BE, Caine VA, Halverson PK. Deficient response to COVID-19 makes the case for evolving the public health system. Am J Prev Med 2020;59(6):887–91.

[43] Kliff S, Sanger-Katz M. Bottleneck for U.S. coronavirus response: the fax machine. *The New York Times*. 2020 July 13, 2020;Sect. Upshot.

[44] American Rescue Plan Act of 2021, Public Law No: 117-2 (2021).

CHAPTER

9

Syntactic interoperability and the role of syntactic standards in health information exchange

Elizabeth E. Umberfield[1,2], *Catherine J. Staes*[3,4], *Teryn P. Morgan*[2,5], *Randall W. Grout*[2,6], *Burke W. Mamlin*[2,6] *and Brian E. Dixon*[2,7]

[1]Division of Nursing Research, Mayo Clinic, Rochester, MN, USA [2]Center for Biomedical Informatics, Regenstrief Institute, Inc., Indianapolis, IN, USA [3]College of Nursing, University of Utah, Salt Lake City, UT, USA [4]Department of Biomedical Informatics, School of Medicine, University of Utah, Salt Lake City, UT, USA [5]Department of BioHealth Informatics, School of Informatics and Computing, Indiana University, Indianapolis, IN, USA [6]School of Medicine, Indiana University, Indianapolis, IN, USA [7]Department of Epidemiology, Richard M. Fairbanks School of Public Health, Indiana University, Indianapolis, IN, USA

LEARNING OBJECTIVES

By the end of this chapter, you will be able to:

- Define syntactic interoperability and describe its role in health information exchange (HIE).
- Describe some of the most common syntactic standards and distinguish their application in health care.
- Describe the process for developing standards in health care.
- Recognize how multiple syntactic standards are used throughout the health information ecosystem to facilitate HIE.
- Identify and describe resources and services used by organizations when they implement syntactic standards.

Health Information Exchange
DOI: https://doi.org/10.1016/B978-0-323-90802-3.00004-6

9.1 Introduction

Successful transactions between disparate information systems require multiple layers of interoperability. In Chapter 8, we defined interoperability and described how an interoperability layer facilitates data exchange between core health information exchange (HIE) services and the many health information system applications that may have a need to send or receive data and information [1,2]. We also defined the three layers of interoperability: foundational interoperability, syntactic interoperability, and semantic interoperability. In this chapter, we more fully describe the concept of syntactic interoperability, covering why syntactic standards are needed, examples of commonly used syntactic standards for HIE, how standards overall are developed, and how syntactic standards are implemented in the real world.

9.2 Defining syntactic interoperability: definition and need

Syntactic interoperability is achieved when multiple information systems discover and access information within transmitted artifacts (e.g., documents, messages) [2,3]. The need for syntactic interoperability became apparent as health information systems proliferated in the 1980s, and syntactic interfaces where each party could decipher the other's artifacts were needed to enable communication between systems. While two systems are linkable with a single interface, the number of interfaces exponentially increases as the number of systems increases. In other words, while two systems require a single interface and 3 systems require only 3 interfaces, 5 systems require 10 interfaces, 10 systems require 45 interfaces, 20 systems require 190 interfaces, and so on. This problem is known as *combinatorial explosion*, and is depicted graphically on the left-hand side of Fig. 9.1 and in the following formula, where n is equal to the number of systems:

$$\text{Number of interfaces} = \frac{n(n-1)}{2}$$

While communication between systems could hypothetically be achieved despite combinatorial explosion, creation of a bespoke syntactic interface or shared language for every combination of two systems is clearly not sustainable when we consider the scale of information systems that exchange data either within or between health care enterprises. For example, a health care enterprise needs to exchange data between an electronic health record (EHR) and myriad interconnected component systems, including lab systems, devices (e.g., electrocardiogram machines, ventilators, etc.), systems that support pharmacy, nursing, nutrition services, etc., regional health information organization, and other ancillary systems.

Syntactic standards address this problem by providing a common structure and syntax for transmitting artifacts between systems. The right-hand side of Fig. 9.1 demonstrates how use of a syntactic standard can reduce the number of unique syntactic interfaces needed

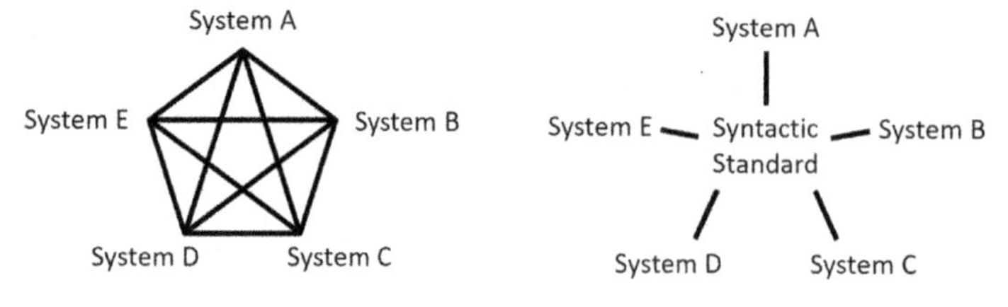

FIGURE 9.1 Side-by-side comparison of the number of syntactic interface connections needed to facilitate syntactic health information exchange between five systems without a syntactic standard ($n = 10$; left) and with a syntactic standard ($n = 5$; right).

to translate between a system's native data structure and standards-based artifacts shared between systems, in this case from 10 to 5.

The structure of an artifact is defined by a *schema*, which is the outline or plan for all artifacts of a given type. A schema defines which elements or parts may be included—including which are required or optional, the type of information contained in each element, the order of elements, and the relationship between elements.

Syntax refers to the set of rules that must be adhered to while expressing information within an artifact, such as a standard message for laboratory data. The rules of syntax are akin to the rules of grammar. Just as a grammatically incorrect sentence can be difficult or impossible for humans to understand, computers require adherence to rules of syntax to understand artifacts. These principles apply to the range of artifacts that require standardization to exchange information between systems, including messages, clinical documents, content for decision support, logic to query an EHR, data models, and others. The most common types of artifacts are messages and documents. Key characteristics of messages and documents are contrasted in Table 9.1.

Let us explore these concepts using an example of sending a potential employer our resume when applying for a job. Foundational interoperability allows us to upload our resume to an online job application website and have it delivered to the intended recipient, provided we use a valid job application URL address. This technical infrastructure is agnostic about the contents of the uploaded document. Syntactic interoperability, on the other hand, provides structure and syntax for the resume to be interpreted by the job application website as well as the human reviewing our resume.

When creating our resume, we place specific information unique to resume documents inside to highlight our unique knowledge, skills, and previous jobs. This information is distinct from other types of documents we might create, such as an essay for a class or an invoice for a client. Syntactic interoperability allows us to explicitly define the type of artifact we are uploading and the nature of its contents using a schema.

In this example, our resume schema might outline five main sections: (1) name and contact information, (2) career goals and objectives, (3) skills we bring to the position, (4) relevant experience, and (5) education and training. The schema for the resume would further define the document's parts, including where address, telephone, and email information should be displayed, where we should list awards we have received, and where we should put professional references, if required. The job application website might provide the schema to us in its description of what is required to be in the

TABLE 9.1 Key characteristics of standardized messages and documents [4].

	Artifacts	
Feature	**Messages**	**Documents**
Communication Function	Between applications	Between people, particularly care providers
Audience	Designed to be machine-readable	Designed to be human-readable
Life Cycle	Temporal (event-driven)	Persistent
Context	Segment: oriented toward the status of a business object	Document-level
Completeness	Fragment	Complete

resume. Alternatively, when we use a software application such as Microsoft Word to create our resume, we can choose to use a *template* which provides a predefined structure in which we added our own specific information.

If we follow the schema provided by the job website, it will be able to parse out our information and use it to apply for multiple jobs for which we are eligible, without needing to retype the information again. Similarly, humans reviewing our resume will be able to quickly find the information they need to examine our skills, knowledge, and abilities when assessing our potential as an applicant. In HIE, we use schemas and templates to create and interpret artifacts that are sent and received by health information systems. Schemas and templates constrain the vast array of possible artifact types and information that could potentially be put into any given artifact. Being compliant with constraints leads to robust and standardized artifacts that facilitate interoperability.

Fig. 9.2 presents examples of abbreviated forms of the same Fast Healthcare Interoperability Resources (FHIR) artifact, written using Extensible Markup Language (XML) and JSON, that adhere to the specifications in the FHIR Patient Resource [3]. This artifact defines a fictional patient's information, including name, date of birth, address, and phone number. It is written in both XML and JSON to demonstrate that artifact content is independent of structure and syntax. It should be noted the FHIR standard allows both formats to be used; the content can be transformed between the two, which can be useful depending on tooling resources, and preferences. In the XML example, *tags*, enclosed in <>, are used to denote each type of information in the section. A similar convention is used in the JSON example, where the name and value are quoted and separated with a colon. Complete FHIR artifacts in health care are much more complex, but they are constructed using these basic "building blocks."

Syntactic interoperability is necessary for discrete information systems to read the artifacts that are sent and received in HIE. Without syntactic standards, an artifact might be sent, but it could not be ingested by the receiving system. Standards provide a framework for tools to be built against, enabling integration of information from multiple sources, increasing efficiency, and yielding options for interacting with transmitted information (e.g., whether to use Microsoft Word, WordPerfect, or Open Office to edit our resume). Tools can leverage the standard syntax to make content easier to read (using indentation, coloring, etc.).

9.3 Common syntactic standards relevant for health information exchange

Multiple syntactic standards exist in health care to exchange different types of information that span content domains. As examples, standards from Health Level Seven International (HL7) range from HL7 version 2 (v2) and FHIR for clinical information, Digital Imaging and Communications in Medicine (DICOM) for radiological imaging, National Council for Prescription Drug Programs (NCPDP) for prescriptions, and X12 for financial data including Health Insurance Portability and Accountability Act (HIPAA)-mandated transactions. In this section, we describe these syntactic standards, including their general purpose and use.

9.3.1 Health Level Seven International standards

Health Level 7 (HL7) publishes the most widely adopted syntactic standards for exchanging clinical and administrative information in the health care domain [5]. The "level 7" in its name refers to the application layer of the Open Systems Interconnection

XML

```
<?xml version="1.0" encoding="UTF-8"?>

<Patient xmlns="http://hl7.org/fhir">
 <id value="example"/>
 <name>
  <use value="official"/>
  <family value="Doe"/>
  <given value="John"/>
 </name>
 <telecom>
  <system value="phone"/>
  <value value="555-555-5501"/>
  <use value="home"/>
 </telecom>
 <gender value="male"/>
 <birthDate value="2001-01-01">

<extension url="http://hl7.org/fhir/Struc
tureDefinition/patient-birthTime">
   <valueDateTime value="2001-01-
01T14:35:45-05:00"/>
  </extension>
 </birthDate>
 <deceasedBoolean value="false">
 <address>
  <use value="home">
  <line value="555 Any Rd."/>
  <city value="Somewhereville"/>
  <state value="State"/>
  <postalCode value="99999"/>
 </address>
<contact>
  <relationship>
   <coding>
<system value="http://terminology.hl7.org
/CodeSystem/v2-0131"/>
   <code value="N"/>
   </coding>
  </relationship>
  <name>
   <family value="Doe"/>
   <given value="Jane"/>
  </name>
  <telecom>
   <system value="phone"/>
   <value value="555-555-5502"/>
  </telecom>
  <address>
   <use value="home"/>
   <line value="555 Any Rd."/>
   <city value=" Somewhereville"/>
   <state value=" State "/>
   <postalCode value="99999"/>
  </address>
  <gender value="female"/>
  <period>
   <start value="2012"/>
  </period>
  </contact>
</Patient>
```

JSON

```
{
 "resourceType": "Patient",
 "id": "example",
 "name": [{
  "use": "official",
  "family": "Doe",
  "given": "John"
 }],
 "telecom": [{
  "system": "phone",
  "value": "555-555-5501",
  "use":"home"
 }],
 "gender":"male",
 "birthDate": "2000-01-01",
 "_birthDate": {
 "extension": [{
"url": "http://hl7.org/fhir/StructureDefi
nition/patient-birthTime",
  "valueDateTime": "1974-12-25T14:35:45-
05:00"
 }]},
 "deceasedBoolean": false,
 "address": [{
  "use": "home",
  "line": "555 Any Rd.",
  "city": "Somewhereville",
  "state": "State",
  "postalCode": "99999",
 }],
 "contact": [{
  "relationship": [{
   "coding": [{
"system": "http://terminology.hl7.org/Cod
eSystem/v2-0131",
    "code": "N"
  }]}],

  "name": [{
  "family": "Doe",
  "given":"Jane"
  }],
  "telecom": [{
   "system": "phone",
   "value": "555-555-5502"
  }],
  "address": [{
  "use": "home",
  "line": "555 AnyWhere Rd.",
  "city": "Somewhereville",
  "state": "State",
  "postalCode": "99999",
  }],
  "gender": "female",
  "period": [{
  "start": "2012"
  }]
 }]
}
```

FIGURE 9.2 Example of an abbreviated message based on the FHIR Patient Resource, written in XML (left) and JSON (right).

(OSI) model, a conceptual model that characterizes and standardizes interactions within a computer system regardless of its underlying technology. The application layer of the OSI model describes functions that typically include synchronizing communication between computer systems [6]. Since the 1980s, HL7 standards have gone through several revisions, from worldwide adoption of HL7 v2 to a worldwide embracing of FHIR for the future of HIE.

9.3.1.1 *HL7 v2 messaging standard*

The HL7 version 2 (v2) messaging standard remains in wide use by health information systems in the United States and worldwide [7]. Successive, incremental improvements to the v2 standard have resulted in clearer, more detailed and documented versions that sought to expand the standard to additional clinical domains while also supporting better normalization. Because of this, the v2 standard is backward compatible, enabling applications to receive and appropriately handle different versions in the v2 family.

HL7 v2 messages are expressed using Encoding Rules 7 (ER7), a syntax which uses segments, fields, and components using a variety of delimiters to encode data [8]. Fig. 9.3 presents a sample Admission, Discharge, Transfer (ADT) v2.3 message, which is one of the most common types of messages. Segments are presented in red and the fields are separated by pipe (|) delimiter. There are other delimiters, such as the carrot (^), used for separating components within fields. Tooling is necessary to parse v2 messages and fully review their content.

One strength of the v2 standard is that it does not overspecify content, allowing implementers to adopt it more easily. Rather, it focuses on what information to send and where to put it instead of specifying exactly how that information is defined. Although the v2 standard has been incrementally improved, many in the health IT world felt it only normalized 80% of a given interface between two systems. This meant that an additional 20% was customized when, for example, an interface was established between a hospital's laboratory information system and that hospital's EHR system. The customization was necessary because many aspects of the v2 standard were inherently designed to be flexible, allowing several "design choices" to be made when implemented.

In addition to being flexible, critics charged that the v2 standard:

- Lacked a consistent data model, meaning that each system could use its own data model, leading to inconsistency across implementations; and
- Lacked clear, well-defined application and user roles, allowing vendors to choose which set of HL7 messages would be supported for a given set of clinical functions.

Despite these limitations, this standard is commonly used today for sharing ADT information, laboratory data, immunization records, electrocardiogram (EKG) results, bone densitometry, and more. 95% of US healthcare

```
MSH|^~\&|GoodEMR|Location1|LIS|Location1|201502042115||ADT^A01|ADT000
01|P|2.3|
EVN|A01|201502042115||
PID|||MRN12345^5^M11||DOE^JOHN^A||19800711|M||C|1 MERIDIAN
STREET^^INDIANAPOLIS^IN^46280|
NK1|1|GOODMAN^CINDY^J|WIFE||||||NK^NEXT OF KIN
PV1|1|I|200^11^01||||006666^GOOD^BARBARA^J.|||SUR||||ADM|A0|
```

FIGURE 9.3 A sample HL7 v2.3 Admission, Discharge, Transfer (ADT) message.

organizations use HL7 v2, and it is implemented in at least 35 countries [7].

9.3.1.2 HL7 CDA document standard

To address the criticisms noted about the v2 messaging standard, the HL7 community created a Version 3 (v3) HL7 standard. The HL7 v3 standard represented a suite of specifications explicitly designed around the HL7 Reference Information Model (RIM), which aimed to serve as a comprehensive, consistent data model and provide a framework for generating HL7 messages. HL7 v3 never achieved the market penetration experienced by the v2 standard [9]. However, the RIM is the backbone for the Clinical Document Architecture (CDA) standard which is used today to share documents between health systems, as well as between providers and patients. CDA is HL7 most widely adopted HL7 v3 standard [9].

HL7 CDA is a document markup standard that specifies the structure and semantics of "clinical documents" for the purpose of exchanging clinical documents between those involved in the care of a patient. In addition, it supports the re-use of clinical data for public health reporting, quality monitoring, patient safety, clinical trials, and more.

CDA documents are encoded in XML. In contrast to the v2 standard described above, the CDA standard defines a clinical document as having six characteristics: (1) persistence, (2) stewardship, (3) potential for authentication, (4) context, (5) Wholeness, and (6) human readability [10]. These characteristics mimic functionality expected when exchanging paper docu ments. Documents contain data (persisting a "snapshot") as it was understood at a particular time [9]. For example, one expects a clinical note or case report to include a human readable summary of clinical content that is signed and dated and clearly identifies the organization responsible for the document (i.e., steward).

All CDA-compliant documents include a standardized *header* that contains metadata about the document (date created, author, organization, etc.) and a standardized *body* composed of sections that can contain a wide variety of clinical content. The type and arrangement of the sections and their related templates are defined in Implementation Guides (IG) published by HL7 [10]. The content of the *body* sections can range from an unencoded payload, such as a PDF, to a fully-encoded HL7 v3 instance of a template. The *body* content depends on the Implementation Guide. For example, there are Implementation Guides for specific Use Cases, such as Public Health Case Reporting and Trauma Registry Data Submission.

The Consolidated-CDA (C-CDA) standard represents a menu of CDA templates which can be used to generate a variety of different clinical notes [11]. The most common types of templates include document-level templates (e.g., History and Physical document), section-level templates (e.g., Physical Exam section), and entry-level templates (e.g., Systolic Blood Pressure entry) [12]. As shown in Fig. 9.4, these templates are building blocks for commonly shared documents, such as a Continuity of Care documents (CCD), Consultation Notes, Diagnostic Imaging Report (DIR), Discharge Summary, History and Physical (H&P), Operative Note, Procedure Note, Progress Note, Referral Note, Transfer Summary, Un structured Document, and Patient Generated Document [13]. The C-CDA implementation guide specifies a library of CDA templates and prescribes their use for given document types, thus simplifying and reducing variation across implementations [11].

Currently, the CDA standard is the primary standard for exchanging clinical documents in the United States. Vendors report exchanging over 500 million C-CDA documents annually in the United States [14], which include all the

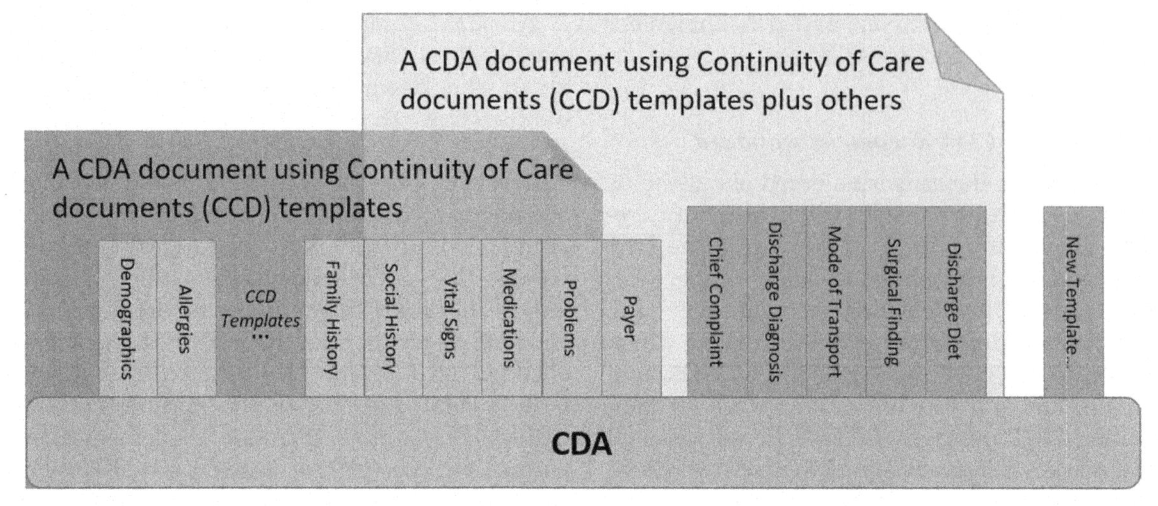

FIGURE 9.4 Templated CDA [12]. Source: *Adapted from HL7 International. HL7 implementation guide for CDA Release 2: consolidated CDA templates for clinical notes [Internet]. 2015. Available from: http://www.hl7.org/ccdasearch/pdfs/CCDA_Volume_One.pdf.*

various types listed above. More recently, in the context of the COVID-19 pandemic, health systems implemented electronic case reporting using the newly-defined CDA standard for an electronic initial case report (eICR). Between May 2020 and November 2021, more than 9600 facilities across the United States started sending COVID-19 electronic case reports to public health using the eICR [15].

Overall, implementations of CDA-based documents have increased over time, particularly motivated by vendor certification requirements; however, researchers have documented ongoing problems with data quality that require enhanced monitoring to ensure the safe exchange of health information [14].

9.3.1.3 *Fast Healthcare Interoperability Resources*

Fast Healthcare Interoperability Resources (FHIR) was developed in the early 2010s in response to the question, "What would health information exchange look like if it started now, using modern approaches?" Their solution builds on the best features of HL7's other syntactic standards and the framework of smartphone "apps." FHIR employs common web technologies (e.g., JSON, XML, application programming interfaces, REST, OAuth) with which developers are already familiar [16]. FHIR is also designed to be compatible with previous HL7 standards through mapping [9]. By leveraging existing standards and common web technologies, FHIR simplifies implementation and enables rapid uptake, therefore advancing HIE [16]. The following are the improvements FHIR presents over previous HL7 standards:

- Implementation of FHIR is designed to be simple and efficient and multiple implementation libraries are available.
- Resources are simple enough to cover a range of use cases but can be extended, modified, or constrained using profiles.
- Specifications are open-access, online, and simply written.
- Serialization formats (e.g., JSON, XML) are human-readable [17].

FHIR serves as a *platform specification*—its resources provide the basis for HIE solutions that provide structure and guidance for the most common or essential data elements. However, FHIR is flexible. Through *integration profiles*, data elements can be added, modified, or constrained to base resources rather than developing new standards [18,19]. In this way, the FHIR specification recognizes that a *one size fits all* approach is not applicable to the wide variability across health care settings.

FHIR has two main components: (1) A content model in the form of *resources* and (2) an *application programming interface (API)* [20]. FHIR resources are individual clinical entities with a specific identity (i.e., a URL), type, structure, and version [21]. For example, the Patient Resource includes demographic and administrative data elements (e.g., contact information) for individuals receiving health services [3]. Resources serve as building blocks that can be combined to meet different use cases [20]. There are 145 resources in FHIR Release 4, that is, the current release and first release to include normative content [22].

The FHIR API is like a library; it defines the rules that applications can use to exchange information with one another [19,21]. FHIR's API follows a RESTful approach (referring to Representational State Transfer), which refers to how information can be easily exchanged using HTTP requests, which are the basis for all website data exchange. FHIR Resources are primarily designed for RESTful HTTP-based implementation. Transactions are performed directly on the RESTful server to obtain resources using a HTTP request/response. A HTTP GET request is sent to the desired Resource Type endpoint, and the response contains the resource. For example, a URL such as https://server/path/Patient might be used to call the Patient Resource.

Developers, implementers, and policy makers largely agree that FHIR demonstrates promise for advancing HIE, and that FHIR will be further developed and implemented for the foreseeable future. Given that the FHIR standard is continually advancing, we recommend exploring the FHIR website to understand the standard's current status and functionality: https://hl7.org/fhir/ [23].

9.3.2 Digital Imaging and Communications in Medicine

DICOM is the most widely adopted standard in the world for the exchange and management of medical images. Since introducing DICOM in 1993, providers have been able to use fully digital images with high resolution instead of physical X-ray films. Using DICOM, images generated by different types of medical imaging devices (e.g., X-ray, computed tomography [CT] scan, magnetic resonance imaging [MRI], ultrasound) can be integrated into picture archiving and communication systems and they can be exchanged in HIE networks. The DICOM standard not only encodes the image but also a set of metadata and attributes that describe the image and can be used by other applications in health care delivery [24].

9.3.3 National Council for Prescription Drug Programs

The NCPDP standardizes electronic exchange of data for prescribing, dispensing, monitoring, managing and paying for medications and pharmacy services [25]. As of 2021, NCPDP has more than 30 published standards.

Three of the most commonly used NCPDP standards include:

1. Telecommunication,
2. SCRIPT, and
3. Manufacturer Rebate.

The NCPDP Telecommunication standard provides a structure to electronically submit third-party drug claims as well as perform eligibility verification and prior authorization. The SCRIPT standard supports transmitting prescription information electronically in support of fulfilling new prescriptions, prescription refill requests, relaying medication history, and transactions for long-term care. To meet this need, the standard defines a structure for information about the prescriber, the recipient of the medication, and the medication. The Manufacturer Rebate standard supports submission of rebate information by Pharmacy Management Organizations to Pharmaceutical Industry Contracting Organizations (PICOs) [26].

9.3.4 X12 standards in health care

Like HL7, X12 is a nonprofit organization that focuses on the development, implementation, and ongoing use of consensus-based, interoperable electronic data interchange (EDI) standards [27]. There exist a variety of X12 standards for various EDI transactions across multiple commercial and noncommercial sectors, including health care. In health care, X12 standards primarily support what is known as the HIPAA 5010 messaging standards. These standards facilitate various administrative data sharing for operational purposes, primarily reimbursement for health services. This set of standards includes the following transactions:

- Submission of billing information for a health care claim,
- Submission of encounter information for a health care claim,
- Check on the status of a health care claim previously submitted,
- Send an Explanation of Benefits remittance advice,
- Make a payment to a health care provider or pharmacy, and
- Inquire about the health care benefits and eligibility associated with a subscriber or dependent.

9.4 How standards are developed for health care

Standards Development Organizations (SDOs) oversee the development and maintenance of standards. SDOs can be private or public organizations. The American Society for Testing and Materials and HL7 International are two important SDOs that develop standards for clinical and administrative information. There are also SDO accreditation organizations, such as the American National Standards Institute, which oversees SDOs in the United States and coordinate standards development with international SDOs so that US products can be used worldwide.

Health Information Organizations (HIOs), such as the Indiana Health Information Exchange (detailed in Chapter 22) and OpenHIE (described in Chapter 8), also play an important role in developing and advancing standards. HIOs often participate closely with SDOs to advocate for standards which align with their own use cases and needs and are essential for testing standards that are under development.

Once the need for a standard is recognized, SDOs recruit and assemble a collaborative team. This team, called a technical committee or working group, is comprised of experts in the area of interest and individuals who represent organizations that will be influenced by the standard. Working group members meet to discuss and develop a draft standard.

Standards can be developed through "bottom up," "top down," or a combination of these approaches and may be classified as "de facto," "de jure," or "ad hoc." Standards that achieve market penetration through organic (bottom up) adoption by industry are said to be de facto or market-driven standards. At the opposite end of the spectrum, standards endorsed or required for use by government authorities are said to be *de jure* "according to the law" standards. Most of the widely used standards today are a combination of these two approaches; for example, HL7's FHIR standard started as a de facto standard and its momentum continues to be driven by the US government [28].

Ad hoc is another classification of standards, developed by group of people or organizations interested in a specific use case. Their informal agreement on a solution for a specific challenge is an *ad hoc* standard. DICOM is an example of a popular *ad hoc* standard for exchanging medical images that resulted from collaborative work between the American College of Radiology and the National Electrical Manufacturers Association.

It is common for the first version of a standard to be referred to as a *Draft* or *Informative Standard*, because it informs the community about an HIE challenge and proposes a solution. The draft standard is distributed among all members of the SDO to be voted upon, usually through a Web-based portal that allows for the balloting of standards. During the balloting period, members can comment on the draft standard and revisions can be made. As revisions are made and balloted, standards are expected to become more stable.

For the FHIR standard, stability is reflected using the FHIR Maturity Model (FMM). Table 9.2 shows the FMM maturity levels and definitions [29,30]. After publication of a Draft version, the standard may be approved for *Trial Use*, meaning that it has been defined to a point that would allow a group of vendors or

TABLE 9.2 Maturity levels as defined by the FHIR Maturity Model (FMM) [29].

Maturity level	Definition (each level builds on prior levels)
0 (Draft)	The resource or profile (artifact) has been published on the current build. This level is synonymous with Draft
1	The artifact produces no warnings during the build process and the responsible working group (WG) has indicated that they consider the artifact substantially complete and ready for implementation. For resources, profiles, and implementation guides, the FHIR Management Group has approved the underlying resource/profile/IG proposal
2	The artifact has been tested and successfully supports interoperability among at least three independently developed systems leveraging most of the scope (e.g., at least 80% of the core data elements) using semirealistic data and scenarios based on at least one of the declared scopes of the artifact (e.g., at a connectathon). These interoperability results must have been reported to and accepted by the FHIR Management Group
3	The artifact has been verified by the work group as meeting the Conformance Resource Quality Guidelines (https://confluence.hl7.org/display/FHIR/Conformance + QA + Criteria); has been subject to a round of formal balloting; has at least 10 distinct implementer comments recorded in the tracker drawn from at least three organizations resulting in at least one substantive change
4	The artifact has been tested across its scope (see below), published in a formal publication (e.g., Trial-Use), and implemented in multiple prototype projects. As well, the responsible work group agrees the artifact is sufficiently stable to require implementer consultation for subsequent nonbackward compatible changes
5	The artifact has been published in two formal publication release cycles at FMM1 + (i.e., Trial-Use level) and has been implemented in at least five independent production systems in more than one country.
Normative	The artifact is considered stable

FHIR, Fast Healthcare Interoperability Resources; *IG*, implementation guide.
Retrieved from HL7 International. Version management policy. Change management and versioning; 2021. https://www.hl7.org/fhir/versions.html.

providers to pilot test its use. After a period when various implementers have trialed the standard and provided feedback, a standard can be revised and approved as *Normative*. The title Normative suggests a final, consensus-based designation that the standard is ready for widespread adoption [29].

Even after a standard becomes normative, it can be further refined or updated for a variety of reasons, such as requirement changes, gaps in the current standard, or expanding the scope of the standard. For example, the HL7 Version 2 messaging standard has been considered normative since the 1990s. Yet this standard continues to be actively used and updated.

Implementing standards is not easy. It is not uncommon for two systems reportedly in compliance with the standard to require additional work to make them interoperable [31]. *Conformance testing* is the process by which implementations of a standard are tested to assess their compliance with the standard. Conformance testing can be performed on individual artifacts (e.g., testing individual instances of Patient or Observation FHIR Resources against a published schema), using an API (e.g., a set of predefined input tested against expected outputs), or directly on client applications [32,33]. National Institute of Standards and Technology is a US government agency designed to promote innovation and competitiveness, in part, through the development and support of Health IT standardization and provides a Health IT Testing infrastructure, which includes testing tools and services for conformance testing [34].

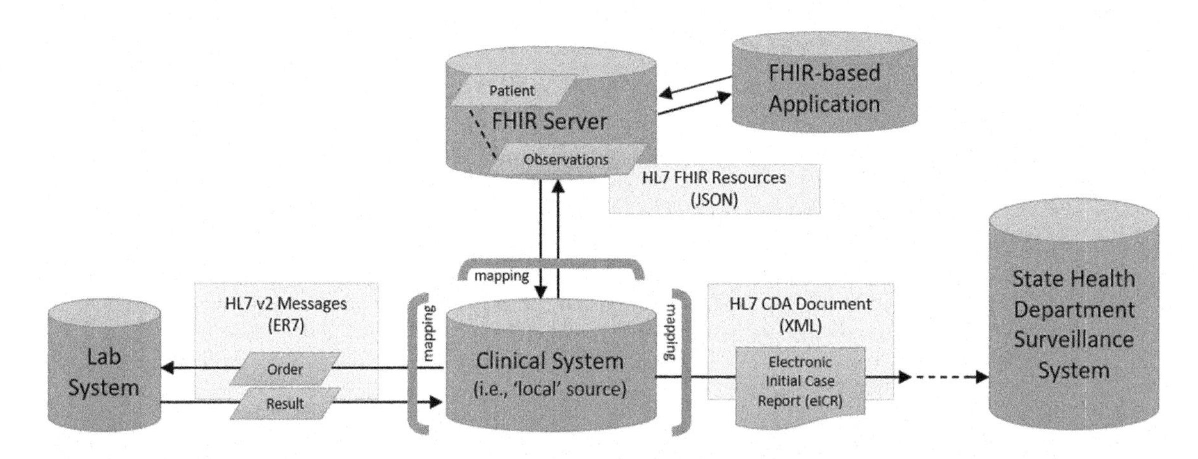

Example of Mappings between a local data source (i.e., EHR or clinical data repository) and the standard exchange formats:					
Data Element	**Sample Values**	**Example table and field names from a local data source**	**V2**	**CDA**	**FHIR Path (Resource.Element)**
Patient's Birth Date	01/01/2000	Person table / DOB	PID.7	<Record target> <PatientRole> <patient> <birthtime>	Patient.birthdate
Patient's Gender	Female	Person table / gender	PID.8	<Record target> <PatientRole> <patient> <administrativeGenderCode>	Patient.gender
Name of lab test performed	Blood lead (ug/dL)	LabResult table / testName	OBX.3	<component> <structured body> <component> <section> <entry...> ...<code>	Observation.code

FIGURE 9.5 Example of how multiple syntactic standards are used throughout the health information ecosystem to facilitate health information exchange.

9.5 How syntactic standards are used and supported in the real world

Given that standards are designed to serve different purposes, a single health system must support use of a variety of standards to send and receive information when carrying out the business of health care.

Data in the EHR are often stored using proprietary methods derived from the vendors' or systems' needs, but interfaces can be used to transform data for exchange. For example, as shown in Fig. 9.5, laboratory data may be shared as an HL7 v2 message from a laboratory and then stored at the health system. These same laboratory results may trigger a clinical decision support (CDS) application based on the FHIR standard. If so, the data may then populate a FHIR-based artifact that becomes an input to a CDS engine with logic that will trigger a message to a provider that an abnormal value was received. Similarly, the laboratory data may be included in a case report implemented as a CDA-based document called an electronic Initial Case Report (eICR) that is then forwarded to a public health system. The same unit of laboratory data can be represented in a pipe-delimited message HL7 v2 message, in XML that conforms to the CDA specifications, or in JSON that conforms to the FHIR standard.

To achieve HIE, implementers require guidance, standards, and tooling tailored to their given use cases. For example, they need: (1) implementation guides, which are documents that outline constraints on top of standards and profiles for a very specific use case; (2) interface engines, technologies designed to implement standards, profiles, and implementation guides, and (3) HIE services, which normalize the transaction of artifacts from one information system to another. Together these resources can be used by implementers to take mature standards and implement them in a community, state, or nation.

9.5.1 Implementation guides

Syntactic standards provide a foundation upon which a specific HIE implementation rests. While necessary, standards alone are not sufficient to achieve interoperability as they are inherently accommodating across a range of use cases. Therefore, for a given use case, standards must be constrained, and guidance must be provided to implementers, which is the purpose of an *implementation guide (IG)*. IGs are usually focused on a narrow use case, such as the electronic ordering of a laboratory test or the electronic reporting of a patient's death.

IGs are often published by SDOs as well as affinity groups such as ministries of health, professional societies, and industry groups. As an example, OpenHIE publishes IGs to provide guidance for HIO architecture, including a range of registries, interoperability architecture, shared health records and terminology services. To implement many of the OpenHIE services described in this book, it is recommended readers consult the IGs available at http://www.ohie.org [35]. While some IGs are open access and free, others require membership or payment for access. The Office of the National Coordinator for Health Information Technology's (ONC) Interoperability Standards Advisory (ISA) also provides IGs for implementing a range of standards, including the *Content/Structure Standards and Implementation Specifications*. These specifications focus on what is needed to achieve syntactic interoperability for a range of use cases [36].

IGs focus on artifact structure and content. The IGs outline what information is required for a given use case, even where it might be generally considered to be optional by the base standard. For example, a field for a patient's race may be required in many US public health use cases, but may be optional in global contexts since some countries do not allow the capture of racial information in EHR systems. For use cases involving FHIR, IGs specify rules for how FHIR resources should be used to meet intended use cases. These IGs provide both content requirements, in the form of logical statements which implementations must conform to, and examples which illustrate how the IG should be applied [37]. IGs defined by the FHIR community are curated by the FHIR Foundation at https://www.fhir.org/guides/registry/ [38].

9.5.2 Interface engines

Implementers need a method by which to interface, or connect, various health IT systems using standards and IGs. An *interface engine* is a mediator technology that supports standard-based implementation of HIE. The engine is software that "listens" for messages on a channel (e.g., think pipeline or roadway), and they can also send messages through a channel to other systems. Typically, interface engines include several different types of input and output channels (e.g., hypertext transfer protocol [HTTP], transmission control protocol [TCP], etc.) and include tools to parse and transform messages then route them where needed, sometimes to multiple output channels. Interface engines also handle queuing of messages when connections are interrupted and the ability to "replay" message when errors have occurred. Enterprise health systems can have hundreds of working parts that need to be integrated. Using standards allows each component to integrate with an interface engine and for that interface engine to manage all the connections.

The interface engine is typically programmed to receive certain types of messages then do something when messages arrive. For example, when electronic laboratory reporting messages arrive, the interface engine could be instructed to pass the message along to the EHR for storage in the patient's medical record. It might also be programmed to forward a copy of the message to the public health department if the result pertained to a disease required to be reported to health authorities (e.g., sexually transmitted infection). This second option might require the interface engine to open the message and inspect its contents. Therefore interface engines are versatile software allowing both simple communication of messages from one system to the next as well as more complex tasks such as interpreting a message and taking an action based on the contents.

Interface engines can also be programmed to translate messages as they pass through. For example, an interface engine might convert HL7 v2 messages to FHIR messages, or vice versa. Other use cases might require transforming an incoming message to a nonstandard version that can be incorporated into a proprietary or legacy system. The potential number of configurations and uses of interface engines is endless given their flexibility and design to support the full spectrum of messages available in the health care domain. Furthermore, as mentioned in Chapter 8, interface engines provide mediation services that combine orchestration and adapter functions. An important design choice in HIEs is whether to implement distinct adapters and orchestrators or use an interface engine. There are several commercial interface engines available in the marketplace, including:

- NexGen Connect [39],
- Lyniate Corepoint and Lyniate Rhapsody [40,41],
- InterSystems Ensemble [42],
- Summit Healthcare Express Connect [43], and
- Infor Cloverleaf Integration Suite [44].

9.5.3 Health information exchange services

To successfully exchange information, one also needs services that will move valid artifacts from System A to System B. In this section of the chapter, we review existing, mature efforts that support HIE implementers' efforts to establish interoperable exchange of information in this way. While some may not consider these initiatives to be true syntactic standards, they provide guidance and support for standardizing transactions, in many ways helping to provide the extra 20% effort needed to achieve interoperability.

9.5.3.1 *Integrating the Healthcare Enterprise*

Integrating the Healthcare Enterprise (IHE) is a nonprofit organization that brings together key stakeholders, including health care subject matter experts (e.g., clinicians, administrators) and health IT vendors, to coordinate interoperability activities. However, IHE does not develop standards. Instead, IHE works with stakeholders to implement already developed standards through a common, standards-based framework (called the IT Infrastructure) that pieces together various standards across the entire OSI model.

Upon its common framework, IHE facilitates collaborative development of implementation guidelines it calls "IHE Profiles" across a range of use cases in health care as well as public health. For example, IHE has developed an RFD (Retrieve Form for Data Capture) profile that uses available standards to query a remote server for a form (e.g., a public health case reporting form), display the form to a user for completion, and then return a completed form to some other health information systems. The IT infrastructure and profiles from IHE are used by more than 160 vendors globally.

9.5.3.2 *eHealth Exchange*

The eHealth Exchange, formerly known as the Nationwide Health Information Network, is the foundation for national health interoperability in the United States. Unlike IHE, the eHealth Exchange is itself an HIE network. The network consists of state and regional HIE networks as well as federal agencies such as the Social Security Administration and Department of Veterans Affairs.

The eHealth Exchange functions as a federated network in which health information is maintained at the source and queried when it is needed. Supporting its transactions is a framework of technical standards carefully selected and supported by the eHealth Exchange. Thus the eHealth Exchange provides HIE services for its members rather than technical infrastructure or data.

The eHealth Exchange was first developed by the Office of the National Coordinator for Health Information Technology (ONC) but is now managed by a nonprofit organization called the Sequoia Project. The Sequoia Project also manages Carequality, a public-private collaborative building consensus among health IT data exchange programs to develop a common interoperability framework enabling seamless exchange among HIE networks.

9.6 Emerging trends

In this section we discuss several emerging trends in the realm of syntactic standards. First, we examine standards that are evolving to support new use cases. Second, we describe a recent US policy which is driving the US's interoperability agenda for the future.

9.6.1 Transferring bulk data: Flat FHIR

Current FHIR implementations focus on transferring small amounts of data through specific requests, often at an individual patient level. However, public and population health, research, and large analytics approaches may require a large data query that would require many small requests in the traditional FHIR approach. The FHIR Bulk Data API, also known as Flat FHIR or Bulk FHIR, defines a FHIR approach to request and transfer large datasets from a FHIR server to an authorized client [45]. In contrast to the typical FHIR RESTful approach, Bulk Data uses an asynchronous request pattern to allow larger queries to run. Briefly, a bulk data client is authorized, then requests an export of data (which can be specified for all data or a subset of patients or data) from the FHIR resource server, and finally receives the location of the bulk data output file when it is ready for download. Though lesser known than the patient-level FHIR API, the population-level FHIR Bulk Data API is also required by the 21st Century Cures Act Final Rule from the ONC for certified health information technology [46]. The FHIR Bulk Data implementation guide is under active development to meet the needed breadth and depth of real-world evidence research, claims and payment data, and population health approaches [47].

9.6.2 Clinical decision support and quality measurement: Clinical Quality Language

Clinical Quality Language (CQL) is a HL7 query language standard that evolved from the Quality Data Model [48]. CQL was developed to unify the expression of logic for Electronic Clinical Quality Measures and CDS [49]. The CQL standard is used to express logic in point-to-point sharing that is both human readable and machine computable. CQL libraries are made up of sets of terms and operations, called "expressions," that can be used to measure patient outcomes and determine clinical actions [50]. For example, an expression like "AgeInYears(start of MeasurementPeriod) ≥ 16" could be used to constrain logic to patients 16 years of age or older. The artifacts generated by using this standard can be developed and published by an organization with expertise in the guidelines or quality measures involved, and then shared with health organizations to implement the standard.

9.6.3 Research: OMOP Common Data Model

Supporting syntactic standardization requires translating data from a system's particular data model into the standard schema. This is more difficult when the data model of a source system varies significantly from the target schema. Fortunately, early work on messaging standards influenced the development of EHRs, and many share similar information models, especially around observational clinical data. Despite this fortune, there are still significant information model differences across EHR systems.

A 2007 mandate for the Food and Drug Administration (FDA) to monitor health data for risks of drugs and other marketed products led to the Observational Medical Outcomes Partnership (OMOP)—a public–private partnership among the FDA, academia, data owners, and pharmaceutical industry that is managed by the National Institutes of Health. OMOP's goal is to create a national program of active drug safety surveillance by using observational data [51]. This work led to development of the OMOP Common Data Model (CDM), a standardized data model upon which reporting and analytic tools could be built and shared. The CDM proved to be a useful model for combining observational databases from disparate EHRs, facilitating syntactic interoperability [52].

Work by OMOP gave birth to Observational Health Data Sciences and Informatics (OHDSI), a large international collaborative community applying open-source data analytic solutions to a wide range of solutions [53]. The OMOP CDM and the shared analytic tools enabled by OHDSI as well as syntactic standards such as FHIR have been used in national programs like All of Us (creating a national cohort of EHR and genomic data) and as the basis for transmitting data to large-scale data warehouses [54,55].

9.6.4 Clinical information models: the Gender Harmony Project

Information models are also useful for informing the enhancement of existing syntactic standards. Standards reflect the developers' understanding and beliefs about the scope of clinical concepts, relationships, and associated attributes that were important for information exchange and shared understanding by computers. However, as society's collective understanding of a concept changes, a standard representing that concept can become outdated quickly and can lead to gaps or differences in representation across standards for a similar clinical topic.

This problem is clearly illustrated by the recent efforts to improve the accurate representation of clinical sex and gender when data are stored in an EHR or shared between health systems. As described by McClure et al., many systems still assume that the HL7 v2 message patient identification segment (PID.8) is the only representation of sex characteristics needed, and that a single, permanent patient value can be prudently applied to care in all situations [56]. However, such an approach does not differentiate sex from gender, nor does it allow for representation of gender fluidity throughout the lifespan. Similar problems are present when exchanging data using CDA-based or FHIR artifacts.

In response, the HL7 Gender Harmony Project community developed a logical model that outlines the data elements, value sets, element attributes, and relationships that clarify information meaning and context and can guide and inform changes within existing exchange standards [56]. The model has five major elements independent of other parts included in an information model for a person [Gender Identity, Sex For Clinical Use (SfCU), Recorded Sex or Gender (RSG), Name to Use (NtU), and Pronouns], and each element has a "duration: validity period" which supports changes over time. If existing standards were enhanced based on a common model, then gaps would be reduced and data transformation between representations would be explicit. This referenced publication describes the Gender Harmony Model and provides a straightforward analysis of the standards described in this chapter relative to documenting a common and important patient concept, and describes the value of a logic model for standards development [56].

9.6.5 Trusted Exchange Framework and Common Agreement

The Trusted Exchange Framework and Common Agreement (TEFCA) is program administered by ONC to establish the minimum infrastructure and governing approach for HIE across the United States [57]. With support from a Recognized Coordinating Entity (RCE), TEFCA plans to establish a network of Qualified Health Information Networks (QHIN) to exchange standard transactions across health system organizations of all shapes and sizes (e.g., small clinic, large hospital). TEFCA is further described in Chapters 3, 6, 7, and 21.

With respect to syntactic interoperability, the RCE will establish syntactic standards which QHINs must conform to execute queries or push data across the network. This will require the RCE to establish conformance testing for QHINs and publish the syntactic standards that will be supported by TEFCA. The current, early draft technical framework for QHINs specifies the use of HL7 C-CDA 2.1 documents for transactions. However, the network anticipates supporting FHIR in future versions. The final version of the technical framework will be published in early 2022. It is not available at the time of writing this chapter.

9.7 Summary

Syntactic standards provide the structure and syntax for interoperable artifacts in HIE. While syntactic standards are necessary, they are not sufficient for achieving meaningful HIE. In addition to use of syntactic standards, semantic standards are also required to enable shared understanding of information shared between systems. Additional effort is necessary to integrate complex health information systems, which requires collaboration among providers, vendors, and other stakeholders. Integration profiles and implementation guides, created by multistakeholder groups, are required to fully connect systems in support of interoperability. Work continues to evolve standards, refine implementation guides, and support implementation of standards in many countries. Development and implementation of robust standards will result in more efficient health systems that support better outcomes for both patients and populations.

Questions for discussion

1. Syntactic standards provide a solution for the combinatorial explosion of interfaces. Describe what steps would be necessary to facilitate exchange of data between two systems without syntactic standards.
2. What are key differences between the three commonly used HL7 standards?
3. What is the process by which an individual or organization can get involved in developing standards with HL7 or integration profiles with IHE?
4. Why are there so many syntactic standards for HIE? What precludes universal development and adoption of a single standard?
5. Why do we need implementation guides? Shouldn't standards be sufficient for achieving interoperability?

Acknowledgments

The authors acknowledge and thank Masoud Hosseini, PhD, who coauthored the corresponding chapter in the first edition of this book, and Clair Kronk, PhD, who peer-reviewed the summary of the Gender Harmony Project. Dr. Umberfield's effort is supported by the National Library of Medicine of the National Institutes of Health under award number T15LM012502. The content of this publication is solely the responsibility of the authors and does not necessarily represent the official views of the National Institutes of Health.

References

[1] Gliklich RE, Dreyer NA, Leavy MB, editors. Registries for evaluating patient outcomes: a user's guide [Internet]. 3rd ed. Rockville, MD: Agency for Healthcare Research and Quality (USA); 2014 [cited 2021 September 28] (AHRQ Methods for Effective Health Care). Available from: http://www.ncbi.nlm.nih.gov/books/NBK208616/.

[2] Healthcare Information and Management Systems Society. Interoperability in healthcare [Internet]. HIMSS; 2020 [cited 2021 September 28]. Available from: https://www.himss.org/resources/interoperability-healthcare.

[3] HL7 International, Patient Administration Work Group. Resource patient – content [Internet]. HL7 FHIR; 2019 [cited 2021 October 7]. Available from: https://www.hl7.org/fhir/patient.html.

[4] Spronk R. HL7 version 3: message or CDA document? [Internet]; 2007 [cited 2021 December 8]. Available from: https://ringholm.com/docs/04200_en.htm.

[5] White P. The evolution of HL7 Standards: V2 to FHIR – Public Health Informatics Research Lab [Internet]. Informatics Innovation Unit: A CDC Technology R&D Lab; 2016 [cited 2021 November 18]. Available from: https://www.philab.cdc.gov/index.php/2016/03/25/the-evolution-of-hl7-standards-v2-to-fhir/.

[6] HL7 International. About Health Level Seven International [Internet]; 2021 [cited 2021 September 28]. Available from: https://www.hl7.org/about/.

[7] HL7 International. HL7 version 2 product suite [Internet]. HL7 standards product brief. [cited 2021 November 18]. Available from: http://www.hl7.org/implement/standards/product_brief.cfm?product_id = 185.

[8] HL7 International. HL7 v2 refactored [Internet]. HL7 v2 + ; 2021 [cited 2021 September 28]. Available from: http://www.hl7.eu/refactored/.

[9] HL7 International. Comparison [Internet]. HL7 FHIR; 2019 [cited 2021 October 7]. Available from: https://www.hl7.org/fhir/comparison.html.

[10] HL7 International. HL7 standards product brief – CDA® Release 2 [Internet]. HL7 International; 2021 [cited 2021 November 17]. Available from: https://www.hl7.org/implement/standards/product_brief.cfm?product_id = 7.

[11] HL7 International. HL7 standards product brief – C-CDA (HL7 CDA® R2 implementation guide: consolidated CDA templates for clinical notes – US Realm) [Internet]. HL7 International; 2021 [cited 2021 November 17]. Available from: https://www.hl7.org/implement/standards/product_brief.cfm?product_id = 492.

[12] HL7 International. HL7 implementation guide for CDA® Release 2: consolidated CDA templates for clinical notes [Internet]; 2015. Available from: https://www.hl7.org/ccdasearch/pdfs/CCDA_Volume_One.pdf.

[13] HL7 International. C-CDA online: a navigation website for C-CDA 2.1 [Internet]. HL7 CDA; 2021 [cited 2021 November 17]. Available from: http://www.hl7.org/ccdasearch/.

[14] D'Amore J, Bouhaddou O, Mitchell S, Li C, Leftwich R, Turner T, et al. Interoperability progress and remaining data quality barriers of certified health information technologies. AMIA Annu Symp Proc 2018;2018:358–67.

[15] Centers for Disease Control and Prevention. Facilities map [Internet]. CDC; 2021 [cited 2021 November 17]. Available from: https://www.cdc.gov/coronavirus/2019-ncov/hcp/electronic-case-reporting/hcfacilities-map.html.

[16] Office of the National Coordinator for Health Information Technology. What is HL7® FHIR? [Internet]; 2021 [cited 2021 October 12]. Available from: https://www.healthit.gov/sites/default/files/page/2021-04/What%20Is%20FHIR%20Fact%20Sheet.pdf.

[17] HL7 International. Introducing HL7 FHIR [Internet]. HL7 FHIR; 2019 [cited 2021 October 7]. Available from: https://hl7.org/fhir/summary.html.

[18] Benson T, Grieve G. Principles of health interoperability: SNOMED CT, HL7 and FHIR [Internet]. Cham: Springer International Publishing; 2016 [cited 2020 August 4] (Health Information Technology Standards). Available from: http://link.springer.com/10.1007/978-3-319-30370-3.

[19] HL7 International. Profiling – FHIR v4.0.1 [Internet]. HL7 FHIR; 2019 [cited 2021 October 29]. Available from: https://www.hl7.org/fhir/profiling.html.

[20] HL7 International. FHIR overview – architects [Internet]. HL7 FHIR; 2021 [cited 2021 October 7]. Available from: https://www.hl7.org/fhir/overview-arch.html.

[21] HL7 International. Base resource definitions [Internet]. HL7 FHIR; 2019 [cited 2021 Dec 6]. Available from: https://www.hl7.org/fhir/resource.html.

[22] HL7 International. Resource index [Internet]. HL7 FHIR; [cited 2021 November 29]. Available from: https://www.hl7.org/fhir/resourcelist.html.

[23] HL7 International. Welcome to FHIR® [Internet]. HL7 FHIR; 2019 [cited 2021 December 8]. Available from: https://hl7.org/fhir/.

[24] Digital Imaging and Communications in Medicine. The DICOM standard [Internet]. DICOM – Current Edition; 2021 [cited 2021 September 28]. Available from: https://www.dicomstandard.org/current.

[25] National Council for Prescription Drug Programs. 2020 [cited 2021 November 29]. Available from: https://ncpdp.org/?.

[26] National Council for Prescription Drug Programs. Standards matrix [Internet]; 2021 [cited 2021 November 29]. Available from: https://www.ncpdp.org/NCPDP/media/pdf/StandardsMatrix.pdf.

[27] X12. About X12 [Internet]; 2016 [cited 2021 November 17]. Available from: https://x12.org/about/about-x12.

[28] Office of the National Coordinator for Health Information Technology. Cures Act Final Rule: standards-based Application Programming Interface (API) certification criterion [Internet]; 2020. Available from: https://www.healthit.gov/cures/sites/default/files/cures/2020-03/APICertificationCriterion.pdf.

[29] HL7 International. Version management policy [Internet]. Change management and versioning; 2021 [cited 2021 September 28]. Available from: https://www.hl7.org/fhir/versions.html.

[30] Office of the National Coordinator for Health Information Technology. FHIR version history and maturity [Internet]; 2021 [cited 2021 October 12]. Available from: https://www.healthit.gov/sites/default/files/page/2021-04/FHIR%20Version%20History%20Fact%20Sheet.pdf.

[31] Oemig F, Blobel B. Compliance or conformance: what should interoperability focus on? Stud Health Technol Inform 2017;237:63–7.

[32] HL7 International. Downloads [Internet]. HL7 FHIR; 2019 [cited 2021 November 17]. Available from: https://hl7.org/fhir/downloads.html.

[33] HL7 International. FHIR conformance testing [Internet]. HL7 FHIR Foundation; 2021 [cited 2021 November 17]. Available from: https://fhir.org/conformance-testing/.

[34] National Institute of Standards and Technology. Healthcare – standards & testing [Internet]. NIST; 2016 [cited 2021 November 17]. Available from: https://www.nist.gov/itl/products-and-services/healthcare-standards-testing.
[35] OpenHIE. OpenHIE; 2021 [cited 2021 October 26]. Available from: https://ohie.org/.
[36] Office of the National Coordinator for Health Information Technology, Interoperability Standards Advisory. Section II: content/structure standards and implementation specifications [Internet]. HealthIT.gov.; [cited 2021 November 30]. Available from: https://www.healthit.gov/isa/section-ii-contentstructure-standards-and-implementation-specifications.
[37] HL7 International. Implementation guide [Internet]. HL7 FHIR; 2019 [cited 2021 November 30]. Available from: https://www.hl7.org/fhir/implementationguide.html.
[38] HL7 International. Implementation guide registry [Internet]. HL7 FHIR Foundation; [cited 2021 November 30]. Available from: https://www.fhir.org/guides/registry/.
[39] NextGen Healthcare. Mirth® Connect [Internet]. NextGen Healthcare; 2021 [cited 2021 October 26]. Available from: https://www.nextgen.com/products-and-services/integration-engine.
[40] Lyniate. Lyniate Rhapsody [Internet]. Lyniate; 2021 [cited 2021 October 26]. Available from: https://lyniate.com/solutions/rhapsody/.
[41] Lyniate Corepoint [Internet]. Lyniate; 2021 [cited 2021 October 26]. Available from: https://lyniate.com/solutions/corepoint/.
[42] InterSystems Corporation. Ensemble integration engine [Internet]. InterSystems; 2021 [cited 2021 October 26]. Available from: https://www.intersystems.com/products/ensemble/.
[43] Summit Healthcare Services. Summit exchange [Internet]. Summit Healthcare; 2021 [cited 2021 October 26]. Available from: https://www.summit-healthcare.com/summit-exchange/.
[44] Infor. Cloverleaf Integration Suite: healthcare interoperability software [Internet]; 2021 [cited 2021 October 26]. Available from: https://www.infor.com/products/cloverleaf.
[45] HL7 International, SMART HealthIT. Bulk Data IG home page [Internet]. HL7 FHIR; 2021 [cited 2021 November 29]. Available from: https://hl7.org/fhir/uv/bulkdata/index.html.
[46] Office of the National Coordinator for Health Information Technology. 21st Century Cures Act: Interoperability, Information Blocking, and the ONC Health IT Certification Program [Internet]; 2020 [cited 2021 November 29]. Available from: https://www.federalregister.gov/documents/2020/05/01/2020-07419/21st-century-cures-act-interoperability-information-blocking-and-the-onc-health-it-certification.
[47] Mandl KD, Gottlieb D, Mandel JC, Ignatov V, Sayeed R, Grieve G, et al. Push button population health: the SMART/HL7 FHIR bulk data access application programming interface. npj Digit Med 2020;3(1):1–9.
[48] Rhodes B, Krauss D. Clinical Quality Language 101 [Internet]. Centers for Medicare & Medicaid Services; 2016. Available from: https://www.youtube.com/watch?v = BETFiQzLb8o.
[49] HL7 International. Clinical Quality Language (CQL) [Internet]. CQL; 2021 [cited 2021 October 7]. Available from: https://cql.hl7.org/.
[50] Rhodes B. Delivering dynamic content: standards and practices in healthcare [Internet]. University of Utah; 2020. Available from: https://hsc.mediaspace.kaltura.com/media/t/0_ga7rvwxz.
[51] Stang PE, Ryan PB, Racoosin JA, Overhage JM, Hartzema AG, Reich C, et al. Advancing the science for active surveillance: rationale and design for the Observational Medical Outcomes Partnership. Ann Intern Med 2010;153(9):600–6.
[52] Overhage JM, Ryan PB, Reich CG, Hartzema AG, Stang PE. Validation of a common data model for active safety surveillance research. J Am Med Inform Assoc 2012;19(1):54–60.
[53] Hripcsak G, Duke JD, Shah NH, Reich CG, Huser V, Schuemie MJ, et al. Observational Health Data Sciences and Informatics (OHDSI): opportunities for observational researchers. Stud Health Technol Inform 2015;216:574–8.
[54] Lynch KE, Deppen SA, DuVall SL, Viernes B, Cao A, Park D, et al. Incrementally transforming electronic medical records into the observational medical outcomes partnership common data model: a multidimensional quality assurance approach. Appl Clin Inform 2019;10(5):794–803.
[55] Klann JG, Joss MAH, Embree K, Murphy SN. Data model harmonization for the All Of Us Research Program: transforming i2b2 data into the OMOP common data model. PLoS One 2019;14(2).
[56] McClure RC, Macumber CL, Kronk C, Grasso C, Horn RJ, Queen R, et al. Gender harmony: improved standards to support affirmative care of gender-marginalized people through inclusive gender and sex representation. J Am Med Inform Assoc [Internet] 2021;. Available from: https://doi.org/10.1093/jamia/ocab196.
[57] Office of the National Coordinator for Health Information Technology. Trusted Exchange Framework and Common Agreement [Internet]. HealthIT.gov.; 2021 [cited 2021 November 29]. Available from: https://www.healthit.gov/topic/interoperability/trusted-exchange-framework-and-common-agreement.

CHAPTER

10

Standardizing health care data across an enterprise

Elizabeth E. Umberfield[1,2], *Jack Bowie*[3], *Andrew S. Kanter*[4,5], *Brian E. Dixon*[1,2] *and Eileen F. Tallman*[1]

[1]Department of Epidemiology, Richard M. Fairbanks School of Public Health, Indiana University, Indianapolis, IN, USA [2]Center for Biomedical Informatics, Regenstrief Institute, Inc., Indianapolis, IN, USA [3]Apelon, Inc., Ridgefield, CT, USA [4]Department of Biomedical Informatics and Epidemiology, Columbia University, New York, NY, USA [5]Intelligent Medical Objects, Inc., Northbrook, IL, USA

LEARNING OBJECTIVES

By the end of this chapter, the reader should be able to:

- Describe the utility of standard reference terminologies in health information exchange.
- Identify factors to consider when selecting context-appropriate terminology standards.
- Describe the process of mapping from local to reference terminologies, as well as identify the types of tools available to assist in mapping.
- Explain why a Terminology Service is important in health information exchange, and describe the process for its implementation.

10.1 Introduction

As described throughout the book, health information exchange (HIE) involves the integration, aggregation, and communication of health data from a variety of distinct sources. As data are exchanged, it becomes a challenge to maintain their original meaning or semantics. Thus, for HIE to achieve semantic interoperability, data from a sending system must be standardized, or normalized, to ensure the receiving system can correctly interpret and use the data it received. This involves clear communication within messages of both the data and the information model from which the data are to be interpreted.

Chapter 9 discussed the importance of standardizing messages and information models. In this chapter, we describe the process of and

Health Information Exchange
DOI: https://doi.org/10.1016/B978-0-323-90802-3.00024-1

challenges inherent in standardizing data within HIE messages. We will examine the concept of a terminology and explain how one terminology can be translated or "mapped" to another. The chapter will further describe the need and use of reference (standardized) terminologies to create semantic interoperability. Finally, we discuss the purpose and implementation of a Terminology Service, which is a set of technical components (e.g., hardware, software) designed to facilitate data standardization and achieve semantic interoperability.

10.2 Role of terminologies in health care

A *terminology* is the body of names (terms and phrases) used with a particular technical application in a subject of study, theory, or profession. Terminologies vary in their purposes, scopes, and structures. This is especially true in health care where there is a high degree of specialization.

While there exists a nearly universal terminology for human anatomy that is taught to a variety of health professions, there is a wide array of specialized terminologies used in health care settings, and these terminologies frequently are designed for single clinical domains. Nursing, for example, has three major terminologies: NANDA International (NANDA-I), the Nursing Interventions Classification (NIC), and the Nursing Outcomes Classification (NOC). The nursing terminologies provide sets of terms to describe nurses' clinical assessments, treatments, and nursing-sensitive patient outcomes, respectively. Other common clinical terminologies include SNOMED CT, the International Classification of Disease (ICD), and the Current Procedural Terminology.

Terminologies in health care support the documentation of observations, treatments, and outcomes that clinicians put in the patient chart—which is increasingly performed using electronic health record (EHR) systems. While there exist a fair number of "major" or standard terminologies like NIC, NOC, SNOMED, ICD, and Logical Observation Identifiers, Names and Codes (LOINC), there are many more terminologies developed for specific purposes.

A *local terminology* is one that is created for a specific purpose by a single organization, such as a laboratory, hospital, clinic, or pharmacy. For example, a local terminology may be used by the laboratory supporting a large health system to provide "user friendly" terms to physicians who order the tests. When physicians interact with their EHR system, they may choose these local terms from dropdown menus or see these terms displayed with results for their patients.

While useful to providers in a particular health system, a local terminology may be difficult to interpret by providers in another health system. For example, Health System A might refer to a glycated hemoglobin (HbA1c) test as "Glycohemoglobin," whereas Health System B may refer to a similar test as "Hemoglobin A1c." While a human clinician can use his or her clinical knowledge and expertise to reason that the two tests likely mean the same thing, computers cannot perform such reasoning in isolation. Therefore, to ensure that meaning or semantics are transferred along with the test results during HIE, clinical documentation in health information systems should use a reference terminology.

A *reference terminology* is a formal, canonical terminology developed and maintained by a national or international standards development organization (SDO). A reference terminology is often referred to as a *standard, terminology standard*, or *standard terminology*.

In reference terminologies, each *concept* (clinical idea) is associated with one or more terms (names) and a code. This code is the unique identifier for the concept. As noted above, there may be many terms or names associated with the same concept, for example, a glycated hemoglobin laboratory test, although one is usually designated the "primary name" to simplify human identification. Because of this structure, standard terminologies are called concept-based terminologies. SDOs and the development of standards is described in Chapter 9.

A concept in a standard terminology can represent a clinical observation (e.g., weight, blood pressure, response to a question asked of a patient), a laboratory result, a clinical diagnosis, or a diagnostic or therapeutic procedure. As described earlier, most concepts, especially those in standard terminologies, are represented by a code and one or more terms. The code is often a unique, numeric identifier that abstractly represents the concept. The term can be a shorthand name or description that is human-readable. For example, a code 12345 might have a primary name of "Hemoglobin A1c.," and a synonym term of "Glycohemoglobin." Some standard terminologies often have multiple axes or hierarchies for each concept to more precisely define them.

Concept codes can be read by computers to consistently identify instances of a given concept each time it occurs and know that those instances are comparable. Similarly, humans ought to be able to read the term/description and understand the nature of the concept that the term represents. As an example, the concept of myocardial infarction is labeled with the SNOMED CT identifier code (SCTID) "22298006" and given the (primary) term "myocardial infarction (disorder)." SNOMED CT also serves as a thesaurus, linking each concept to a list of human-readable synonyms which might be used to express the same idea. Example synonym terms for "myocardial infarction (disorder)" include "cardiac infarction" and "heart attack" [1].

In addition to a typical hierarchical structure of concepts, machine-interpretability of concepts in many health care terminologies are also supported by *ontologies* which formally specify classes of entities (represented by concepts) and relationships between them [2]. Ontology files specify the rules of inference and inheritance, enabling computers to extract the contextual meaning (i.e., the *semantics*) of terms and interact with that information in ways similar to those of human users [3].

In addition to being a body of concepts and terms, SNOMED CT has an ontological basis in which parent and child classes of each concept are asserted. For example, "myocardial infarction (disorder)" (SCTID: 22298006) has a parent class of "Disease (disorder)" (SCTID: 64572001) and a child class of "Mixed myocardial ischemia and infarction (disorder)" (SCTID: 428196007). This should be understood as "Mixed myocardial ischemia and infarction (disorder)" is a type of "myocardial infarction (disorder)" which is a type of "Disease (disorder)." Additional information about myocardial infarctions is expressed through ontological attributes, including where in the body it is located or its morphology (see Fig. 10.1). While it is outside the scope of this chapter to fully describe the role of ontologies, it is important to understand that ontologies play a significant role in machine interpretation of the semantics (i.e., meaning) of the terms defined within each terminology.

10.3 Standard terminologies in health care

The use of reference terminologies is the foundation for facilitating semantic interoperability—maintaining data's original meaning during HIE. Standardized, reference terminologies accomplish this by providing a structured, comparable technical language that enables the data to have meaning outside of the originating system. As a result, comparability of data can allow for accurate and consistent measurement, aggregation, analysis, and reporting of information. Terminology standards also allow data reusability, allowing standardized terms to be stored as a single concept and used multiple ways in a variety of applications [5].

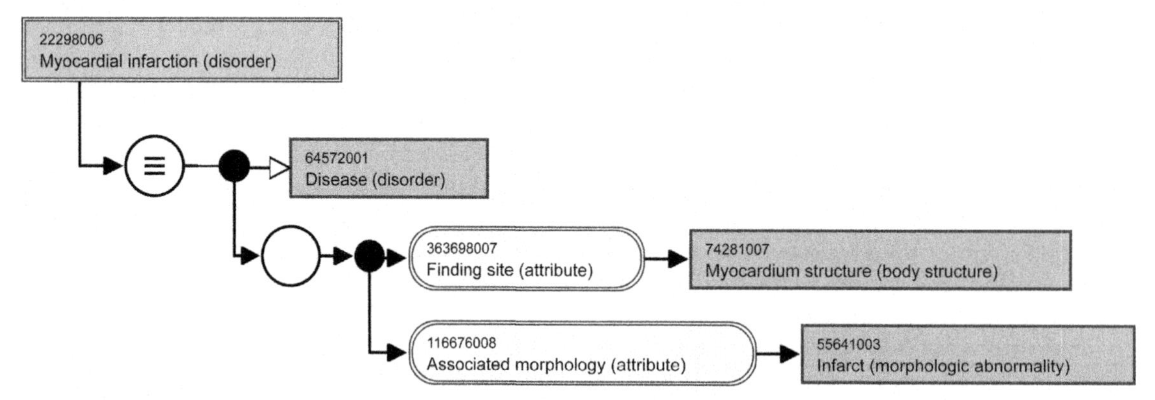

FIGURE 10.1 Representation of the term "Myocardial infarction (disorder)" (SCTID: 22298006) in terms of its stated parent class and attributes [4]. *Source*: Screenshot taken from the SNOMED CT Browser.

Examples of standard terminologies in health care are presented in Table 10.1. While additional reference terminologies exist, we include those most commonly used in HIE transactions within the United States. For a comprehensive description of available terminology standards and their relative level of maturity and usage, the reader is referred to the Interoperability Standards Advisory published annually by the US Office of the National Coordinator for Health Information Technology (ONC) [6].

Terminology standards are typically revisited and expanded on an annual basis. However, updates can be driven by population trends, community requests, or national objectives, such as those described by Healthy People [7]. For example, LOINC initiated a collaboration with the Centers for Disease Control and Prevention (CDC) to update its terminology due to the COVID-19 pandemic [8]. The terminology evolved multiple times since early 2020, adding new terms as COVID-19 laboratory tests, including antigen and antibody tests, were created by manufacturers around the world. ICD-10 also released updates for COVID-19 ahead of schedule to keep pace with the rapidly evolving global health event [9].

Although global reference terminologies like SNOMED CT are relatively comprehensive, there is no single terminology that encompasses all concepts found in the health care domain. A given HIE network, including enterprise HIE networks and vendor-based HIE networks, will likely need to adopt and use multiple terminologies to meet their varied data needs—including diagnoses, procedures, laboratory testing, medications, and vaccinations. Covering all these subdomains likely requires at least three reference terminologies. And since some nations have specific requirements from their Ministries of Health, it is likely most health systems and HIE networks will need to adopt and use 5–7 reference terminologies.

10.4 Selection of standard terminologies for health information exchange

Given the variety of standard terminologies, HIE leaders must determine which terminology standard(s) should be selected. Moreover, as described above, in some cases it will be necessary to select more than one standard vocabulary to achieve the goals of an HIE use case.

TABLE 10.1 Commonly used standard terminologies in the US health care system.

Terminology	Full name	Domain	Responsible organization
CPT	Current Procedural Terminology	Billing (Outpatient and Office Procedures)	American Medical Association (http://www.ama-assn.org)
CVX	Clinical Vaccines Administered	Vaccines (Active and Inactive)	US Centers for Disease Control and Prevention (https://www2a.cdc.gov/vaccines/iis/iisstandards/vaccines.asp?rpt = cvx)
ICD	International Classification of Diseases	Diseases and Injuries	World Health Organization (http://www.who.int)
LOINC	Logical Observation Identifiers, Names and Codes	Clinical Results (e.g., Lab Tests, Vital Signs)	Regenstrief Institute (http://www.loinc.org)
RxNorm	RxNorm	Drugs (Clinical)	US National Library of Medicine (http://nlm.nih.gov/research/umls/rxnorm/)
SNOMED CT	Systematized Nomenclature of Medicine – Clinical Terms	Clinical Content (Electronic Health Records)	International Health Terminology Standards Development Organisation (http://www.snomed.org)
NDC	National Drug Code	Drugs (Finished and Unfinished List for FDA)	US Food and Drug Administration (FDA) (https://www.accessdata.fda.gov/scripts/cder/ndc/index.cfm)

The process of selecting terminology standard(s) for a given HIE service or context of use requires consideration of several factors [10], including:

- Underlying health needs and priorities of the health system,
- Overall goals and objectives of the HIE or specific HIE service,
- Types or categories of data to be exchanged among a network of systems, and
- Workflow which will generate the data to be exchanged or in which data will be queried.

The goals and objectives for a given HIE service or use case (context of use) are the primary driver for which terminology standard(s) are to be selected. For example, the goal for an HIE or an initial service may be to improve childhood vaccination rates in a low-income population. A HIE use case may be to report the proportion of children who have received all required vaccinations by age 5 at a given point-in-time within every low-income neighborhood in a geographic area to prioritize targeted interventions. This use case requires a standard terminology that can adequately capture the case definition and has good coverage of the intervention being tracked (injectables and vaccines). Given these requirements, a candidate terminology to consider would be National Drug Code (NDC) maintained by the US Food and Drug Administration. The NDC includes all drugs manufactured, prepared, propagated, compounded, or processed for commercial distribution, including injectables and vaccines. If this use case were outside the United States, a different standard terminology, based on that country's medication delivery system, might be more appropriate.

The entire NDC catalog includes much more breadth than what is necessary for the vaccination use case. Therefore the HIE might consider selecting a *value set*, a subset of concepts drawn from a standard vocabulary, instead of the entire NDC. Numerous value sets have been predefined by various authorities, including the US CDC and the US National Library of Medicine (NLM). The CDC maintains a collection of value sets used for a series of public health HIE use cases [11], and the NLM maintains values sets for clinical quality measures [12].

In addition to the context of use and the scope of data for exchange, HIE leaders must consider the workflow that either generates the data to be exchanged or how the data will be requested. In this case, given the static nature of the query by a public health authority, we consider the workflow around how the data are generated. Administration of vaccines are performed by nursing staff and included in their documentation at a clinic. NDC terms, however, are voluminous and complex, and many NDC identifiers are similar to one another. This makes clinical documentation using NDC terms challenging for nurses and physicians. Therefore HIE leaders may need to implement an *interface terminology* in addition to NDC, a standard terminology.

An *interface terminology* is one that is user-facing (or in the case of health care, provider-facing) rather than being concept-based, and consists of a set of words, terms, or phrases used in a point-of-care application that have documented associations, called "mappings," to concepts in a standard terminology. Thus user documentation can use the interface terms, while the underlying health information system, for example, an EMR, can store both the verbatim entry and its associated concept representation. The interface terminology may be a locally based terminology, or it could be a national or international reference terminology; however, reference terminologies are rarely presented to end users to select from in clinical workflows.

Most often interface terminologies are locally based and mapped to (associated with) entries in one or more reference terminologies, thus achieving both ease-of-use and standardization. Of note, if workflows use interface-reference maps, the use of a subset—rather than the complete standard—occurs at the interface terminology level rather than the reference terminology level.

Additionally, decisions regarding terminology selection should be made with long-term use in mind. Frequent changes to the selected terminology and term mappings (see Section 10.6 below) can be expensive and time-consuming. Such changes also can result in a loss of historical data compatibility.

Finally, technical, political, cultural, and economic factors must be considered when selecting a standard. This is necessary to ensure the standard's feasibility and sustainability in each HIE's unique context. To help guide this process, it may be beneficial to seek out information on successful implementation in similar settings [13]. In other cases, policy may dictate or guide selection processes.

In the United States, ONC publishes an annual Interoperability Standards Advisory [6] that provides guidance on the selection of available terminology standards recommended for use in various contexts. As part of the 21st Century Cures Act, ONC established the United States Core Data for Interoperability (USCDI), which is a standardized set of data elements or data that has been aggregated by a common theme or use case [14]. It provides guidance about EHR data sharing to prevent information blocking and aims to improving national-level HIE [15]. A good illustration of the USCDI involves the addition of data elements designed to codify the social determinants of health (see Box 10.1). Other nations often create similar lists that may provide guidance or outline required terminologies in those countries.

10.5 Current use of standard terminologies

As previously described, a wide variety of reference terminologies are in a mature state of development and are readily available for use in health information systems [19]. Historically, despite availability, actual use in the real world

BOX 10.1

What do terminologies codify? The case of social determinants.

When selecting a terminology, it is important to consider the domain or collection of concepts terminologies are attempting to codify. One example is the strongly desired, but not well-captured, social determinants of health (SDOH). In 2021 ONC released its latest version of the USCDI [14] which expanded its content to include SDOH data such as sexual orientation, updated race/ethnicity categories, and identify SDOH interventions. Many standard terminologies have value sets that aim to capture SDOH data. One example is the 'Z' codes provided by ICD-10 [16], which address problems related to social environment, upbringing, and occupational exposure to risk factors, among others. Additionally, LOINC has developed a set of SDOH terms [17] that is divided into subgroups (e.g., community, environment, education, etc.) based on guidance from the National Academy of Medicine.

As they are captured and analyzed, SDOH standardized terms have the potential to describe patients' social needs, the effect they have on health outcomes, and improve care contexts for those patients and their communities [18]. For more information on SDOH data exchange, including commonly used terminologies, see Chapter 19.

is inconsistent and limited, and local terms remain highly prevalent in many nations. There is evidence that this is changing, at least in the United States where interoperability and use of terminology standards have been incentivized through polices such as Meaningful Use and now Promoting Interoperability (see Chapter 3 for details on these policies). For example, Bhargava et al. [20] studied LOINC use at the VA between 1999 and 2018 and found that in 2018, 85% of lab tests and 99% of lab results had assigned LOINC, reflecting a 2.78-fold increase since 1999. The experience in the VA might be different from other health systems within the United States. Previous research in nonfederal hospitals found the use of reference terminologies to be well under 50% [21,22]. Moreover, use may be limited if the terminology does not provide comprehensive functionality for a use case [23] or if user support is lacking. Park et al. [24] found several barriers to use including limited technical support, insufficient governance, and lack of local vendor capacity.

There can be many reasons why terminology standards fail to be implemented widely. In many instances, this is because the local requirements for documentation or workflow did not align with the standard, or the standard required complicated technology which was not implementable by the developers or users. It may also be the case that stakeholders do not perceive a value to implementing a reference terminology (e.g., lack of business drivers). For example, in Israel when HIE expanded from the largest Health Maintenance Organization (HMO) to the rest of the nation, smaller HMO and hospital networks decided to adopt the local terminology used by the predominant HMO. It is only recently that the nation decided to move toward the use of reference terminologies. To facilitate implementation of reference terminologies, and to address the ongoing challenge of situations like the one in Israel, a complex and resource-intensive linking process of terms and concepts from one terminology to another, called mapping, may be necessary for implementation of the selected HIE standards.

10.6 Mapping

Linking terms from one terminology to another is a process called *mapping*. Mapping can be defined as the development of correspondences between the concepts or terms in two different terminologies [10]. In mapping, the *source term* is the origin of the map (i.e., the dataset from which one is mapping). The *target term* is that in which the relationship, or equivalence, is being defined [25]. In other words, the target term is that into which the source term is being translated. For example, mapping can be done to link terms from an interface terminology to a reference terminology. In this situation, the interface terminology would be considered the source, and the reference terminology the target.

It is important to note that while the use of mapping to a target terminology facilitates downstream data analysis and communication from a repository, both the original (verbatim) data element and the mapped (equivalence) element should be saved to maintain fidelity to the original clinical information.

10.6.1 Equivalence

It should also be noted that mapping does not mean equivalence. Terminologies are developed by different groups, at different times, often for different applications (use-cases). Each of these groups tend to have their own "world-view" which inevitably is passed on to their work product. Due to these idiosyncrasies, mapping does not always result in a 1-to-1 linkage from the source term to the target. Instead, many types of equivalence, or correspondence, can be observed [13,25,26], including:

- **1-to-1 exact**, where a single source term is mapped to a single target term with identical clinical meaning;
- **1-to-1 approximate**, where a single source term is mapped to a single target term with similar but not identical clinical meaning;
- **1-to-many**, where a single source term is mapped to multiple target term with similar clinical meaning; and
- **Many-to-1**, where multiple source terms are mapped to a single target term with similar clinical meaning.

Variations and combinations of these may also occur. An illustration of the various types of mapping equivalence is presented in Fig. 10.2.

At times, it may occur that a source term may not be translatable or "mapped" to a target term, resulting in an *orphan term*. Such an occurrence may be due to various causes, which have been elucidated by Lin and colleagues [27], including:

- No equivalent concept for the source term exists in the target term;
- The source term has an ambiguous meaning, and this lack of meaning precludes any linkage into a meaningful target term;
- The source term is overly specific, preventing linkage to a less-specific target term;
- The data are narrative "free" text with no meaning outside a specific clinical case; or
- The source term is institution-specific, such as one related to internal processing procedures, and therefore may have no meaning outside its specific setting.

10.6.2 Mapping process

The process of mapping between two terminologies is iterative, complex, and can be labor-intensive. It requires consideration of the characteristics of the two terminologies being mapped and, much like selection of terminology standards, it is context-specific and highly dependent on the use case that requires HIE.

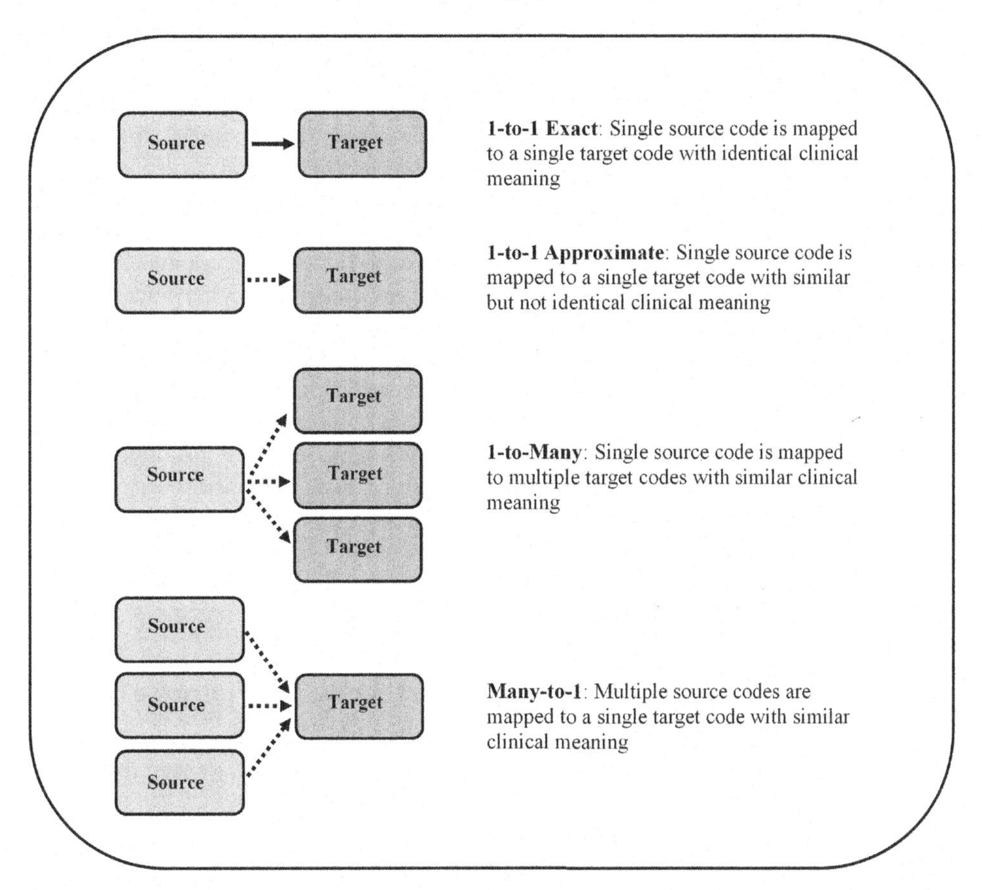

FIGURE 10.2 Types of mapping equivalence.

Furthermore, variations in interpretation of data standards are possible, requiring significant effort to harmonize approaches prior to implementation [28]. For this reason, it is essential to establish a set of mapping rules to guide the entire process prior to undertaking subsequent steps [29,30] in order to ensure an efficient and effective process. The American Health Information Management Association published a set of best practices that offer guidance on mapping that might be of use [25].

Use of previously developed maps when possible is recommended, as this greatly reduces internal map development and maintenance burdens on the HIE [10]. A variety of mapping tools developed by SDOs, government entities, and commercial institutions are available for use [25]. It must be noted, however, that mapping cannot be fully automated [31]. Human review by subject matter experts (SMEs) is required to identify differences in granularity between source and target terms. These differences cannot yet be deciphered by a computer [32]. Finally, most participants in HIE networks have some locally developed interface terminologies or ad hoc dictionaries [29] that must be mapped to the HIE network's selected standards, and as such, local mapping will still be required.

A common requirement for mapping involves translation from precoordinated interface terms (commonly used clinical phrases or concepts) and postcoordinated reference terminologies (which require multiple reference concepts to capture the entire meaning of the source concept). Classifiers are available to assist in postcoordination, but this is an area of substantial effort if the interface terminology being used as a source does not already provide a reference terminology map for each precoordinated concept [33].

Use of predefined interface terminologies which include associations from clinically friendly precoordinated terms to commonly used reference concepts can dramatically reduce individual mapping efforts. In the United States, most acute and primary care facilities leverage this type of interface terminology in one or more dictionaries within their EHRs. Using shared, professionally curated maps may provide more accurate results [34], since differences in structures and granularity between the reference codes may be better understood by teams specifically trained for the creation, and maintenance, of these maps. This strategy is highlighted in Box 10.2, which details how a researcher used mapping to identify patients with a rare disease.

Regardless of mapping strategy used, all maps require SME review and curation before finalization to ensure accuracy and completeness [10]. For example, most maps involve some interpolation, as they may not be one-to-one. This requires SMEs to interpret and make value judgments on the maps. If the terminology or value set includes specialty terms, such as procedures used in cardiology, then the SME review should involve appropriate clinical expertise (e.g., cardiologists). In addition, due to the dynamic nature of health care, such as the development of new laboratory tests, identification of new diseases, and advent of new procedures, no clinical map can be static. It will need to be revisited and revised over time.

10.6.3 Fitness for purpose

Broadly, *fitness for purpose*, or data appropriateness, is the extent to which a target

BOX 10.2

Using mapping to identify patients with rare conditions.

The information that comes from standardized data can help identify problems in population health and community characteristics that were previously unknown or not well studied, especially where small sample sizes are common. For example, Alkhayyat [35] leveraged ICD-9-CM diagnostic codes and RxNorm prescription drug orders mapped to SNOMED-CT to find that patients with Celiac disease are at increased risk of having multiple psychiatric diseases. Celiac disease has a prevalence of only 1% in the western population, and the investigators needed access to 50 million patient billing inquiries to find approximately 110,000 patients. Using available mappings from SNOMED-CT to ICD-9-CM and RxNorm codes enabled the study team to use Celiac disease concepts in the reference terminology to identify patients with disease inclusion criteria available in claims data using the other two terminologies. This approach was efficient, enabling completion of the project in a timely fashion and with a relatively small budget. Furthermore, the use of a national claims database linked to SNOMED-CT concepts enabled investigators to make use of data from all 50 states with a large enough sample size and with a high degree of confidence.

terminology can meet the needs of an intended use case [36]. In the context of mapping, it refers to the degree that a real-world objective can be represented by a potential reference terminology. The National Library of Medicine's Unified Medical Language System is the coordinating body responsible for confirming fit-for-purpose maps [37]. A strong fit-for-purpose between mapped terminologies creates automatic, lossless translation.

Fitness for purpose should especially be considered in the context of secondary data use. Data encoded with standard terminologies may have a strong fit-for-purpose in their originating clinical setting, but a weak fit-for-purpose for other use cases. Secondary use of EHR data will have a strong fit-for-purpose if the data accurately and reliably address a research question that is asked [36] or serve a specific decision-making function [38]. Consider, for example, whether EHR data could be fit-for-purpose if used by a public health agency to learn about disease screening behaviors in the community. In this case, an epidemiologist may be evaluating rates of sexually transmitted infection (STI) diagnosis in the community within a certain timeframe. The epidemiologist has EHR data that contain ICD-10 diagnostic codes, but a preliminary analysis shows the providers primarily used a general term (e.g., "Contact with and (suspected) exposure to infections with a predominantly sexual mode of transmission") when encoding STI diagnoses. These terms may fail to indicate a clear, specific STI diagnosis (e.g., chlamydia) and therefore have a weak fit-for-purpose for this intended use case. If the health agency does not care about specific STI diagnoses, this dataset might indeed have a good or reasonable fit-for-purpose. This is one example of why it is imperative to capture data at the highest level of specificity possible so that those data elements can be transformed to provide the necessary granularity for different secondary use cases. In the above example, the EHR might have used a clinically-friendly terminology including terms like "gonococcal urethritis" or "chlamydial prostatitis" which were encoded with more general ICD codes during data extraction or billing. This terminology then might provide more specific maps, or perhaps maps to multiple code systems, useful for subsequent analysis.

10.7 Terminology Services

In Chapter 8 we introduced the OpenHIE architectures, which includes a *Terminology Services* component. This component consists of server software and management tools, server and operating system software, database software, and associated hardware [10]. It integrates and manages terminology standards and definitions, including terminologies, ontologies, dictionaries, code systems, value sets, and mappings, across an HIE network or enterprise. Terminology Services (TS) provides a centralized resource for key data structures that can ensure incoming data are normalized and stored using defined standards. It also provides a set a common service interfaces, or application programming interfaces, so that terminologies and other data structures can be accessed in a reliable, reproducible way. Terminology services can be focused either on central curation and distribution of interface and reference terminologies that are pushed out to the point of service, or the services can be used to dynamically translate point of service local or interface terms to reference concepts for storage.

The choice of architecture is beyond the scope of this chapter, but both options have their advantages and disadvantages. Standardized reference terminologies available in the point of service systems allow for sharing of data collection objects, clinical decision support, and reporting objects. Dynamic translation allows for more flexibility in point of service systems and other HIE components which can use these services to normalize clinical data. Both architectures allow for consistent measurement, aggregation, analysis, evaluation, and reporting of information. Factors to be considered in the choice include speed and reliability of network communications, sophistication of the end-user (point of care) systems, and level of support available by a central service.

Terminology Services enable compliance with national standards for health care delivery. Ultimately, the result is an accurate exchange of information among members of the HIE community, including laboratories, clinics, pharmacies, hospitals, imaging centers, and public health entities. This exchange can enhance health care coordination and improve patient care decisions. The use of Terminology Services is illustrated in Box 10.3, which highlights how West African nations used TS in combination with other services discussed in other chapters of this book to improve communication across the health sector.

In practice, terminology services are used by HIE applications such as an EHR or a laboratory information system, informaticists, and health professionals [41]. HIE applications use TS to conduct queries. Before returning concepts associated with the target (end-user request), the HIE application validates, normalizes, looks up, and translates the target. Informaticists use TS for importing and exporting local target code associations and value sets. As end-users, health professionals use HIE applications that make use of terminology services [41].

BOX 10.3

Using the Terminology Service to improve the exchange of critical health information in West Africa.

The Ebola Crisis in 2014 and the COVID-19 outbreak in 2020 overwhelmed health sectors and created an urgent need for West Africa to share up-to-date information that helped health workers care for their patients and health officials gain and share insights from real-time reports. But even in less turbulent times, members of the West African health system sought ways to find out how to communicate better and faster [39].

To meet their demands, they began using applications that facilitate two-way communication between the ministries of health and health workers (mHero); help track, manage, and plan their health workforce (iHRIS); and identify and reconcile duplicate facility records across data sets (Facility Match). This has improved coordinated response in health emergencies [39].

The OpenHIE architecture and open data exchange standards in combination with FHIR standards helped make this possible. The applications used three registries (Health Worker, Client, and Facility Registries) and the Terminology Service component of the architecture. The Terminology Service component helped streamline exchange activities by providing the central source for terminologies, ontologies, and value sets required to normalize the information being exchanged. That information is normalized across five dimensions: (1) who received health service, (2) who provided health service, (3) where was the service received, (4) what care was received, and (5) what products were involved in treatment [40]. These five dimensions contain the most relevant information needed by health care teams across health facilities at the point of care and as real-time information for reporting from health ministries. Overall, the application of the terminology service helped to improve the exchange of information for the health sector in West Africa.

Prior to adopting a terminology service, an HIE network should consider its maturity level as a part of organizational strategy. Terminology services with lower levels of maturity are in earlier phases of development and are unlikely to improve interoperability. OpenHIE describes the following five stages of terminology service maturity: (1) Nascent, (2) Emerging, (3) Shared Electronic Reference, (4) Digital Subscription, and (5) Institutionalized [42]. These stages are described in Fig. 10.3.

10.7.1 Implementation of Terminology Services

The implementation of TS within an HIE network is a multistep process that begins with an assessment of available resources and the development of a project plan. To do so, the following types of activities must be addressed [10]:

- Choosing, acquiring, installing, and configuring software and hardware.
- Identification of the local and proprietary terminologies currently in use by the network, and selection of the (target) standard terminologies to be the basis of the future HIE.
- Populating the Terminology Service with the required dictionaries and terminologies.
- Mapping of existing dictionaries, data collection objects and reports to standardized dictionaries and terminologies as required.
- Enhancing the point-of-care systems, insurance systems, and/or national registry systems that will interact with the TS so that they can communicate with the Terminology Service through the Interoperability Layer of the architecture.
- Documenting the technical information required to support the system.
- Testing the system to ensure that it is operating as planned.
- Developing and implementing policies and procedures required to support the system and business processes, and training users

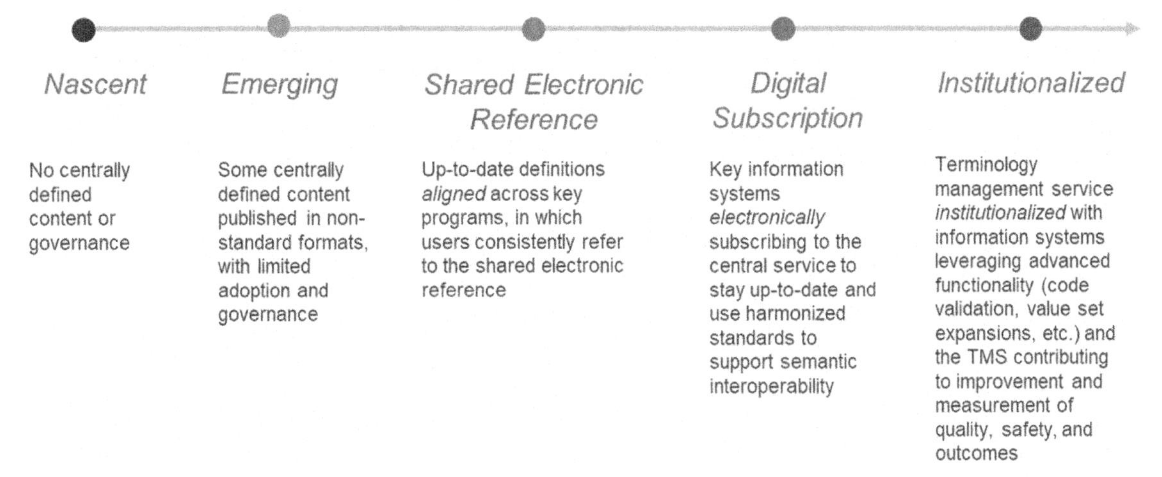
Terminology Services Maturity Model
Nascent
Emerging
Shared Electronic Reference
Digital Subscription
Institutionalized
No centrally defined content or governance
Some centrally defined content published in non-standard formats, with limited adoption and governance
Up-to-date definitions aligned across key programs, in which users consistently refer to the shared electronic reference
Key information systems electronically subscribing to the central service to stay up-to-date and use harmonized standards to support semantic interoperability
Terminology management service institutionalized with information systems leveraging advanced functionality (code validation, value set expansions, etc.) and the TMS contributing to improvement and measurement of quality, safety, and outcomes

FIGURE 10.3 Terminology Services Maturity Model [42]. Source: *Screenshot taken from the OpenHIE Terminology Service Community Wiki.*

on these topics. These include processes for system maintenance and backup as well as processes such as loading dictionary and terminology updates and resolving potential conflicts and inconsistencies between update data sets.

Next, these activities will be discussed more specifically. At the start of the implementation process, it is necessary to select and implement TS software and hardware based on economic, technical, and standard-specific considerations. The software needs, the high-level system constraints, and the architecture will drive hardware needs. These considerations are examined in the following sections.

After the software and hardware have been put into place, the next step is to load the interface terminologies, reference terminologies, and mappings that were identified using methods discussed earlier in this chapter. This should then be followed by establishing, testing, and verifying the interfaces between HIE components to ensure the connections required to support use cases and workflows are effective. Finally, all software used should then be tested and validated to ensure the TS can maintain and support the required terminologies, and that the interactions with other Open HIE architecture components and interfacing systems are supported [10].

10.7.2 Terminology Service support

Implementation of a Terminology Service is just the beginning. Once in place, ongoing, iterative support is necessary to meet the needs of the evolving health network. Common types of support include:

- **Operations support**: This includes the development and maintenance of policies and procedures that are necessary to support business and technical processes for the Terminology Service. It may also comprise tasks such as evaluating adherence to the selected terminology standards.
- **Terminology support**: Standards are modified and improved over time. Medical science is constantly evolving with new therapies, interventions, and diagnoses, such as COVID-19, entering the field. All of these advancements must be codified and integrated with existing data sets. Newer versions of standards may impact previous mappings due to new concepts, retired concepts, or structural changes [43]. Because of this, TS must have an ongoing analysis of impact of any terminology or mapping changes. In addition, the Terminology Service should maintain a history (versions, effective dates, etc.) of all the terminologies supported, so that references to historical data can be normalized and longitudinal analyses performed.
- **Help desk support**: As more and more users and organizations utilize TS, it may become important to identify, document, and triage responses to types of requests from the various users. For each request, it may be necessary to track who requested it, why it was requested, and when it was requested. Detailed information of how the issue was resolved should also be documented for reference purposes.
- **Training of support personnel**: Successful implementation of the support plan is grounded in effective training of all personnel charged with overseeing it.

10.7.3 Evaluation of Terminology Services

Once implemented with necessary support services in place, it becomes essential to conduct ongoing evaluation of the HIE network's TS to ensure efficiency and effectiveness of the operation. Appropriate timing of these evaluations will be determined by the HIE, depending on need as well as data and resource availability. For example, they may be conducted annually, quarterly, or on a real-time basis. Varying aspects of the service can be assessed, including but not limited to: frequency of code use; correctness of methods of code validation; frequency, types, and causes of errors; and prevalence of redundancy/over-coding [10]. Any concerns or areas of weakness regarding these features or others should be referred to administrators for correction.

10.8 Emerging trends

The growth of national and international data-reporting and disease surveillance efforts, led by organizations such as the World Health Organization [44], Nongovernmental Organizations, and other funding groups, has amplified the importance of the collection of standardized data. While previously health systems could "get by" with data inconsistently or locally coded, these large-scale efforts demand clinical data consistency only possible through the use of strong reference data standards.

Data standards have matured substantially over the last decade, in no small part due to the growing cooperation among SDOs, as well as adoption of standards on a national level [45]. As such, substantial progress toward harmonization and practical applications has occurred. From here, continued growth in several areas is anticipated, including genetic data standardization [46], bidirectional public health data transfer [47], and the development of metadata standardization for interoperability of systems that include heterogeneous interacting components [45,48–50]. Another emerging area is the management, curation, and distribution of value sets, such as those available from the US NLM [12] and HL7 [51]. Additionally, as standards continue to be implemented, evaluation of their ability to achieve harmonization must be conducted to ensure their real-world effectiveness [52]. Changing regulations will also continually require data to be synchronized with new regulatory expectations [50].

In addition to data standards, interface (communication) standards have increased

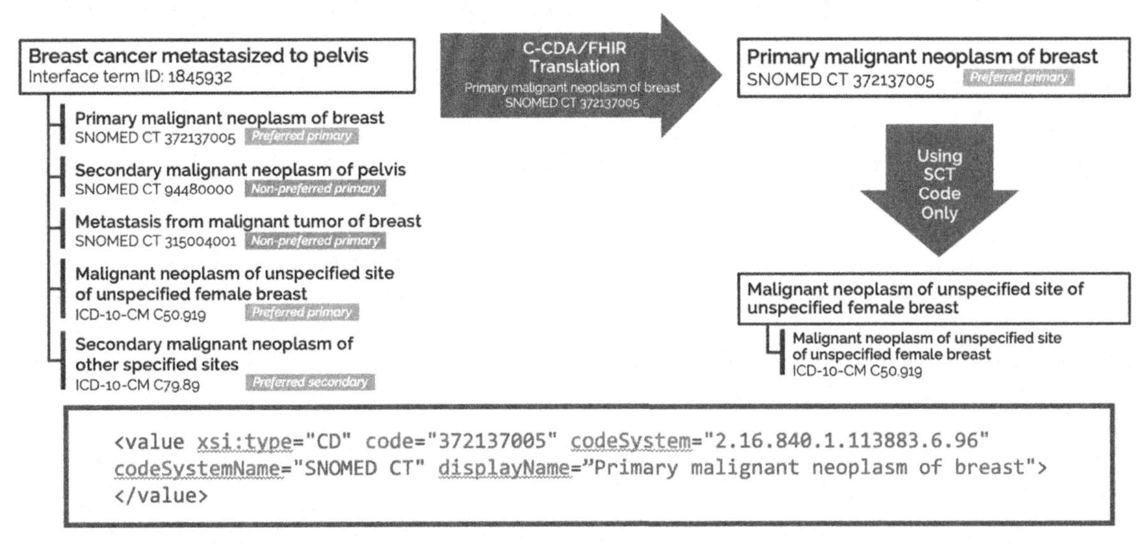

FIGURE 10.4 Representation of the frequent loss of clinical specificity when transferring data with C-CDA/FHIR.

their focus on terminology and semantic consistency. Organizations such as Health Level Seven (HL7) [53] and Integrating the Healthcare Enterprise (IHE) [54] have identified specific use-cases and profiles to address terminology query, normalization, and mapping. It is expected that this focus will continue and new interface protocols will need to be supported by Terminology Services implementations [55].

There is a growing recognition that current Consolidated-Clinical Document Architecture (C-CDA) and Fast Healthcare Interoperability Resources (FHIR) resources do not provide sufficient granularity of meaning to drive more complex use cases. The existing one concept-one code model does not take into account that clinical medicine often requires complex concepts and postcoordination. The example in Fig. 10.4 shows how a complex concept like "Breast cancer metastasized to pelvis" would be translated using C-CDA or FHIR. Transfer of postcoordinated expressions, such as this example, in a reliable and understandable way is currently an effort underway within HL-7. However, this would require both sender and receiver to understand how to do the postcoordination.

Even after agreement is reached on standardizing postcoordinated or complex expressions, the use of services which assist senders to decompose precoordinated clinical terms into these standardized resources and back again will likely be needed.

10.9 Summary

Data standardization is an ongoing challenge but key to facilitating semantic interoperability in HIE. Through the use of reference standards, including thoughtful and complete mapping of local terminologies to these standards, effective exchange of clinical data between various entities in the health care ecosystem can occur, allowing for accurate and consistent measurement, analysis, and communication of information. The implementation of standards and Terminology Services is a complex undertaking that requires consideration of context-specific economic, political, social, and technological factors. Despite challenges, the field of data standardization is currently at a stage of rapid advancement due to increasing cooperation and international guidance. While much work remains, the future is promising for widespread semantic interoperability.

Questions for discussion

1. Reference terminologies are the foundation of semantic interoperability in an HIE network. Describe some of the potential beneficial outcomes that result from having comparable, structured language among the differing systems participating in the HIE network.
2. What considerations must be taken into account when selecting an HIE terminology standard? Should the entire standard be utilized or only a subset?
3. Describe some types of equivalence that may be observed when mapping. What might cause a source code to go unmapped?
4. What is the purpose of a Terminology Service? What considerations must be taken into account when selecting the appropriate software and hardware of the Terminology Service?
5. Terminology Services require ongoing, iterative support and assessment. Explain why continuous evaluation and updates are necessary.

Acknowledgments

The authors acknowledge and thank Jennifer Alyea, PhD, MPH, who coauthored the corresponding chapter in the first edition of this book.

References

[1] SNOMED International. SNOMED – 5-step briefing. n.d. [cited 2021 July 16]. Available from: <https://www.snomed.org/snomed-ct/five-step-briefing>.

[2] Noy N, McGuinness D. Ontology Development 101: a guide to creating your first ontology. Knowledge Systems Laboratory; 2001. p. 32.

[3] Berners-Lee T, Hendler J, Lassila O. The semantic web: a new form of web content that is meaningful to computers will unleash a revolution of new possibilities. Scientific American; 2001.

[4] Rogers J, Bodenreider O. SNOMED CT: browsing the browsers. In: KR-MED 2008: Representing and sharing knowledge using SNOMED; 2008 May 31–June 2; Phoenix, AZ.

[5] Zafar A, Dixon BE. Pulling back the covers: technical lessons of a real-world health information exchange. Stud Health Technol Inform 2007;129(Pt 1):488–92.

[6] Office of the National Coordinator for Health Information Technology. 2021 Interoperability Standards Advisory reference edition [Internet]. Washington, D.C.: U.S. Department of Health and Human Services; 2021. Available from: <https://www.healthit.gov/isa/sites/isa/files/inline-files/2021-ISA-Reference-Edition.pdf>.

[7] Office of Disease Prevention and Health Promotion. Objectives and data [Internet]. U.S. Department of Health and Human Services; n.d. [cited 2021 Aug 9]. Available from: <https://health.gov/healthypeople/objectives-and-data>.

[8] Regenstrief Institute. 2020 LOINC annual report [Internet]. Indianapolis, IN; 2020 [cited 2021 Jul 19]. Available from: <https://loinc.org/annual-reports/year-2020/>.

[9] Centers for Medicare & Medicaid Services. 2020 ICD-10-CM [Internet]. Baltimore, MD; 2020. Available from: <https://www.cms.gov/Medicare/Coding/ICD10/2020-ICD-10-CM>.

[10] OpenHIE. OHIE Terminology Services: planning and implementation guide; 2014 [cited 2015 Jun 15]. Available from: <https://ohie.org/terminology-service/>.

[11] Centers for Disease Control and Prevention. PHIN vocabulary access and distribution system (VADS) Atlanta, GA; 2021 [updated Dec 5, 2018]. Available from: <https://phinvads.cdc.gov/vads/SearchVocab.action>.

[12] U.S. National Library of Medicine. Value Set Authority Center (VSAC). Bethesda, MD; 2012 [updated Oct 25, 2021]. Available from: <https://vsac.nlm.nih.gov/>.

[13] Cimino JJ, Hayamizu TF, Bodenreider O, Davis B, Stafford GA, Ringwald M. The caBIG terminology review process. J Biomed Inform 2009;42(3):571–80.

[14] Office of the National Coordinator for Health Information Technology. United States Core Data for Interoperability (USCDI) [Internet]. 2021 [cited 2021 Aug 5]. Available from: <https://www.healthit.gov/isa/united-states-core-data-interoperability-uscdi#uscdi-v2>.

[15] Hatt N. What you need to know about the new ONC and CMS Healthcare Interoperability and Information Blocking Rules [Internet]. Madison, WI: RedoxEngine; 2020. Available from: <https://www.redoxengine.com/blog/what-you-need-to-know-about-the-new-onc-and-cms-healthcare-interoperability-and-information-blocking-rules/>.

[16] Centers for Medicare & Medicaid Services. Using Z codes: the Social Determinants of Health (SDOH) data journey to better outcomes [Internet]. 2021. Available from: <https://www.cms.gov/files/document/zcodes-infographic.pdf>.

[17] Regenstrief Institute. Social Determinants of Health [Internet]. n.d. Available from: <https://loinc.org/sdh/>.

[18] Gallego E. Consensus-driven standards on Social Determinants of Health [Internet]. 2021. Available from: <https://confluence.hl7.org/pages/viewpage.action?pageId = 76153059&preview = /76153059/118980865/Gravity%20Overview_ONC%20Workshop%2020210713.pdf>.

[19] Bodenreider O. Biomedical ontologies in action: role in knowledge management, data integration and decision support. Yearb Med Inf 2008;67–79.

[20] Bhargava A, Kim T, Quine DB, Hauser RG. A 20-year evaluation of LOINC in the United States' largest integrated health system. Arch Pathol Lab Med 2020;144(4):478–84.

[21] Dixon BE, Siegel JA, Oemig TV, Grannis SJ. Electronic health information quality challenges and interventions to improve public health surveillance data and practice. Public Health Rep 2013;128(6):546–53.

[22] Dhakal S, Burrer SL, Winston CA, Dey A, Ajani U, Groseclose SL. Coding of electronic laboratory reports for biosurveillance, selected United States hospitals, 2011. Online J Public Health Inform 2015;7(2):e220.

[23] Drenkhahn C, Ingenerf J. The LOINC content model and its limitations of usage in the laboratory domain. Stud Health Technol Inform 2020;270:437–42.

[24] Park H-A, Yu S-J, Jung H. Strategies for adopting and implementing SNOMED CT in Korea. Healthc Inform Res 2021;27(1):3–10.

[25] Bronnert J, Clark J, Cook J, Fenton S, Scichilone R, Williams M, et al. Data mapping best practices. J AHIMA 2011;82(4):46–52.

[26] De Suman. 8 steps to success in ICD-10-CM/PCS mapping: Best practices to establish precise mapping between old and new ICD code sets. Journal of AHIMA 2012;83(6):44–9 In press.

[27] Lin MC, Vreeman DJ, McDonald CJ, Huff SM. A characterization of local LOINC mapping for laboratory

tests in three large institutions. Methods Inf Med 2011;50(2):105–14.
[28] McCarthy DB, Propp K, Cohen A, Sabharwal R, Schachter AA, Rein AL. Learning from health information exchange technical architecture and implementation in seven beacon communities. EGEMS (Wash DC) 2014;2(1):1060.
[29] Abhyankar S, Demner-Fushman D, McDonald CJ. Standardizing clinical laboratory data for secondary use. J Biomed Inform 2012;45(4):642–50.
[30] Vreeman DJ, McDonald CJ. Automated mapping of local radiology terms to LOINC. AMIA Annu Symp Proc 2005;2005:769–73.
[31] Saitwal H, Qing D, Jones S, Bernstam EV, Chute CG, Johnson TR. Cross-terminology mapping challenges: a demonstration using medication terminological systems. J Biomed Inform 2012;45(4):613–25.
[32] National Library of Medicine. ICD-9-CM Diagnostic Codes to SNOMED CT Map. [Internet]. 2018. Available from: <https://www.nlm.nih.gov/research/umls/mapping_projects/icd9cm_to_snomedct.html>.
[33] Cimino JJ. Desiderata for controlled medical vocabularies in the twenty-first century. Methods Inf Med 1998;37(4–5):394–403.
[34] Burrows EK, Razzaghi H, Utidjian L, Bailey LC. Standardizing clinical diagnoses: evaluating alternate terminology selection. AMIA Jt Summits Transl Sci Proc 2020;2020:71–9.
[35] Alkhayyat M, Qapaja T, Aggarwal M, Almomani A, Abureesh M, Al-Otoom O, et al. Epidemiology and risk of psychiatric disorders among patients with celiac disease: a population-based national study. J Gastroenterol Hepatol 2021;36:2165–70.
[36] Reynolds MW, Bourke A, Dreyer NA. Considerations when evaluating real-world data quality in the context of fitness for purpose. Pharmacoepidemiol Drug Saf 2020;29(10):1316–18.
[37] Bowman S. Coordinating SNOMED-CT and ICD-10: getting the most out of electronic health record systems. J Am Health Inf Manag Assoc 2005;76(7):60–1.
[38] Barbazza E, Klazinga NS, Kringos DS. Exploring the actionability of healthcare performance indicators for quality of care: a qualitative analysis of the literature, expert opinion and user experience. BMJ Qual Saf 2021;30.
[39] OpenHIE. Systematizing communication channels to support health messaging needs in West Africa and beyond [Internet]. 2021. Available from: <https://ohie.org/impact-stories/systematizing-communication-channels-to-support-health-messaging-needs-in-west-africa-and-beyond/>.
[40] OpenHIE. OpenHIE architecture & standards [Internet]. 2021 [updated Sept. 29]. Available from: <https://wiki.ohie.org/pages/viewpage.action?pageId = 8454157>.
[41] Thomas J. Terminology Services community documentation: integration of TS use case examples [Internet]. Open HIE; 2014. Available from: <https://wiki.ohie.org/display/SUB/Integration + of + TS + Use + Case + Examples>.
[42] OpenHIE. Terminology Management Maturity Model [Internet]. 2018 [updated September] Available from: <https://wiki.ohie.org/display/SUB/Terminology + Service + Community?preview = /9437189/32408821/Terminology_Services_%20Maturity%20Model-2018.pptx>.
[43] Wade G, Rosenbloom ST. The impact of SNOMED CT revisions on a mapped interface terminology: terminology development and implementation issues. J Biomed Inform 2009;42(3):490–3.
[44] World Health Organization. Surveillance in emergencies [Internet]. n.d. Available from: <https://www.who.int/emergencies/surveillance>.
[45] Richesson RL, Chute CG. Health information technology data standards get down to business: maturation within domains and the emergence of interoperability. J Am Med Inform Assoc 2015;22(3):492–4.
[46] Deckard J, McDonald CJ, Vreeman DJ. Supporting interoperability of genetic data with LOINC. J Am Med Inform Assoc 2015;22(3):621–7.
[47] National Committee on Vital and Health Statistics. Electronic standards for public health information exchange [Internet]. 2014. Available from: <http://www.ncvhs.hhs.gov/>.
[48] Fenton S, Giannangelo K, Kallem C, Scichilone R. Data standards, data quality, and interoperability (updated). J AHIMA 2013;84(11):64–9.
[49] Marcos C, González-Ferrer A, Peleg M, Cavero C. Solving the interoperability challenge of a distributed complex patient guidance system: a data integrator based on HL7 Virtual Medical Record standard. J Am Med Inform Assoc 2015;22(3):587–99.
[50] HIMSS Health Information Exchange Committee. The future of HIE: HIMSS HIE thought leadership brief [Internet]. 2012. Available from: <http://www.himss.org/>.
[51] HL7. Value sets defined in FHIR – FHIR v0.0.82 [Internet]. 2014 [cited 2015 Jul 31]. Available from: <http://www.hl7.org/implement/standards/fhir/terminologies-valuesets.html>.
[52] Gold MR, McLaughlin CG, Devers KJ, Berenson RA, Bovbjerg RR. Obtaining providers' 'buy-in' and establishing effective means of information exchange will

be critical to HITECH's success. Health Aff (Millwood) 2012;31(3):514–26.

[53] HL7 International. Introduction to HL7 Standards [Internet]. 2015 [cited 2015 Jul 17]. Available from: <http://www.hl7.org/implement/standards/index.cfm>.

[54] IHE International. IHE resources [Internet]. 2015 [cited 2015 Jul 17]. Available from: <http://www.hl7.org/implement/standards/index.cfm>.

[55] HL7. FHIR: Terminology Service [Internet]. 2015 [cited 2015 Jul 10]. Available from: <http://hl7.org/implement/standards/fhir/2015Jan/terminology-service.html>.

CHAPTER

11

Shared longitudinal health records for clinical and population health

David Broyles[1], *Ryan Crichton*[2], *Bob Jolliffe*[3], *Johan Ivar Sæbø*[3] *and Brian E. Dixon*[4,5]

[1]Marion County Public Health Department, Indianapolis, IN, USA [2]Jembi Health Systems, Cape Town, South Africa [3]Department of Informatics, University of Oslo, Oslo, Norway [4]Department of Epidemiology, Richard M. Fairbanks School of Public Health, Indiana University, Indianapolis, IN, USA [5]Center for Biomedical Informatics, Regenstrief Institute, Inc., Indianapolis, IN, USA

LEARNING OBJECTIVES

By the end of the chapter, the reader should be able to:

- Identify and describe the differences between an electronic medical record, electronic health record, and a shared heath record;
- Explain the role of a shared health record in a health information exchange;
- List and describe the components of a shared health record;
- Discuss the role and benefits of a health management information system within a health information exchange;
- Define a population health indicator;
- Identify and describe application domains for a health management information system;
- Define a database management system;
- Compare the implications of implementing a shared health record using an electronic health record system versus a database management system; and
- Discuss emerging trends likely to shape the evolution of shared health records and health management information systems.

11.1 Introduction

Health care systems are organized differently around the globe. Systems vary in the proportion of care delivered by public versus private facilities, in their emphasis on primary, secondary,

Health Information Exchange
DOI: https://doi.org/10.1016/B978-0-323-90802-3.00025-3

and tertiary care, in the levels and sources of funding, by the populations they serve, in the burden of disease faced by their populations, and in the level of development of the environments of human and technological infrastructure. Nevertheless, there is consensus that health information systems have a pivotal role to play in improving quality and efficiency in all of these contexts [1], though the nature of such technological systems as well as the roles and relative importance of their individual components and their sequence of emergence will be conditioned by socio-political, historical, and geographical realities.

Electronic medical record (EMR) systems can streamline the delivery of health care within an individual organization by archiving, monitoring, and facilitating operations [2]. These systems assemble a digital representation of patient's legal medical record within a single health organization or network [3]. A patient's EMR contains information such as medical history, immunization records, physician notes, laboratory test results, and vital signs. In the fragmented health care system of the United States, many autonomous health networks coalesce to provide care for an individual patient [4]. Consequently, it should not be assumed that the EMR from an individual organization contains a complete medical history for an individual patient. Key pieces of a patient's medical history such as a diagnosis or laboratory result that occurred in a different health network may not be available to a physician providing care.

In contrast, an *electronic health record (EHR)* system is designed to promote continuity of care across numerous health care networks within a region through collaborative data sharing [5]. An EHR system consolidates health datasets that were collected from an array of different sources into a person-centric health record in order to provide a more complete and longitudinal portrayal of an individual's medical history [3,6]. However, this information may only be useful within the network of collaborating organizations. A national or regional health information exchange (HIE) must be able to harmonize the clinical information that is being collected from multiple EHR systems into a single shared, longitudinal health record. These comprehensive, longitudinal records are intended to decidedly enhance the quality and productivity of health care through reductions in medical errors, decreased redundancies in testing, and averted costs [7–10]. In additional, longitudinal records can be aggregated to provide population-level indicators of health outcomes to support health policy, disease surveillance, health systems management, and clinical research.

11.2 Shared longitudinal records for clinical health

The OpenHIE model discussed in Chapter 8 includes a component system called the *Shared health record (SHR)* that compiles a longitudinal, person-centric record across a patient's many clinical encounters for access by the organizations participating in HIE. The SHR system provides a permanent, centralized repository to store and manage the health information shared by the heterogeneous information systems of a regional or national HIE network. Contributing applications could include anything from an enterprise EHR system to a small-scale mobile application (recall the point-of-service applications from the OpenHIE model).

The SHR component of an HIE network facilitates a variety of interactions between the internal components and external point-of-service applications with the goal of supporting the delivery of clinical care. The SHR enables point-of-service applications (e.g., EMRs or pharmacy information systems) to store key clinical data such as a summary of care, laboratory test results, or vitals. The SHR can manage both structured data that is reconcilable with standard exchange formats (e.g., discrete clinical observations) and unstructured data such as a digital image with associated patient information. In addition, point-of-service systems can update existing patient records in the SHR with new information while preserving a version history. However, the data stored in the SHR should be restricted to include only information that is deemed relevant for sharing within the implementing nation or region [11]. The SHR should not necessarily contain a complete dump of information from all point-of-service systems in the nation or region, but rather contain relevant information that when shared gives a complete view of a patient's medical history and health. Table 11.1 provides a list of some of the pertinent types of clinical data that are often stored in a SHR.

An SHR also enables client services to retrieve clinical information from the repository as needed to improve the delivery of care. The SHR can provide end users with a complete longitudinal medical history for a particular patient. In addition, client systems can query the SHR to retrieve a partial subset of a patient's medical history that has been restricted to a specific time frame or a unique type of observation. For example, a physician caring for a patient with a high diastolic blood pressure may want to know if the elevated blood pressure is a trend or just an isolated occurrence to determine the appropriate approach for treatment. The physician could acquire this information by querying the SHR to retrieve a list of the patient's blood pressure during each previous encounter.

An SHR is also designed to semantically understand certain sections of the information that it receives from point-of-service systems. This is enabled through the use of standardized representations of the clinical information, which support semantic descriptions of the data in the SHR. It is important for the SHR to semantically understand certain clinical information for a few main reasons. First, this

TABLE 11.1 Common data elements included in a shared longitudinal health record.

Data type	Description
Structured data	Demographics
	Clinical observations
	Care summaries
	Allergies
	Prescribed medications
	Laboratory results
	Immunizations
	Medical histories
	Mental health assessments
	Nutritional assessments
	Action plans (care plans)
	Quality of life indicators
Unstructured data	Medical imaging documents (e.g., X-rays)
	Narrative text (e.g., progress notes)

enables the SHR to produce and return an accurate summary of a patient's clinical history, and second it enables population health indicators to be produced more easily. Aggregating all blood pressure measurements, for example, allows trending and integrated presentation to the clinician. Finally, semantic understanding of clinical information enables other, secondary uses (reuse) of the clinical data, such as medical research or real-world evidence generation.

11.3 Shared longitudinal records for population health

In addition to improving the delivery of individual clinical care, sharing longitudinal health records also cultivates opportunities to improve health outcomes at the population level [12,13]. The OpenHIE model described in Chapter 8 contains a component called the health management information system (HMIS) that stores and distributes cumulative population level information. The HMIS supports management or administration of a health system, as well as public health functions, and it contains a wide range of aggregate level data. The HMIS aggregates individual clinical records that are shared within an HIE to generate indicators that characterize the health of the underlying population at the provider, facility, state, or national level. In addition, the HMIS should contain data on human resource distribution, population figures, service availability, and service quality such as the efficiency of the supply chain. This enables the HMIS for added value analysis of the aggregated clinical data. The information in the HMIS is available for reporting purposes and is intended to improve the administration and development of public health programs rather than the delivery of clinical care [12]. Aggregated health information can benefit the health of a society by enhancing surveillance capacities, promoting advancements in medical research, and supporting the development of effective health policies.

11.3.1 Population health dashboards and indicators

The aggregation of individual clinical records through the HMIS can drive the use of dashboards featuring health indicators that can improve understanding of community health status. A *dashboard* is a data visualization tool that provides at-a-glance views of data and information, especially key metrics or performance indicators, that drive decision-making processes in organizations. Dashboards are quite popular outside of health care, analyzing manufacturing productivity data or aggregating sales data across a team or company. Health indicator dashboards rocketed into popularity during the COVID-19 pandemic. The Johns Hopkins University COVID-19 Dashboard [14] is the most prominent example, yet there are several others including an enterprise dashboard at the University of California San Diego Health System [15] and a statewide HIE dashboard created by the Regenstrief Institute [16]. Dashboards can be implemented as standalone information system components, or they can be functions within a system like an EHR or the HMIS.

A *health indicator* is a metric that is routinely reported to provide insight into the characteristics of a population or the performance of a program [17]. An accurate assessment of the current health status of the population and influential factors within the community is essential for elevating the overall health of the community. Important health indicators may constitute clinical outcomes (e.g., mortality rates for cancer) or the prevalence of important health risk factors such as obesity or smoking. These health indicators can be leveraged to drive public health action such as policy changes or interventions to address significant health issues [18]. Programs such as Healthy People 2030 [19] define health indicators to call attention to crucial public health issues (e.g., increasing prevalence of diabetes), institute goals for improving the issue (e.g., reduce the hospital admission rate for older adults with diabetes, reduce the number of diabetes cases diagnosed yearly), and then evaluate progress toward those goals (e.g., compare baseline rates with future rates).

11.3.2 Disease surveillance

The global COVID-19 pandemic, as well as other threats to population health globally, including Ebola virus (EBV), influenza (H1N1), Middle East respiratory syndrome (MERS-CoV) and severe acute respiratory syndrome (SARS), illustrates the importance of building capacities within countries to detect the presence of infectious diseases at an early stage of an outbreak [20,21]. Compiling information from individual clinical records can provide insight into the patterns and trends of disease throughout a population [12,22]. Syndromic surveillance systems, for example, involve the exchange of emergency department encounter data to public health authorities in real-time, enabling epidemiologists to assess population trends in respiratory and gastrointestinal diseases [22,23]. During the COVID-19 pandemic, multiple HIE networks integrated data on laboratory-confirmed cases as well as hospitalizations following infection, providing public health authorities real-time status on how many people were infected and had severe disease [16,24,25]. Fig. 11.1 illustrates the dashboard from the Regenstrief Institute built on top of the Indiana HIE network featuring hospitalizations due to COVID-19 along with population indicators based on race, age, and sex. These data informed where public health authorities set up testing sites as

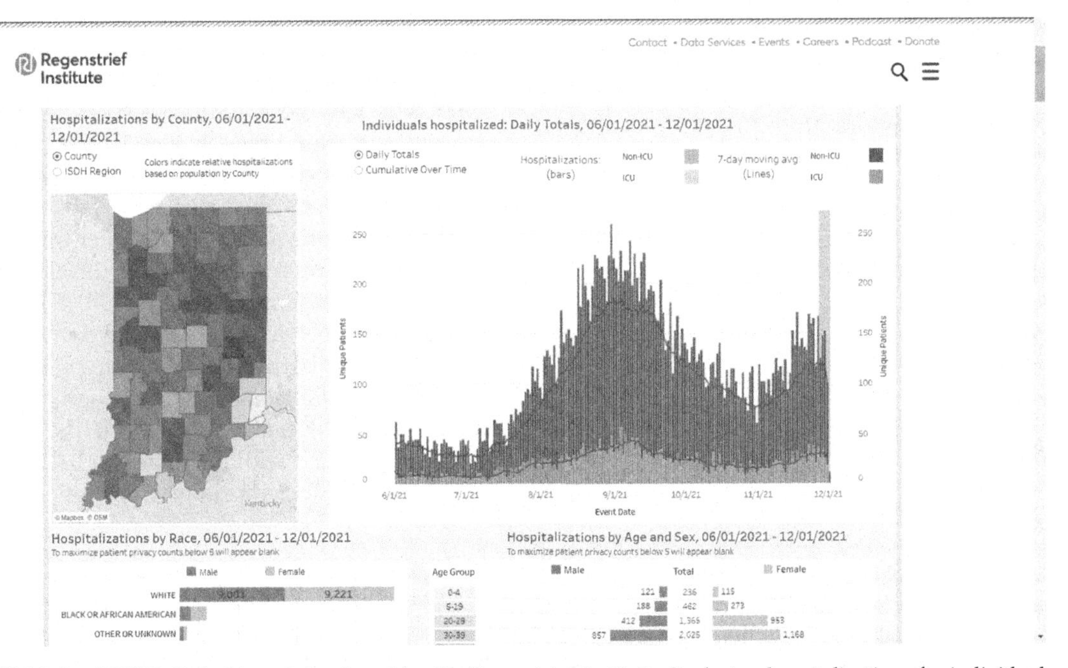

FIGURE 11.1 COVID-19 dashboard developed by the Regenstrief Institute displaying hospitalizations for individuals with positive SARS-CoV-2 infection along with population strata based on race, age, and gender.

well as vaccination clinics once vaccines were available [26]. Shared EHRs from Regenstrief and the Indiana HIE further supported the U.S. Centers for Disease Control and Prevention in tracking the effectiveness of vaccines longitudinally by integrating data from immunization registries with hospitalization data on individuals testing positive for COVID-19 [27–29].

Integrating data from the SHR and HMIS with traditional surveillance strategies, such as vital records (e.g., birth records, death certificates), can provide a more complete picture of the prevalence and spatial distribution of important diseases [12,23,30,31]. This includes chronic disease, including diabetes, hypertension, and HIV. HIE networks often receive newborn screening laboratory results, enabling longitudinal tracking of individuals diagnosed with sickle cell disease and other rare conditions. Currently the CDC is working with medical centers and HIE networks to leverage data from a SHR to measure the prevalence and incidence of diabetes in children as well as young adults [32]. Integrated disease surveillance enhanced with SHR and HMIS components, if widely implemented and adopted, would be transformative to public health surveillance practice [33].

11.3.3 Medical research

Available, semantically interoperable information contained in the SHR and HMIS could be leveraged to advance medical research [13,18,34]. Analysis of the cumulative clinical data that are available in the HMIS can be especially useful for the generation of hypotheses and when performing comparative assessments [7]. Currently, population health in the United States is predominantly assessed through nationally funded health surveys such as the National Health Interview Survey (NHIS) [7,12,35]. The information collected in these surveys is self-reported, and may be unreliable or lack critical information [7]. Incorporating the cumulative information from the HMIS that was collected as a part of routine care can complement and strengthen the value of existing data sources [7].

SHRs also have the potential to identify eligible participants for clinical trials [12]. Clinical trial participants have traditionally been recruited through advertisements, notices, or contacting physicians [12]. A SHR system can be designed to simplify the process by adding optional alerts that can be relayed to candidates eligible for clinical trials by their physicians [12]. The Indiana Health Information Exchange, described in Chapter 22, is the only HIE known to routinely leverage its SHR for study recruitment, observational research, and comparative analyses.

11.4 Implementation

Due to differences in organizational needs and health information infrastructures, the most appropriate solution for the implementation of a SHR will vary across HIE networks and nations as well as over time. In some cases, an EHR-based solution (e.g., use an off-the-shelf EHR product) may be the most acceptable approach for implementing a SHR, while other implementations may require that a SHR is developed on a database management system (DBMS) platform with tailored services for that HIE network. For a SHR to be supportive of the requirements of consumers and local contexts, a thorough assessment of the goals, systems, data, standards, and challenges associated with the pertinent health system should be conducted prior to implementation.

11.4.1 SHR implemented as an EHR

The OpenHIE model implements the SHR system as an independent component within a larger infrastructure. The interoperability layer (IL; described in Chapter 8) receives transactions from the disparate point-of-service systems exchanging information, and facilitates the interaction between the internal components of the HIE. The OpenHIE infrastructure includes client registry (Chapter 12), health worker registry (Chapter 14), and facility registry (Chapter 13) components to verify that the patients, providers, and facilities involved in a transaction request are known to the HIE. A complete shared record must also reconcile the unique terminologies and coding used by different point-of-service applications interacting with the HIE [36]. The OpenHIE uses a terminology service to map local codes to the standardized internal format (see Chapter 10).

The SHR component of OpenHIE was developed on a modified version of an EHR platform called OpenMRS (http://www.openmrs.org) to serve as the centralized repository for the storage and management of clinical data within the OpenHIE infrastructure. The capacity to manage discrete values effectively, and a powerful API, made OpenMRS a favorable SHR solution for OpenHIE [11]. OpenHIE provides three different types of modules that facilitate the processing and storage of data using the OpenMRS platform including interface modules, a content handler module, and processing modules (depicted in Fig. 11.2). The interface modules provide service interfaces that enable an external application to access the data in the SHR. A content handler module is used to receive data from the service interfaces, and pass the information on to the proper processing module for storage. Processing modules provide the capacity to decipher information in a specific format so that it can be stored in or retrieved from the OpenMRS system. For example, a robust HIE may require a processing module that accommodates Health Level Seven (HL7) version 2 documents, processing modules for multiple types of clinical document architecture (CDA) documents, and a processing module that supports unstructured documents. Fig. 11.2 illustrates the architecture of the components that would enable OpenMRS to be implemented as the SHR for OpenHIE.

The flexibility of the OpenHIE architecture permits implementers to replace or expand the storage model supporting the SHR as necessary. The most appropriate EHR platform for a SHR may vary based on the requirements and idiosyncrasies of the particular implementation [37–39]. Potentially more than one data storage model could be used for a single SHR. For example, OpenMRS could manage the discrete data within the SHR while OpenXDS could manage the document store. The following EHR platforms could also be considered for use as a SHR:

- OpenXDS (github.com/jembi/openxds/),
- OpenEMR (open-emr.org),
- OSCAR (oscar-emr.com),
- OpenVista CareVue (Medsphere), and
- OpenMRS (openmrs.org).

Enterprise EHR systems, including but not limited to Epic (Verona, WI) and Cerner (Kansas City, MO), could also serve as a SHR. Most comprehensive EHR systems manage both discrete data and document stores using components on the proprietary, commercial platform. This option might be best for enterprise HIE networks. Community and national HIE networks may find it challenging to implement an enterprise EHR as the SHR if there are different EHR solutions used by providers across the region or nation.

11.4.2 SHR implemented as a database

A SHR can be operationalized as a database instead of an EHR system to provide a method of storing, organizing, and managing the clinical records. In this case, a *DBMS* would be used to empower users or other applications to interact

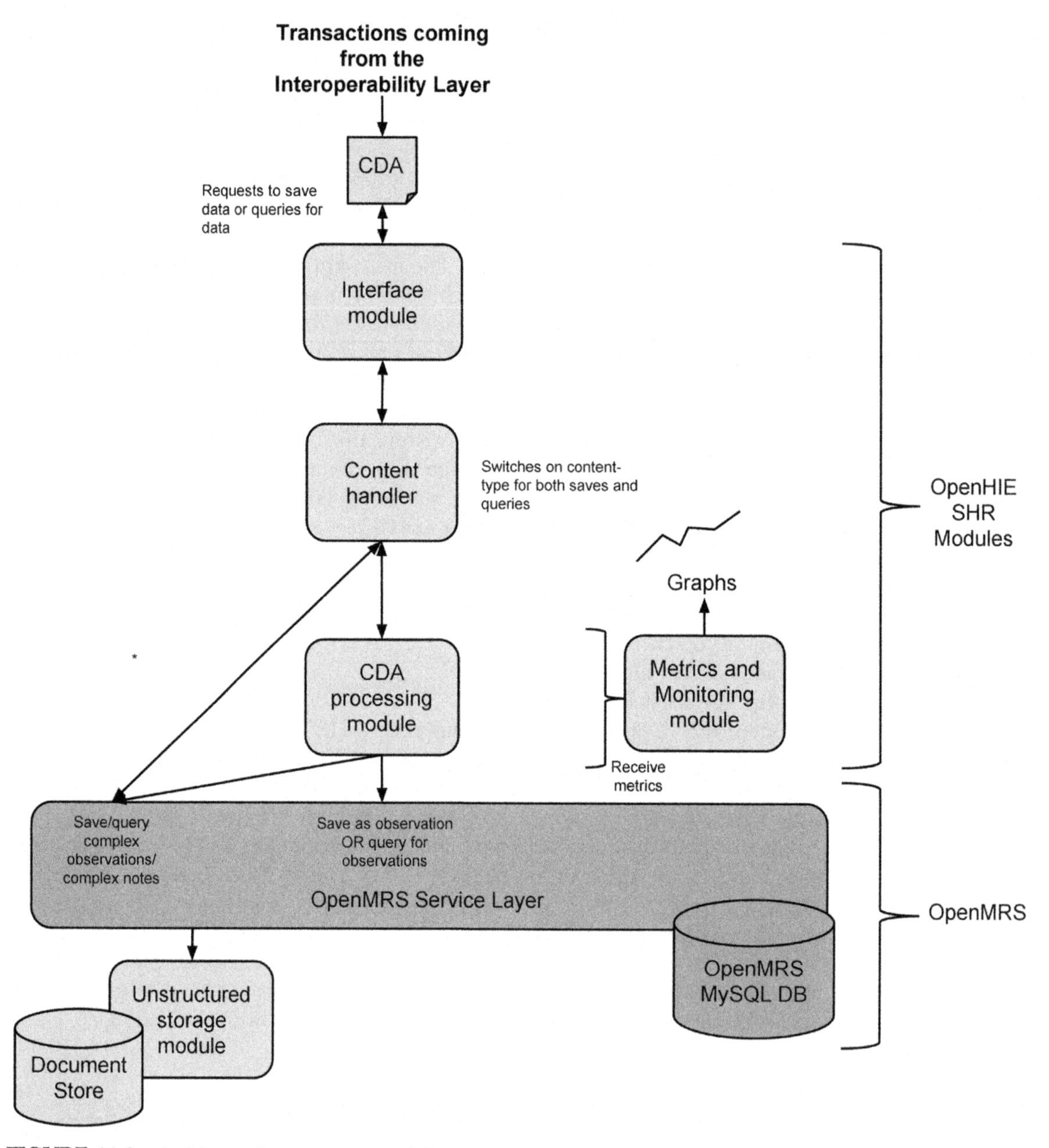

FIGURE 11.2 Architectural representation of the components of the shared health record as they could be implemented using the OpenMRS software.

with the SHR. A DBMS allows users or applications to perform tasks such as saves, queries, and updates to the database. Relational database management systems (RDBMSs) and NoSQL DBMSs are two of the most common DBMS models [40].

11.4.2.1 *Relational database management system*

A RDBMS model manages a database by allowing users to define and ascertain relationships between multiple tables within a repository. A standard language called Structured Query Language (SQL) is used to communicate with and manipulate the database [40,41]. SQL allows users to perform complex queries and analysis with relatively basic syntax [41]. A relational database has tables that consist of rows that represent records and columns that contain descriptive characteristics such as heart rate, age, or gender. Assigning a unique identifier to each row enables the table to be linked to rows from other tables in the database that share the same identifier. For example, if a researcher needed to combine a table that contained patient heights with a table that contained patient weights in order to calculate BMI, an SQL statement could be written to link the two tables together by matching the unique patient identifier from each table.

However, using a RDBMS to manage and store clinic databases has some limitations that must be considered. A RDBMS does not easily support documents such as medical imagery or free text [40,42]. In addition, clinical databases often contain a large number of fields that primarily remain unpopulated [40]. A RDBMS managing a SHR with an excessive number of blank fields may experience substandard performance and inefficiencies [40].

11.4.2.2 *Not only SQL DBMS*

The limitations of relational databases led to a demand for an alternative approach to database management [40]. There has been a recent shift toward the use of NoSQL data stores to manage large clinical databases [40]. NoSQL stands for "Not only SQL" and refers to a category of DBMSs that were developed with a contrasting approach to traditional relational databases [40]. NoSQL DBMSs do not depend on predefined relationships for the management and storage of clinical data, which allow faster processing [40]. NoSQL also supports structures such as key-value, document, and graph in addition to relational databases [40]. This flexibility allows a NoSQL DBMSs to manage the diversity of formats associated with medical data more easily than a traditional RDBMS. In addition, NoSQL DBMSs enable horizontal scaling to increase system capacity if the need arises [40,43]. Horizontal scalability describes the capability of the DBMS to disburse the data and workload among multiple servers [43]. However, there are also some drawbacks to NoSQL DBMSs. RDBMSs are able to complete transactions without losing data or being corrupted with more reliability than NoSQL DBMSs [40].

11.4.3 HMIS implemented as data analysis platform

The implementation of a HMIS system within a HIE requires the standardization of indicators, an appropriate software platform, and methods of collecting and evaluating the quality of the data from a variety of sources. The indicators included in the HMIS must be standardized to facilitate meaningful comparison across health facilities, geographic areas, and over time. Indicator definitions and codes must be consistent throughout the HIE [38] to enable interoperability between the systems exchanging health information [44]. There should also be cohesion of the aggregated data from the facility level on up to the national level [38].

A challenge facing HMIS/EHR interoperability is the lack of development of mature data exchange standards in this domain—certainly in comparison with other domains of HIE. In 2009, the World Health Organization (WHO) led an effort to develop a standard called SDMX-HD for representing indicators and aggregate datasets [38,45] aimed primarily at global health reporting. The SDMX-HD standard never saw significant uptake. Therefore indicator definitions must be predetermined and specified between senders and receivers. While this facilitates data exchange, it would not constitute the definition of interoperable.

Also in 2009, the HL7 consortium published the first edition of a standard for quality indicator reporting from EHR systems called QRDA (Quality Reporting Document Architecture). QRDA documents are contained within HL7 CDA documents (see Chapter 9) and include a type (QRDA category 3) designed specifically for the representation of aggregate data. QDM (Quality Document Model) is an information model that facilitates extraction of clinical data from an EHR using a standardized format to enable electronic quality performance measurement [46]. QRDA together with QDM provides standards-based building blocks for automatic extraction of quality data—including aggregated indicators [47].

From the HMIS perspective, there are two major challenges with QRDA. The first is that it is premised on the fact that the data originate in an EHR (hence its encapsulation as a clinical document). The HMIS described in this chapter has its origins in a context of use where EHR systems have been thin on the ground. Aggregate health data messages could originate in an HL7 compliant EMR system, but they are just as likely to be mined from the logistics management system for cold chain management data or from simple community health worker mobile phone applications. Second, QRDA is designed primarily to facilitate the exchange of U.S. Centers for Medicare and Medicaid Services (CMS) quality indicators from eligible hospitals and providers under the Promoting Interoperability program [48]. As depicted in Fig. 11.3, data specifications

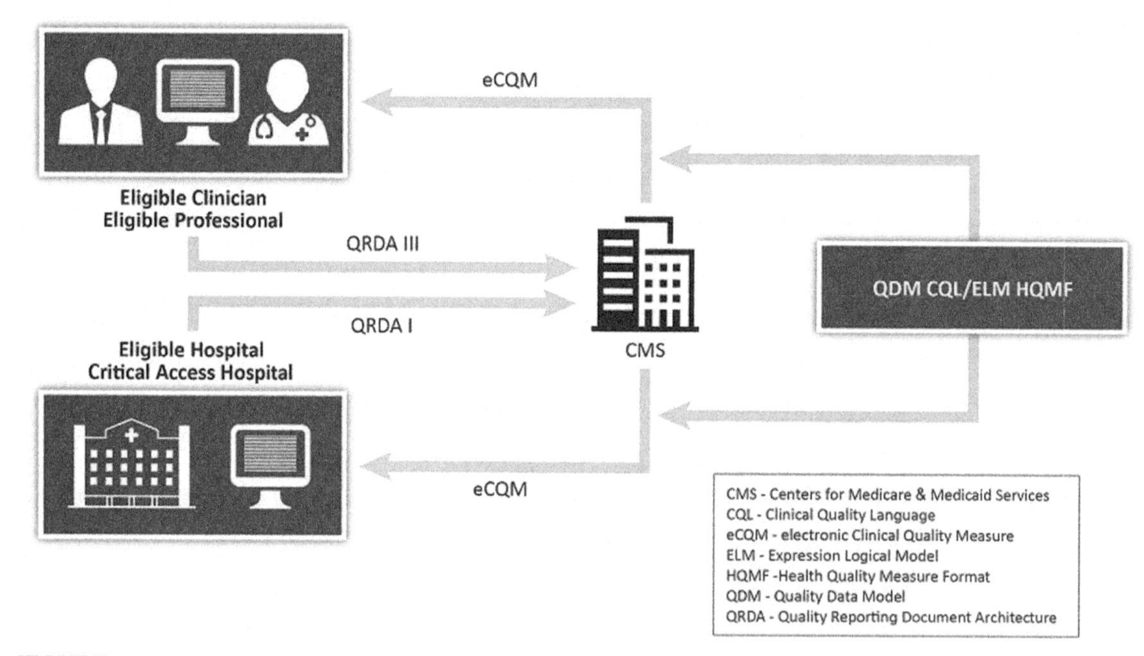

FIGURE 11.3 Representation of how the U.S. Centers for Medicare and Medicaid Services transmits structured quality measure definitions to hospitals and providers and how those organizations communicate calculated indicators back to the federal agency [48]. The figure illustrates how aggregate population-level data can be shared within an HIE network.

for CMS-based quality measures are communicated electronically to hospitals and provider EHRs using the electronic Clinical Quality Measure standard. After calculating the indicators, QRDA messages are sent to CMS. Level I documents from hospitals contain patient-level information, whereas Level III documents from providers contain aggregate indicators. This method works for granularly defined clinical quality indicators, such as the proportion of individuals with diabetes who received their annual eye exam for prevention if diabetic retinopathy. However, it is unclear how well it may work with broader, nonclinical measures of population health.

For these reasons, the HMIS community within OpenHIE is actively developing a new profile in the QRPH (Quality Research and Public Health) committee of IHE [49] called ADX (Aggregate Data Exchange). ADX is not a CDA document, owing more of its ancestry to SDMX-HD. In fact, ADX relies upon public health jurisdictions to publish their reporting definitions using SDMX. Then hospitals and other facilities report their data in ADX using tuples, a model more consistent with semantic web standards. EHR systems, which can and do produce QRDA, should be readily able to map that content onto ADX (though the reverse mapping would not be possible). Development of ADX to date has largely focused on DATIM4U DHIS2 [50], a platform designed for reporting HIV-related population health indicators from multiple nations to PEPFAR, the program in the United States that funds HIV diagnosis, treatment, and management globally.

The software platform that is used to collect, manage, and dispense aggregated health information for a HMIS can be a DBMS or a more flexible and customizable open-source model [38]. The OpenHIE HMIS was built on an open-source platform called the District Health Information Software 2 (DHIS2). DHIS2 enables implementing nations or regions to tailor the HMIS system to meet their requirements without the need for extensive programming [38]. The aggregated information captured by the SHR is imported into the DHIS2 system to produce reports on a regular basis that can be disseminated through the HIE [38].

Of major importance to DHIS2 is the flexibility to also rely on manual data entry, since the HMIS should contain a wide range of data for combinatorial analysis. In many developing countries, an OpenHIE architecture may not be supported by interoperable software applications, and data beyond the clinical encounter at facility level is collected through a wide range of paper-based forms. An excellent example of this is Tanzania [51], which has implemented several components of an HIE infrastructure including DHIS2 as an HIMS along with a health facility registry (see Chapter 13) and an IL (see Chapter 8). These three components support operational management of health facilities in the nation, informing the ministry of a facility's operating status and enabling information exchange (e.g., bed availability, inpatient mortality, revenue) from the nation's seven specialty hospitals. These components, while not anywhere the scale of countries like Israel (Chapter 31), Taiwan (Chapter 30), or Denmark (Chapter 28), establish an important foundation of HIE upon which the nation can develop over time.

Because there are different maturity levels, it is important that the HMIS, given its importance for overall health service management, is able to function as a wholly or partly independent electronic system. The variation in contexts around the world calls thus not only for standardization of data exchange, but also for flexibility in data collection to respond to a mix of electronic and manual processes. Furthermore, the HMIS is a critical component for a nation's incremental process toward a digital health infrastructure "that aligns with the country's broader e-Government policies...guided by requirements and standards" [51].

11.4.4 Data quality challenges to implementation

In order for the HMIS to provide a reliable method of measuring population health outcomes and evaluating the performance of public health programs and policies, it is critical that data quality is assessed effectively [52]. Poor data quality stems from several factors, including limited use of data, poor design of data entry systems and workflows, and increasingly an overload of data without support for translating them into actionable information.

A high degree of data quality can be attained by regulating processes, identifying the underlying sources of errors, and correcting processes to eliminate failures as data are entered into EHR systems or directly into the HMIS [53]. A quality assessment should consider the data itself, the use of the data, and the collection process [52]. Many health care organizations have adopted a total quality management (TQM) approach to consistently improve the quality of their data [53,54]. The TQM approach pursues quality improvement through the continuous refinement of existing systems and processes based on evaluations and feedback [54]. While originally used in the business sector, TQM is now adapted for use in health care [53].

Studies reveal significant challenges in realizing the automatic extraction of indicators from EHR [55,56] in practice. This stems partly from a dominant institutional logic of EHR implementations driven by the needs of transactional use case requirements rather than quality reporting and the related consequences in completeness and quality of data. A study from the Netherlands [55], for example, shows that the accuracy of indicator data derived from EHR is not necessarily better than that which was obtained from paper registers. This result is also consistent with what the authors have seen in implementations in Rwanda and has been described in India [57]. A large international study found that data completeness and quality are associated with standardization and design of forms, relevance of indicators, and a local information culture, rather than the technology applied in data collection [58,59]. The results are also consistent with other studies examining the quality of data in EHR-captured clinical documentation [60] as well as HIE transactions [61,62]. With the increasing focus on quality reporting from EHR in OECD countries coupled with the continued growth of EHRs in countries of the global South, we can expect these challenges to receive greater and urgent attention.

11.5 Emerging trends

The creation and management of SHR and HMIS components within HIE infrastructures are likely to both influence and be influenced by three global trends. First, postpandemic many states and nations seek to translate dashboards designed for COVID-19 into tools that will guide efforts to address other public health priorities. Second, the advancement of learning health systems that enable learning feedback loops using real-world evidence on a national scale will benefit from SHRs and real-time calculation of population level indicators. Finally, efforts to better understand and use the social determinants of health will benefit from HIE components that can efficiently and effectively gather information across a wide range of nonclinical, disparate sources. Furthermore, these movements are likely to influence design changes to the SHR and HMIS as they evolve.

11.5.1 Postpandemic infrastructure redesign

Influenced by the Johns Hopkins dashboard [14], many US states and nations, as well as regional authorities such as the Africa CDC, created COVID-19 dashboards [63]. These dashboards published daily updates on infections, hospitalizations, and/or deaths due to COVID-19. Several dashboards also published detailed information about ICU (intensive care unit) utilization as well as hospital bed capacity. Some dashboards presented updated information on racial, ethic, and other subpopulations disproportionately affected by COVID-19. As the world prepares for SARS-CoV-2 to become endemic, many hospital systems, public health authorities, and researchers seek to translate the public's interest in population health dashboards to other diseases, including diabetes, HIV, suicide, and obesity. The hope is that these dashboards could help bolster research, innovation, and support for mitigating other diseases that significantly impact morbidity and mortality across the globe.

The dashboards for COVID-19 were possible due to emergency public health orders and an *esprit de corps* that enabled large-scale integration of lab, hospitalization, mortality, and research data into SHR and HIMS infrastructures in public health agencies with collaboration from industry, universities, and nongovernmental organizations. The challenge facing nations is how to translate these nontechnical factors into a global focus on diabetes or another condition. Furthermore, how can SHR and HMIS infrastructures and dashboards designed for an infectious disease like COVID-19 evolve to support chronic diseases like diabetes and injuries like self-harm whose data requirements are unique? Although challenging, ongoing public health modernization and information infrastructure rebuilding efforts present an opportunity for data visualization efforts on top of SHR and HMIS platforms.

11.5.2 Learning health systems

The National Academy of Medicine (NAM) advocates for learning health care system that harnesses real-world evidence to provide patients with the best possible care, and then capture the results of evidence-based care delivery in order to enhance future treatment [64,65]. Physicians are currently forced to treat patients through medical procedures and pharmaceuticals that have a relatively small amount of evidence, mostly from clinical trials, to document their effectiveness [66]. Yet, many nations (mostly high-income) have robust adoption of EHR systems that could be leveraged to generate real-world evidence to enable the optimization of treatment strategies for conditions such as cancer or coronary artery disease [66]. Moreover, advanced analytics and artificial intelligence (AI) methods could leverage real-world data from EHR systems to generate evidence and predict how patients might do under various treatment strategies [67]. Supplying physicians as well as patients with information based on real-world evidence could make a substantial difference health outcomes [66].

Efforts to create learning health systems benefit from SHR and HMIS components and HIE as these components help states and nations capture real-world data for evidence generation. Furthermore, learning health system needs shape the evolution of SHR and HMIS components. Many learning health system initiatives are just now emerging, and their data needs are similar in nature to traditional observational and comparative research. Yet, given the broad scope of the NAM's vision, these efforts are likely to expand dramatically in the next 5–10 years. As they expand, data and analytical needs will morph, especially given the influence of AI, which may require changes to the scope of both the SHR and HMIS components as we might envision them today.

11.5.3 Social determinants of health

The Robert Wood Johnson Foundation (RWJF) seeks to promote a "culture of health" that considers the impact of factors beyond clinical care on the collective health of a community or nation as a whole [68]. Social determinants, such as income level, educational attainment, family environment, and crime rate, have a significant influence on both health outcomes and health disparities [68]. The increasing availability of large, up-to-date clinical datasets that bridge organizational boundaries, such as those in a SHR or HMIS, enables analyses that can reveal patterns of health outcomes and their underlying factors [69].

However, such analyses require integration of not only clinical data but also individual-level data from sources well beyond the health system. These sources include nongovernmental organizations, such as community-based service providers like churches, food pantries, and after-school programs. As discussed in Chapter 19, capturing these data in EHR systems and integrating them into HIE infrastructures is challenging. As efforts like those described in Chapter 19 evolve, new data types will be added to Table 11.1 and the requirements for the SHR and HMIS components will be updated. Yet, these components hold significant promise for achieving the visions set out by RWJF and others for national health systems that wholly address the health and well-being of populations rather than just focus on "sick care."

11.6 Summary

Patient care is a multifaceted process that can involve a range of tasks such as personal consultations, blood tests, and X-rays. As a result, clinical data are collected in many different formats including structured observations, image documents, transcribed notes, and laboratory results. This information often resides in numerous heterogeneous information systems. The ability to successfully assemble the data that are stored in disparate formats and systems into a single, integrated and longitudinal patient health record can benefit the individual patient, the health care organizations participating in the HIE, and the community as a whole. A SHR simplifies interoperability between information systems by providing a centralized repository that stores the information moving throughout the HIE in order to improve the quality and efficiency of clinical care. Shared, longitudinal health records can also be aggregated at the population level through systems like an HMIS, and subsequently distributed through an HIE to promote the advancement of community health outcomes through policy changes, surveillance, and research.

Questions for discussion

1. Which organizations and roles benefit from shared, longitudinal health records in a health system? What benefits do these stakeholders receive from access to SHRs?
2. How would the implementation of a SHR system in the United States differ from an implementation in other countries around the world?
3. What advantages does a HMIS component offer over traditional sources of health indicator data such as population-based surveys?
4. What are some of the benefits of NoSQL DBMS in comparison to a RDBMS for managing clinical data?
5. Under what conditions would an SHR not make sense for an HIE network to implement?
6. Why is data quality critical to both the SHR and HMIS components of an HIE network?
7. How might the SHR and HMIS components evolve following the COVID-19 pandemic?

References

[1] Walsham G, Sahay S. Research on information systems in developing countries: current landscape and future prospects. Inf Technol Dev 2006;12(1):7–24.

[2] Dixon BE. A roadmap for the adoption of e-health. e-Service J 2007;5(3):3–13.

[3] Office of the National Coordinator for Health Information Technology. What are the differences between electronic medical records, electronic health records, and personal health records? Washington: U. S. Department of Health and Human Services; 2019 [updated May 2, 2019; cited 2021 December 2]. Available from: https://www.healthit.gov/faq/what-are-differences-between-electronic-medical-records-electronic-health-records-and-personal.

[4] Coiera E. Building a National Health IT System from the middle out. J Am Med Inform Assoc 2009;16 (3):271–3.

[5] Knaup P, Bott O, Kohl C, Lovis C, Garde S. Electronic patient records: moving from islands and bridges towards electronic health records for continuity of care. Yearb Med Inf 2007;34–46.

[6] Katehakis DG, Sfakianakis SG, Kavlentakis G, Anthoulakis DN, Tsiknakis M. Delivering a lifelong integrated electronic health record based on a service oriented architecture. IEEE Trans Inf Technol Biomed: Publ IEEE Eng Med Biol Soc 2007;11(6):639–50.

[7] Miriovsky BJ, Shulman LN, Abernethy AP. Importance of health information technology, electronic health records, and continuously aggregating data to comparative effectiveness research and learning health care. J Clin Oncol: Off J Am Soc Clin Oncol 2012;30(34):4243–8.

[8] Gand K, Richter P, Esswein W. Towards lifetime electronic health record implementation. Stud Health Technol Inform 2015;212:225–32.

[9] Krist AH. Electronic health record innovations for healthier patients and happier doctors. J Am Board Family Medicine 2015;28(3):299–302.

[10] Gunter TD, Terry NP. The emergence of national electronic health record architectures in the United States and Australia: models, costs, and questions. J Med Internet Res 2005;7(1):e3.

[11] Mamlin BW, Biondich PG, Wolfe BA, Fraser H, Jazayeri D, Allen C, et al. Cooking up an open source EMR for developing countries: OpenMRS – a recipe for successful collaboration. AMIA Annu Symp Proc 2006;529–33.

[12] Kukafka R, Ancker JS, Chan C, Chelico J, Khan S, Mortoti S, et al. Redesigning electronic health record systems to support public health. J Biomed Inf 2007;40 (4):398–409.

[13] Wu AW, Kharrazi H, Boulware LE, Snyder CF. Measure once, cut twice–adding patient-reported outcome measures to the electronic health record for comparative effectiveness research. J Clin Epidemiol 2013;66(8 Suppl):S12–20.

[14] Center for Systems Science and Engineering. COVID-19 Dashboard Baltimore: Johns Hopkins University; 2020. Available from: https://gisanddata.maps.arcgis.com/apps/opsdashboard/index.html#/bda7594740fd40299423467b48e9ecf6.

[15] Reeves JJ, Hollandsworth HM, Torriani FJ, Taplitz R, Abeles S, Tai-Seale M, et al. Rapid response to COVID-19: health informatics support for outbreak management in an academic health system. J Am Med Inf Assoc 2020;27(6):853–9.

[16] Dixon BE, Grannis SJ, McAndrews C, Broyles AA, Mikels-Carrasco W, Wiensch A, et al. Leveraging data visualization and a statewide health information exchange to support COVID-19 surveillance and response: application of public health informatics. J Am Med Inf Assoc 2021;28(7):1363–73.

[17] Office of Disease Prevention and Health Promotion. About healthy people 2015. Available from: http://www.healthypeople.gov/2020/About-Healthy-People.

[18] Menachemi N, Collum TH. Benefits and drawbacks of electronic health record systems. Risk Manag Healthc Policy 2011;4:47–55.

[19] National Academies of Sciences E, Medicine, Health, Medicine D, Board on Population H, Public Health P, et al.. Copyright 2019 by the National Academy of Sciences. All rights reserved Criteria for selecting the leading health indicators for healthy people 2030. Washington, DC: National Academies Press (US); 2019.

[20] WHO Ebola Response Team. Ebola virus disease in West Africa–the first 9 months of the epidemic and forward projections. N Engl J Med 2014;371 (16):1481–95.

[21] Paterson BJ, Durrheim DN. The remarkable adaptability of syndromic surveillance to meet public health needs. J Epidemiol Glob health 2013;3(1):41–7.

[22] Coletta MA, Ising A. Syndromic surveillance: a practical application of informatics. In: Magnuson JA, Dixon BE, editors. Public health informatics and information systems. Cham: Springer International Publishing; 2020. p. 269–85.

[23] Dixon B. Applied public health informatics: an eHealth discipline focused on populations. J Int Soc Telemed eHealth 2020;8(e14):1–8.

[24] Snowdon J, Kassler W, Karunakaram H, Dixon BE, Rhee K. Leveraging informatics and technology to support public health response: framework and illustrations using COVID-19. Online J Public Health Inform 2021;13(1).

[25] Dixon BE, Holmes JH. Section editors for the IMIA yearbook section on managing pandemics with health informatics. Manag Pandemics Health Inf Yearb Med Inform 2021;30(1):69–74.

[26] Hansotte E, Bowman E, Gibson PJ, Dixon BE, Madden VR, Caine VA. Supporting health equity through data-driven decision-making: a local health department response to COVID-19. Am J Public Health 2021;111 (S3) S197-s200.

[27] Thompson MG, Stenehjem E, Grannis S, Ball SW, Naleway AL, Ong TC, et al. Effectiveness of Covid-19 vaccines in ambulatory and inpatient care settings. N Engl J Med 2021;385(15):1355–71.

[28] Embi PJ, Levy ME, Naleway AL, Patel P, Gaglani M, Natarajan K, et al. Effectiveness of 2-dose vaccination with mRNA COVID-19 vaccines against COVID-19-associated hospitalizations among immunocompromised adults - nine states, January–September 2021. Morb Mortal Wkly Rep 2021;70(44):1553–9.

[29] Bozio CH, Grannis SJ, Naleway AL, Ong TC, Butterfield KA, DeSilva MB, et al. Laboratory-confirmed COVID-19 among adults hospitalized with COVID-19-like illness with infection-induced or mRNA vaccine-induced SARS-CoV-2 immunity - nine states, January–September 2021. Morb Mortal Wkly Rep 2021;70(44):1539–44.

[30] Comer KF, Grannis S, Dixon BE, Bodenhamer DJ, Wiehe SE. Incorporating geospatial capacity within clinical data systems to address social determinants of health. Public Health Rep 2011;126(Suppl 3):54–61.

[31] Magnuson JA, Hopkins R, McFarlane TD. Informatics in disease prevention and epidemiology. In: Magnuson JA, Dixon BE, editors. Public health informatics and information systems. Cham: Springer International Publishing; 2020. p. 239–58.

[32] DiCAYa Network. Welcome to DiCAYA network. New York: NYU Long Island School of Medicine and NYU Grossman School of Medicine; 2020 [updated 2021 Jan 26; cited 2021 Dec 2]. Available from: https://www.dicaya.org/home.

[33] McNabb SJ, Conde J, Ferland L, Macwright W, Okutani S, Park M, et al. Transforming public health surveillance. Elsevier; 2015.

[34] Blonde L, Khunti K, Harris SB, Meizinger C, Skolnik NS. Interpretation and impact of real-world clinical data for the practicing clinician. Adv Ther 2018;35 (11):1763–74.

[35] Centers for Disease Control and Prevention. About the National Health Interview Survey Atlanta: U.S. Department of Health & Human Services; 2020 [updated September 16, 2020; cited 2021 Dec 2]. Available from: https://www.cdc.gov/nchs/nhis/about_nhis.htm.

[36] Dixon BE, Vreeman DJ, Grannis SJ. The long road to semantic interoperability in support of public health: experiences from two states. J Biomed Inf 2014;49:3–8.

[37] Mohammed-Rajput NA, Smith DC, Mamlin B, Biondich P, Doebbeling BN. OpenMRS, a global medical records system collaborative: factors influencing successful implementation. AMIA Annu Symp Proc 2011;2011:960–8.

[38] Braa J, Kanter AS, Lesh N, Crichton R, Jolliffe B, Saebo J, et al. Comprehensive yet scalable health information systems for low resource settings: a collaborative effort in sierra leone. AMIA Ann Symp Proc / AMIA Symp AMIA Symp 2010;2010:372–6.

[39] Seebregts CJ, Mamlin BW, Biondich PG, Fraser HS, Wolfe BA, Jazayeri D, et al. The OpenMRS implementers network. Int J Med Inf 2009;78(11):711–20.

[40] Lee KK, Tang WC, Choi KS. Alternatives to relational database: comparison of NoSQL and XML approaches for clinical data storage. Computer Methods Prog Biomed 2013;110(1):99–109.

[41] Jamison DC. Structured Query Language (SQL) fundamentals. Current protocols in bioinformatics / editoral board, Andreas D Baxevanis [et al.]. 2003; Chapter 9: Unit9.2.

[42] Cios KJ, Moore GW. Uniqueness of medical data mining. Artif Intell Med 2002;26(1–2):1–24.

[43] Cattell R. Scalable SQL and NoSQL data stores. ACM SIGMOD Record 2011;39(4):12–27.

[44] WHO Regional Office for the Western Pacific. Developing health management information systems: a practical guide for developing countries. World Health Organization; 2004.

[45] The Global Health Observatory. Indicator metadata registry list Geneva. World Health Organization; [cited 2021 Dec 2]. Available from: https://www.who.int/data/gho/indicator-metadata-registry.

[46] eCQI Resource Center. QDM - quality data model. Washington, DC: U.S. Department of Health and Human Services; [updated Nov 16, 2021; cited 2021 Dec 3]. Available from: https://ecqi.healthit.gov/qdm.

[47] Fu Jr. PC, Rosenthal D, Pevnick JM, Eisenberg F. The impact of emerging standards adoption on automated quality reporting. J Biomed Inform 2012;45(4):772–81.

[48] eCQI Resource Center. QRDA - quality reporting document architecture. Washington, DC: U.S. Department of Health and Human Services; 2021 [updated Dec 2, 2021; cited 2021 Dec 4]. Available from: https://ecqi.healthit.gov/qrda.

[49] Integrating the Healthcare Enterprise. Aggregate data exchange 2019 [updated Nov 4; cited 2021 Dec 4]. Available from: https://wiki.ihe.net/index.php/Aggregate_Data_Exchange.

[50] Shivers JE. Workflow - DATIM4U ADX (Aggregate Data eXchange) process: OpenHIE; 2018 [updated Mar 7, 2018; cited 2021 Dec 4]. Available from: https://wiki.ohie.org/display/projects/Workflow + - + DATIM4U + ADX + %28Aggregate + Data + eXchange%29 + Process.
[51] Nsaghurwe A, Dwivedi V, Ndesanjo W, Bamsi H, Busiga M, Nyella E, et al. One country's journey to interoperability: Tanzania's experience developing and implementing a national health information exchange. BMC Med Inform Decis Mak 2021;21(1):139.
[52] Chen H, Hailey D, Wang N, Yu P. A review of data quality assessment methods for public health information systems. Int J Environ Res Public Health 2014;11:5170–207.
[53] Dixon BE, Rosenman M, Xia Y, Grannis SJ. A vision for the systematic monitoring and improvement of the quality of electronic health data. Stud Health Technol Inform 2013;192:884–8.
[54] Kim PS, Johnson DD. Implementing total quality management in the health care industry. Health Care Superv 1994;12(3):51–7.
[55] Dentler K, Cornet R, Ten Teije A, Tanis P, Klinkenbijl J, Tytgat K, et al. Influence of data quality on computed Dutch hospital quality indicators: a case study in colorectal cancer surgery. BMC Med Inform Decis Mak 2014;14:32.
[56] Garrido T, Kumar S, Lekas J, Lindberg M, Kadiyala D, Whippy A, et al. e-Measures: insight into the challenges and opportunities of automating publicly reported quality measures. J Am Med Inform Association 2014;21(1):181–4.
[57] Jolliffe B, Mukherjee A, Sahay S. Heterogeneous interoperable systems as a strategy towards scaling: the case of hospital information systems in India. The 12th International Conference on Social Implications of Computers in Developing Countries (IFIP Working Group 94) 2013. p. 456-66.
[58] Day LT, Sadeq-ur Rahman Q, Ehsanur Rahman A, Salim N, Kc A, Ruysen H, et al. Assessment of the validity of the measurement of newborn and maternal healthcare coverage in hospitals (EN-BIRTH): an observational study. Lancet Glob Health 2021;9(3):e267–79.
[59] Shamba D, Day LT, Zaman SB, Sunny AK, Tarimo MN, Peven K, et al. Barriers and enablers to routine register data collection for newborns and mothers: EN-BIRTH multi-country validation study. BMC Pregn Childbirth 2021;21(1):233.
[60] Liaw ST, Chen HY, Maneze D, Taggart J, Dennis S, Vagholkar S, et al. Health reform: is routinely collected electronic information fit for purpose? Emerg Med Austr 2012;24(1):57–63.
[61] Dixon BE, Siegel JA, Oemig TV, Grannis SJ. Electronic health information quality challenges and interventions to improve public health surveillance data and practice. Public Health Rep 2013;128(6):546–53.
[62] Dixon BE, McGowan JJ, Grannis SJ. Electronic laboratory data quality and the value of a health information exchange to support public health reporting processes. AMIA Annu Symp Proc 2011;2011:322–30.
[63] Ahmed K, Bukhari MA, Mlanda T, Kimenyi JP, Wallace P, Okot Lukoya C, et al. Novel approach to support rapid data collection, management, and visualization during the COVID-19 outbreak response in the World Health Organization African Region: development of a data summarization and visualization tool. JMIR Public Health Surveill 2020;6(4):e20355.
[64] Institute of Medicine Roundtable on Evidence-Based Medicine. The National Academies Collection: reports funded by National Institutes of Health. Leadership Commitments to Improve Value in Healthcare: Finding Common Ground: Workshop Summary. Washington, DC: National Academies Press (US) National Academy of Sciences; 2009.
[65] Institute of Medicine. The learning health system and its innovation collaboratives 2011. Available from: https://www.iom.edu/~/media/Files/Activity%20Files/Quality/VSRT/Core%20Documents/ForEDistrib.pdf.
[66] Robert Wood Johnson Foundation. Creating a rapid-learning health system 2014 Available from: http://www.rwjf.org/content/dam/farm/reports/program_results_reports/2014/rwjf72101.
[67] Kasthurirathne SN, Ho YA, Dixon BE. Public health analytics and big data. In: Magnuson JA, Dixon BE, editors. Public health informatics and information systems. Cham: Springer International Publishing; 2020. p. 203–19.
[68] Robert Wood Johnson Foundation. Building a culture of health 2014. Available from: http://www.rwjf.org/content/dam/files/rwjf-web-files/Annual_Message/2014_RWJF_AnnualMessage_final.pdf.
[69] Plough AL. Developing new systems of data to advance a culture of health. eGEMs (Generat Evid Methods Improve Health Outcomes) 2014;2(4):9.

CHAPTER

12

Client registries: identifying and linking patients

Cristina Barboi[1,2], *Brian E. Dixon*[1,2], *Timothy D. McFarlane*[3] *and Shaun J. Grannis*[4]

[1]Department of Epidemiology, Richard M. Fairbanks School of Public Health, Indiana University, Indianapolis, IN, USA [2]Center for Biomedical Informatics, Regenstrief Institute, Inc., Indianapolis, IN, USA [3]Family and Social Services Agency, State of Indiana, Indianapolis, IN, USA [4]Indiana University School of Medicine, Indianapolis, IN, USA

LEARNING OBJECTIVES

At the end of the chapter, the reader should be able to:

- Define a client registry and describe why such registries are essential for in health information exchange.
- Detail common strategies for implementing a client registry.
- Discuss common challenges encountered when implementing a client registry.
- Highlight the critical role a unique identifier plays in implementing a client registry.
- Distinguish between the common methods of patient matching.

12.1 Introduction

Uniquely identifying patients is an essential task for both the delivery and administration of healthcare and doing so accurately is deceptively difficult, yet crucial to delivering the right care to the right patient. Patient data moving within and between organizations, as in the case of health information exchange (HIE), further motivates a need to accurately describe who these data represent.

Simply transmitting (or routing) information from point A to point B does not require knowing about whom the information pertains. Participants in HIE networks, however, seek not only to move information about the network but also to create services that aggregate information about patients and populations to support a

Health Information Exchange
DOI: https://doi.org/10.1016/B978-0-323-90802-3.00008-3

range of tasks in clinical and public health. These services rely on **patient-centric data**: a set of data (e.g., diagnoses, prescriptions, visits, demographics, symptoms) pertaining to a single, unique individual who has utilized the health system. Patient-centric data are often scattered across multiple facilities, including healthcare organizations and providers, pharmacies, urgent care clinics, and mental health professionals, where each institution or system typically uses proprietary identifiers that are largely meaningless outside of the assigning organization.

Fully functional, patient-centric HIE services must uniquely identify individuals through record linkage. Community-based HIEs (defined in Chapter 1) need to link patient records across multiple health systems, and private HIEs (defined in Chapter 1) need to link patient records across facilities within their network or enterprise. In many cases, a single hospital or clinic also needs to link records across different sources, including clinical laboratory, radiology, pharmacy, and admitting services. Furthermore, record linkage is not unique to the healthcare environment.

In 1946 Dunn first described *record linkage* as a method of bringing together pages in the book of life [1]. By the 1950s record linkage was used in matching vital records for individuals and families [2]. Today, record linkage is ubiquitous with applications in business (e.g., mailing lists), research (e.g., database management and merging), government agencies (e.g., US Census) [3] healthcare, reconstruction of historical populations, law enforcement (crime, fraud detection), and national security [4]. The process of record linkage has various names throughout user communities; epidemiologists and statisticians call it *record linkage*, while others call the same concept *record matching*, *entity disambiguation*, *object identification*, *object isomerism*, and *entity reconciliation* [5].

At a larger scale, record linkage is necessary for knowledge discovery needed in clinical care. Integration of separate, patient-centric data sources facilitates timely access to an individual's continuum of health while also adding a rich data source to improve health through clinical and population research, as well as public health. Regardless of the use, all data are patient-centric and at some point, the identity of the patient must be determined. Even in countries where citizens are assigned a national identifier, there remains a need to ensure the unique identity of an individual among the myriad fragmented information systems that collectively represent a person's electronic health record (EHR).

A *client registry* (*CR*), illustrated in Fig. 12.1, is a patient-centered and purpose-driven software application designed to support uniquely identified individuals who receive healthcare services from multiple sites and collate these records into a single, longitudinal health record at the point of care [5]. Client registries facilitate the process of record linkage for HIE networks.

This chapter begins by introducing techniques used for identifying patients within organizations, followed by an overview of the key elements of client registries. The main components of client registries are [6]:

- database management system,
- master patient index,
- demographic data validation and standardization processes,
- record indexing, searching, and blocking,
- process for comparison of record pairs,
- decision model/classification (discerns if a record pair is a match, nonmatch, possible match),
- measurement tools (maintain matching performance criteria), and
- graphical user interface.

After examining client registries, we examine emerging trends likely to shape record linkage and CRs in the future. By the end of this chapter, readers should understand the components of CRs, their role in facilitating HIE, and the challenges when implementing and operating CRs.

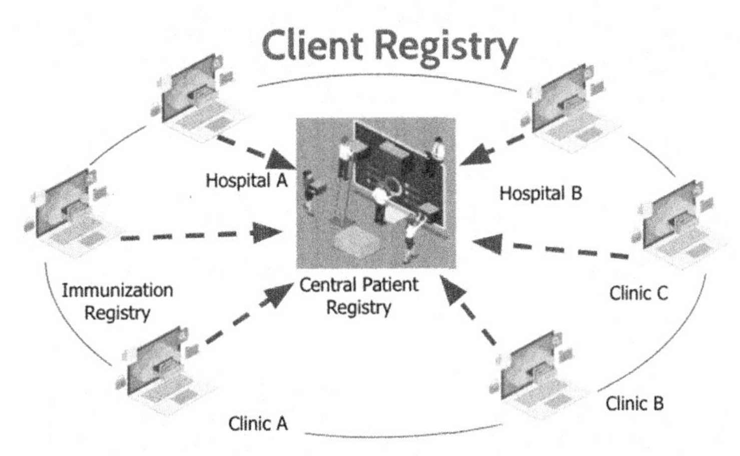

FIGURE 12.1 Illustration of a client registry, a central software application that captures identifying data on individuals from multiple health information systems.

12.2 Patient identifiers

Much of the information maintained in EHR systems pertains to patients—or clients who receive healthcare services from a clinic or hospital. To effectively manage information about patients, EHR systems must assign and use patient identifiers, such as a medical record number (MRN), when performing tasks such as creating a new record, updating an existing record, or deleting a record. Identifiers (or IDs) ensure that the correct record is added, updated, or deleted. "Patient matching" and "patient identification" are often used interchangeably but are two different processes. Matching involves linking a single patient to their unique records from a prior encounter; whereas, "patient identification is the process of correctly associating a patient to appropriately intended interventions and communicating information about the patient's identity accurately and reliably throughout the continuum of care" [7].

Linking or matching patients to the right record is paramount to avoiding harm and delayed medical care, eliminating the cost associated with duplicate of medical testing, and reducing the financial burden associated with correcting mismatched and duplicate records. Patient identifiers not only physically identify patients, but also enhance the accuracy of the identification process.

Patient identifiers can be thought of as belonging to two general classes:

1. a unique code or set of codes specifically designed to uniquely identify a patient in a system, or a personal unique identifier—UPI and
2. an aggregate set of demographic and related attributes used to describe a patient uniquely, such as gender, date of birth, address, etc., or quasi-identifiers—QID.

Whether utilizing existing or creating new patient identifiers, it is prudent to understand the context in which the identifiers will be deployed.

Strategies that rely upon unique identifiers vary based on the country of implementation and availability of certain identifiers, such as a national health ID number or national ID number. If a national ID exists, it is important to understand the attributes of the identifier. Are all individuals given an identifier at birth, or later in life? Does every person, including immigrants, possess an identifier?

Within the context of each country, demographic attributes vary based on naming conventions, geographic data (e.g., village vs city), and other cultural practices. Additionally, the collection of certain demographic attributes may be more complete based on cultural differences (e.g., withholding for privacy), healthcare infrastructure, and the presence of civil registration systems. Adding to the difficulty, the format, completeness, and accuracy of demographic attributes often vary between organizations, even within the same region, state, or country.

Due to both the assortment of available identifiers and inconsistent use of these identifiers across healthcare institutions, for both unique codes and demographic attributes, there exists a need to understand how identifiers are created, what makes a good identifier (i.e., ideal attributes), and what identifiers are currently available?

As will be detailed, the CR uses a combination of unique identifiers and quasiidentifiers—demographic attributes—to establish patient identity.

12.3 Unique patient identifiers

Allocating UPI is a method for standardizing patient identification also to protect sensitive medical information by maximizing the likelihood that only appropriate data for the intended unique individual is integrated. A UPI should be easily read and recognized by all healthcare organizations, support the exchange of data between healthcare organizations, and should be valid only in the context of health information. The UPI can be a number, a biometric measure, a smart card, or any other digital identity method [8].

A unique ID requires a sequence allocation sufficiently large to cover the entire population over time, theoretically for as long as the number will be in use. Sequencing schemes available for development of a UPI generally fall into three numbering systems: (1) serial, (2) derived, and (3) composite.

1. In serial numbering systems, one individual is assigned a number from a central location. These numbers are automated and do not assimilate any nonunique characteristics of the individual. England's National Health Service number is an example of serial numbering system, with some added functionality [9].

2. As the name suggests, derived numbering systems create a number based on, or derived from, a personal trait of the individual. In contrast to serial numbering, assignment of a derived number can take place anywhere but runs the risk of failing to be unique when derived from a personal trait which is shared by other individuals.

3. Composite numbering systems assign part of the number from a central location and the other part is derived from personal traits, thus represents a combination of the serial and derived systems [10].

Regardless of the allocation methodology, errors can occur during entry, transcription, and preparation. Check digits limit errors by inserting one or more nonidentifying numbers or characters within the UPI that are checked against an algorithm to validate the number [11,12]. Check digits improve accuracy of identifiers during data entry and retrieval, improving the reliability and accuracy of patient identification.

12.3.1 Attributes of ideal identifiers

Much of the concern around utilizing a universal identifier for healthcare, particularly in the United States, is fear of malicious intent in the event of a data breach. The only true way to prevent the possibility of confidentiality breaches is to exclude personal information, such as name, social security number (SSN), and date of birth, and to eliminate the possibility of linking the healthcare identifier to databases that contain personal information [13]. At the time of writing, and for the foreseeable future, no identifier exists which will perfectly ascertain all individuals uniquely across the entire healthcare landscape; at least not one that is neither physically invasive (e.g., implanted device) nor invasive of a citizen's right to privacy.

Healthcare identifiers are often assigned within individual information systems (e.g., laboratory, radiology) as well as organization-wide (e.g., MRN). However, as discussed, these identifiers are meaningless outside of the domain in which they operate. One solution to this identity challenge is to establish a unique identifier that crosses organizational boundaries. The American Society for Testing and Materials (ASTM), which is a standards development organization accredited by the American National Standards Institute (ANSI), describes 30 criteria which should be used to evaluate the efficacy of a candidate identifier [14]. Meeting all the proposed criteria would lead to a UPI that achieves the following: positively identifies patients, automatically links and collates patient records from disparate electronic sources, creating a longitudinal care record; protects patient's personal health information and privacy; and effectively minimizes the cost of patient record management.

No identifier exists which could meet all the criteria proposed by the standard, because some ideal attributes conflict with each other. For example, a ubiquitous and easily accessible identifier may not adequately preserve privacy. The following is a description of selected ideal UPI attributes; for succinct definitions and examples, refer to Table 12.1.

- A *unique* identifier, by definition, can never be associated with more than one individual. That is, once assigned, the possibility of another person being assigned the same number must be eliminated, or infinitely minuscule.
- A *ubiquitous* identifier is available and accepted across the healthcare spectrum. For example, a nonubiquitous identifier would identify a patient for a hospitalization but not the subsequent primary care visit. Ubiquity also requires the identifier to be durable and made readily available at the time of service.
- *Unchanging*. For an individual identifier to be effective, every individual should have an identifier that applies only to that

TABLE 12.1 Attributes of ideal unique personal identifiers.

Attribute	Description	Examples
Unique	An identifier which can only be associated with a single individual or entity.	Fingerprints, retinal scans, DNA, national identifiers
Ubiquitous	A durable and constantly available identifier which is accepted across the healthcare spectrum.	Name, date of birth, sex, eye color, smart cards, fingerprints, retinal scans
Unchanging	The identifier is permanently associated with the individual and will not change over time.	Date of birth, sex, DNA
Uncontroversial	The potential for malicious use of the identifier must be limited.	Identifier not derived from personal attributes such as serial numbering system.
Uncomplicated	The identifier should be simple to implement, use, and recall.	SSN
Inexpensive	The implementation and maintenance should be reasonable within the context of healthcare costs.	Existing identifiers—name, date of birth, sex, SSN

individual and does not change over time. This requires foresight on the part of the issuing agency because enough numbers must be generated to support the population throughout the lifespan of the identifier.
- *Uncontroversial.* The identifier should help minimize the opportunities for crime and abuse and should not contain substantive information about the individual. Similarly, the various stakeholders must perceive the identifier to be minimally invasive. The subjectivity of what is and is not invasive makes universal acceptance difficult, if not impossible.
- *Uncomplicated.* An identifier or identifier system that is not practical to implement or that does not meet the requirements of administrative simplification must be deemed unacceptable.
- *Inexpensive.* The costs of implementation and use of the identifier must be within an acceptable range. Analysis of costs across all healthcare settings should be considered including, patients, providers, payers, and government agencies. For example, it has been estimated that a national health identifier implemented in the United States would cost between $4.9 and $12.2 billion to deploy and $1.5 billion per year, which many view as unsustainable [15].

The Health Insurance Portability Accountability Act of 1996 (HIPAA) recognized the need to uniquely identify patients for managing care and administrative purposes, thus proposing a unique health identifier for all individuals, with the provision that "is not derived from or related to information about the individual" [16]. In 2020 the US senate removed the 22-year-long ban on the use of federal funds for the development of deployment of a National Patient identifier. In 2019 the private sector (Experian) has announced the development of the technological infrastructure for a UPI maintained in a master patient index and a Universal Identity Manager supporting interoperability for everyone that has ever received medical care or utilized a pharmacy in the United States, based on the National Council for Prescription Drug Programs (NCPDP) telecommunication standards and SCRIPT standards.

Uncertainties remain concerning the appropriation process and political controversies related to security and invasion of privacy posed by a national patient identifier; a national patient ID repeal bill is waiting in Congress.

12.3.2 Social security number

The SSN has been advanced as a candidate for a UPI in the United States because it is theoretically unique, ubiquitous, and unchanging, most adults can recite it from memory and would not require additional infrastructure to implement (i.e., inexpensive and uncomplicated). However, in reality, the SSN is sometimes shared by multiple individuals, not all people are eligible for an SSN, in rare circumstances, an individual may possess more than one SSN, SSNs are not universally available at birth, and there is no legal protection for maintaining SSN confidentiality in nongovernment organizations [17]. Using the SSN also comes with controversy, largely because of its universality. At its inception, the SSN was for use only within the context of the Social Security program and intended to identify an account, not a person. Currently, the SSN has become tightly linked to an individual's credit score, banking, health insurance records, government activities, among other things, and is now largely viewed as a nonconfidential identifier [18].

The SSN is incorporated in healthcare to a great extent and is frequently included in patient matching algorithms. When SSN is used as a health identifier, generally patients report the associated numbers; when the card is requested, since it does not contain a picture or biometrics, it is impossible to confirm if the person using the card is the one to whom the card was issued. Unfortunately, the SSN is routinely used for illegal purposes in the United States. For this reason, the federal government, numerous states, third-party payors, and the Federal Trade Commission are attempting to restrict the use and disclosure of the SSN or have replaced it with their own unique identifiers. Currently, Medicare has removed SSN-based Health Insurance Claim Numbers from Medicare cards and is using Medicare Beneficiary Identifiers for Medicare transactions. The prospects of using SSN as a UPI in the United States are declining. Furthermore, its use in healthcare is declining [19].

12.3.2.1 *Biometric identifiers*

Biometric identifiers are distinctive, measurable characteristics used to label and describe individuals, such as fingerprints, iris scans, voice recognition, and facial shapes. Behavioral biometrics identify humans through their interaction with technology [7]. Biometrics offer unique, ubiquitous, and relatively unchanging identifiers. In the developed nations, implementation of biometrics has been scarce, mainly because of concerns with privacy and the potential for law enforcement to use these data [20]. However, underdeveloped nations often lack universal coverage by civil registration systems leading to an identification problem that reaches far beyond healthcare. Recent technological advances are allowing cheaper, more accurate identification using biometric indicators such as fingerprints and iris scans. In a report for the Center for Global Development, Gelb and Clark [21] found that 160 countries have deployed biometrics to address the identity gap covering more than 1 billion people.

While highly discriminating, biometric identifiers do not eliminate the need for sophisticated matching algorithms to uniquely identify an individual. Measurements of a person's fingerprint or iris can vary over time in the same person due to changes in age, environment, disease, stress, and occupational factors, as well as hardware variabilities, for example, sensor calibration and age of the device. In the case of fingerprints, any single individual can produce several distinct images depending on the angle of depression, pressure, presence of dirt, moisture, and sensor characteristics [22]. Certain biometrics are not well captured in certain patient populations, thus increasing disparities when these characteristics are used for identification; moreover, biometrics are difficult to capture and subject to change during child development [7].

The presence of biometric data does not implicitly support HIE since different healthcare organizations may use different types of biometrics or store data in formats incompatible with each other. Acquisition of biometric data is also expensive, and any physical damage to a biological identifier makes it unusable.

In the United States, the collection, use, and transfer of biometric data without the consent of the individual is protected by privacy laws in 27 states. Furthermore, once biometric data are hacked, the individual's identity is permanently compromised. For many reasons, biometric identifier usage for uniquely identifying patients and enabling HIE is quite limited.

12.3.3 International unique patient identifiers

UPIs have been developed and implemented in low, middle, and high-income countries. Specific use cases for implementing a UPI in Denmark, Botswana, Kenya, Brazil, Malawi, Ukraine, Thailand, and Zambia are discussed in a UNAIDS whitepaper addressing developing and using individual identifiers for health services including HIV [23]. Chapter 28, which profiles Denmark, also describes the Danish UPI that enables nationwide HIE.

As of 2020, the following countries used a National Identifier as a patient identification number: in Europe—England, Wales, Denmark,

Estonia, Slovenia, Spain, and Ireland; and outside Europe—New Zealand, Israel, Thailand, South Korea, and China. In Singapore, nonresidents, without an identity card represents 28% of the population; thus, the National Registration Identity card is not ubiquitous enough to be used as a UPI [7]. Countries like Slovenia and Australia have a unique health identifier linked to a unique national identifier [24]. Both case studies on Israel (Chapter 31) and Taiwan (Chapter 30) discuss the national health identifiers used in those nations and their role in facilitating HIE.

Although no single identifier currently exists with each of the ideal attributes, Fig. 12.2 depicts the degree to which the examples discussed meet the expectations of an ideal identifier. As will be discussed, a key strength of the CR is the ability to utilize multiple identifiers through matching algorithms to positively identify a patient, that is, the CR does not rely on the necessity to produce an ideal UPI; however, when a UPI is available, matching efficiency is improved.

UPIs hold promise for simplifying patient identification, but even in the case a UPI is in use, it will be necessary at times to match patients using other attributes, such as demographics, when a UPI is unavailable at the time of service (e.g., forgotten card, emergency situations). Similarly, if temporary identification must be issued, the matching authority will need to use other identifiers, such as demographics, to link a patient's UPI to the temporary ID to prevent record fragmentation. In general, the implementation of a UPI will improve the accuracy of matching procedures but will not replace the need for demographic attributes.

12.4 Client registries

A CR or a **Master Patient Index** reconciles patient identities from multiple sources, consolidating multiple records across organizations belonging to the same individual enabling more complete integration of data associated with that individual. For a single patient, a CR attempts to solve the following problems: record deduplication within a single healthcare system and record

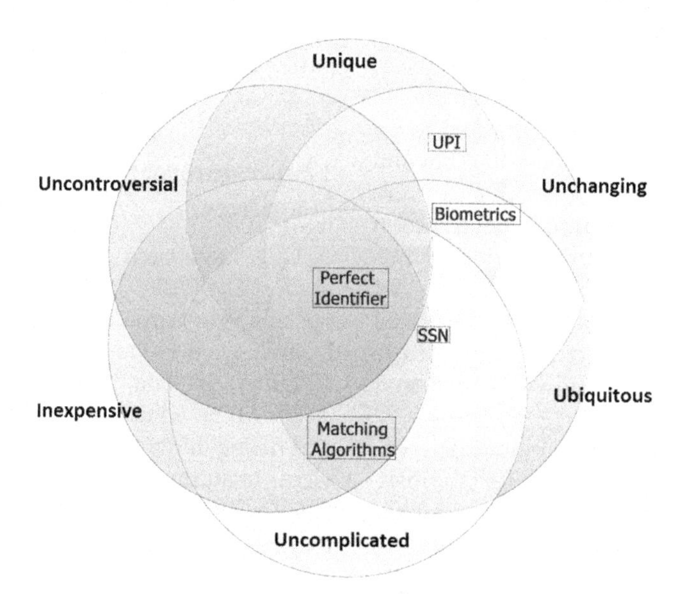

FIGURE 12.2 The ideal attributes of unique personal identifiers, highlighting where commonly used identifiers exist within this framework. *UPI*, Unique patient identifier; *SSN*, social security number.

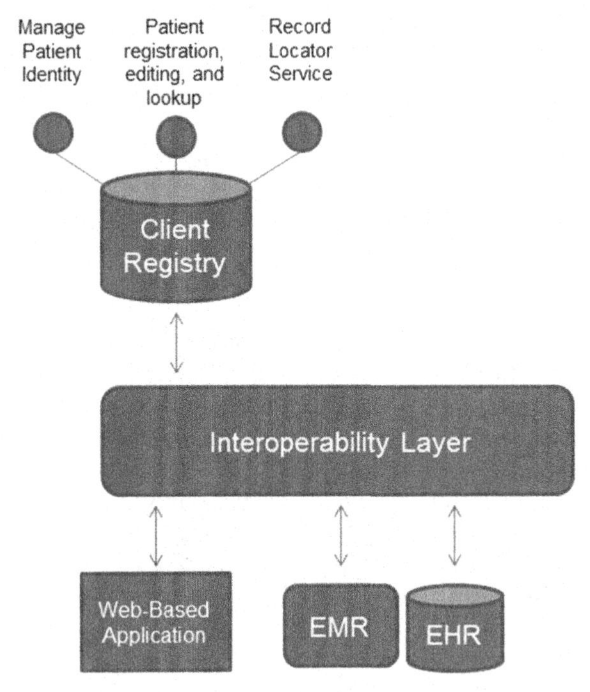

FIGURE 12.3 The client registry architecture within the OpenHIE model. *EMR*, Electronic medical record; *EHR*, electronic health record.

linkage across systems. At a population level, CRs are essential for public health outcome monitoring, case-based surveillance, and information exchange among disparate healthcare systems. A CR does not capture clinical data as in the case of a shared health record. Instead, a CR contains:

- **Patient, system identifiers**
- **Demographic information**—date of birth, place of birth, patient's name, gender, addresses, marital status, telephone number/email addresses, multiple birth status/order, death status/date
- **Relationships**
  - o Mother/father/next of kin
- **Facility the patient demographics came from**

A CR operates by adjudicating demographic attributes and other personal identifiers from each data supplier (e.g., hospitals, clinics) to create a single record for each patient within the HIE. Fig. 12.3 demonstrates how the CR fits into the scheme of an HIE model. Organizational EHR systems and point-of-care applications interact with the CR through the interoperability layer allowing users to retrieve, add, and edit patient records. Once positive identification is made, the CR associates each patient's records with an enterprise unique identifying number called **the EUID** in the enterprise **master patient index (MPI)**.

12.5 The Enterprise Master Patient Index

The **Enterprise Master Patient Index (EMPI)** is a patient database used by healthcare organization to maintain correct and consistent medical data across various departments that enables timely, accurate and accessible healthcare information. Patients are assigned unique identifiers that represent them across all organization's systems clinical, financial, and administrative.

To further explore the need for unique patient identification and record linkage, let us consider a scenario applicable to both clinical and population health. Consider the scenario (Fig. 12.4) in which a 9-year-old girl child named Jill receives her immunizations at a vaccine clinic; she also receives other care such as regular checkup, laboratory tests, in a primary care clinic. When Jill visits her pediatrician, will the vaccinations records be available to her doctor?

Sharing healthcare records can be a challenge in a complex environment where there are multiple systems across multiple healthcare institutions, and each institution and/or system has a different way to identify their clients. Even in environments where citizens are assigned national identification cards, there is still a need to ensure the unique identity of an individual among the myriad of fragmented information systems which collectively represent a person's health record. If Jill is also visiting a sports medicine clinic, will the provider have access to the information present in Jill's chart?

Linking records on the same patient to create an integrated and complete medical record is accomplished by an **EMPI**. The EMPI software assigns a unique identifier to each patient and ensures that the patient is represented only one time within the enterprise EHR system or private HIE. But what if Jill has to visit the emergency department (ED) within another, competing healthcare system? Each healthcare organization's MPI associates its own unique identifier with patient data; thus, a single patient may have several "unique" MPI identifiers, one within each organization where care occurred. Each facility record belongs to an enterprise record created by the EMPI and two facility records of the same patient belong to the same EMPI enterprise record. An enterprise record contains its own set of patient demographics called the Single Best Record, which is calculated from the demographics data of its facility records. The EMPI generates a unique patient ID, called an EUID, for each enterprise record.

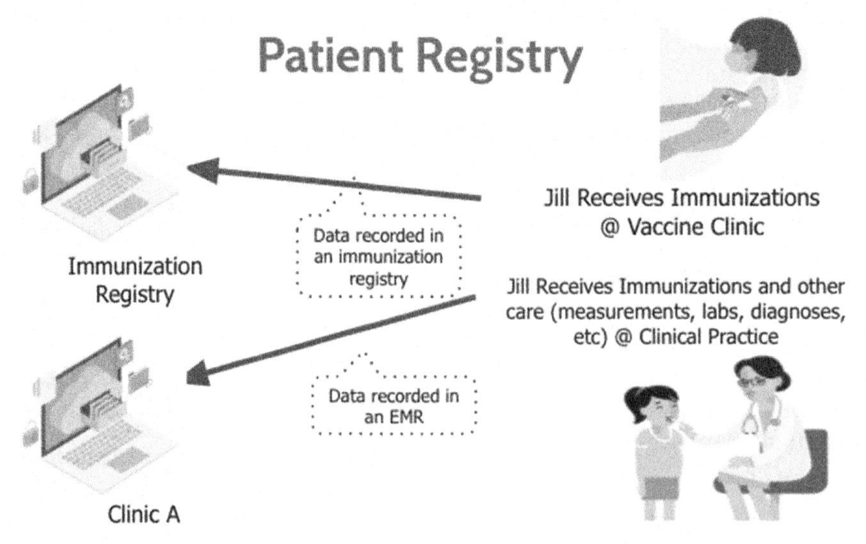

FIGURE 12.4 Illustration of the patient registry. Each facility in which Jill receives care will store a record of the care delivered in its own information system. These transactions will be linked to Jill using an identifier within that system.

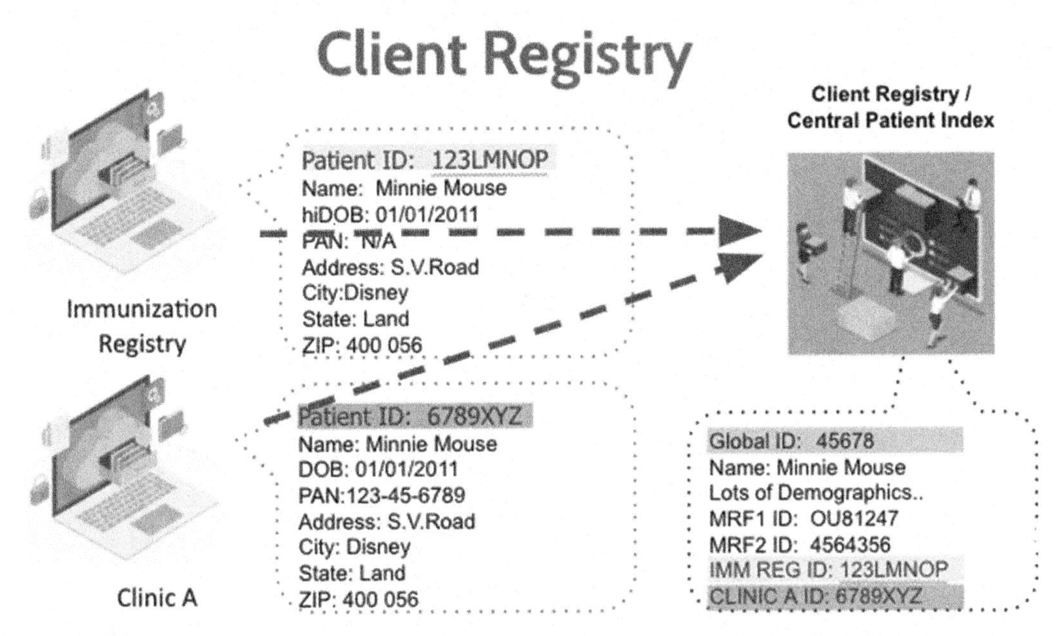

FIGURE 12.5 Illustration of the client registry. The immunization registry and Clinic A both maintain a unique patient identifier for Minnie Mouse. These identifiers are shared with the client registry, which maintains a global identifier that links all source identifiers together for Ms. Mouse.

This process is illustrated in Fig. 12.5. In this illustration, the patient's name is Minnie Mouse. Ms. Mouse has her immunization records stored in the state's immunization registry, and she receives primary care at Clinic A. Each facility has a unique patient ID for Ms. Mouse, highlighted in blue and green in the figure. These identifiers are linked to an EUID, called the Global ID and highlighted in red, as well as other demographics pertaining to Ms. Mouse.

The lack of a shared identifier across organizations makes integrating patient data difficult. For example, if Jill visits an ED outside her usual integrated healthcare system, data about the visit would not be integrated into the EHR system record utilized by her pediatrician, and her doctor would not have access to the ED information, unless the healthcare organizations share a common HIE platform. Through a CR, patient's identifying information (e.g., ID numbers, names, birth date) would be identified and the records linked using patient matching algorithms.

The EMPI uniquely identifies and links each of Jill's specialty care visits, because they are within the same network or enterprise, but data from an ED visit outside the usual integrated healthcare system would remain in a silo if an HIE network was not available. Thus, to link data across the healthcare ecosystem within a state or nation, we must rely upon an assemblage of existing identifiers.

In the context of the CR, the EMPI acts as the controller for all other local identifiers that may be associated with the patient, including one or more MRNs assigned by individual facilities and MPI identifiers assigned by integrated healthcare networks; this relationship is depicted in Fig. 12.6. The EMPI of the CR, therefore, bridges the gap for interorganizational patient identification, allowing creation

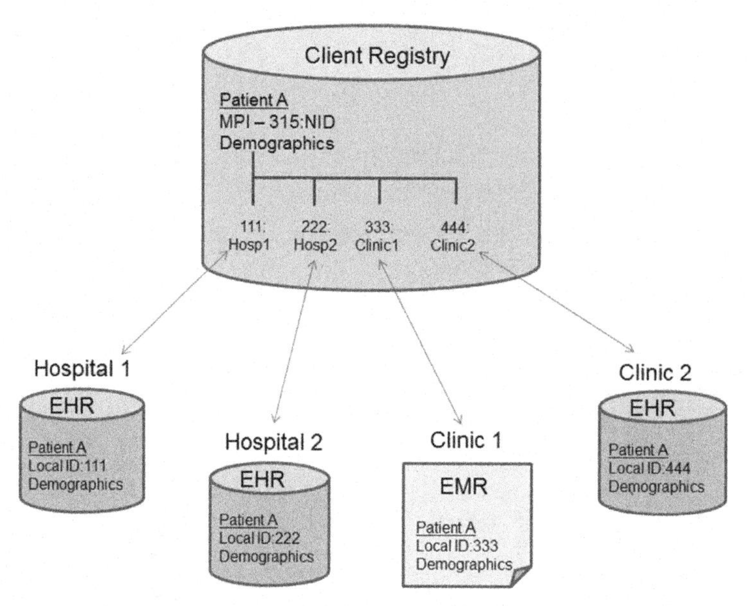

FIGURE 12.6 The relationship between the client registry and source systems (EMR, EHR) of participating organizations within an HIE network. *EMR*, Electronic medical record; *EHR*, electronic health record.

and maintenance of a patient-centric records that contain all clinical information regardless of the source. Unlike an MPI, an EMPI can provide extensive data stewardship capabilities to maintain the integrity of the patient record.

The relationship between each organization and the CR is depicted in Fig. 12.6. Each hospital and clinic identify the patient using a set of demographic attributes and identifiers (e.g., name, SSN, date of birth) and a local, unique code identifier (e.g., MRN, MPI), which are shared with the CR. As will be discussed later in this chapter, the data shared from hospital and clinic information systems are subjected to a matching algorithm that establishes positive patient identity and links any new record to any previous records in the CR, when applicable. If the patient is new to the HIE, the CR assigns a new MPI for future record linkage. Once an MPI has been established, the CR becomes the source of truth for identity of individuals.

For the CR to resolve patient identities, facilities must send sufficiently discriminating demographic attributes. Examples of common data elements used for resolving identity are listed in Table 12.2. As the source of truth about identity, the CR can communicate with myriad EHR systems and point-of-service applications to update and sync patient identity data for future encounters. A strength of the CR is the ability to perform linkage of patient demographics when the patient is registered with slightly different

TABLE 12.2 Example of attributes for patient identification within the client registry.

Local patient identifier	Social security number
Patient name	Facility identifier
Date of birth	Universal identifier, if applicable
Sex	Admission date
Race	Discharge date
Ethnicity	Service type
Address	

demographic attributes because of receiving care from multiple sites. For example, a hypothetical diabetic patient, Bob, could still be identified if his podiatrist included last name, date of birth, and sex, while his endocrinologist included first and last name, SSN, and address.

Establishing the identity of a patient within the CR and communicating this identity consistently across participating organizations enable the implementation of a **record locator service (RLS)**. The RLS queries HIE records to identify all locations where a patient may have data. This is particularly useful for rapid retrieval if a clinician is seeking a specific piece of information, such as a primary care physician searching for an emergency room discharge summary [13].

Accuracy of the CR matching is substantially impacted by data quality. If data used for matching are incomplete, inaccurate, or inconsistent, matching algorithm performance will suffer. Because the goal is to match based on a collection of demographic attributes and personal identifiers, multiple incomplete or inaccurate identifiers decrease the confidence of positive patient identification. While poor identifying data quality can arise from any point in the care process, the patient registration process is essential to ensure robust data are captured. The next section will discuss common data-related errors as well as solutions in the form of metadata and standards (i.e., data format), after which the discussion shifts to how the CR handles inconsistent data across participating organizations and common approaches to algorithmic patient matching used by the CR. After COVID-19, there is significant focus on improving the capture of patient race, ethnicity, and other key demographic data in EHR systems during patient registration processes [25]. These efforts will enhance not only population health activities within hospitals and clinics but also when shared with a CR in the context of HIE the ability of public health agencies to improve population health and well-being at the community level (Box 12.1).

12.6 Data quality

Inadequate data quality is either due to incomplete or inaccurate data recording. Data quality represents a challenge for CR, because the integration of healthcare data largely depends on matching several personal identifier attributes, including demographics. The accuracy and reliability of the CR is largely determined by data captured at the point-of-care. This is particularly challenging, yet important, when an organization first joins the HIE network and their historic patient data must be cleaned prior to being exported. Often organizations do not have the resources or the foresight to effectively prepare these data, leading to future matching difficulties. However, as will be discussed in the next section, the CR may standardize incoming data to improve identity resolution and facilitate integration of patient data.

Errors affecting data quality typically occur during data collection, entry, and query. Poor data quality is the result of collecting incorrect data due to the lack of patient recall, or incorrect assumptions, observations, recordings made by the medical personal (e.g., race); the absence of data is the outcome of simply failing to collect relevant patient demographics. Often, recording errors take one of the following forms: (1) phonetic misrepresentations, (2) typographical inaccuracies, and (3) morphological confusion [26].

A brief review of each recording error follows:

1. A phonetic error occurs when a spoken word or name has multiple "correct" handwritten representations. For example, a woman named Lindsey who lives on Neely Avenue represents at least 35 phonetically similar but incorrect combinations: Lindsy, Lindsay, Linsea, Lyndsey, Lyndsay, Lyndsy, Lynzay, who lives on Neeley, Nealy, Nealey, Kneely, or Kneeley.

BOX 12.1

Highlights an example from the nation of Myanmar. The story of Myanmar demonstrates how the implementation of a CR for a specific use case laid the foundation for future HIE across the nation in multiple areas of healthcare delivery. Implementation of the CR further positioned Myanmar to expedite its registration process for immunization against COVID-19.

In 2016 Myanmar faced a challenge of fragmented data across its >100 HIV and Tuberculosis (TB) clinics. Each clinic used the open source EHR system OpenMRS (openmrs.org) to manage patient data, but the clinics did not have a method for sharing patient data with one another or the Ministry of Health (MOH). This meant that when national statistics for HIV and TB cases were calculated, individuals who received care in more than one clinic were counted more than once. At the time, the nation did not have a national healthcare identifier, compounding the problem.

In a collaboration between the MOH, the clinics, and SantéSuite, a digital health vendor, the nation implemented SantéMPI as a CR to manage patient identity information among HIV/TB clinics. The identity management solution, along with the implementation of national unique health ID, established a foundation for connecting and sharing patient level-data across multiple systems, including OpenMRS, vital statistics (DHIS2), and clinic registration systems.

Key benefits of the CR solution for Myanmar included:

- The MPI generated high quality, discrete data at the point-of-care whose strategic impact "rippled upward" across all levels of the health system;
- The ability of SanteMPI's technology architecture to leverage and support existing investments in both hardware and software, both legacy and more modern systems;
- The MPI's role as strategic foundation building block for operationalizing HIE; and
- National unique ID as critical success factor to achieving Universal Healthcare (see Chapter 15 for more information).

Because the nation established a foundation for HIE using the CR and national patient ID, during the COVID-19 pandemic Myanmar quickly pivoted to establish its national vaccination campaign. The immunization registry at MOH was integrated with the CR, enabling preregistration for COVID-19 vaccines. More than 25,000 per day were registered within the first 2 weeks of the vaccination campaign. The CR further supported the generation of "proof of vaccination" cards while also checking identity to ensure patients received the appropriate dose regimen.

The nation of Myanmar is well positioned to continue expanding its HIE efforts given a foundation that enables unique identification of patients across clinics as well as immunization records. Additional digital health strategy goals in the future could expand HIE efforts in inpatient, emergency, and primary care settings.

2. Typographical errors are another common recording error that occurs as a result of omitted, inserted, or transposed characters (e.g., Lndsey, Linndsey, and Lnidsey, respectively).
3. Characters that appear similar, such as the number 0 (zero) and capital letter O or lowercase L and capital I, can be mistakenly interchanged leading to a morphological error [26].

Although errors are more numerous during data entry, a provider querying the HIE for a patient may encounter similar errors as those committed during data entry, thus failing to locate the patient's data. For example, a clinician may mistakenly search for "B0b" instead of "Bob" when entering the first name of our hypothetical patient with diabetes.

Erroneous or omitted data will continue to be a challenge in patient identification but can be limited by (1) providing adequate and continuous training for staff that register patients and (2) establishing a data quality monitoring program to identify and resolve problems. The CR provides solutions to data recording errors through the implementation of phonetic transformations and string comparators, which will be discussed in more detail later in Section 12.8.

In contrast to errors related to data entry, which are at least in theory preventable, data accuracy may not be as amenable to improvement by adherence to procedures and standards alone. Personal traits are often unstable, such as address, employer, marital status, and surname. In the United States, in 2019, 16.3/1000 women were married and 7.6/1000 women got divorced, which are likely to result in a number of demographic changes to the individuals involved [27]. Furthermore, roughly 9% of the United States population changes their address each year [24]. Since patients are not required to update providers when a change occurs, it is imperative to request updates at each point-of-care encounter. Demographic updates should be communicated to the CR and subsequently sent out to other organizational EHR systems to maintain consistent identification.

The differences in culture may also impact the semantic meaning, or interpretation, of patient data. For example, Hispanic cultures may use multiple family names. Consider the daughter of a Hispanic couple named Carlos Lopez and Isabella Gonzalez, Maria Lopez Gonzalez. Maria's name should be entered as either Maria Lopez or Maria Lopez Gonzalez, but not Maria Gonzalez [26]. Other cultural practices to consider include: (1) the order of names (surname listed before given name), (2) usage of particles (e.g., de, da, dos) and hyphens or other special characters in names, (3) religious names, and (4) different practices of listing date of birth (DD/MM/YYYY vs MM/DD/YYYY) [28]. In some cases, an encounter may correctly match to an individual, but the data were generated from a different person, such as the case in identity theft and when individuals share identifiers.

Handling of the missing data can be challenging. Removing records with missing data can introduce bias; imputation of missing data through a regression model or other model technique can add additional errors to the data. Estimating the missing value based on values of other variables in the sample is also difficult, since most quasiidentifiers are strings. To handle missing data, the value of the match weight of the field containing the missing data can be redistributed to the matching fields, and the nonmatch weight of the missing data field be redistributed to the other nonmatching fields. Another solution is imputing the match status of the field containing the missing value based on the matching status of the other fields compared. These two options outperform setting the missing fields weight set at zero [29]. Generally, organizations that match across large data sets have automated standardization processes in place to prevent errors or identify errors post hoc for resolution by humans.

12.7 Metadata and standards

Performing data standardization both in terms of formats (capitalization) and values (i.e., street to st) reduces unnecessary variations in the data and significantly improves automatic linkage; nonstandardized EHR data can result in match rates as low as 50% within the same healthcare system. Address and name standardization improve matching sensitivities by 4.5% and 0.6%, respectively [30]. Standardizing and cleaning the data through a data processing pipeline that adds standardization rules iteratively over time support the linkage process [30].

As discussed throughout this book, interoperability is achieved through universal and consistent implementation of standards, including HL7 or X12 for data transactions (refer to Chapter 9). The same need exists for patient identification. The healthcare industry needs to develop and adhere to standards for the various data fields used to identify patients, or at the very least provide adequate descriptions of fields (also referred to as metadata). Although syntactic data field standards exist, such as MM/DD/YYYY for date of birth, usage may differ from one EHR system to another. Furthermore, the meaning or semantics of data may differ by organization and the individual entering the data. Consider the example of Ms. Maria Lopez-Gonzalez. By name alone, it is quite possible that she could be entered into an EHR system using at least four permutations of her first and compound last names. The lack of precise standardization can hinder accurate linkage of disparate records originating from the same patient, resulting in incomplete data sharing and fragmented records.

In addition to coding standards, the linkage of patient records is facilitated by the following: controlling the type of data allowed in a field (e.g., only numbers for a laboratory result), parsing out components, and standardizing attributes. For example, addresses may be parsed into street number, street name, city, zip code, country, etc., and standardized by mapping different inputs (e.g., road, rural route, rd) into one commonly stored abbreviation, RD [31].

Parsing components may help complete missing or incorrect data fields. For example, if an error was made in the spelling of city, the street name, street number, and zip code can be used to resolve the error. Another commonly encountered example is the storage of patient sex. Male could be stored as M, 0, 1, or 2 and female as F, 0, 1, or 2, depending on the protocols established at the registering organization. Some description of these data (metadata) would need to accompany an HL7 message, but these data can rather simply be converted to a standardized format for identification purposes within the CR. Although, to fully achieve interoperability, the generating facility should transmit these data in a standardized form (e.g., ISO IEC 5218) such that the CR would be able to receive and interpret data without instructions. ISO/TC 215 (International Organization of Standards technical committee) has more than 200 international standards for semantic, technical, and functional interoperability that supports information exchange [31]. The Office of the National Coordinator for Health Information Technology (ONC) has partnered with standard development organizations and the US postal service to create a unified, industry-wide address specification standard for patient matching in the Project US@ [29].

Fast Healthcare Interoperability Resources (FHIR) is an HL7 standard that supports the exchange of health information electronically, by aligning data exchange requirements for quality measurement and reporting with interoperability standards used in other healthcare exchange methods. Organizations like Integrating the Healthcare Enterprise (IHE) create interoperability profiles, such as the Patient Master Identity Registry (PMIR), that describe a collection of coordinated FHIR-based identity management resources and transactions. PMIR details methods for querying, saving, and updating patient identity using FHIR Patient Resources such as identifier, and links to other instances of identities [32]. This profile is intended for FHIR-only configurations without other underlying standards for patient master identity management.

12.8 Algorithmic matching

A core function of the CR is applying matching algorithms to determine whether the client

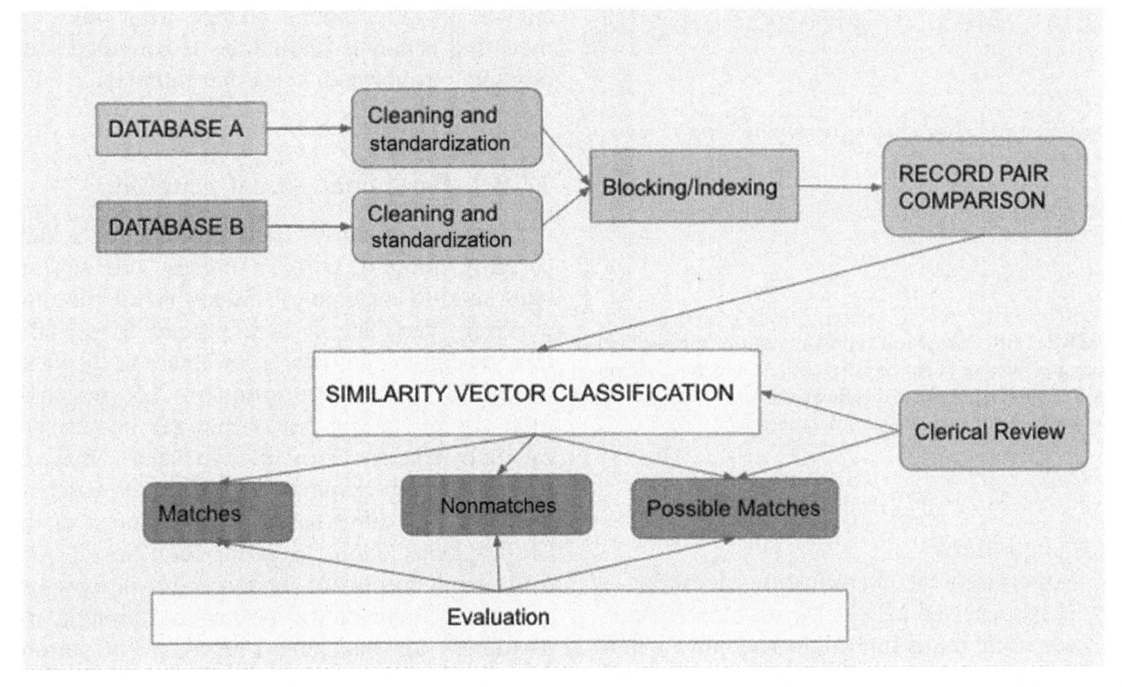

FIGURE 12.7 A detailed overview of the processes involved in CR operations. A CR not only executes algorithmic matching but also implements data cleaning and standardization processes that include blocking and indexing to support record linkage prior to computation in which pairs are evaluated.

(patient) already exists in the registry, subsequently linking records regardless of the source, when applicable. This process is illustrated in Fig. 12.7 and described further in the remainder of this section. The CR can accommodate differences between data sources by the following sequential processes:

1. preparing (cleaning) data;
2. using programs that detect errors and deviations (field comparators);
3. separating likely matches from unlikely matches (blocking);
4. configuring matching algorithms and creating record pair vectors;
5. applying decision models to the comparison vectors to classify record-pairs as reflecting the same individual or entity; and
6. measuring the performance of the decision models.

Generally, patient matching methods can be described as deterministic, probabilistic, statistic, **machine learning (ML)** based, or combinations [29]. Fig. 12.8 provides a simple representation of matching methodologies with increasing complexity from left to right.

Methods of algorithmic matching include [29]:

1. Deterministic matching—exact matching on a single unique identifier; exact 1–1 matching assumes the identifier is recorded without error.
2. Probabilistic matching (Fellegi and Sunter)—calculates match weights for attributes, Bloom filters, naïve Bayes.

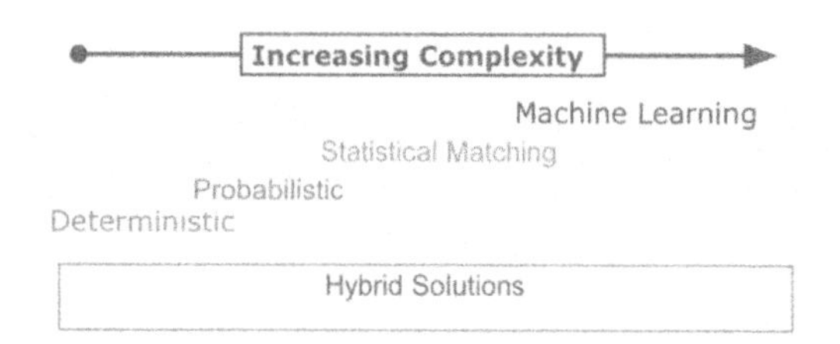

FIGURE 12.8 Graphical representation of the sophistication spectrum of client registry patient matching techniques. The least sophisticated techniques are on the left with the most sophisticated techniques on the right.

3. ML algorithms
   - Supervised ML classification methods
   - Unsupervised ML—*k*-means clustering, semantic matching (highest quality when multiple similarity measures are aggregated to create a single measurement system), similarity measurement.
4. Statistical matching: propensity score matching, regression-based matching, nearest neighbor.
5. Hybrid methods—referential matching.

In the absence of a UPI, matching can be accomplished using unique identifiers or quasiidentifiers. Unlike algorithms that rely on UPIs, which are fundamentally simple by comparison, matching methods that use demographic attributes are more complex and rely upon sufficient data quality (e.g., accuracy, completeness) of multiple attributes and, intuitively, the accuracy of the matching algorithm increases with the number of (high quality) identifiers used [33]. Using an improperly tuned algorithm may result in a higher rate of duplicate records; therefore, it is recommended that the HIE develop a process to determine the appropriate matching scheme. Furthermore, because patient attributes as well as populations change over time, CR matching schemes should be reexamined, and possibly recalibrated, at regular intervals.

12.8.1 Basic concepts of matching

Common identifiers such as names, SSN, date of birth, address, parent's names, and sex are often used as matching variables. When choosing matching variables, it is important to consider their discriminating power, or ability to distinctly identify a patient. For example, SSN possesses more discriminatory power than sex because sex can only take the form of two values, male or female. The discriminatory power of matching variables will differ based on the context of the CR implementation. In some countries, a relatively small number of given names will represent a large segment of the population, limiting the usefulness for matching purposes. Put simply, any CR implementation is highly specific to the population encapsulated by the HIE network and cannot simply be replicated in other contexts.

The decision rule, or match determination, is established by the algorithm and the matching variables selected. A pair is evaluated based on the prescribed decision rule, which will delineate the pair as a match, a possible match, or a nonmatch. Possible matches that lack sufficient information to enable the decision rule to assign the pair to the match or nonmatch group typically require human review, or they are simply labeled as a nonmatch when the cost of human review is prohibitive. The resulting matched pairs will fall into one of the following four groups [34]:

1. true match—the decision rule matched records which are indeed the same person.
2. false match—the decision rule matched records which are not the same person.
3. true nonmatch—the decision rule correctly did not match records which are not the same person.

4. false nonmatch—the decision rule incorrectly matched records which are not the same person.

The ability of the CR to reliably identify pairs as matching or nonmatching is critically dependent upon a balance between data quality and matching algorithms. A simple algorithm with complete and standardized data will perform well, but as data degrades more sophisticated algorithms will be necessary. In general, high-quality data are preferred over a sophisticated algorithm. The data preparation phase is where the CR addresses the concerns of heterogeneity of data, as discussed in previous sections, by parsing and transforming (standardizing) potential matching variables.

12.8.2 Field comparison methods

The occurrence of typographical and phonetic errors limits the ability to compare two strings for exact matches. If matching, or blocking, depended on exact character matches, the algorithms may erroneously exclude true matches due to variant spellings or transposed keystrokes. Several coding systems have been created which loosen the constraints around the argument and allow approximate agreement between fields. For example, a "fuzzy match" may be employed to apply semantic logic or allow some range of disagreement among fields, such as date of birth (e.g., within 3 months) or a name which agrees on a defined number of characters (e.g., Alex Smith vs Alexander Smith).

Several phonetic transformation systems are available that limit the disruption caused by errors from similar sounding words and match these homophones even though minor variations in spelling, such as the following: the New York State Identification and Intelligence System (NYIIS), soundex, metaphone, and double metaphone.

Approximate string comparators, such as Levenshtein edit distance, Jaro-Winkler comparator, and longest common subsequence, act to improve matching efficiency by computing a comparator score, or measure of similarity, between the strings of two records within a field. If the comparator score exceeds a specified threshold, the two records are considered a match. Grannis et al. [35] demonstrated that Jaro-Winkler can achieve sensitivities exceeding 97%, which is approximately 10% greater than requiring exact matches for linkage.

The details of the algorithms are beyond the scope of this text, but readers who are interested in comparators are referred to the appendix of Gill's *Methods for automatic record matching and linkage and their use in national statistics* [36] for a nice review of methodology and applications of phonetic transformations as well as the article by Grannis et al. [35] for a review of approximate string comparators.

12.8.3 Blocking

Blocking methods reduce the number of candidate record comparison pairs to a feasible number based on a limited number of shared attributes. As potentially each record in one data set must be compared to all records in a second data set, the number of record pair comparisons grows quadratically with the number of records to be matched, creating an imbalance problem. This approach is computationally infeasible for large data sets. To reduce the number of possible record pair comparisons, traditional record linkage techniques work in a blocking fashion, that is, they use a record attribute (or subset of attributes) to split the data sets into blocks. The Standard Blocking (SB) method clusters records into blocks where they share the identical blocking key [6]. A blocking key is defined to be composed from the record attributes in each data set. **Blocking** is a technique of data reduction, which can filter unlikely matching pairs before record matching. Blocking methods directly affect the sensitivity of matching if the true matching pairs are not in the same block, and indirectly influence specificity—a better reduction ratio of the number of record pair comparisons allows more computationally intensive comparators to be employed [37].

Multiple methods have been attempted in search for the best technique besides traditional blocking approaches, including clustering techniques, canopy clustering, bigram indexing, and locality-sensitive hashing (LSH)-based approaches—"shingling," transitive LSH, and *k*-means LSH (can be used in privacy preserving record linkage). All these methods differ in terms of computational complexity, recall, precision, reduction ratio, and privacy-related issues [37].

Imagine the scenario where an organization newly joins the HIE and, based on their EMPI, has 100,000 unique patients in their private database. Say, for instance, the CR contains 1,000,000 unique patients. Likely some of the 100,000 patients from the organization are already uniquely identified within the CR from encounters at other organizations. Therefore each unique record in the organization's EMPI must be compared to each unique record in the CR's MPI, leading to (100,000 × 1,000,000) 100 billion possible pairs to evaluate. A naïve approach would attempt to make these computationally infeasible comparisons. To increase the efficiency of the matching process, regardless of the matching algorithm to be deployed, records are often considered for comparison only if they match on a few specific identifiers, such as the last four digits of SSN or zip code combined with age. The data sets are then separated into blocks, or subsets, and candidate matches are only evaluated within each block.

People perform blocking to assist them in daily tasks. For example, if you are searching the phone book for Timothy McFarlane, you may first mentally block based on those with the last name beginning with Mc, then the first name Tim or Timothy. Intuitively, this process is much more efficient than starting at the A's and searching each name until you find the one for which you are looking. CR blocking fields should be those which are least prone to recording errors, have high discriminatory power, and have uniform distributions in the population [38]. Generally, it is advisable to perform multiple passes of blocking, with different blocking criteria, to catch false nonmatches, or, missed matches that failed to agree on the previous blocking criteria [39].

12.8.4 Decision models

12.8.4.1 Deterministic matching

Also known as heuristic, rule-based, exact, and all-or-none algorithms, deterministic matching techniques typically use a set of rules based on either exact matching of two records or the use of field comparators and phonetic transformations for near matching. Deterministic models are best when both records contain a field that is highly discriminatory. A unique identifier-organization-specific MRN, and to a lesser degree SSN, represents examples of fields often used in deterministic matching. In fact, most information systems implement a basic deterministic matching algorithm using exact (MRN or SSN) or partial matching (name and DOB) [40]. However, basic deterministic models are severely limited by the quality and completeness of data and by the discriminatory power of the identifier. Accuracy can be improved by first matching on a ubiquitous and highly discriminatory identifier (e.g., SSN) and then further confirming with additional ones such as sex, name, and date of birth [41]. Complex deterministic algorithms may incorporate partial identifiers (e.g., zip code, first letter of the last name), phonetic codes, transposition of elements (e.g., date of birth), similarity scores, or distance-based measures [33].

Because of the need for precision and accuracy, and heterogeneous nature of data across entities, purely deterministic algorithms are not typically well suited for a CR. Even in instances where UPIs have been distributed nationwide, such as in the United Kingdom, it is advisable to supplement with additional patient traits [42].

12.8.4.2 Probabilistic matching

Probabilistic methods calculate a match weight (a score) that represents the likelihood that two records belong to the same individual. The most widely adopted method was developed by Fellegi and Sunter [43], based on the ideas introduce by Newcombe et al. [2], which draws from maximum likelihood theory to produce probabilities that two records represent the same person. The Fellegi and Sunter algorithm determines field weights based on log-likelihood ratios to determine record similarity. The likelihood ratios are estimated rather than calculated and are constructed using estimated conditional probabilities of observing agreement on each matching variable; the "m-probability" of agreement on an identifier, given two records belong to the same individual and the "u-probability" of agreement, given the records belong to different individuals [33]. If these scores are greater than an appointed upper threshold, they are deemed a true match; if they fall below a lower threshold, they are deemed a true nonmatch; and if they are in between the thresholds, the pair represents a possible match. Although in practice possible matches often require human review, more sophisticated decision rules have been shown to perform at a high level when human intervention is not feasible. Probabilistic matching of anonymized/pseudonymized data sets is currently performed using indirect and proxy identifiers with the ability to enhance deterministic linkage methods [44].

12.8.4.3 Machine learning–based linkage methods

In ML, a training set of data is used to "teach" a classification algorithm, such as a decision trees, support vector machines, ensemble methods, random forest, or conditional random fields. The probabilities of a match given a particular agreement pattern across the fields are determined on the training set; subsequently, new pairs of records are assigned the match probability based on probability of the agreement fields consistent with a match [29].

Supervised ML methods can classify each record pair individually, as a cluster, or can take the *collective entity resolution techniques* approach that consider the relationship between records in the classification step and seek the optimal linkage solution [4]. Clustering can overcome problems related to nontransitivity of the matched pairs. Unsupervised ML is mostly employed in linkage situations where multiple records of the same individual or group of individuals need to be linked. Based on calculated similarities between the compared records, all records that correspond to the same individual or group of individuals are inserted into one cluster in a database [33]. Semantic matching determines if two strings of text represent related concepts based on a known set of linked concepts against which the two strings of text can be compared. The similarity measure is based on how "close" or how frequently the two strings are in the map of known concepts. Semantic matching is of highest quality when multiple similarity measures are aggregated to create a single measurement system [29].

Theoretically, ML models can achieve high accuracy and sensitivity in matching records; the performance depends on the data quality and availability of a training data sets and computing power.

12.8.4.4 Statistical matching

Statistical matching, or data fusion, is a model-based approach that merges records based on the similarities between the variables observed in multiple data sources. In statistical matching, information from both data sets is used to determine a joint density of the combined records [45]. When comparing two variables from different data sets, if there are not have enough appropriate comparison fields for probabilistic record linkage, then statistical matching can be used to link the most appropriate records to each other [29].

12.8.4.5 *Hybrid methods of record linkage*

Combinations of deterministic and probabilistic methodology have been used with increased linkage accuracy [46]. Hybrid approaches to record linkage increase linkage accuracy and outperform the independent probabilistic and deterministic methods performance [46].

Referential matching is an example of hybrid record linkage that combines probabilistic algorithms with big data and ML technologies. This approach matches demographic data to a continuously updated reference database (credit reporting and public utilities) that contains more than 300 million identities spanning the entire US population, each identity containing demographic data spanning a 30-year history. Referential matching cloud-based plug-ins can match duplicates flagged by EMPI and EHRs for manual review. This method is limited in matching records of children, undocumented immigrants, or homeless population [7].

12.8.4.6 *Privacy preserving record linkage*

Privacy preserving record linkage (PPRL) is an increasingly popular matching method implementing techniques that maintain patient privacy while still reconciling a person's identity across multiple data sources. PPRL removes direct identifiers and quasiidentifiers by applying cryptographic hash functions to the identifiable data, which obfuscates a direct connection to the original data. The hashed data are passed to the indexing step where statistical linkage keys, secure multiparity computation, and bloom filters are implemented [47]. A two-party protocol involves only the two data owners who wish to link their data; a three-party protocol involves a trusted third party that conducts the linkage. In a multiparty protocol, more than two databases are linked. For the linkage process to occur, the two parties interested in the linkage share their file with the other or share the data with a third party that performs the match and returns the linked pairs [29].

12.8.5 Linkage quality metrics

Linkage errors can manifest as missing data, measurement error and misclassification, unrepresentative sampling, or combinations. False links occur when different individuals share the same identifiers or where identifiers are not sufficiently discriminative. Missed links can occur due to recording errors, genuine changes over time, or where missing or insufficiently distinguishing identifiers prevent a link from being made. The level of linkage error depends on the quality and completeness of the identifying data available within a data set and can occur irrespective of the linkage methods employed. In all linkage methods, some choice must generally be made about an evidentiary threshold for classifying record pairs as links or not. Decisions about classifying record pairs usually consider the likelihood of both false (where records belonging to different individuals are linked together) and missed (where records belonging to the same individual are not linked) links, but the balance between the two error types will depend on the requirements of the data.

Linkage accuracy is typically a trade-off between sensitivity or recall (the proportion of true matches that are correctly identified), specificity (the proportion of true nonmatches that are correctly identified), and precision or the positive predictive value (proportion of assigned links that are true matches).

The performance of a decision rule can be simply quantified by:

- Sensitivity $= \frac{\text{True Match}}{\text{True Match + False Nonmatch}}$

  = The true-positive rate (aka recall) and

  1−sensitivity = false-negative rate

- Specificity $= \frac{\text{True Nonmatch}}{\text{True Nonmatch} + \text{False Match}}$

  = The true-negative rate and

  1−specificity = false-positive rate

A false negative occurs when a pair of records match in reality but the decision rule declared them as a nonmatch. On the other hand, a false positive occurs when two truly nonmatching records are erroneously linked together. In healthcare, it is usually desirable to control the rate of false positives because erroneously linking together data from two different patients may result in significant morbidity and mortality from inappropriate treatments. False negatives may lead to incomplete information regarding medical conditions, medications, or allergies, but these errors are analogous to the fragmented nature of healthcare without HIE, and therefore perceived by many as less severe [15].

It is not possible to eliminate all false positives, because there is an inverse relationship between false negative and false positive rates—as one measure decreases, the other increases proportionately. That is, there is no free lunch—one can only achieve a false positive rate of 0% by allowing nearly 100% of false negatives. This concept is illustrated in Fig. 12.9 by two distributions; the top represents the distribution of pairs which are actually the same entity, the bottom represents the distribution of pairs which are truly not the same entity, and the area underneath the curves represents the true positive rate and true negative rates. Despite the give-and-take relationship of false positives and negatives, the CR will typically utilize enough reliable and stable matching variables to limit false positives. Implementers of CR's must set a balance between the two errors by tuning the threshold/s, which indicate a match based on the available data within the context of their implementation.

While more complex linkage algorithms can better discrimination between true matches and true nonmatches, there is generally an

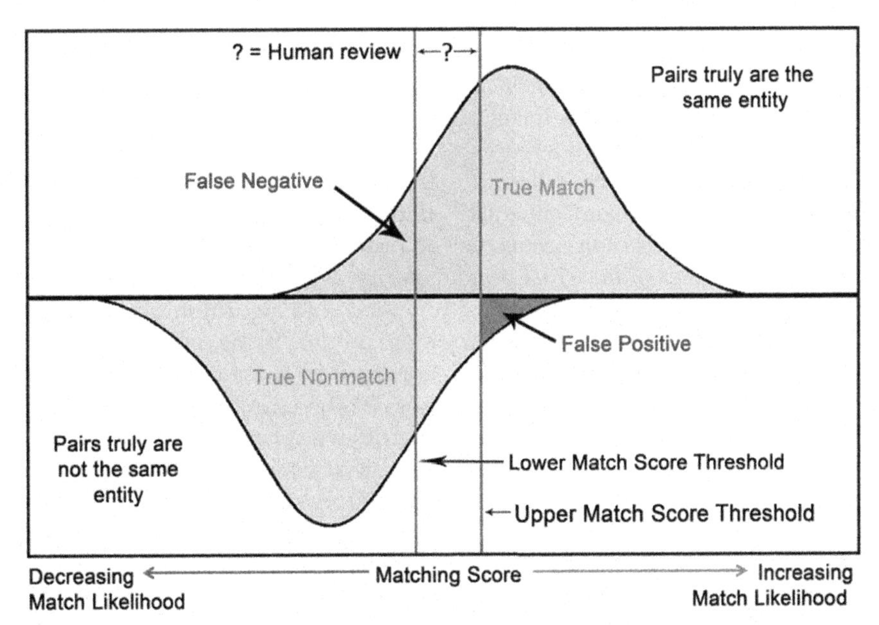

FIGURE 12.9 Decision rules and results of probabilistic matching techniques. Illustration of the balance between *matching likelihood*, *false positive matches*, and *false negative matches* and the trade-off between sensitivity or *recall* (proportion of true matches correctly identified) and *precision* or the positive predictive value (proportion of assigned links that are true matches).

inescapable trade-off between precision and recall (or any other ways of measuring false links and missed links) among any uncertain links that cannot be classified as definite matches or definite nonmatches.

An optimal single threshold may be chosen to either minimize the sum of errors (false links + missed links) or minimize the net effect of errors (false links − missed links). The *F*-measure (the harmonic means of precision and recall: $f = (2 \times \text{precision} \times \text{recall})/(\text{precision} + \text{recall})$) is a metric used in the context of data linkage for deriving a single number measure of linkage quality. However, the *F*-measure depends on the match rate of the different linkage classifiers used, and therefore, it is not recommended in the context of evaluating data linkage quality [48]. It has recently been suggested that F^* a transformation of *F* has better interpretation and applicability [48].

Decisions on the most appropriate classification of record pairs are ideally made on a study-by-study basis, depending on the likely effects of linkage errors and any arising bias for a particular analytical output. If linkage is conducted without knowledge of the intended analysis or to support multiple analyses, then the linkage outputs must support a range of preferences about linkage error. This can only be achieved by retaining less-than-certain links and generating link-level measures of agreement or accuracy (e.g., match weights or estimates of marginal precision) for use by analysts. With these outputs, end-users can effectively tune linkage algorithms and implement sensitivity analyses without requiring access to identifiers.

12.8.6 Biases in record linkage

Linkage errors can lead to information bias and selection bias. The source of information bias comes from missing data, misclassification of categorical variables, and measurement error of quantitative variables.

Since differential record linkage is well recognized and data quality determines the probability of linkage, populations at risk for having records with poor data quality, mostly underrepresented groups, have a higher error rate in the linked data [49]. Most of the data standardization techniques have been developed in an English-centric linguistic cultural context; therefore, when applied to non-English data (i.e., names), these methods may introduce bias. Thus far, in the linkage process, the gender classification is restricted to two options, nonaccounting for the transgender or nonbinary individuals. Records of women, whose last name has changed after marriage or divorce, have a lower chance of matching, if the algorithm relies on the last name.

When implementing ML algorithms for record linkage, one must recognize that they are prone to incorporating the biases of their human creators. Also, these algorithms are trained and tested on data sets that may not be representative of the population where they are implemented, thus giving rise to outcome biases [50].

12.8.7 User interface

Users interact with CR through a **graphical user interface (GUI)**, which is a platform for data presentation and interpretation of performance measurements. The GUI allows users to specify the matching attributes, searching method, and algorithmic parameters of the decision model. Some interfaces give access to a comparison function to appraise the effectiveness of the searching methods through various metrics—i.e., *pair completeness* (number of actual matched record pairs in the reduced comparison space) and *reduction ratio* (relative reduction in the size of the comparison space). The comparison function also gives users the ability to determine the performance of the decision model by displaying the calculated *accuracy* (percentage of correctly classified record pairs) and *completeness* (ratio of number of matched record pairs by the decision model to the total number of record pairs known in the data). Through the interface, most users also have the option to manually review the record pairs when the automatic processes are not possible.

12.9 Emerging trends

12.9.1 Data quality

As indicated throughout this chapter, data quality has a significant effect on record linkage accuracy. To improve and simplify linkage, focus must be placed on the data gathering process. From a technical level, data may be improved by implementing standards for data capture (e.g., HL7, SNOMED). However, standardization alone will not alleviate all data entry errors or omissions. One method of enhancing data gathering is to continually train personnel for data collection and entry. Once trained, accountability can be established by keeping an error log and remediating users when errors occur. Additionally, users can be incentivized to be more thorough during the data collection and entry process.

12.9.2 Biometrics

Biometric identifiers have yet to gain acceptance in many developed nations, despite the technology becoming more affordable and amenable to daily use. Currently biometrics are used in healthcare largely to identify employees (e.g., doctors, nurses, staff) when they login to use a health IT system.

As societies becomes more acquainted with biometrics, such as using a fingerprint to unlock their cellular phone, these identifiers may gain acceptance for use in patient identification and record linkage. Although the adoption of biometrics is sparse, they have great potential for becoming unique identifiers due to their availability, not necessarily adoption, in mobile and smart technologies handled by patients. Leveraging existing technologies present in patients' hands can assist healthcare organizations with the deployment of biometrics, such as facial recognition from selfies and fingerprints, turning them into ubiquitous identifiers. Yet significant policy, technical, and literacy work will be necessary to unleash the power of biometrics present in mobile technologies for use in HIE to uniquely identify patients.

12.9.3 Hybrid matching algorithms

Hybrid matching algorithms, associated with privacy preserving linkage methods, supported by cloud computing resources represent future solutions to CR for many healthcare organizations with variable financial and infrastructure resources.

12.9.4 Location intelligence

Location intelligence through geocoding and address verification authenticates address information in real-time thus avoiding duplicate records. Location intelligence is efficient in appending geocode coordinates to medical records processing millions of addresses per hour. Location intelligence is one of the most promising tools in maintaining the accuracy of patients' home address.

12.9.5 Patient engagement

Empowering patients with access to personal data and personal medical records can drive the accuracy of data present in records. There is evidence that control and maintenance of data quality by patients can improve the accuracy of the demographic information [51]. Leveraging information from personal mobile technologies can confirm patients' identities and update or correct existing information. Taking a patient-centered approach to record matching can overcome clerical errors and utilize patient-generated data for improved record matching.

12.9.6 National strategic framework for identity matching

The COVID-19 pandemic uncovered significant flaws in patient identification with implications on patient safety and healthcare delivery. The inability to match patients with their records impedes HIE and coordination of care; produces delays and duplicate care; and raises the cost of healthcare. In 2017 the American College of Surgeons, American Health Information Management Association, College of Healthcare Information Management Executives, Intermountain Healthcare, and Premiere Healthcare Alliance formed the Patient ID-Now coalition [52]. The coalition released a report entitled "Framework for a National Strategy on Patient Identity" that addresses, among other issues, patients' identification and record matching [53]. Unfortunately, the success of this plan is under the control of politicians and their divided views on patient identity legislation; presently, such legislation is unlikely to succeed, leaving the problem of patient identification to local governments and healthcare organizations.

12.10 Summary

Healthcare data are generated from numerous clinical sites, often by different EHR systems. Each organization has its own method of uniquely identifying patients, but these identifiers are incapable of identifying patient records from outside organizations. Currently, no single unique patient identifier is capable of spanning the entire healthcare environment, and record linkage must rely upon multiple patient attributes and identifiers. The CR handles inconsistent completeness and quality of identifying data by standardizing incoming data and employing statistical matching algorithms to link data from separate organizations for the same patient. Once identified, a single, unique identifier (the EUID) is associated with the patient, allowing HIE networks to create and maintain patient-centric records and services. When implementing CR, healthcare organizations have to consider the level of fragmentation within the system, the quality and timeliness of acquired data, the health information systems infrastructure, and human resources available for data storage, retrieval, client identity verification, and tracking. To fulfill their clinical and administrative role, support population health management, clinical decision-making, quality improvement, and clinical research, CR must be connected to an HIE network.

Questions for discussion

1. Compare and contrast SSN, biometric identifiers, and voluntary universal health identifiers in terms of the seven ideal unique patient identifier attributes discussed in this chapter.
2. Discuss the impact data quality has on CR patient matching. Is it preferable to have a sophisticated algorithm or high-quality data?
3. How do client registries limit the number of potential matches before deploying matching algorithms? Describe how this is achieved.
4. What are the differences between deterministic and probabilistic matching algorithms? Is one preferred to the other?
5. What are the major barriers to a national patient ID in the United States? Do you think the United States might ever change its approach given the success of national IDs used in other nations?

References

[1] Dunn HL. Record linkage. Am J Public Health Nations Health 1946;36(12):1412–16.

[2] Newcombe HB, Kennedy JM, Axford SJ, James AP. Automatic linkage of vital records. Science. 1959;130 (3381):954–9.

[3] Herzog TH, Scheuren F, Winkler WE. Record linkage in Wiley interdisciplinary review. Computational Statistics 2010;2(5):535–43. Available from: https://doi.org/10.1002/wics.108.

[4] Christen P. Data linkage: the big picture. Harv Data Sci Rev 2019;1. Available from: doi:10.1162/99608f92.84deb5c4.

[5] Singla P, Domingos P. Entity resolution with Markov logic. Sixth international conference on data mining (ICDM);. IEEE; 2006. p. 572–82.

[6] Winkler WE. Encyclopedia of machine learning and data mining. In: Christen P, editor. Record linkage. Boston, MA: Springer; 2017.

[7] Riplinger L, Piera-Jiménez J, Dooling JP. Patient identification techniques—approaches, implications, and findings. Yearb Med Inf 2020;29(1):81–6.

[8] Van Houten JP, Brandt CA. Universal patient identification: what it is and why the US needs it. HealthAffairs; 2021.

[9] Department of Health. The operating framework for the NHS in England 2012–2013. London, England: Department of Health; 2011.

[10] Gill L. Methods for automatic record matching and linkage and their use in national statistics. Norwich: National Statistics. Her Majesty's Stationary Office; 2001.

[11] Wild WG. The theory of modulus N check digit systems. Computer Bull 1968;12:308–11.

[12] Fernandes L, Schumacher S. Universal health identifiers: issues and requirements for successful patient information exchange. IBM Software; 2010.

[13] Markle Foundation Working Group on Accurately Linking Information for Health Care Quality and Safety. Linking health care information: proposed methods for improving care and protecting privacy; 2005.

[14] ASTM E1717-07. Standard guide for properties of a universal healthcare identifier (UHID). West Conshohocken, PA: ASTM International; 2013.

[15] Hillestad R, Bigelow J, Chaudhry B, Dreyer P, Greenberg M, Meili R, et al. Identity crisis: an examiniation of the costs and benefits of a unique patient identifier for the U.S. health care sysyem. Santa Monica, CA: RAND Corporation; 2008.

[16] U.S. Department of Health & Human Services. November 26, 2012. Health information privacy, guidance regarding methods for de-identification of protected health information in accordance with the health insurance portability and accountability act (HIPAA) privacy rule. Retrieved from: https://www.hhs.gov/hipaa/for-professionals/privacy/special-topics/de-identification/index.html

[17] U.S. Department of Health and Human Services. White paper on unique health identifier for individuals. Washington, DC; 1998 (revised 2011).

[18] Fernandes L, O'Connor M. Patient identification in three acts. J AHIMA / Am Health Inf Manag Assoc 2008;79(4):46–9 quiz 51–2.

[19] Culbertson A, Goel S, Madden MB, Safaeinili N, Jackson KL, Carton T, et al. The building blocks of interoperability. A multisite analysis of patient demographic attributes available for matching. Appl Clin Inform 2017;8(2):322–36.

[20] Prabhakar S, Pankanti S, Jain AK. Biometric recognition: security and privacy concerns. IEEE Security Priv 2003;1(2):33–42.

[21] Gelb A, Clark J. Identification for development: the biometrics revolution. Center for Global Development; 2013.

[22] Pato J, Millett L. Biometric recognition: challenges and opportunities. Washington, DC: The National Academies Press 2010.

[23] Beck E, Santas X. Developing and using individual identifiers for the provision of health services including HIV. Montreux, Switzerland: UNAINS; 2009.

[24] Mills S, Lee JK, Rassekh BM, Zorko Kodelja M, Bae G, Kang M, et al. Unique health identifiers for universal health coverage. J Health Popul Nutr 2019;38(Suppl 1):22.

[25] National Commission to Transform Public Health Data Systems. Charting a course for an equity-centered data system: Robert Wood Johnson Foundation; 2021 [updated Oct 1; cited 2022 Mar 27]. Available from: https://www.rwjf.org/en/library/research/2021/10/charting-a-course-for-an-equity-centered-data-system.html.

[26] Dimitropoulos L, Grannis S, Banger AK, Harris DH. Privacy and security solutions for interoperable health information exchange. Chicago, IL: RTI International; 2009.

[27] Bureau UC. US marriage and divorce rates by state: 2009 & 2019; 2020.

[28] HIMSS Patient Identity Ingertity Work Group. Patient identity integrity whitepaper; 2009.

[29] Asher J, Resnick D, Brite J, Brackbill R, Cone J. An introduction to probabilistic record linkage with a focus on linkage processing for WTC registries. Int J Environ Res Public Health 2020;17(18). Available from: doi:10.3390/ijerph17186937.

[30] Grannis SJ, Xu H, Vest JR, Kasthurirathne S, Bo N, Moscovitch B, et al. Evaluating the effect of data standardization and validation on patient matching accuracy. J Am Med Inf Assoc 2019;26(5):447–56.

[31] International Standards Organization. STANDARDS BY ISO/TC 215. 2021. Accessed 13 June 2022. Available at https://www.iso.org/home.html
[32] Commitee IT. IHE IT Infrastructure Technical Framework Supplement Patient Master Identity Registry (PMIR). IHE International; December 11, 2020.
[33] Harron K, Doidge JC, Goldstein H. Assessing data linkage quality in cohort studies. Ann Hum Biol 2020;47(2):218–26.
[34] Winkler W. Matching and record linkage. Washington, DC; 1993. Available from: http://www.census.gov/srd/papers/pdf/rr93-8.pdf.
[35] Grannis SJ, Overhage JM, McDonald C. Real world performance of approximate string comparators for use in patient matching. Stud Health Technol Inform 2004;107(Pt 1):43–7.
[36] Gill L. Statistics GBOfN. Methods for automatic record matching and linkage and their use in national statistics. Office for National Statistics; 2001.
[37] Steorts R, Ventura SL, Sadinle M, Fienberg SE. A comparison blocking method for record linkage. arXiv:1407.3191; 2014.
[38] Jaro M. Advances in record-linkage methodology as applied to matching the 1985 Census of Tampa, Florida. J Am Stat Assoc 1989;84:414–20.
[39] Mason CA, Tu S. Data linkage using probabilistic decision rules: a primer. Birth Defects Res A Clin Mol Teratol 2008;82(11):812–21.
[40] Bartschat W, Burrington-Brown J, Carey S, Chen J, Deming S, Durkin S, et al. Surveying the RHIO landscape. A description of current RHIO models, with a focus on patient identification. J AHIMA / Am Health Inf Manag Assoc 2006;77(1) 64a-d.
[41] Grannis SJ, Overhage JM, McDonald CJ. Analysis of identifier performance using a deterministic linkage algorithm. Proceedings/AMIA annual symposium; 2002.p. 305–9.
[42] Lichtner V, Wilson S, Galliers JR. The challenging nature of patient identifiers: an ethnographic study of patient identification at a London walk-in centre. Health Inform J 2008;14(2):141–50.
[43] Fellegi IP, Sunter SB. A theory of record linkage. J Am Stat Assoc 1969;64(328):1183–210.
[44] Blake HA, Sharples LD, Harron K, van der Meulen JH, Walker K. Probabilistic linkage without personal information successfully linked national clinical datasets. J Clin Epidemiol 2021;136:136–45.
[45] Gessendorfer J, Beste J, Drechsler J, Sakshau JW. Statistical matching as a supplement to record linkage: a valuable method to tackle nonconsent bias? J Off Stat 2018;34:909–33.
[46] Ong TC, Duca LM, Kahn MG, Crume TL. A hybrid approach to record linkage using a combination of deterministic and probabilistic methodology. J Am Med Inf Assoc 2020;27(4):505–13.
[47] Vatsalan D, Sehili Z, Christen P, Christen E. Privacy-preserving record linkage for big data: current approaches and research challenges. In: Zomaya A, Sakr S, editors. Handbook of big data technologies. Springer; 2017. Available from: https://doi.org/10.1007/978-3-319-49340-4_25.
[48] Hand DJ, Christen P, Kirielle N. F*: an interpretable transformation of the F-measure. Mach Learn 2021;110(3):451–6.
[49] Lariscy JT. Black-White disparities in adult mortality: implications of differential record linkage for understanding the mortality crossover. Popul Res Policy Rev 2017;36(1):137–56.
[50] Kasthurirathne S, Grannis SJ. Analytics. In: Finnell JT, Dixon BE, editors. Clinical informatics study guide: text and review. 2nd ed. Cham, Switzerland: Springer Nature Switzerland AG; 2022.
[51] Rudin RS, Hillestad R, Ridgely MS, Qureshi NS, Davis JS, Fischer SH. Defining and evaluating patient-empowered approaches to improving record matching. Rand Health Q 2019;8(3):3.
[52] Patient ID Now Coalition. Patient ID Now Homepage 2021 [cited 2022 Apr 2]. Available from: https://patientidnow.org/.
[53] Patient ID Now Coalition. Framework for a national strategy on patient identity. Chicago, IL: AHIMA; 2021 [cited 2022 Apr 2]. Available from: https://catalog.ahima.org/view/251156390/.

CHAPTER

13

Facility registries: metadata for where care is delivered

Brian E. Dixon[1,2], *Scott Teesdale*[3], *Rita Sembajwe*[4], *Martin Osumba*[5] *and Eyasu Ashebier*[6]

[1]Department of Epidemiology, Richard M. Fairbanks School of Public Health, Indiana University, Indianapolis, IN, USA [2]Center for Biomedical Informatics, Regenstrief Institute, Inc., Indianapolis, IN, USA [3]Resolve To Save Lives, New Orleans, LA, USA [4]Global Public Health Impact Center, RTI International, Atlanta, GA, USA [5]Global Public Health Impact Center, RTI International, Nairobi, Kenya [6]John Snow, Inc., Addis Ababa, Ethiopia

LEARNING OBJECTIVES

By the end of this chapter, the reader should be able to:

- Define the concept of a health facility registry (FR).
- Define the concept of a master facility list.
- Differentiate between a master facility list and health FR.
- Explain the value of health facility registries in supporting health systems.
- Discuss various methods of generating unique identifiers for healthcare facilities.
- Recommend FR signature and service domain components based on local context.
- Describe how metadata enable facility data integration and harmonization.

13.1 Introduction

In the previous chapter, we discussed how to identify each unique individual to link patient-centric data, answering the question: who do these data represent? The focus now shifts to identifying and describing the facilities where care is delivered. A facility can be defined "as a concept which represents multiple dimensions of care delivery location" including its name, location, clinical services,

Health Information Exchange
DOI: https://doi.org/10.1016/B978-0-323-90802-3.00032-0

organizational hierarchy, capacity, and infrastructure [1]. Healthcare delivery is scattered among thousands of facilities, and the rapid pace of evolution in the healthcare environment results in frequent changes to facility services, resources, staffing, and ownership. Facilities can also be closed or de-certified from offering a procedure or set of service, and sometimes the closure can be temporary. In the absence of regular, systematic identification and description of facilities, it is difficult, if not impossible, for stakeholders to grasp the complete nature of services in a community or country.

Comprehensively identifying facilities establishes a connection for linkage of secondary data and a means of primary data collection, which enables the determination of factors that may be used for health system decision-making and planning, such as what care services are provided, how services are funded, population access to care, quality of services, and the state of healthcare infrastructure [2]. Accurate identification of facilities further supports care referrals as well as the calculation of routine health indicators [3,4].

Although related, it is important to note that the facility where care is delivered and the provider of said care are, in fact, distinct. Many providers, of different specialties, will deliver services at a single facility, and a single provider may practice at multiple facilities. Furthermore, business processes make distinguishing between providers and facilities acutely important. For example, identifying a provider at a given facility does not provide insight as to the conditions and resources of the facility in which they practice, nor would it detail all of the services offered at the facility. Identification of health workers, including providers, is the focus of Chapter 14.

13.2 Facility registry background

Integrated and interoperable health information systems are critical to improve the quality and continuity of healthcare. Improved data sharing among electronic health (eHealth) tools can serve to reduce both redundancy and cost associated with each system. Despite the potential value of health information exchange (HIE), many eHealth systems continue to be highly fragmented. One example of this challenge can be observed among systems that collect and store separate lists of health facilities with divergent levels of standardization, curation, quality, and completeness. For example, in a study of the Ugandan health system, researchers found that several nongovernmental and faith-based organizations complied their own lists of available health facilities to use when referring clients [4]. Similarly, district health officers maintained their own lists of facilities in their district. Each list varied with respect to the details and attributes captured about the facilities.

Registries are fundamental to addressing the challenges related to normalizing reference datasets and facilitating interoperability. The purpose of a **health facility registry (FR)** is to act as the central authority to collect, store, and distribute an up-to-date and standardized set of health facility data electronically to organizations across the health system (e.g., Ministry of Health, hospitals, clinics, nongovernmental organizations). The resulting current, canonical facility dataset stored in the registry is called a **master facility list (MFL)** and is the key to linking disparate data sources. Currently most MFLs, if they exist, are stored as word processing or spreadsheet documents whose structure varies from one organization to the next.

While closely related, an FR can be understood as the interoperable technology that manages and shares facility data, while an MFL is the standardized data stored in the registry. Accordingly, an FR acts as a source of truth to collect, store, and share facility data. To further differentiate between the FR and MFL, refer to Fig. 13.1, a basic conceptual model of an FR, and Fig. 13.2, a depiction of

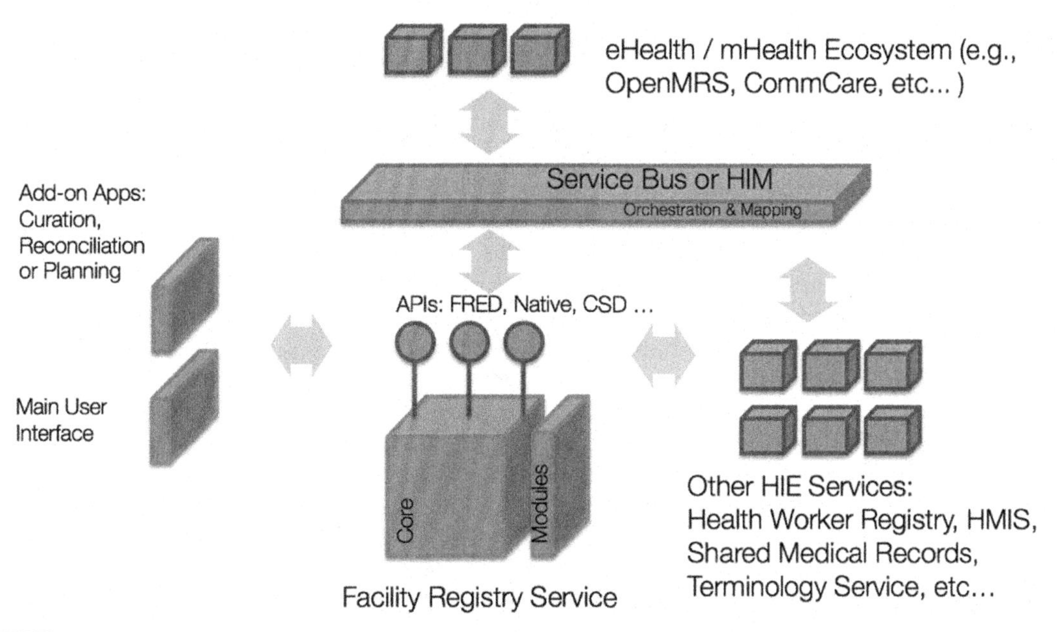

FIGURE 13.1 Facility registry conceptual model. Source: *Figure provided by the OpenHIE facility registry community.*

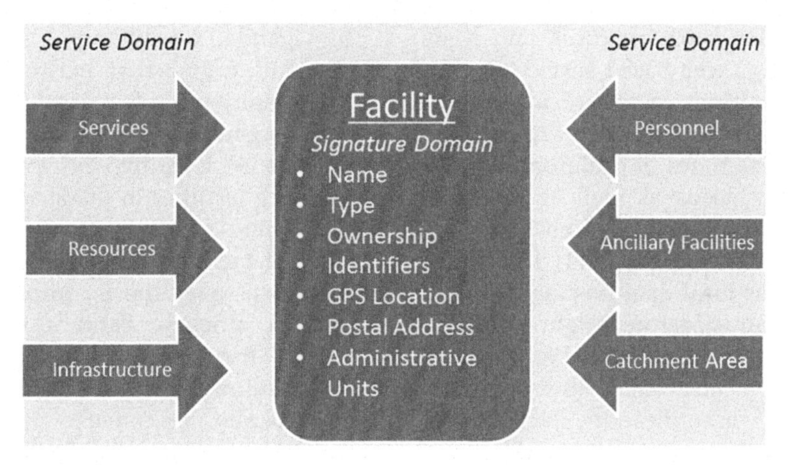

FIGURE 13.2 Master facility list domains and data elements.

the data stored in the MFL. As Fig. 13.1 details, the FR includes the technical infrastructure necessary to integrate MFL data with external information systems (e.g., eHealth point of service applications), user interfaces (UI), and applications to facilitate data contribution and consumption. On the other hand, the simple schema of the MFL displayed in Fig. 13.2 pertains only to the facility-related data. These data are the primary focus of this chapter; however, core FR functionalities are introduced.

13.3 Implementation of a health facility registry

From a technical point of view, an FR is relatively simple. The difficulties with implementation are typically sociopolitical; feasibly balancing the needs and interests of private, public, and governmental entities (e.g., donor influence) as well as consumers is complex. Thus health facility data collection, storage, and use should mirror the diversity of the organizations and individuals consuming the data.

The strategy for implementing an FR is heavily influenced by local contexts, largely because healthcare administration, healthcare infrastructure and governance, and resources for developing the registry will differ by country, region, or state. The first step of the process is to understand the landscape, stakeholders, and assets for the planned implementation area. Do all facilities have some form of electronic data storage (e.g., health information system data hosting infrastructure), and if so, is connectivity (e.g., web-based services) available? Are there current means of identifying facilities, and if so, what gaps need to be filled by the FR? Two examples of preliminary work to document user needs as well as the local context of use can be found in published studies from Nigeria [3] and Uganda [4]. If facilities or the ministry has local data hosting capabilities, then local infrastructure might be leveraged. If local hosting is not available, then the HIE would need to host data. Similarly, if an existing facility identification scheme is defined, it can be codified electronically. Otherwise, a scheme would need to be developed before it could be implemented using an HIE network.

The key to any successful implementation is understanding stakeholder needs and motivations. Because an FR may span a diverse network of stakeholders, with various types of information systems, it is critical to unite entities interested in facility data to ensure concordance of data standardization, thus promoting interoperability and benefits. Local stakeholders may hold the key to understanding what data sources or assets are already established and available for amalgamation into the registry. In Uganda, researchers found that the various approaches for developing the MFL for the Ministry of Health used inconsistent data attributes [4]. Moreover, the nation uses two different methods for uniquely identifying health facilities. This scenario led to confusion as to which data should be prioritized for inclusion in the FR.

Requirements of the FR must be established to address what the registry will achieve and how it will operate. Requirements should be the result of a collaborative effort between FR implementers and key stakeholders. The requirements will be met by appointing data specifications based on both existing metadata and data collected specifically for the purposes of the FR, when necessary.

In Uganda, researchers examined requirements and found that existing paper MFLs used by many providers as well as nongovernmental organizations were incomplete and inaccurate [4]. Existing work processes favored only listing facilities in the local area as well as public clinics and hospitals. Many private healthcare facilities were not included in the existing lists, even those compiled by Ministry of Health officials. Patients themselves also compiled their own MLFs to help family, friends, and neighbors seek care when needed. The disparate, fragmented lists of facilities often meant nearest facilities were overlooked and patient care suffered.

Development of an FR should be an iterative process to recognize, prioritize, and address stakeholder needs or use cases, as well as add new stakeholders or use cases as they develop over time. The iterative process allows the registry to grow by continuously adding entities that provide or consumer facility data, maximizing value to the healthcare community.

Nigeria conducted a series of one-on-one and group consultations to develop FR use cases with stakeholders [3]. The group discussions enabled implementers to validate, and stakeholders agree on, the most important steps in developing the system.

13.4 The value of facility registries

The FR serves as a consistent list across all information systems that track healthcare activity and therefore should serve as a reference for point-of-service applications to facilitate care coordination by managing, for example, referrals and tracking of patient services [5]. As the demand for data-driven decision-making has increased, so has the need to understand where facilities are and what services are available in governing, planning, strengthening, and monitoring the healthcare environment. Facility-based data enables researchers and planners, from both governmental and nongovernmental agencies, to monitor and evaluate how factors like service availability and delivery, health workforce, health information systems, medical products and technologies, financing, and leadership are related to improved health outcomes, responsiveness, social and financial risk protection, and improved efficiency [6]. It further allows for improved resource distribution within a nation [4]. Health services research also depends on identification of specific facilities to analyze how idiosyncratic nuances in governance, policies, leadership, etc., translate into services and outcomes.

The MISSION Act of 2018 enables greater access to care outside of the US Department of Veterans Affairs (VA) health system [7]. Each legislative component in the law requires facility identification. Outside, non-VA facilities need to be identified for care coordination as well as billing purposes, and health services researchers will need to identify VA facilities for evaluation and quality improvement (QI) of eHealth systems [8].

In addition to use by professionals and policy makers, facility registries can be made publicly available for patients to find a facility that matches their healthcare needs. For example, the US Health Resources and Services Administration publishes their facility data warehouse online [9]. The website allows users to find health facilities by name or by entering an address to display nearby facilities with Google maps.

13.4.1 Care coordination

Due to the nature of healthcare professional specialization and relatively limited interaction with patients, each provider may be cognizant of only a small piece of the complexity of a patient's overall health status, leading to fragmented perspectives of patient health [10]. This is particularly true in the case of treating and managing chronic diseases, which may require several specialists and frequent encounters in emergency departments (ED) and hospitals. Bringing together each specialized view of patient's health status, through care coordination, allows for a complete and up-to-date medical history and can improve patient outcomes [11].

An FR provides the means by which care for a patient can be coordinated across the health system. A study by O'Malley et al. [12], which surveyed US physicians, office staff, chief medical officers, electronic medical record (EMR) vendors, and US national experts, found the perception that implementation and use of an EMR facilitates within-office care coordination but not coordination between clinicians or settings (facilities). A survey by Schoen et al. [13] revealed that external care coordination is a challenge in multiple nations. This is because eHealth tools, such as EMRs, are necessary but insufficient, because information systems often lack interoperability [14].

As discussed throughout the book, HIE operates to resolve the discordance between the languages of information systems through application of standards to assimilate data from disparate sources into a shared and longitudinal record (see Chapter 11). This process brings together the specialized views of patient health but still does not ensure coordination. Furthermore, the contemporary healthcare consumer is mobile. A study in the United States found that 40% of ED patients that lived in one state possessed data at multiple institutions, and the majority of EDs shared patients with more than 80 other EDs, putting to rest the commonly held belief that "all healthcare is local" [15].

For primary care physicians to facilitate coordination with and between specialists, emergency care, and hospital encounters, they must be able to accurately identify the location and contact information for where all care is delivered, whether within or across healthcare facilities. In Chapter 29, we profile an example of how HIE can be used to facilitate care coordination within the VA health system. A component of the HIE described in the case study involves identification of the non-VA hospital or ED in which a Veteran was treated. This enables primary care to understand where care was provided and where a follow-up call or message might be needed to gather details about the non-VA encounter.

13.4.2 Quality improvement

Quality, according to the Institute of Medicine, is "the degree to which health services for individuals and populations increase the likelihood of desired health outcomes and are consistent with current professional knowledge" [16]. Under this working definition of quality, QI consists of obtaining measurable improvement in healthcare services and the health outcomes of those receiving services, with the operative word being measurable [9]. At the facility level this may consist of projects that improve some workflow process or implementing clinical decision support for access to up-to-date clinical practice guidelines. However, both the scope of QI projects and measurable results often differ from facility to facility; therefore standardization of quality assessment and improvement is often lacking. It is important to understand how healthcare facilities are improving at an aggregate level in order to achieve national and global goals for health services (e.g., primary cancer prevention) and health outcomes (e.g., surveillance and control of communicable diseases). Currently, few countries possess the data necessary to strengthen their health services by evaluating the quality of health services and monitoring temporal changes [17,18]. Of course, crucial to the process is the ability to comprehensively identify all facilities where patient care is delivered.

The FR maintains the MFL, which establishes a standardized identification process and regular point of contact for each facility. Once established, the FR provides an avenue for accurate data collection and analysis over time, as well as improvement in data harmonization by linking different databases pertaining to the same facility. These data may be used to assess goals at any scale, such as access to health services goals set forth by Healthy People 2030 [19].

13.4.3 Public health

During a public health crisis, a short amount of time could mean the difference between containing the spread of a disease and catastrophic sequelae impacting millions of lives. The ability to identify and communicate with health facilities for information dissemination, coordination, assessment, and utilization of facility-based resources is crucial to rapid response and control of communicable disease outbreaks and other public health emergencies (e.g., natural disasters) [20]. For example, nine out of ten individuals, if susceptible (i.e., unvaccinated or never exposed), who come into close contact with a measles patient will subsequently develop measles [21].

Intuitively, rapid response to suspected measles cases is pivotal to preventing widespread transmission. Consider the outbreak of measles tied to Disney theme parks in Southern California where 39 measles cases occurred among park patrons between December 17th, 2014 and December 20th, 2014. By February 8th, 2015 an additional 86 cases from seven states (mostly California) and three countries were identified as linked to this outbreak, demonstrating the ease at which the disease is transmitted even among a largely vaccinated population [22]. The threat of catastrophic outbreaks of communicable disease is much greater in many developing nations, where the causative organisms are more common and healthcare infrastructure is often deficient, thus specifically highlighting the need to know where facilities are located and what services they can handle during a public health emergency. More information on the role of an FR during a large-scale public health emergency like the COVID-19 pandemic is discussed in Box 13.1.

Identifying facilities remains suboptimal in many nations, even in the United States. Prior to COVID-19, a study by Dixon and colleagues [24] found the data field indicating the name of the submitter (e.g., physician, hospital, or clinic) in electronic laboratory messages sent for routine communicable disease reporting were complete for only 57.4%–66.5% of transactions, and the address of the submitter was complete for only 84.6% of transactions [24]. Incomplete facility data can impede the ability of public health professionals to perform surveillance and manage a disease outbreak or public health emergency in a timely and effective manner.

A study by Batteiger et al. [25] used facility information to examine where populations sought diagnosis and treatment of sexually transmitted diseases. Using the information, the team hoped public health agencies could target specific facilities for education programs with providers to improve adoption of CDC-recommended treatment guidelines. Furthermore, public health agencies could use the information to identify where subpopulations (e.g., pregnant women, men who have sex with men) might be recruited into public health programs aimed at reducing disease burden in the community. Researchers found that facility information was available on just 63.3% of females and 81.2% of males [25] despite widespread adoption of EHR systems in the community. Facility information would be useful and could support public health programs if it were more generally available in electronic systems.

13.5 Components of a facility registry

An FR consists of primarily an MFL and the functional components to facilitate contribution to and consumption of the MFL (Fig. 13.1). However, what constitutes a facility in the MFL will vary based on contextual factors and stakeholder needs. After assessing such requirements for the MFL, the HIE can define or customize the following attributes of the MFL as depicted in Fig. 13.2:

- Data specification—technical specification document outlining the data elements to be included in the signature and service domains that define a facility.
- Signature domain—collection of attributes which identify both private and public facilities.
- Service domain—information about the facility with respect to infrastructure, workforce, and/or types of services offered.

In the remainder of this section of the chapter, we briefly introduce the functionality of a FR then discuss the MFL attributes, offering

BOX 13.1

Facility management during the COVID-19 pandemic.

Early on in the COVID-19 pandemic, it became clear that limited hospital resources (e.g., intensive care beds, ventilators, oxygen) were needed to treat severely impacted patients. Tracking hospital resource utilization was critical to enabling redistribution of resources from the national stockpile in the United States as well as guiding patients to the nearest available hospital for treatment [23]. However, public health agencies struggled to keep up with the status (e.g., open, closed, on diversion) of health facilities, especially hospitals. Agencies were also challenged to understand how many intensive care beds in a facility could be staffed, which became a variable that changed daily as clinical staff also became infected and needed to be quarantined. Moreover, routine reporting on hospital status and resources was a manual, resource-intensive process for most hospitals. This is illustrated in Fig. 13.3, which shows facility status in the metropolitan area of Atlanta. The facilities in orange are closed, and the facilities in yellow are impacted but open. In multiple waves of the COVID-19 pandemic, hospitals filled to capacity and diverted patients to facilities further away from patients' homes. The situation necessitated clinicians to call facilities in other states, sometimes over 300 miles away, to find an available bed.

While the map is helpful in geospatially identifying closed facilities, the data behind this system are manually entered by hospital staff each day. In many hospitals, there was confusion as to who should be responsible for collecting the various data required by public health authorities. Those collecting the data could spend hours each day validating information that came from multiple information systems within the hospital. Furthermore, operational status could change between shifts, such that data entered into the system 6 hours ago were no longer accurate.

The COVID-19 pandemic therefore underscored the importance of facility data and the need for a FR. However, the pandemic also demonstrated that existing information systems and data collection processes are woefully inadequate to handle a large-scale pandemic or disaster [23]. HIE would enable routine, automated data capture into an FR that would be enhanced with visualization tools like the one depicted in Fig. 13.3. However, without interoperability, the systems are likely to be outdated and unhelpful in the context of a large-scale event [14].

guidance on their design and implementation. We further reference two examples of FR implementations in the countries of Rwanda and Tanzania. The FR in these countries utilized the open-source reference implementation, Resource Map [26]. Resource Map was developed by InSTEDD, a nonprofit technology organization that focuses on solutions which support health, safety, and sustainable development.

13.6 Facility registry functionality

Similar to other registry components, the functionality of an FR will depend on the needs of stakeholders in a given context. The functionality will iteratively evolve over time as the scope of the registry is expanded. Regardless of scope, several core FR functionalities exist, and are presented in Table 13.1.

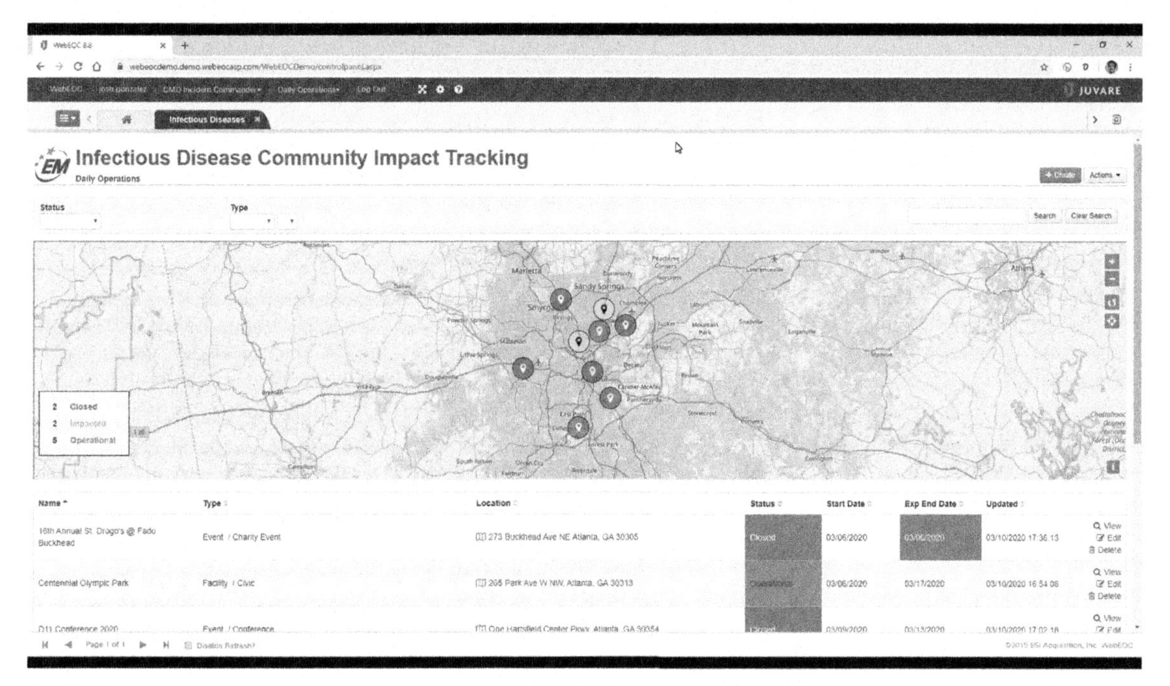

FIGURE 13.3 Screenshot from the Juvare application, illustrating how facility registry data can be geographically represented allowing users to at-a-glance view free/busy facilities.

Briefly, the FR functional components include the following:

- Managing the MFL by adding, editing, deleting fields and records;
- Creating custom queries through free text searches, filtering, and grouping;
- Importing and exporting data in various formats for ease of contribution and/or consumption;
- Geospatial mapping of the physical location and attributes of facilities;
- Integrating or interfacing an FR with other systems or applications, using SOA or application programming interfaces (APIs), for interoperability and graphical user interfacing (see Chapter 8); and
- Managing user authentication for MFL access and layering authorization for MFL capabilities (e.g., read/write).

The user stories in Table 13.1 are all examples of successfully implemented FR requests from various stakeholders in Rwanda and Tanzania, and further elucidate how the same functionality can be implemented to serve various needs based on the context.

Although there are many functions that could be implemented in an FR, OpenHIE has defined a set of minimum functional requirements [27]. Most of these functions are recommended, allowing maximum flexibility for the FR to evolve over time as nations evolve their HIE and digital health infrastructures. However, the international collaboration does specify the following functions as required for facility registries:

- The system shall support the ability to create, define, and evolve the attributes and associated data dictionary for a registry.

TABLE 13.1 User stories of core facility registry functionalities.

Facility registry function	User story for facility registry functions
Managing the master facility list (MFL)	• Collecting and storing a MFL so that users and systems can access and update trustworthy facility information. • Easily editing and adapting the data dictionary of the facility data to remain agile as system requirements change. • Creating fields with single and multiple select lists that can predefine the options available for user selection.
Searching, Filtering, and Grouping	• Finding a facility by looking up a specific name, identifier, or other field. • Filtering facilities by multiple attributes, such as ownership and facility type, to determine the catchment area served by the area managed by the user. • The ability to view a group of facilities based upon their administrative zone. • Identifying empty fields in order to curate and complete data as needed.
Importing and Exporting	• Exporting a list of facilities into a spreadsheet for use outside the FR. • Importing data contained in CSV format to quickly get started with an existing list.
Mapping and Visualization	• Establishing the ability to find facilities and visualize administrative zone boundaries. • Establishing the ability to measure the distance between facility locations on a map. • Distinguishing different types of facilities from one another graphically while looking at a map (e.g., hospitals from medical clinics, one partner from another)
Integration and application programming interface (API)	• Establishing the ability to consume and provide data between the registry and other systems using an API. • Specifying codes to fields, and to options in lookup fields, so that the information exposed in APIs have a stable schema that is not dependent on labels and internationalization. • Creating a notification mechanism around changes to data, metadata, permissions, etc.
Authentication and Authorization	• Creating accounts, managing credentials, resetting passwords, etc. • Specifying public collections/layers, to allow for public users to perform searches, and access the API for specified. • Specifying explicit permissions for users to view and/or edit data in different layers.

- The system shall support the ability to create, define, and maintain multiorganizational hierarchies of facilities and related geo-objects.
- The system shall support the ability to set up and manage users, permissions for reading data, writing data (posting, validation, publishing), viewing data, and system administration.
- The system shall support the ability to do bulk imports.

13.7 Data specification

A data specification document is a technical tool describing the MFL data elements or the information to be managed in the FR. This is a similar concept to a data dictionary where the contents and format of data elements in the system are documented. Critical to the process of data specification is input from a representative group of stakeholders who will use the FR. A number of recommendations for data specification have been proposed but stakeholder input and iterative development are necessary to ensure the FR is responsive to the users' needs and applicable to the local context. The basic layout of a specification document includes:

- *Variable Name*—The short name and/or the database code used to describe the data element.
- *Definition*—A simple description of the data element, along with any relevant context.
- *Data Type*—Predefined data types are helpful to understand the formatting associated with a data element. Some common data types that have been used in other facility registries include: text, numeric, yes/no, select one, select many, hierarchy, date, site, user, identifier, email, and phone.
- *Hierarchy or List Metadata*—Hierarchical, single, and multiple select data elements will have additional categorical or leaf metadata which should also be documented in the data specification.
- *Data Rules*—A description of constraints or conditions that should be applied to a data elements to improve accuracy and clarity. A single select variable, numerical, text field, or a specific algorithm for an identifier such as the Luhn algorithm.
- *Data Source*—A description of the individual, group, and system where this information is generated from. Often a FR will collect partial updates from other systems and it is helpful to understand the source of each data element.
- *Standards*—Documenting any semantic standards or common code sets used as metadata. Documenting these will help with interoperability with other systems.

OpenHIE recommends that countries use the MFL resource guide from the WHO [28]. Specifically, OpenHIE recommends that the FR support the collection of data for the following minimum facility attributes dataset [27]:

- Signature domain
  - Facility name
  - Facility type (e.g., hospital, clinic, mobile clinic, lab, pharmacy)
  - Facility ownership/managing authority
  - Facility physical address
  - Facility contact information
  - Record date
  - Operational status
  - Administrative level/areas
  - Geographic coordinates
  - Facility unique identifier
- Service domain
  - Type of services offered—Lab, HIV, TB, etc.
  - Human resource for health, numbers by cadre
  - Opening and closing times
  - Common and mapped identifiers per location
  - Details on infrastructure—power, water, etc.

These domains and data elements are described in further detail below.

13.7.1 Signature domain

The signature domain is a collection of attributes which identify both private and public facilities. In many cases, such as facility name, a single attribute is not sufficient for canonical identification. However, implementation of a unique identifier will, in most cases, provide sufficient discriminatory power for positive facility identification. Recommendations of exemplar data elements by the Health Facility Assessment Technical Group and World Health Organization (WHO) are described Table 13.2, but may not be applicable in all countries or contexts [18,28].

To respond to the need for current and standardized facility data, the OpenHIE Facility Registry Community recommends proven tools, processes, technologies, and core functional

TABLE 13.2 The signature domain: suggested data fields from the World Health Organization [18] and Health Facility Assessment Technical Working Group [29].

Attribute	Description	Suggested data rules
Date of data collection	The date is invaluable when examining time trends and combining datasets.	Standardized entry based on countries' preferred presentation.
Health facility country registration code or unique identifier	If a district, state, or national ID exists it should be associated with all data from a facility. This ID is the authoritative and unequivocal facility identifier and acts as the primary key to link data sources.	Should be unique, not vary over time, and be assigned in the same manner for all facilities within the country.
Facility name	The official (full) name of the facility.	A text field for the legal name of the facility, free of abbreviations, and with proper punctuation.
Facility type	The classification of the facility. Example: acute care hospital, clinic, free standing emergency room, long-term care, etc.	Standardization will vary by country of implementation. A central authority (e.g., Ministry of Health) should provide facilities with a structured list for selection.
Facility ownership	Examples: military, private, government.	Standardization will vary by country of implementation. A central authority (e.g., Ministry of Health) should provide facilities with a structured list for selection.
Facility location/ address and contact information	The physical location of the facility. Other pertinent information includes main telephone and fax number, main email address, name of director and director's contact information.	Standardization will vary by country of implementation. The address should be given to the lowest possible administrative level and parsed into subparts (e.g., street name, street number, ZIP, state/provenance).
Administrative units	Refers to the facilities location in terms of district, provenance, census tract, etc. This is useful for differentiating facilities with identical or similar names.	Avoid including facility name in the field and indicate designated level in hierarchy (e.g., 0 = national, 1 = provincial, 2 = district).
Geographical coordinates	The physical coordinates of the facility.	Implementation should reflect the preferred national coordinate system. Generally latitude and longitude recorded in decimal degrees referencing the WGS84 system is often preferred.
Operational status	The operational status of the facility, such as operational, closed, licensed, pending licensure, etc.	Each country should provide operational statuses based on regulatory and licensing bodies.

requirements to implement facility registries. These resources have been derived from existing reference implementations in Tanzania and Rwanda, among others. As an example of the signature domain, the Rwanda health facility registration form is presented in Fig. 13.4. Although the structure of the form could be used in many contexts, the content will differ

1. Identification			
Health Facility Name :		FOSA ID: (HMIS unit only)	
Type of health facility :	☐ National Referral Hospital (HNR) ☐ Provincial Referral Hospital (PH) ☐ District Hospital (HD) ☐ Health Center (CS) ☐ Health Post (PS) ☐ Dispensary (DISP) ☐ Community Dispensary (FOSACOM)	☐ Prison Clinic (PRIS) ☐ Medical Clinic (CLIN) ☐ Military Hospital (HM) ☐ District Pharmacy (DP) ☐ Mutuelle/CBHI section (MU) ☐ Blood Bank (BB) ☐ Other, Specify : .	
Status :	☐ Active : ☐ Planned, specify probable opening date : ☐ Closed :		
Category:	☐ Public ☐ Agrée ☐ Private ☐ Community owned ☐ Parastatal (e.g. Military, Police, Prison, State run dispensaries)		
Date inaugurated :			
Name of titulaire/director :		NID #	
email of titulaire/director:		Cell phone #	
Name of primary referral/reporting facility[1]			
Implementing partner organization:			
2. Geographic Coordinates			
Province:		Latitude:	
District:		Longitude:	
Sector:		Catchment area population (list villages in section 5):	
Cell:		Source of population data :	
Village:		Year of population estimate :	
PO box:			
Street:		Number	Complement

FIGURE 13.4 Identifying facilities with the Rwanda Health Facility Registry Form signature domain.

based on each country's facility nomenclature and hierarchical structure.

13.7.2 Service domain

The service domain contains information about the facility in terms of infrastructure, workforce, and types of services offered. Ideally these data should depict a more granular view of the facility, allowing for assessments of the facility's resources, understanding if the needs of the facility catchment area are being met, and planning for the future in terms of staffing and infrastructure. A catchment area is the population which a given facility routinely serves. For example, if there are four facilities in a particular district of a malaria endemic country and only one offers malarial prophylaxis, diagnosis, and treatment they may be overwhelmed by patients, from both an infrastructure and staffing point of view. Identifying the gap in services offered will allow for policy makers to make educated decisions about resource allocation.

4. Services offered (check all services that are offered)					
03		**Clinical services**	06		**Pharmacy**
0301		Primary Outpatient Curative Consultation (CPC)	0601		Pharmacy
0302		Hospitalization	07		**Prosthetics and Medical devices**
0303		Emergency care	0701		Prosthetics
0304		Dentistry	0702		Other medical devices
0305		General Ophthalmology	08		**Complementary actions to promote health**
0306		Integrated Management of Childhood Illness	0801		Hygiene and environmental health
0307		Management of gender violence	0802		Medico-Legal documentation
0308		Mental Health Services	0803		Pre-marital Consultation
0309		Physical therapy	0804		Vector and Zoonosis control
0310		Nutritional Rehabilitation	0805		Epidemiological Surveillance and Response
0311		Cardiovascular care and treatment	02		**Diagnostic services**
0312		TB care and treatment	0201		Laboratory
0313		Care and treatment for persons living with HIV/AIDS	0202		Voluntary Counseling and Testing
0314		Diabetes care and treatment	0203		Ultrasound
0315		Other Non Communicable disease (NCD) care and treatment	0204		Medical Imagery (x-ray)
0316		Management of dystocic pregnancies	01		**Health promotion and prevention**
0317		Post-abortion care	0101		Ante-natal consultation
0318		Deliveries - high risk	0102		Behavior Change Communication/Health Education
0319		Deliveries – normal	0103		Community mobilization
0320		Newborn care	0104		Family Planning
04		**Surgical services**	0105		Post Natal Consultation
0401		Major surgical interventions	0106		Growth Monitoring/Nutrition Surveillance
0402		Minor surgical interventions	0107		Vaccination
05		**Organ transplants and Blood transfusions**	0108		Psychosocial support
0501		Blood bank	0109		General Health Promotion Activities
0502		Organ transplants			

FIGURE 13.5 Capturing facility health service availability with the Rwanda Health Facility Registry Form.

The services offered section in the Rwandan health facility registration form is provided as an example in Fig. 13.5. In this case, data are captured using simple Boolean (yes/no) responses by asking respondents to check all services that apply. Types of services are binned as clinical, surgical, organ transplants and blood transfusions, pharmacy, prosthetics and medical devices, complementary actions to promote health, diagnostic, and health promotion and prevention. As one can see in Fig. 13.5, this is a simple method for collecting detailed data regarding services rendered at the facility.

The data regarding facility infrastructure can be at a high level, such as having inpatient or maternity beds, or described in more detail by including the types of rooms and beds, vehicles own by the facility, physical barriers for infection control and personal protective equipment, and facility sanitation, among other things. The data elements captured regarding infrastructure are largely country-specific. In Rwanda, and other developing countries, it is pertinent to collect fundamental information that may not be relevant to developed countries, such as facilities' power source (if applicable), water source, internet connectivity, modes of transportation, and X-ray capabilities (Fig. 13.6). In addition to basic services, such as X-ray and laboratory testing, stakeholders of developed countries may be more interested in advanced technologies, such as digital imaging, clinical decision support, Da Vinci surgical robotics, smart patient rooms, and robotic drug dispensing.

The final data element captured in the service domain relates to the types and number of staff the facility employs. Although more detailed data may be available from the health worker registry, as will be discussed in Chapter 14, it is important to maintain an aggregated list of

3. Infrastructure			
Number of rooms (clinical and administrative) :		Number of Patient beds:	
Transport available : (and functional)	# of ambulances # of cars # of motorcycles	Principal Water Source:	☐ National piped water supply ☐ Local piped water supply ☐ Protected well ☐ Open well ☐ Surface water (river, lake, etc.) ☐ Rain water reservoir ☐ Water Truck ☐ No regular water source
Principal Electricity Source :	☐ National Grid ☐ Generator, specify KVA : ☐ Solar panels ☐ No electricity		
Cold chain:	# of functional refrigerators/freezers:	Computers :	# functioning
Communication: (belonging to FOSA)	☐ Fixed Telephone N° ☐ Mobile Telephone N° ☐ Radio	Internet Connection:	☐ Cell Modem ☐ Fixed Line (ADSL, fibre) ☐ Satellite (VSAT) ☐ Wireless (WIMAX, etc.) ☐ No internet connection

FIGURE 13.6 Assessment of facility infrastructure using the Rwanda Health Facility Registry Form.

personnel for each facility for emergency preparedness and assessing facility-specific workforce needs. A nonexhaustive list of proposed data elements for the service domain is listed in Table 13.3.

We now discuss two sets of candidates that an HIE or country might consider when considering the design of its MFL. The first set is derived from a report by the WHO. The second comes from a US-based case study involving HIE to improve disability determination.

13.8 Creating unique identifiers

The long-term goal of the FR should be to develop and uniformly implement unique identifiers for facilities. Furthermore, as discussed above, it is often challenging to uniquely identify facilities by their names alone. Many techniques are available for generating and assigning unique facility identifiers for the signature domain. Regardless of the method employed, manual generation is discouraged because of the increased likelihood of error and duplication. The intent is to create and disseminate a standardized, unique identifier which serves as the primary, authoritative and unequivocal identifier for a given facility. Thus, once assigned, the identifier must be permanently attached to a facility regardless of changes in physical location, ownership, and name.

13.8.1 World Health Organization candidate identifiers

Three types of identifiers are described in a WHO report on creating MFLs, each with their own merits and pitfalls: integer codes, facility codes, and universally unique identifiers (UUID) [18]. An example of a fourth unique identifier is the facility identification number used in the Tanzania, Africa, FR.

13.8.1.1 Integer codes

Integer codes are automatically generated and managed by a central authority. The numbers generated are considered information free because they do not contain any facility-specific attributes, such as an administrative unit prefix. For this reason, integer codes can stand the test of time when facilities relocate or alter their affiliations, and they are guaranteed

TABLE 13.3 Possible facility-specific data elements for services, infrastructure, and workforce for the service domain.

Services offered	Infrastructure	Workforce
• General Clinical Services (Inpatient/Outpatient Care)	• Types of Rooms	• Primary care physicians
• Malaria Diagnosis and Treatment	• Types of Beds	• Specialist physicians
• TB Diagnosis, Care and Treatment	• Ambulances	• Subspecialist physicians
• Cardiovascular Care and Treatment	• Cars	• Physician assistants
• HIV/AIDS Prevention	• Motorcycles	• Nurse practitioners
• HIV/AIDS Care and Treatment	• Sterilization and Infection Control	• Nurses
• Therapeutics	• Referral Point	• Radiology technicians
• Prosthetics and Medical Devices	• Source of Energy	• Laboratory technologists
• Health Promotion and Disease Prevention	• Mobile Networks	• Respiratory therapists
• Diagnostic Services	• Source of Water	• Midwives
• Reproductive and Child Health Care Services	• Toilet Facility	• Clinical nursing assistants
• Growth Monitoring/Nutrition Surveillance	• Toilet Remarks	• Medical assistants
• Oral Health Service (Dental Services)	• Waste Management	
• ENT Services		
• Emergency Preparedness		

to be unique when generated by a central authority. When implemented in decentralized architectures, a range of numbers can be assigned to each administrative unit. For example, District A corresponds to combination of three integers from 000 to 100 and district B is represented by 101 to 200.

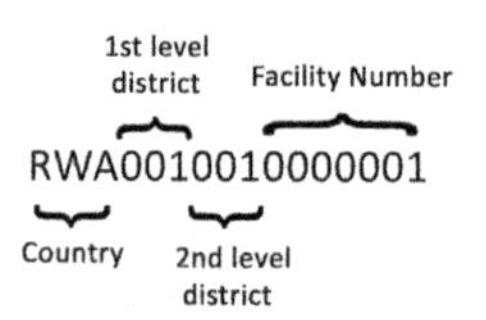

FIGURE 13.7 Components of a facility code.

13.8.1.2 *Facility codes*

Identifiers containing a combination of numbers and letters that frequently include some piece of facility-specific information, which may or may not be human readable, are referred to as facility codes. For example, the code in Fig. 13.7 can be segmented into three letters for country code, followed by three numbers for the first administrative district, the next three identify the lower-level district, then a series of numbers identifying the facility. The primary difficulty of facility codes is they would need to be updated if a facility was to move or the country restructured their districts.

13.8.1.3 *Universally unique identifiers*

Also known as globally unique identifiers, UUID represent a standard identifier that is ubiquitous throughout computer applications. UUIDs are a 128-bit value—for example, 261a7f40-1f9f-11e5-adfc-0002a5d5c51b—that can be uniquely generated by a standard algorithm regardless assigning entity's location. As such, UUIDs are well suited for decentralized architectures where no central issuing authority is designated.

13.8.1.4 *The Tanzanian facility identifier number*

The Tanzanian FR identifies facilities using an auto-generated sequential number allocated to each facility when it is added to the MFL. It is generated by the central FR and provided back to the health community for subsequent use, replacing the old registration ID. The ID follows the format: xxxxxx-y, where xxxxxx is a six digit numeric code, and y is a one digit check digit, generated via the Luhn algorithm. The Luhn algorithm, an ISO standard, is a modulus 10 "double-add-double" algorithm which is used to generate check digits in numerous identification systems including the US Centers for Medicare and Medicaid Services (CMS) National Provider Identifier (NPI) [30].

13.8.2 Other candidates for creating unique identifiers

In search of unique identifiers for facilities in a US-based HIE, Dixon et al. [1] considered the following candidates: object identifiers (OIDs), NPIs, and health industry numbers (HIN).

13.8.2.1 *Object identifiers*

OIDs are globally unique identifiers for objects in a distributed system, and they are an alternative to UUIDs. Many healthcare networks and facilities in the United States already possess OIDs, as they are required for HL7 CDA-based HIE transactions in compliance with MU to identify assigning authorities in messages. Unfortunately, OIDs are sometimes re-used within a given health system network of facilities. Therefore, to be effective, unique OIDs would need to be created and maintained at a health system level making maintenance of an MFL for a community or nation challenging as health systems expand and contract.

13.8.2.2 *National provider identifiers*

Created by CMS, NPIs uniquely identify providers, but providers frequently practice at multiple medical facilities. CMS also allows healthcare organizations and facilities to request NPIs, so an alternative approach would be to require facilities to obtain an NPI if it did not already have one. However, many medical centers are large campuses composed of numerous and variable buildings, clinics, private offices, and other care delivery units. The NPI of a medical center can apply to multiple physical locations that vary greatly in the type(s) of care delivered (e.g., intensive, acute, rehabilitation, chronic, long-term residential). Therefore there would have to be consensus on the level of granularity of the lowest denominator NPI.

13.8.2.3 *Health industry numbers*

The HIN is a unique identifier used in electronic data interchange transactions among healthcare trading partners for supply chain management [31]. These identifiers are maintained by the Health Industry Business Communications Council, an accredited international standards development organization which uses multiple sources to identify human healthcare facilities and assign each a unique identifier. A database of HIN identifiers is available for licensing. Current HIN licensees are predominantly pharmaceutical companies, medical device manufacturers and wholesalers [32]. To date, there has been no use of the HIN database within HIEs despite the list of licensees including so-called data intermediaries.

The identifier chosen to uniquely represent facilities should reflect stakeholder consensus as well as governance and healthcare structures. Beyond unique identification, the FR provides the technology to standardize and manage data that describe the facility and will be the focus for the remainder of the chapter. The 2014 Ebola virus outbreak in West Africa represents a prime example of the requisite need for data which goes beyond facility identification. It is essential to quickly ascertain facilities with personnel capable of handling the deadly potentially deadly virus and also have the infrastructure required to protect healthcare workers and other patients (e.g., full body coverage and isolation rooms). Identifying well-equipped facilities allows public health to act fast in establishing centers to immediately provide care and prevent further transmission of the virus.

13.9 Data sources for constructing the master facility list

Limiting expenditures in the healthcare environment is often a top priority for policy makers. Therefore those implementing an FR should use existing data sources when possible. The initial goal in creating an FR should be to compile a complete MFL for the country or service area. If a MFL is already in place, this should be used to populate the FR. Even in the case where no MFL exists, most countries will have some type of facility list, with varying degrees of completeness and frequency of updates.

An MFL is often governed by the country's Ministry of Health, although the list may be generated by a separate licensing regulatory body or health management information system, such as the International Health Information Systems Programme supported by the University of Oslo [33]. In the United States, several sources of facility data exist, including but not limited to the CMS NPI, the Health Resources and Services Administration's health center data warehouse, the Social Security Administration (SSA), and governmental public health agencies. Further, disease-specific registries (e.g., cancer, HIV, tuberculosis) may provide facility information where each patient received care.

Existing surveys, while not necessarily comprehensive, will assist in populating the MFL as well as obtaining additional service domain data. Examples of surveys include, the WHO Service Availability and Readiness Assessment and the Service Provision Assessment by the US Agency for International Development [34,35].

As should be apparent by now, it is unlikely that a single source will populate all of the data elements desired, establishing the need to link data on a facility from multiple databases. The common identifiers in the signature domain of the MFL provide a mechanism to link disparate data sources to obtain more complete data for the services domain. However, just as the case in linking client-level data, in most cases, facility databases will not be inherently interoperable establishing the need for metadata and standards within the FR.

13.10 An example from the US social security administration

In 2010 approximately 18.7%, or 56.6 million civilian, noninstitutionalized US citizens reported a communicative, mental, or physical disability to the US SSA [36]. The SSA determines disability and awards benefits, including health insurance benefits, through a sequential process that incorporates the medical, legal, and vocational aspects of disabilities [37]. As a part of the claim submission process, individuals submitting claims are required to list the name and addresses for all healthcare providers and facilities from which they received care and theses reported facilities should match healthcare records. Needless to say, the existing paper-based system is considered by researchers, the Institute of Medicine, and SSA advisory board to be inefficient, often incomplete, and outdated [38,39]. Therefore, in 2010, SSA partnered with the Regenstrief Institute

(RI) to facilitate evaluation of submitted claims using a statewide HIE. RI utilized the HL7 continuity of care document (CCD) standard (based on the Clinical Document Architecture or CDA) to populate a comprehensive EHR using information from various healthcare facilities [1].

In total, between May 2012 and June 2013, RI received over six million encounter transactions and delivered 7732 CCDs to SSA. However, SSA noticed the facility names contained within the CCDs differed from the claimant submissions and were uninterpretable by SSA case reviewers. Some facilities would include a full name (e.g., "xyz clinic"), while others would be cryptic, such as "NORTH." For example, "WKRANC" represented a hospital cardiology service, a university hospital was simply named "UH," and the surgical ward at a hospital was represented as "B2." Furthermore, the majority of transactions (60.4%) did not provide any value in the CCD field designated for facility identification.

When examining the issue, RI noted that HL7 CCD specifications allow virtually any information to represent a facility. Facilities can be represented by both free-text as well as coded elements, yet the codes can be locally developed and maintained. In one case, a large 20 hospital health system used more than 9000 distinct facility identifiers, uniquely identifying every campus, floor, unit, and bed in its network. Other examples included different facility identifiers depending on the information system (e.g., laboratory, pharmacy, radiology, etc.) which transmitted the message [1]. Clearly, such facility identifiers are not useful to SSA, nor would they be useful for a FR.

This study highlights one of many use cases for a unique and universal facility identifier in the United States and that current systems not only lack standardized identifiers needed for interoperability but are frequently uninterpretable and impossible to map to standards for data linkage. In order to support care coordination, public health, QI and assurance, research, policy making, and other use cases, the various stakeholders must agree and implement a standardized method for identifying facilities. Once the data specifications are agreed upon, an FR can be tasked with maintaining these data.

13.11 Mapping disparate facility data

Because disparate facility data like those highlighted in the SSA case study exist in multiple nations, there are efforts to help nations reconcile facility codes. Facility Match is an example of a tool for identifying, reconciling, and synthesizing duplicate or incomplete facility records across multiple datasets [40]. Originally developed for DATIM, a PEPFAR funded Project, the Facility Match tool takes disparate facility lists and allows users to reconcile facilities into a single MFL. For example, users could reconcile a list of public health facilities from a district health office with a list of health facilities in a country maintained by an NGO. A ministry might reconcile all lists from its district health offices across the country. The resulting MFL, once exported from the tool, could become the canonical MFL for a district or nation.

The Facility Match tool has been used in Ethiopia (Box 13.2) to reconcile and maintain facility data. Other nations have used DHIS2 to create and maintain their MFL. Other nations have built custom applications for creating and maintaining their MFL. There are also efforts at the regional level to map facilities across borders. For example, the African Society for Laboratory Management hosts an online resource map that maintains and visualizes a laboratory facility list for the continent [41]. The LabMaP program asks nations to voluntarily submit information on its laboratories with a goal of mapping laboratory capacity in the region.

BOX 13.2

A case example from Ethiopia: updating the master facility registry.

Ethiopia is Africa's oldest independent country and the continent's second largest in terms of population with over 117 million people. Although the nation is considered a low resource or developing country, it has one of the fastest growth rates in the world, and the nation seeks to be middle income by 2025.

Currently Ethiopia operates its second MFR. Initially, the nation sought to adopt the global good Resource Map as its first MFR (see Fig. 13.8). The original scope outlined by the Federal Ministry of Health included technical requirements and customizations that required workarounds (e.g., custom code or programming, workflow adaptations for FR users), resulting in an implementation in which the tool was utilized in a nonstandard way. The workarounds resulted in performance gaps, because the customization forced the software to work in a way in which it was not designed. A less than ideal workflow due to the workarounds frustrated users, and this prompted the nation to review and revise the technology stack upon which the MFR is developed and maintained.

Because Ethiopia decided to update its technology stack, it also decided to pursue moving to the Fast Healthcare Interoperability Resources (FHIR) standard during its redesign. Moving to FHIR was essential as the MFR is a shared service in Ethiopian eHealth Architecture (Fig. 13.9) and the nation desired to ensure a standards-based approach was adopted. As depicted in the figure, Master Facility Registration is a core service for the national health ICT infrastructure. FHIR ensures the service can interoperate with point-of-service ICT systems across the country.

The new technology stack (Fig. 13.10) features three components that enable FHIR-based queries of the MFR from other applications part of the Ethiopian eHealth Architecture. First, the backend database for the MFR is now hosted using PostgreSQL, an open source database management system. A customized API using .NET Core facilitates queries using the FHIR standard and provides an interface to the UI component for management of the MFR. The final component is the UI, developed using Angular, an open-source web application framework. The UI component allows authorized users at the Ministry of Health to update the MFR, such as adding new facilities or editing details about an existing facility.

Implementation challenges

An implementation challenge for Ethiopia was the variety of health information systems previously implemented by various partners (e.g., NGOs) in the recent past. The myriad systems implemented nationally made it challenging to populate the MFR with facility information. Because DHIS2 is widely implemented across Ethiopia, the nation selected it to serve as the primary source of MFR data when constructing the MFR. Data from additional information systems were reconciled using Facility Match, an open-source software tool from IntraHealth that identifies and synthesizes health facility records from multiple sources [40]. Missing facilities had to be entered manually using the new UI component.

Following implementation, Ethiopia designated DHIS2 to be the primary recipient of data from the new MFR. Each night, a scheduled process updates DHIS2 with new information from the MFR. This enables users of DHIS2 to have current, up-to-date MFR data at their fingertips. This benefits the whole country as DHIS2 is used widely throughout Ethiopia.

Another challenge when building the MFR was collecting accurate geospatial information

BOX 13.2 (*cont'd*)

on facilities. The Ministry of Health attempted to capture geo-coordinates for facilities by reconciling the consolidated, clean list of facilities with Geographical Information System data collected from Ethiopian Geospatial Agency. However, only 25% of facilities registered in the MFR could be matched. As a workaround, the nation developed an Open Data Kit (ODK) form that field staff could use to collect geolocation data at the district level which could later be imported into the MFR. ODK is a set of open-source applications that allow creation of questionnaires (using the Xform standard) that can be completed using mobile devices or tablet computers with the data entered stored centrally for use by backend systems.

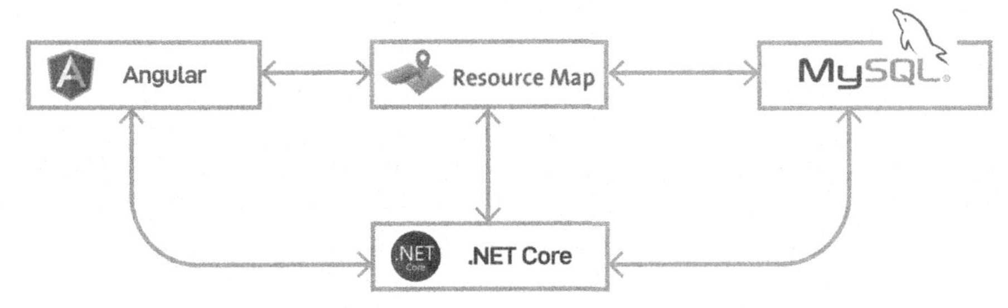

FIGURE 13.8 Previous design of Ethiopian Master Facility Registry.

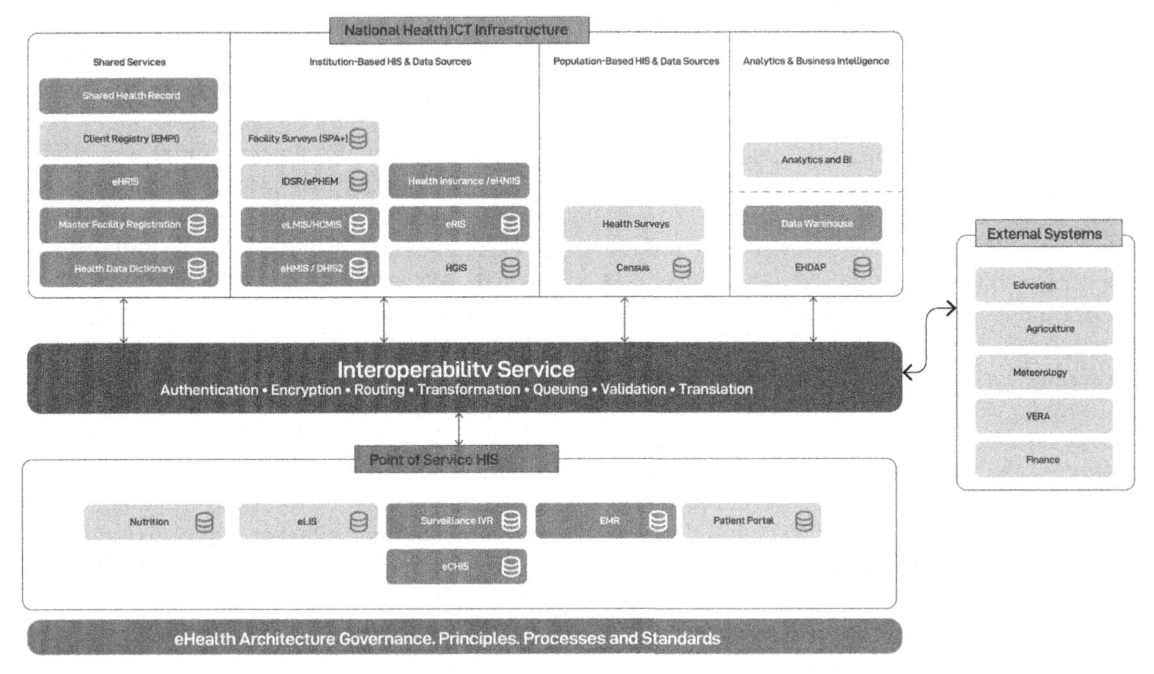

FIGURE 13.9 Current eHealth Architecture in Ethiopia.

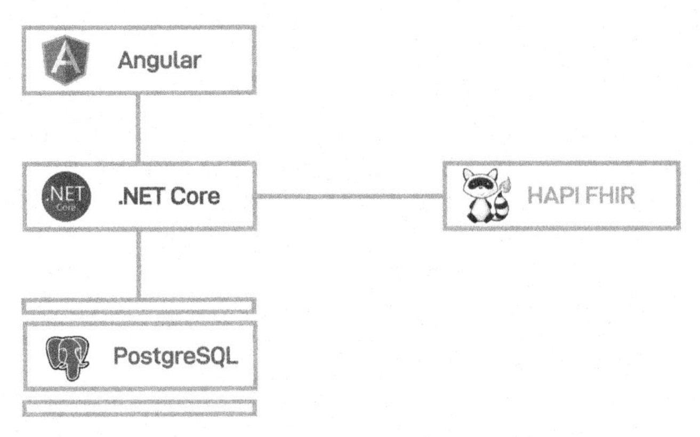

FIGURE 13.10 Current design of Ethiopian Master Facility Registry.

13.12 Emerging trends

Coming out of the COVID-19 pandemic, multiple nations are looking to strengthen their public health infrastructure for the future. Infrastructure enhancement includes investments in health information technologies, including HIE. A critical component of an enhanced public health infrastructure is an FR. If a state (e.g., Indiana, California) or nation could develop a comprehensive FR, it could better identify capacity and capabilities for health service provision within its jurisdiction during a public health crisis. Routine data electronically shared between clinics and hospitals with ministries of health about bed availability, staffing, resources (e.g., ventilators, PPE), and services offered (e.g., intensive care, radiology) could reduce health worker burden and enable rapid response. Even in times of noncrisis it would help public health authorities assess capacity, such as assessing whether the region contains any OB-GYN desserts. Routine assessment would aid in planning the location of the next district hospital or redeployment of specialists or the location of a new telemedicine service.

It is recommended that health systems examine their existing MFL processes and procedures, and plan for the development and implementation of an FR. Data elements such as bed capacity, specialty services offered, and staffing should be considered in addition to the data described in this chapter as typical in existing FR implementations. Times have changed, and the FR for the future likely needs additional information to aid in situational awareness during a crisis. Regardless, national digital health (or eHealth) strategies should include a roadmap toward the use of an FR for public health, QI, and care coordination. The FR could play a central role in strengthening the resilience of the health system as well as preparedness for the next major population health threat.

Integrating the Healthcare Enterprise (IHE) hosts an international profile entitled Care Services Discovery (CSD) that aims at facilitating the exchange of facility data (along with organizational and provider information) [42]. This profile supports querying of a MFL (called the Care Services Directory) to return information on a given facility. A Care Services InfoManager looks for updated information facilities and finds available care services at facilities that can be returned to the application that queries for information. There are subcomponents that allow for querying whether a given provider is free or busy for the purposes of scheduling. The profile was last updated in 2016 but is available for Trial Implementation. Furthermore, IHE created a new profile in 2021 focused on making

CSD information available on mobile platforms using FHIR [43]. Nations should consider whether either of these profiles might make sense for implementation to connect their MFL to the broader health IT application ecosystem. This would extend the MFL and FR, opening greater possibilities to support the use cases described in this chapter.

13.13 Summary

Healthcare facilities are scattered by both geography and scope. Providing access to services, in times of emergency or routine care, and strengthening appropriate and timely delivery of healthcare require the capacity to identify facilities in an area as well as enumerate their menu of services and capabilities. A FR provides the technical infrastructure to develop and manage a MFL for identification, integration of data from various sources, and communication with information systems to harmonize facility data across the healthcare environment.

Questions for discussion

1. Compare and contrast the different protocols for developing unique facility identifiers. Which method would be preferable for a rapidly developing and changing healthcare environment? Which would be preferable for a well-established environment?
2. How can facility registries achieve true interoperability? What are some barriers to interoperability of facility-related data?
3. Discuss why it is important to go beyond facility identification and collect facility services and infrastructure or resources.

Acknowledgments

The authors acknowledge and thank Eduardo Jezierski, former CEO of InSTEDD, for his contributions to the Implementation Guide for the OpenHIE Facility Registry [44], which served as a primary reference for this chapter. The authors further acknowledge Timothy D. McFarlane, MPH, PhD, graduate from the Indiana University Richard M. Fairbanks School of Public Health who principally authored the first edition of this chapter. The revised chapter leverages his work, even though he declined to participate as an author.

References

[1] Dixon BE, Colvard C, Tierney WM. Identifying health facilities outside the enterprise: challenges and strategies for supporting health reform and meaningful use. Inform Health Soc Care 2014;40(4):319–33.

[2] Ritz D, Althauser C, Wilson K. Connecting health information systems for better health: leveraging interoperability standards to link patient, provider, payor, and policymaker data. Joint Learning Network for Universal Health Coverage; 2014.

[3] Makinde OA, Azeez A, Adebayo W. Potential use cases for the development of an electronic health facility registry in Nigeria: key informant's perspectives. Online J Public Health Inform 2016;8(2):e191.

[4] Mpango J, Nabukenya J. A qualitative study to examine approaches used to manage data about health facilities and their challenges: a case of Uganda. AMIA Annu Symp Proc 2019;2019:1157–66.

[5] Rose-Wood A, Heard N, Thermidor R, Chan J, Joseph F, Lerebours G, et al. Development and use of a master health facility list: Haiti's experience during the 2010 earthquake response. Glob Health Sci Pract 2014;2(3):357–65.

[6] World Health Organization. Everybody's business: strengthening health systems to improve health outcomes, WHO's framework for action. Geneva: WHO; 2007.

[7] VA MISSION Act of 2018, Pub. L. No. 115-182 (June 6, 2018).

[8] Dixon BE, Haggstrom DA, Weiner M. Implications for informatics given expanding access to care for veterans and other populations. J Am Med Inform Assoc 2015;22(4):917–20.

[9] Health Resources and Services Administration. Quality improvement. Washington, D.C.: U.S. Department of Health and Human Services; 2011 [cited 2021 Dec 13]. Available from: https://www.hrsa.gov/sites/default/files/quality/toolbox/508pdfs/qualityimprovement.pdf.

[10] Office of the National Coordinator for Health Information Technology. Improve care coordination. Washington, D.C.: U.S. Department of Health and

Human Services; 2014 [updated 2017 Sep 15; cited 2021 Dec 13]. Available from: http://www.healthit.gov/providers-professionals/improved-care-coordination.
[11] Dixon BE, Embi PJ, Haggstrom DA. Information technologies that facilitate care coordination: provider and patient perspectives. Behav Med Pract Policy Res 2018;8(3):522–5.
[12] O'Malley AS, Grossman JM, Cohen GR, Kemper NM, Pham HH. Are electronic medical records helpful for care coordination? Experiences of physician practices. J Gen Intern Med 2010;25(3):177–85.
[13] Schoen C, Osborn R, Squires D, Doty M, Pierson R, Applebaum S. New 2011 survey of patients with complex care needs in eleven countries finds that care is often poorly coordinated. Health Aff (Millwood) 2011;30(12):2437–48.
[14] Madhavan S, Bastarache L, Brown JS, Butte AJ, Dorr DA, Embi PJ, et al. Use of electronic health records to support a public health response to the COVID-19 pandemic in the United States: a perspective from 15 academic medical centers. J Am Med Inform Assoc 2021;28(2):393–401.
[15] Finnell JT, Overhage JM, Grannis S. All health care is not local: an evaluation of the distribution of Emergency Department care delivered in Indiana. AMIA Annu Symp Proc. 2011;2011:409–16.
[16] Institute of Medicine (US) Committee on Quality of Health Care in America. Crossing the quality chasm: a new health system for the 21st century. Washington, DC: National Academies Press (US); 2001.
[17] World Health Organization. Monitoring and evaluation of health systems strengthening: an operational framework. Geneva: World Health Organization; 2010.
[18] World Health Organization. Creating a master health facility list. Geneva: World Health Organization; 2012.
[19] Giroir BP. Healthy people 2030: a call to action to lead America to healthier lives. J Public Health Manag Pract 2021;27(Suppl 6):S222–4.
[20] Reeder B, Revere D, Hills RA, Baseman JG, Lober WB. Public health practice within a health information exchange: information needs and barriers to disease surveillance. Online J Public Health Inform 2012;4(3).
[21] Centers for Disease Control and Prevention. Measles (Rubeola). Atlanta, GA: National Center for Immunization and Respiratory Diseases, Division of Viral Diseases; 2020 [updated 2020 Nov 5; cited 2021 Dec 13]. Available from: http://www.cdc.gov/measles/hcp/index.html.
[22] Zipprich J, Winter K, Hacker J, Xia D, Watt J, Harriman K. Measles outbreak – California, December 2014–February 2015. MMWR. 2015;64 (06):153–4.
[23] Dixon BE, Caine VA, Halverson PK. Deficient response to COVID-19 makes the case for evolving the public health system. Am J Prev Med 2020;59 (6):887–91.
[24] Dixon BE, McGowan JJ, Grannis SJ. Electronic laboratory data quality and the value of a health information exchange to support public health reporting processes. AMIA Annu Symp Proc. 2011;2011:322–30.
[25] Batteiger TA, Dixon BE, Wang J, Zhang Z, Tao G, Tong Y, et al. Where do people go for gonorrhea and chlamydia tests: a cross-sectional view of the Central Indiana population, 2003–2014. Sex Transm Dis 2019;46(2):132–6.
[26] InSTEDD. Resource Map. 2011 [cited 2022 Feb 18]. Available from: http://resourcemap.instedd.org/en.
[27] OpenHIE. OpenHIE Facility Registry (FR). 2021 [cited 2022 Feb 18]. Available from: https://guides.ohie.org/arch-spec/openhie-component-specifications-1/openhie-facility-registry-fr.
[28] World Health Organziation. Master Facility List Resource Package: guidance for countries wanting to strengthen their Master Facility List. 2018 [cited 2022 Feb 18]. Available from: https://www.who.int/healthinfo/MFL_Resource_Package_Jan2018.pdf?ua = 1.
[29] Health Facility Assessment Technical Working Group. The signature domain and geographic coordinates: a standardized approach for uniquely identifying a health facility. Chapel Hill, NC: Carolina Population Center, University of North Carolina; 2007.
[30] Department of Health and Human Services. 45 CFR part 162 HIPAA administrative simplification: standard unique health identifier for health care providers; final rule. Washington, D.C.: Federal Register. 2004 [cited 2021 Dec 13]. Available from: https://www.cms.gov/Regulations-and-Guidance/Administrative-Simplification/NationalProvIdentStand/downloads/NPIfinalrule.pdf.
[31] Health Industry Business Communications Council. The health industry number system. Phoenix, AZ: Health Industry Communications Council; 2021 [cited 2021 Dec 13]. Available from: http://www.hibcc.org/hin-system/.
[32] Health Industry Business Communications Council. Health Industry Number System (HIN) Authorized Licensees. Phoenix, AZ: Health Industry Communications Council; 2021 [updated 2021 Dec 3; cited 2021 Dec 13]. Available from: https://www.hibcc.org/wp-content/uploads/Current-HIN-Authorized-Licensees.pdf.
[33] University of Oslo. Health Information Systems Programme (HISP). Oslo, Norway: Department of Informatics, University of Oslo. 2011 [updated 2021 May 5; cited 2021 Dec13]. Available from: http://www.mn.uio.no/ifi/english/research/networks/hisp/.

[34] The Demographics & Health Survey (DHS) Program. SPA overview. Rockville, MD: U.S. Agency for International Development; 2021 [cited 2021 Dec 13]. Available from: https://dhsprogram.com/methodology/Survey-Types/SPA.cfm.

[35] World Health Organization. Service availability and readiness assessment (SARA). 2021 [cited 2021 Dec13]. Available from: https://www.who.int/data/data-collection-tools/service-availability-and-readiness-assessment-(sara)?ua = 1.

[36] Brault MW. Americans with disabilities: 2010. U.S. Department of Commerce. Washington, D.C.: U.S. Census Bureau Economics and Statistics Administration; 2012. p. 70–131.

[37] Social Security Advisory Board. Aspects of disability decision making: data and materials. Washington, D. C.: U.S. Social Security Administration; 2012 [cited 2021 Dec 13]. Available from: https://www.ssab.gov/research/disability-decision-making/.

[38] Ni P, McDonough CM, Jette AM, Bogusz K, Marfeo EE, Rasch EK, et al. Development of a computer-adaptive physical function instrument for Social Security Administration disability determination. Arch Phys Med Rehabil 2013;94(9):1661–9.

[39] Institute of Medicine. Improving the social security disability decision process. In: Stobo JD, McGeary M, Barnes DK, editors. Committee on Improving the Disability Decision Process: SSA's Listing of Impairments and Agency Access to Medical Expertise. Washington, D.C: The National Academies Press; 2007.

[40] IntraHealth International. Facility match: global open facility registry. 2022 [cited 2022 Feb 18]. Available from: https://www.facilitymatch.net/.

[41] African Society for Laboratory Medicine. Laboratory Mapping Program (LabMaP). 2022 [cited 2022 Feb 18]. Available from: https://aslm.org/what-we-do/labmap/.

[42] Integrating the Healthcare Enterprise. Care Services Directory. 2016 [cited 2022 Feb 18]. Available from: https://www.ihe.net/uploadedFiles/Documents/ITI/IHE_ITI_Suppl_CSD.pdf.

[43] Integrating the Healthcare Enterprise. Mobile Care Services Discovery. 2021 [cited 2022 Feb 18]. Available from: https://www.ihe.net/uploadedFiles/Documents/ITI/IHE_ITI_Suppl_mCSD.pdf.

[44] OpenHIE. OpenHIE health facility registry implementation guide. 2015 [cited 2022 Feb 18]. Available from: https://docs.google.com/document/d/1KaUPHQRiZ-9hQ59Irp56oKayvVZbkWngTYkl2AZdafhw/view.

CHAPTER

14

Health worker registries: managing the health care workforce

Nora J. Gilliam[1], *Dykki Settle*[2], *Luke Duncan*[2] *and Brian E. Dixon*[1,3]

[1]Department of Epidemiology, Richard M. Fairbanks School of Public Health, Indiana University, Indianapolis, IN, USA [2]PATH, Seattle, WA, USA [3]Center for Biomedical Informatics, Regenstrief Institute, Inc., Indianapolis, IN, USA

LEARNING OBJECTIVES

By the end of this chapter, the reader should be able to:

- Define a health worker.
- Identify sources of health worker data and describe the limitations of their use.
- Define a health worker registry.
- List and describe potential uses for a health worker registry in the context of health information exchange.
- Explain the process of developing a minimum data set for a health worker registry.
- Identify syntactic and semantic standards to support a health worker registry.

14.1 Introduction

As described in earlier chapters, registries play an important role in health information exchange (HIE). Client registries, for example, facilitate patient-level data transfer and allow for continuous, longitudinal patient care across episodic health care encounters (Chapter 12). Facility registries (FRs) provide a central authority to store, manage, and share health facility identification, services, and resource data across a community, state, or nation (Chapter 13). Here we present another type of registry—the health worker registry (HWR)—as an additional component of HIE networks for use across myriad contexts by multiple stakeholders.

Health Information Exchange
DOI: https://doi.org/10.1016/B978-0-323-90802-3.00026-5

The health care field consists of workers from a variety of professions, including clinical workers such as physicians and nurses, but also health sector and facility managers, pharmacists, pharmaceutical supply chain workers, ambulance drivers, and even volunteer community health workers (CHWs), to name a few. Harmonization of information about health care workers—such as licensure and employment data—across these various fields can allow for efficient workforce planning, regulation, management, identification of worker shortages, emergency response preparation, and improved coordination of care. However, the current patchwork of data sources and variations in content often preclude their use for these purposes. In this chapter, we discuss how the inclusion of an HWR within an HIE can help to address this gap and maximize information gained from the available health worker data sets.

14.2 Need for coordinated health care worker data

Health care is a multifaceted field consisting of a diverse and multidisciplinary workforce. Indeed, the definition of who is a "health worker" is broad and extensive. According to the World Health Organization (WHO), health workers are "all people engaged in activities whose primary intent is to enhance health" [1]. Given this inclusive definition, it is evident that health care workers are a diverse group with a variety of approaches to providing patient care. Physicians, physician assistants, nurses, nurse practitioners, CHWs, health sector managers, pharmacy warehouse employees, and ambulance drivers—these are just a few of the many health care workers in the field today [2]. But who are these individuals? Where and when were they trained? Where do they work now? Tracking such information has proven to be difficult.

Data on health care workers are currently available from a variety of disparate sources. In the United States, extensive data from state licensure records and surveys as well as professional organizations are available [3]; however, these are often inconsistent from source to source. For example, the North Carolina Health Professions Data System collects licensed health care provider data through a collaboration between a university-based policy center, state professional licensing boards, and an Area Health Education Centers program [4]. Some data, such as gender, birth year, home address, graduation year, school of attendance, and practice setting, are collected on all licensed professionals. Other data, such as place of birth and clinical practice area, are collected for some but not others. Additionally, data for health care workers who do not require licenses—such as medication aides, geriatric aides, and feeding assistants—are collected through an entirely separate system via North Carolina's Division of Health Service Regulation Health Care Personnel Registry Section [5]. Given the variety of sources and data collection methods, barriers to aggregation and analysis are inevitable. Internationally, similar challenges are present, with employment data often housed within a country's Ministry of Health (MOH), and licensure data often housed within professional councils and medical licensure boards [6]. As such, whether in an entire country or within an enterprise such as an HIE network, developing a single source of health worker data has proven to be a challenging and complex undertaking.

While challenges exist, efforts to create a master and canonical list of health workers can yield substantial benefits [2,3,6]. Access to such coordinated data can allow for efficient workforce planning. It can provide verification of employment, education, and other training. It can aid in understanding the geographic distribution of health professionals to identify areas of abundance as well as areas of shortages, allowing for worker deployment into areas of need for specific types of care. This would further be useful during an infectious disease outbreak where human resources might need to be redeployed based on morbidity and mortality of disease, such as during the 2014 West Africa Ebola outbreak and the SARS-CoV-2 (COVID-19) pandemic that each filled hospital wards in some areas but not others. Similarly, registries can be used to perform payroll analyses for reallocation of limited resources for under- or uncompensated workers [7].

A master list of health care workers would also allow for rapid identification and communication between health care professionals for emergency responses purposes, such as a regional outbreak or global pandemic. Additionally, such a list would allow for ease of referrals between providers, facilitating effective and comprehensive patient care. A canonical list would also support provider attribution or identifying a primary care provider for a given patient in a given context (e.g., which provider delivered the majority of preventative services). Finally, making this list available to other health information systems would support interoperability and comparability of information across systems. For example, calculation of quality indicators or performance indices would be possible by physician, nurse, or allied health professional instead of clinic or hospital level only. Given the potential utility, a single, canonical registry with complete and current data on all health workers is a valuable component of an HIE.

14.3 Health worker registries

A **health worker registry (HWR)** is defined as a central, authoritative information system that captures, stores, and maintains the unique identities of health workers using a predefined, canonical minimum data set [6]. A **minimum data set (MDS)** is a canonical list of names, definitions and sources of data elements needed to support a specific purpose. In the context of an HWR, an MDS should contain the smallest, most basic set of data necessary to answer critical health workforce questions, including:

- How many practitioners do we have?
- Where are they practicing?
- Who is providing patient care?
- What types of care are practitioners providing?

Minimum data sets facilitate the establishment of national databases with consistent core data elements covering demographic, educational, credentialing, and practice characteristics of health professionals. In the United States, several Health Professions Minimum Data Sets [3] are defined and maintained by the Health Services Resources Agency (HRSA).

Because there can exist numerous lists of health workers within a state or country, a HWR seeks to merge various lists in accordance with a governance policy to be established by HIE stakeholders. The policy should ensure that as data are merged, the HWR creates a superset of health worker identities to enable de-duplication across available, individual data sets. WHO provides guidance on development of such policies as part of its national health workforce accounts [8].

14.4 Health worker registries within a health information exchange

As noted, an HWR serves as a container for authoritative information on health workers within a nation or enterprise. In an HIE, an HWR component must easily communicate with other parts of the system, just as a client registry (Chapter 12) and facility registry (Chapter 13) must do (see Fig. 14.1). The HWR allows data to be shared and queries to be

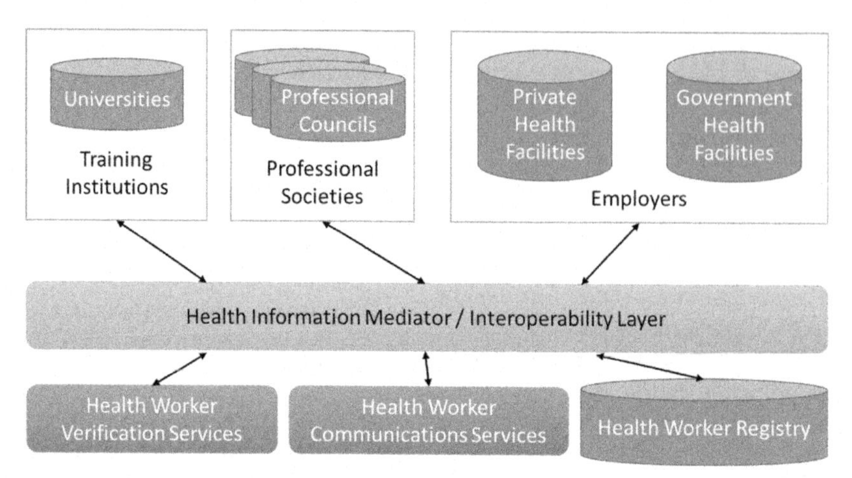

FIGURE 14.1 Illustration of the OpenHIE Architecture highlighting the health worker registry and point of service applications that potentially interface with the registry. Source: *Adapted from OpenHIE. OpenHIE health worker registry implementation guide [Internet]. 2016 [cited 2022 Mar 29]. Available from: https://docs.google.com/document/d/1b7ZQz3NWjoqmLcgmee_tNDiXrj4Y6urDmT7dBqCI6d4/view.*

conducted by a variety of client systems consisting of computer and human users, including mobile health (mHealth) tools, such as clinical decision support or health service directory apps, electronic medical record systems, training information systems, human resources information systems (HRIS), licensure and qualification systems, health management information systems, and health workforce observatories, which cooperative organizations designed to promote, develop, and sustain a knowledge base for health-related human resources in a region [6]. Ultimately, any source system in the HIE should report the MDS for health worker data from the system it manages to the HWR, and any client system should be able to query the HWR for any information defined by the MDS.

Despite its potential usefulness, an HWR is generally considered to be a "nice to have" component in the United States and therefore not implemented by most HIE networks. The closest analogs to an HWR in US-based HIE networks are Health Information Service Providers (HISPs) created as part of the DirectTrust [9,10]. However, this analogy is very weak as described below.

The DirectTrust specifies a method for medical providers, government organizations, vendors, and others to send authenticated, encrypted health information directly to known, trusted recipients over the Internet [11]; a method often referred to as secure electronic mail (email) for providers or Direct Secure Messaging. HISPs are the entities responsible for delivering messages between senders and receivers. HISPs must therefore create and maintain email addresses for each sender and receiver, whom are most often licensed health workers. For example, the Indiana Health Information Exchange (IHIE) created a Direct email address for each of its more than 40,000 Docs4Docs providers to help comply with meaningful use regulations in the United States [12]. The email addresses were yet another data element added to the MDS IHIE maintains for its Docs4Docs service. The list of health care providers participating in a HISP, therefore, is similar in concept to an HWR because it requires maintaining an MDS about each provider. However, HISP lists are incomplete and often represent only those providers who subscribe to a specific HIE service like Docs4Docs; therefore HISPs should not be considered true HWRs.

Inclusion of an HWR within US-based HIEs requires consideration of economic factors. For example, should an HIE wish to offer an HWR service for a fee, this would require the participation of clients such as state governmental and professional organizations to ensure access to robust, timely data, thereby justifying the expenditure of scarce financial resources. Additionally, an HWR would compete with existing workforce management systems and therefore must demonstrate cost-effectiveness to gain buy-in of HIE participants. As such, much work remains to make this an appealing and economical option.

Internationally, creating and maintaining an HWR has proven to be quite effective and feasible, at least for public sector health workers. In many countries, data (for at least the public sector workforce) are centralized within a national MOH, which could make coordination less daunting. Collaboration between countries in a region (e.g., East Africa, Europe) might allow for more feasible development of HRIS when funding and investment of resources are present. The West Africa Health Organization, the health arm of the Economic Community of West African States (ECOWAS), supported the deployment of HRIS systems in West African countries during the early part of the last decade [13]. The Kenya MOH, as another example, collaborated with the Zambia MOH to provide technical and regulatory support for development of a Zambian HRIS. Because of this partnership, development of the Zambian HRIS took less than half as long to setup compared to the length of the setup of the more veteran Kenyan HRIS [14,15]. The Republic of Serbia implemented its Register of Employees in 2021, registering nearly 4000 health workers (most of whom work in private health settings) within the first five months [16].

There is strong interest in utilizing open-source HIE systems for development of HWRs, especially outside the US IntraHealth International, with support from USAID, curated iHRIS as an open-source health workforce information systems software to be used by other nations for a variety of needs including management and regulation of health care workers, analysis of an entire health workforce for planning needs and interventions, and tracking and managing licensure practice of health care workers [17]. iHRIS also offers the opportunity for upkeep of HWRs for a nation to analyze distribution of resources. The Ministry of Public Health within the Democratic Republic of Congo utilized iHRIS for updating accurate representations of health care workers on payroll in order to reallocate funds to under- or uncompensated workers [7]. In countries with MOH consisting of federated units similar to the fragmented system in the United States, smoother coordination may not be plausible. Fragmented, nongovernmental organizations (NGOs) can also provide a significant portion of health workers in a nation, similarly making construction of an HWR complex.

Despite their complexities, HWRs have proven to be valuable components to the implementation of national eHealth strategies. Box 14.1 profiles the nation of Tanzania, which recently updated its HWR after a decade. The newer version is well integrated into is national eHealth architecture, and the expanded Human Resource for Health Information System (HRHIS) includes data on professionals working in public, private, and faith-based organizations.

In addition to serving human resource management needs, HWRs are also important for communications with health workers, especially during public health emergencies. For example, HWRs played a critical role in supporting rapid dissemination of information to health workers during the 2014 Ebola outbreak (see Box 14.2).

14.5 Existing minimum data sets

As previously mentioned, an MDS is the cornerstone to the development of an HWR. An MDS identifies which data to collect from

BOX 14.1

An updated health worker registry for Tanzania.

In alignment with its National Digital Health Strategy, Digital Health Investment Roadmap, Tanzania Health Enterprise Architecture, and Human Resource for Health and Social Welfare Strategic Plan, the Tanzania Ministry of Health recently (January 2022) implemented a new, updated HRHIS. The system serves as the national HWR. The implementation of the new system is detailed in a report from the Ministry of Health [18].

The system is a major improvement over the previous HWR and possesses the two key advantages. First, the system fully supports modern application programming interfaces (APIs) that enable retrieval from multiple back-end systems, including databases maintained by training institutions and professional societies. Second, the system facilitates access to the full range of health professionals working in the nation, including public-sector employees who are directly paid by the government as well as private and faith-based health facility workers who collectively provide up to 16.3% of health services in the nation.

An important aspect of planning for the new system included mapping the full lifecycle of professional careers in health services and their associated data flows. Fig. 14.2 represents the various stages of a career in health and the touchpoints with registration, updating, and termination in the HWR. The lifecycle includes training, an important first step in a health professional's career. It is during training when an individual first enters the HWR. As they are fully trained and licensed, their record is updated as they enter full-time employment. When they leave employment, their status is updated, and they are de-registered from the HWR. The system further captures information on continuing professional education and development. The authors note the model is comprehensive and generalizable to every nation.

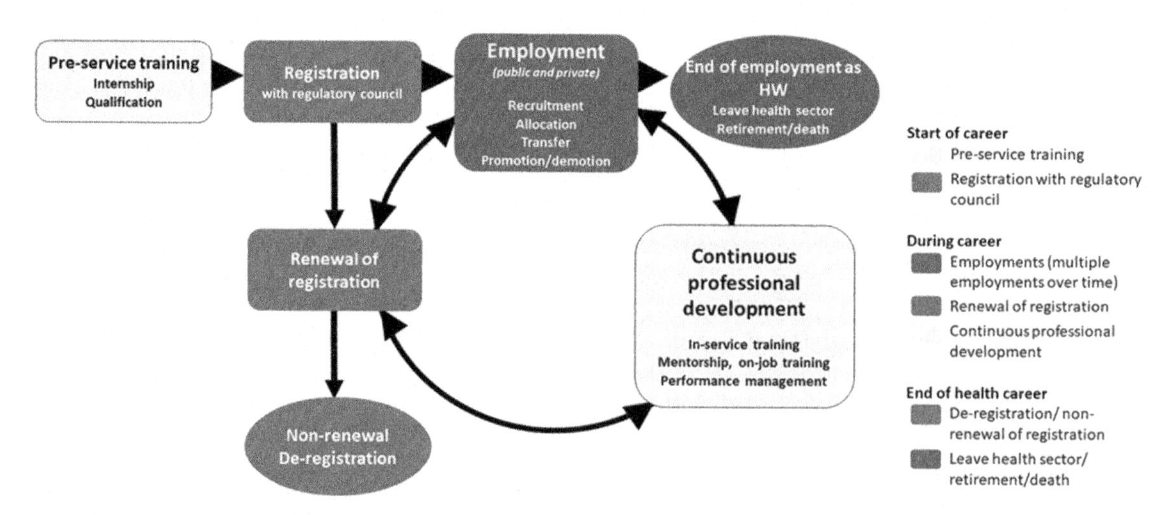

FIGURE 14.2 Tanzania health worker "lifecycle" and associated data flows [18]. The diagram represents important preimplementation planning that precedes development of a health worker registry. Source: *Image used with permission from the Tanzania Ministry of Health.*

BOX 14.2

Leveraging a health worker registry during a public health emergency.

Timely and accurate communication between health care workers is particularly essential during an emergency response such as the COVID-19 pandemic. Thus utilizing technologies able to disseminate information rapidly to health care workers within a health care system has proven to be important part of emergency preparedness.

mHero was created by a partnership between UNICEF and IntraHealth International in response to the West African Ebola outbreak to support health-sector communication via mobile phone devices between MOH and health care workers. mHero is a technology that links existing technologies in efforts for interoperability and thus communication between users of these technologies.

Existing technologies needed to allow for rapid communication include an HWR that provides contact information and a notification tool that can alert these contacts. By linking iHRIS through OpenHIE and RapidPro (see Fig. 14.3), a clinical notification tool linked to any form of mobile device, the data from the HWR were accessed to deliver pertinent messaging to be then used in real-time. mHero was so successful during the Ebola outbreak, that Liberia continued to develop this platform for ongoing systematic communication.

Direct linkage of health care workers to centralized information can allow for alerting workers of a particular geographic area and for preventing the spread of miscommunication not from official sources. Optimizing mHero the years following the Ebola outbreak proved to be a great investment; Liberia and several other countries then deployed linking technology mHero in respond to the COVID-19 pandemic. Investing in a HWR, especially for rapid dissemination of information to health care workers within this HRIS, can be life-saving.

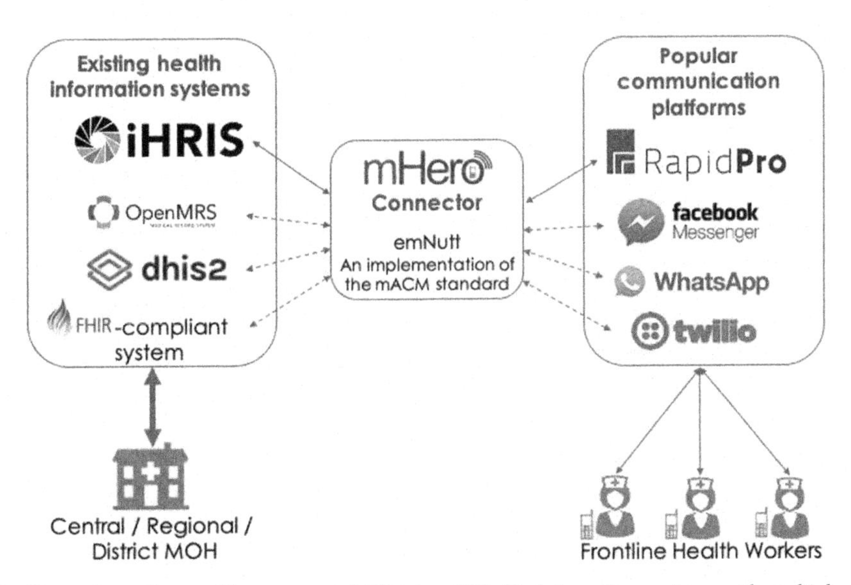

FIGURE 14.3 Illustration of how mHero connected Ministry of Health information systems with multiple communications platforms to support response to Ebola in West Africa. Source: *Image used with permission from IntraHealth International.*

both the public and private sectors [6]. In the United States, HRSA currently maintains minimum data sets for several professions [3], including dental hygienists, licensed professional counselors, nurses, occupational therapists, pharmacists, physical therapists, physician assistants, physicians, psychologists, and substance abuse/addiction counselors. However, each MDS is distinct and separate from the others, and they are not coordinated within an HWR. Additionally, the degree to which data collection and implementation is complete varies by state. As such, gaps remain and efforts to improve coverage continue.

WHO strongly supports the establishment of health care workforce MDSs and HWRs [2]. The organization has provided guidance to inform the process throughout the world [2]. Within this context, numerous international efforts for MDS development for a variety of health care workers have already been undertaken from Australia to Mozambique [19–22].

One example of a successful MDS and HWR is South Africa. In 2019 the National Department of Health and CDC partnered with HISP, a NGO that supports integration of information systems through open standards and data exchange mechanisms [23], to create a HRIS for the country. The solution involved development of a HWR called the "Human Resources for Health Registry," which functions as a data warehouse using health worker data collated from multiple source systems. Each source contains different puzzle pieces regarding health workers. Using a HAPI FHIR-based approach, the MDS is parsed into the HWR. Data are then aggregated into a database, which is connected to DHIS2 and custom analytics solutions for visualizing and reporting data on the nation's health workers. To date, more than 70,000 public health care worker records are stored in the HWR [24].

14.6 Creation of minimum data sets

The creation of an MDS for an HIE is a process that requires substantial stakeholder input [2,6]. In many cases, it will be necessary to conduct interviews of source system participants in order to identify data elements that currently exist or elements that users desire to have collected. From there, it is necessary to link the identified data elements to previously established use cases and user stories for the HIE. This will ensure the scope of the MDS matches what users need with the most appropriate set of data elements.

To determine whether a data element should be included in an MDS, a good rule of thumb is the 80/20 rule. This states that if an element will be used by at least 80% of the source or client systems, it should be part of the MDS. Possible data fields to consider for inclusion are demographic, contact, employment, education, and license/certification information [2,6], with others included as indicated by user needs.

14.7 Standards to support the minimum data set

As with any component of an HIE, interoperability is the goal. To accomplish this, an MDS must follow a set of standards. For example, standardized data lists that provide a reference terminology must be adopted in order to ensure the data can be effectively analyzed [6]. These lists are typically available through a Terminology Service (see Chapter 10). In addition to using reference terminologies, component interaction or technical standards must also be selected [6], including those for Terminology Services, such as Sharing Valuesets, Codes, and Maps (SVCM)[1] [25] and

[1] IHE intends to replace the current SVCM implementation guide, Revision 1.2, in 2022 as an updated FHIR Implementation Guide. The newer document was not available at the time of publication.

TABLE 14.1 Common health worker and health services data standards.

Standard	Full name	Responsible organization
ANSI/HL7 V3 HCSPDIR, R1-2010	HL7 Version 3 Standard: Healthcare, Community Services, and Provider Directory Service	HL7 (http://www.hl7.org)
CSD	Care Services Discovery	Integrating the Healthcare Enterprise (IHE) (http://www.ihe.net)
mCSD	Mobile Care Services Discovery	IHE (http://www.ihe.net)
FHIR	Fast Health Care Interoperability Resources	HL7 (http://www.hl7.org)
VHDIR	Validated Healthcare Directory	HL7 Patient Administration Group (http://www.hl7.org/Special/committees/pafm)
HPD	Health Care Provider Directory	IHE (http://www.ihe.net)
ISO 21091:2013	Health Informatics – Directory Services for Healthcare Providers, Subjects of Care and Other Entities	International Organization for Standardization (ISO) (http://www.iso.org)

Sharing Value Sets [26]. Standards for health worker and health services data must also be selected. Descriptions of some such standards are included in Table 14.1.

In addition to Terminology Services, WHO defined a standard MDS format for use "by ministries of health to support the development of standardized health workforce information systems" [27]. The Global MDS serves as an international standard for HRIS. In 2017 researchers in Zimbabwe developed a methodology to compare existing HRIS to the Global MDS standard [28]. Through use of iHRIS, it was demonstrated that rapid adoption and standardization of HWR MDS is feasible in low-to-middle-income countries (LMICs) [8].

We note that unfortunately the standards for health worker data have not evolved much since the first publication of this chapter in 2016. This is an area for further work, especially as new health worker classes are established. For example, since the original publication of this chapter, CHWs have become more common in the United States as well as LMICs. These workers are not typically considered licensed health professionals, and they may therefore be excluded from traditional health care worker lists. Similarly, caregivers in the home, including children caring for aging parents, may not be considered health care workers. International standards may need to be updated to incorporate the full breadth of individuals who participate in health and wellness care for individuals outside of health care facilities (e.g., home, community).

14.8 Emerging trends

As nations rebuild their infrastructures following the COVID-19 pandemic, there is a critical need to develop or strengthen HWR technologies, including systems like iHRIS as well as mHero, in preparation for the next public health disaster. During a regional outbreak or global pandemic, it is imperative that public health authorities have the capability to identify health workers and where they are deployed. The COVID-19 pandemic required ambulatory services to be shut down with many of those workers redeployed to inpatient units and hospital facilities to triage incoming patients as well as staff beds. Elective surgeries were canceled, again redeploying the nurses and nonphysician workers to those facilities with higher acuity patients. Long-term care settings as well as hospitals also lost staff due to infections and quarantine, requiring auxiliary staff to work, including individuals retired from medicine or nursing. These system challenges could be better managed using integrated HWR systems. Moreover, contact information for HWRs could facilitate rapid communication of situational reports to frontline workers, enabling them to be informed. Perhaps this might have helped frontline workers to have genuine information from the WHO rather than misinformation from the Internet [29].

14.8.1 A health care provider directory for the United States

In 2016 the US Office of the National Coordinator for Health Information Technology initiated a project to create a national resource to include "a broad set of provider data that supports a variety of healthcare directory use cases." [30] This initiative has supported the development of the HL7 Validated Healthcare Directory (VHDir) based on the FHIR Version 4.0 standard [31]. Although not released for implementation, the design is exciting for the promise of HWRs in the United States. There exist a number of FHIR resources enumerated already, including Practitioner (e.g., primary care doctor, nurse, diabetes educator) and Care Team (a group of practitioners that provide coordinated care for a patient). Practitioner resources require at minimum a name and indicator of whether or not the relationship with the patient is active. These resources can also include digital certificates as well as service endpoints, including those for the DirectTrust. There are also resources for Location and Organizations, concepts more relevant to FRs, and would enable FRs and HWRs to work together to enumerate health workforces in a given state, region, or health system.

In addition, the Sequoia Project has initiated work on an implementation guide for a health care directory [32]. The guide is focused on the service endpoints supported by Sequoia, including the eHealth Exchange and Carequality. Although promising, the current version of the guide (0.0.1) has not been updated since 2017 and targets a now outdated release of the FHIR standard.

14.8.2 Health worker registries support operational health system needs

Beyond outbreak scenarios, this chapter outlined several routine health care operational areas that would also benefit from up-to-date, integrated HWR components operating as part of an enterprise, statewide, or national HIE network. Human resource management is critical, and routine assessment of care deserts (e.g., obstetrics desert, midwife desert) could help health system decision-makers to identify where providers are lacking. Moreover, HWR components could support better transitions of care and provider attribution by identifying who cares for patients during an encounter. Real-world evidence on care processes could guide learning health systems on where breakdowns occur, and which members of team could better support patient care delivery.

Given that most HWRs are limited to the public health workforce, nations should consider policy options or financing levers that could expand capture and monitoring of private health workers. Registries that capture private health workforce metrics could be used to further measure and improve national strategies that seek to implement universal health care access in alignment with WHO's sustainable development goals. Furthermore, private worker data could be used to assess where private health workers are located to complement reports on public health worker deployment, even if nations cannot control where private health care workers are deployed.

14.8.3 Registries for community health workers

Going forward, more nations are likely to establish registries for CHWs, or integrate CHW data into existing HWRs. In 2017 Uganda established the first and only known CHW Registry (CHWR) to register, track, and manage CHWs [33]. These important frontline health workers are a crucial link to patients in villages, given that just 12% of the Ugandan population lives in an urban center. Some CHWs are organized into teams that are deployed in villages to support maternal and child health services, including childhood vaccination [34]. Others are facilitators for primary care for HIV patients who live hours away from the nearest health facility. Following a pilot of the CHWR in 11 health districts by IntraHealth International, the MOH expanded the registry to an additional 23 districts.

The CHWR in Uganda is used for a variety of important management operations, including generation of reports on workforce density, succession, incentives, training, and program design to drive decision-making [33]. For example, NGOs and health facilities that use village health teams are required to register the CHWs in the registry. Reports are used to identify which teams are qualified to recruit new CHWs. Data are also used to identify which teams could be deployed to address a localized measles outbreak. The registry is also useful in analyzing training needs for CHWs.

In the future, as CHWs become more commonplace in LMICs and other nations, monitoring who is providing health services, which health services are provided using nonlicensed professionals, and the level of training CHWs receive will become important for health systems. Specialized HWRs for CHWs, or updating the MDS to include CHW-specific metadata, is likely to be a focus of HIE efforts. Furthermore, standards development organizations may also wish to review whether existing syntactic and semantic standards can accommodate CHW data in support of these initiatives.

14.9 Summary

The health care field consists of a variety of workers from diverse specialties. Through the harmonization of numerous health worker data sets from varying sources, the development of an HWR utilizing an MDS within an HIE can allow for efficient and effective workforce planning and coordination. Challenges in the development of HWRs exist, particularly due to a patchwork of disparate data sources. However, the potential benefits of HWR likely justify their development and use in both United States and international efforts to support a range of services that allow health systems to assess and adapt to a rapidly changing health care landscape.

Questions for discussion

1) What are some of the major challenges in creating an HWR for an HIE? How do these vary by country?
2) Describe some of the benefits of implementing a health worker registry. Provide examples of situations where an HWR might improve workforce efficiency.
3) Who are some of the potential users of a HWR? Who may provide the data?
4) What considerations must be taken into account when developing a MDS? Who should participate? What data fields should be included?
5) How might future changes in health care influence the usefulness of HWRs?

Acknowledgment

The authors acknowledge the efforts of Jennifer M. Alyea, MPH, PhD, a graduate of the Indiana University Fairbanks School of Public Health, who principally authored the first version of this chapter during her studies. Dr. Alyea has since graduated from the doctoral program in epidemiology and declined to be an author in this edition. However, this edition leverages her incredibly strong research and content. The authors further acknowledge Dr. Carl Leitner who also coauthored the first edition of this chapter while an employee at IntraHealth International.

References

[1] World Health Organization. Health workers [Internet]. 2006 [cited 2021 Sep 14]. Available from: http://www.who.int/whr/2006/06_chap1_en.pdf.
[2] World Health Organization. Human resources for health information system: minimum data set for health workforce registry [Internet]. 2015 [cited 2021 Sep 14]. Available from: http://www.who.int/hrh/statistics/minimun_data_set.pdf?ua = 1.
[3] National Center for Health Workforce Analysis. Explore health workforce data policy [Internet]. Health Resources & Services Administration; 2022 [cited 2022 Mar 29]. Available from: https://bhw.hrsa.gov/data-research/explore-health-workforce-data-policy.
[4] Cecil G. Sheps Center for Health Services Research, University of North Carolina at Chapel Hill. North Carolina Health Professions Data System (HPDS) [Internet]. Sheps Center; n.d. [cited 2021 Sep 14]. Available from: https://www.shepscenter.unc.edu/programs-projects/workforce/projects/hpds/.
[5] North Carolina Department of Health and Human Services. NC HCPR: about the N.C. Health Care Personnel Registry Section [Internet]. 2011 [cited 2021 Sep 14]. Available from: https://www.ncnar.org/about.html.
[6] OpenHIE. OpenHIE health worker registry implementation guide [Internet]. 2016 [cited 2022 Mar 29]. Available from: https://docs.google.com/document/d/1b7ZQz3NWjoqmLcgmee_tNDiXrj4Y6urDmT7dBqCI6-d4/view.
[7] Likofata Esanga JR, Viadro C, McManus L, Wesson J, Matoko N, Ngumbu E, et al. How the introduction of a human resources information system helped the Democratic Republic of Congo to mobilise domestic resources for an improved health workforce. Health Policy Plan 2017;32(suppl_3):iii25–31.
[8] World Health Organization. Policy Brief – national health workforce accounts: the knowledge-base for health workforce development towards Universal Health Coverage [Internet]. WHO; 2015 [cited 2022 Mar 29]. Available from: https://www.who.int/hrh/documents/15376_WHOBrief_NHWFA_0605.pdf.
[9] DirectTrust. Homepage [Internet]. n.d. [cited 2022 Mar 29]. Available from: https://directtrust.org/.
[10] Morris G, Afzal S, Bhasker M, Finney D. Provider directory solutions: market assessment and opportunities analysis [Internet]. Office of the National Coordinator for Health Information Technology; 2012 [cited 2022 Mar 29]. Available from: https://www.healthit.gov/sites/default/files/provider_directory_-solutions_final.pdf
[11] DirectTrust. What we do [Internet]. n.d. [cited 2022 Mar 29]. Available from: https://directtrust.org/what-we-do.
[12] Indiana Health Information Exchange. Docs4Docs [Internet]. n.d. [cited 2022 Mar 29]. Available from: https://www.ihie.org/onecare/#d4d.
[13] Odusote K, Bales C, Dwyer S, Settle D. Technical Brief – West Africa's regional approach to strengthening health workforce information. CapacityPlus and IntraHealth International; 2012 [cited 2022 Mar 29]. Available from: https://www.intrahealth.org/sites/ihweb/files/attachment-files/west-africa-regional-approach-strengthening-health-workforce-information.pdf.
[14] Were V, Jere E, Lanyo K, Mburu G, Kiriinya R, Waudo A, et al. Success of a South-South collaboration on Human Resources Information Systems (HRIS) in health: a case of Kenya and Zambia HRIS collaboration. Hum Resour Health 2019;17(1):6.
[15] Waters KP, Zuber A, Willy RM, Kiriinya RN, Waudo AN, Oluoch T, et al. Kenya's health workforce information system: a model of impact on strategic human resources policy, planning and management. Int J Med Inform 2013;82(9):895–902.
[16] Krstić M, Milić N. Development and implementation of a register of employees in the healthcare system of the Republic of Serbia. Glas Javnog Zdravlja 2022;96(1):6–17.
[17] IntraHealth International. iHRIS health workforce information systems software [Internet]. [cited 2021 Sep 12]. Available from: https://www.ihris.org/about.
[18] Tanzania Ministry of Health. Report on the improved human resource for health information system. 2022 [cited 2022 Apr 8]. Available from: TBD.
[19] Middleton S, Gardner G, Gardner A, Della P, Gibb M, Millar L. The first Australian nurse practitioner census: a protocol to guide standardized collection of information about an emergent professional group. Int J Nurs Pract 2010;16(5):517–24.
[20] Chen C, Baird S, Ssentongo K, Mehtsun S, Olapade-Olaopa EO, Scott J, et al. Physician tracking

in sub-Saharan Africa: current initiatives and opportunities. Hum Resour Health 2014;12:21.

[21] Rural Health Workforce Australia. Resources [Internet]. 2022 [cited 2022 Mar 29]. Available from: http://www.rhwa.org.au/resources2.

[22] Waters KP, Mazivila ME, Dgedge M, Necochea E, Manharlal D, Zuber A, et al. eSIP-Saúde: Mozambique's novel approach for a sustainable human resources for health information system. Hum Resour Health 2016; 14(1):66.

[23] HISP. About us [Internet]. n.d. [cited 2022 Mar 29]. Available from: https://www.hisp.org/?page_id = 1989.

[24] HISP. Human Resource Information Systems (HRIS) for South Africa [Internet]. 2021 [cited 2022 Mar 29]. Available from: https://www.hisp.org/?p = 3015.

[25] Integrating the Healthcare Enterprise. IHE IT infrastructure technical framework supplement: sharing valuesets, codes, and maps (SVCM) [Internet]. 2020 [cited 2022 Mar 29]. Available from: https://www.ihe.net/uploadedFiles/Documents/ITI/IHE_ITI_Suppl_SVCM.pdf.

[26] Integrating the Healthcare Enterprise. IHE IT infrastructure technical framework supplement: sharing value sets (SVS) [Internet]. 2021 [cited 2022 Mar 29]. Available from: https://profiles.ihe.net/ITI/TF/Volume1/ch-21.html.

[27] World Health Organization. Human resources for health information system: minimum data set for health workforce registry [Internet]. 2015 [cited 2022 Mar 29]. Available from: https://apps.who.int/iris/handle/10665/330091.

[28] Waters KP, Zuber A, Simbini T, Bangani Z, Krishnamurthy RS. Zimbabwe's Human Resources for health Information System (ZHRIS) – an assessment in the context of establishing a global standard. Int J Med Inform 2017;100:121–8.

[29] Cuan-Baltazar JY, Munoz-Perez MJ, Robledo-Vega C, Perez-Zepeda MF, Soto-Vega E. Misinformation of COVID-19 on the Internet: infodemiology study. JMIR Public Health Surveill 2020;6(2):e18444.

[30] Ryan C. Healthcare Directory Initiatives. Washington, DC: Office of the National Coordinator for Health Information Technology; 2019 [updated Jun 25; cited 2022 Apr 8]. Available from: https://oncprojectracking.healthit.gov/wiki/display/TechLabSC/Healthcare + Directory.

[31] HL7. Validated Healthcare Directory: HL7 International – Patient Administration Work Group. [cited 2022 Apr 8]. Available from: http://build.fhir.org/ig/HL7/VhDir/.

[32] Sequoia Project. Sequoia Project healthcare directory implementation guide. 2017 [cited 2022 Apr 8]. Available from: https://carequality.org/SequoiaProjectHealthcareDirectoryImplementationGuide/.

[33] Liu A, Ballard M, Oliphant N, Bhavsar M, Ebener S, Kerubo, et al. Implementation support guide: development of a national georeferenced community health worker master list hosted in a registry. UNICEF; 2021 [cited 2022 Mar 29]. Available from: https://www.unicef.org/media/113081/file/National-Georeferenced-Community-Health-Worker-Master-List-Hosted-in-a-Registry-2021.pdf.

[34] IntraHealth International. Uganda takes major steps to professionalize community health workforce [Internet]. 2018 [cited 2022 Mar 29]. Available from: https://www.intrahealth.org/news/uganda-takes-major-steps-professionalize-community-health-workforce.

CHAPTER

15

Healthcare finance data exchange: toward universal health coverage

Nimish Valvi[1], *Katie S. Allen*[1,2], *Carl Fourie*[3] and *Brian E. Dixon*[1,2,4]

[1]Center for Biomedical Informatics, Regenstrief Institute, Inc., Indianapolis, IN, USA [2]Department of Epidemiology, Richard M. Fairbanks School of Public Health, Indiana University, Indianapolis, IN, USA [3]Program for Appropriate Technology in Health (PATH), Seattle, WA, USA [4]Department of Veterans Affairs, Health Services Research & Development Service, Center for Health Information and Communication, Indianapolis, IN, USA

LEARNING OBJECTIVES

By the end of the chapter, the reader should be able to:

- Describe the concept of universal healthcare as defined by the World Health Organization.
- Define claims processing and describe its role in the health system.
- Discuss the role of health information exchange in supporting the processing of claims and achievement of universal healthcare goals.
- List and describe two examples of nations that have implemented HIE technologies in support of claims processing.

15.1 Introduction

Healthcare financing is a vital component of a robust healthcare structure and is achieved through a variety of means, with variation throughout the world. Financing of healthcare is complex and comprehensive, including all items related to "mobilization, accumulation, and allocation of money to cover the health needs of the people" [1]. This means that the financing scheme must cover all aspects of the healthcare process, including infrastructure (e.g., buildings, equipment, information systems), administration, and the clinical staff and supplies.

Driven in part by the World Health Organization (WHO) Sustainable Development Goals (SDGs), there has been a focus on Universal Health Coverage (UHC). UHC is not a method of

Health Information Exchange
DOI: https://doi.org/10.1016/B978-0-323-90802-3.00014-9

finance, but rather a goal to have all individuals receive health services they need without undue financial hardship [2]. However, the underlying finance schemes are a vital aspect of achieving UHC. Financial models for achieving UHC vary from country to country, but typically adopt some form of either compulsory insurance or socialization of the healthcare system as the underlying finance scheme. In other words, healthcare services are paid for by an organization (e.g., insurance company, government), guaranteeing reimbursement for the clinician or clinic that delivered the service without requiring a cash payment from the patient.

Even with variation in finance schemes a country can choose from, all systems rely on the processing of healthcare claims as part of implementation. Claims can be thought of as an invoicing system, where the provider (e.g., a hospital, physician) requests payment for the services (e.g., healthcare visit, treatments) they complete on behalf of the patient. Ultimately, the payor (e.g., insurance company, government) then pays the invoice. However, this can be a complicated process requiring negotiation of payments and debate over what treatments are covered. This complexity gives rise to a process that can cause long delays and high expense, especially as many countries seek to minimize the administrative costs associated with healthcare financing schemes.

Health information exchange (HIE) technologies create efficiencies in the processing of healthcare claims, thereby reducing the time and costs involved in the process. Managing the core business processes of enrolling beneficiaries, policy renewals, filing, and processing claims digitally creates more efficiency, thereby reducing costs. Handling the claims process remains a challenge for many nations, and even more so for Low-and-Middle Income Countries (LMICs). However, many nations, especially LMICs, lack the resources to design, procure, and maintain their own health insurance information systems.

In this chapter, we explore HIE in the context of nations that are implementing UHC policies, requiring robust information systems to facilitate insurance operations. We will also examine claims processing in high income as well as LMIC nations, focusing on how the health information systems are utilized to facilitate healthcare finance.

15.2 Role of claims in health information exchange to achieve universal health coverage

Universal health coverage (UHC) is defined by the WHO as "all people [having] access to the health services they need, when and where they need them, without financial hardship" [2]. One of the WHO SDGs seeks to increase the number of people with access to essential health services by 1 billion individuals by 2030. A primary mechanism to achieve UHC within a nation is through policy in which citizens are required to enroll in an insurance program. These policies are referred to as mandatory, compulsory, or universal health insurance programs [3]. The architecture is made of software components that make it possible for health data to be shared across information systems between facilities, across regions, or countries. For example, the United States passed the Affordable Care Act of 2010 in an attempt to achieve UHC. This law required citizens to purchase healthcare insurance through their employers or a "marketplace" facilitated by the government. The law further expanded access to free health insurance for children.

Multiple nations have adopted or implemented **compulsory insurance laws** or programs over the past decade. In 2019 the following countries passed UHC legislation: Egypt, South Africa, the Philippines, Uzbekistan, Zambia, and Mali [3]. These nations are just some of the 115 member states part of the WHO UHC Partnership [3], which seeks to increase the adoption and implementation of UHC programs across the globe.

A key component of the WHO strategy for achieving UHC goals involves health information systems. Information technologies support a range of healthcare and HIE services as described throughout this book. In addition, information systems facilitate fundamental processes in mandatory insurance programs, including claims processing.

Health insurance information systems are core components to achieve UHC as they facilitate the exchange of data between payers (insurance programs) and healthcare providers. They must exchange data (membership, eligibility, claims, and payments) that are the core business functions of health finance. Connecting clinical systems to public health systems is important for health surveillance; it also helps health systems to know if the services are reaching the entire population.

15.2.1 What is claims processing?

Claims processing in healthcare is the foundation for any public or private insurance provider. This is the point where the entity (e.g., insurance company, government) begins to process medical data on the premise of delivering on an agreement and commitment to its customers by reviewing and approving filed claims. Individuals, employees, and businesses invest in the insurance process, the healthcare provider sends a medical claim for the services rendered and thus ensures a rightful compensation for the healthcare provider, and the insurance pays for the covered benefits.

Prior to healthcare claims being sent electronically, claims were transmitted by the US Postal Service. The limitation was that the postal service could not prescreen the claims for errors. This archaic system was replaced, and claims are now managed with software, which send and receive a large amount of electronic claim information.

Without the use of information exchanges, claims processing is a manually intensive, expensive, and causes lengthy delays in payment. Healthcare costs are an important issue for all countries and one way of controlling costs is to limit administrative and managements costs. For example, in the United States, the premium paid for individual market plans must spend 85% of the premiums on direct medical services, thus limiting the payer to 15% to cover for administrative and overhead costs, as specified under the Affordable Care Act [4].

15.3 Claims processing in the United States and Europe

Claims processing happens in four broad steps:

1. Submission: In the medical billing process, submitting a claim is an important step. This step determines the amount of reimbursement a healthcare provider will receive from the insurance firm that receives the submitted claim. Submitting a claim without errors determines the provider's clean claim percentage, which ensures less time in the accounting process and timely payment. A higher clean claim percentage ensures the profitability of a healthcare practice.
2. Adjudication: After the submission of the claim, the insurance company reviews the claim and the financial obligation it has for the payment to the healthcare provider. This process is called as claim adjudication. In this step, the insurance company may decide to either pay the claim in full, deny the claim, or revise the amount that needs to be paid to the provider. If the insurance company decides to reduce the payment to the provider, the insurance company has adjudicated that the billed service is not appropriate for the diagnosis or the procedure. Thus accurate coding for the service is essential for accurate reimbursement.
3. Payment: The adjudicated amount by the insurance company is reimbursed to the healthcare provider based on negotiated rates for the services.

4. Settlement: the insurance company prepares a statement of the services that were billed by the provider, the amount that was paid by the insurance company, and send the statement to the individual for any out-of-pocket expenses that the individual might owe for the services.

This general process can vary, depending on the country, insurance program, or plan. In nations with socialized medicine, this process might happen in the background, and the individual receiving care might not see some of these steps or be aware they occur.

The next section will take a more detailed look at claims systems in several countries, highlighting a variety of implementations and processes.

15.3.1 United States

In the United States, insurance companies use both manual and automated verification for the adjudication of claims. After adjudication is complete, the insurance company decides how much it is willing to pay for the claim based on negotiated rates. Automated systems use specialized methods to capture the information from medical claim forms such as HCFA/CMS-1500 or UB-04. These processes by automated systems use precise extraction technology to ensure high accuracy and accountability to review customer billing, accounting, and healthcare data. Once captured, the data are electronically submitted to a claims service (Fig. 15.1), which serves as a clearinghouse for claims as they are routed to insurance companies for adjudication. Examples of claims services include Waystar, Optum, Experian Health, Infinix Healthcare, and Office Ally.

Each year the US medical industry spends $4.5 billion on claim submissions; thus administrative transactions account for approximately 13% of the total healthcare spending [5]. Therefore claims processing is an expensive

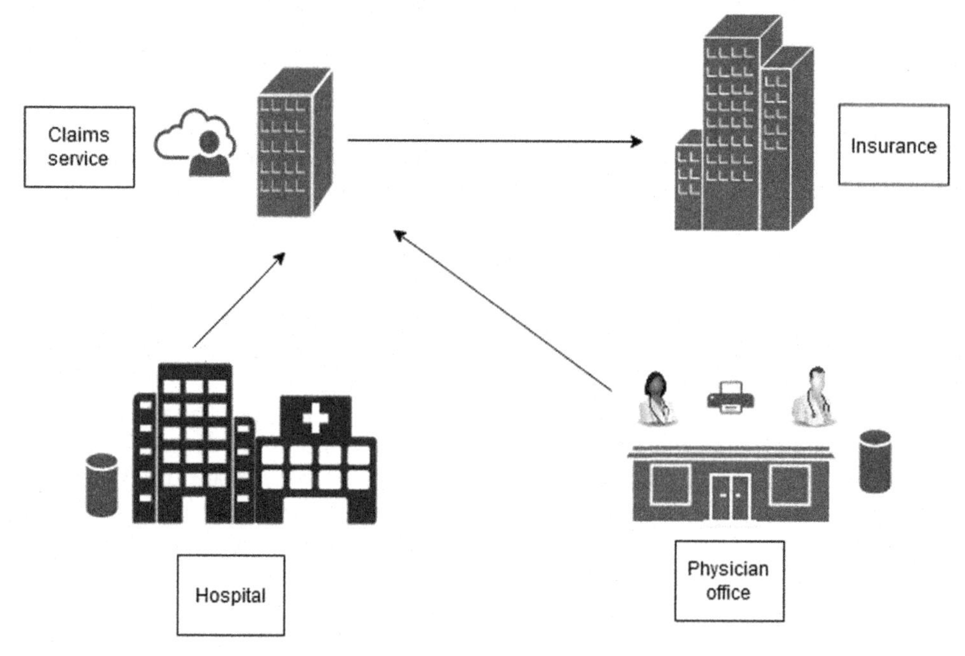

FIGURE 15.1 Information flow for submitting insurance claims in the United States.

undertaking for both health insurers and providers. Effective claims management is complex and goes beyond processing and paying claims—companies are looking for ways to increase customer interactions and manage medical costs. The steps for claims processing and areas for automation are described in Table 15.1.

Digitizing the claims process from data input to claims payment is one way to address the rising costs, but it also will increase accuracy and efficiency. Over the past few years there has been interest in the use of self-learning algorithms in healthcare and claims processing [6,7]. However, a few ethical concerns have been raised with the introduction of biases in these algorithms, which may violate the norms of justice and equality [8]. This phenomenon is known as **algorithmic bias** and defined as "the outputs of an algorithm benefit or disadvantage certain individuals or groups more than others without a justified reason for such unequal impacts" [9]. Although full digitalization approach is not yet realistic, portions of the claim process have used existing technologies as consumers have become comfortable with digital transactions. Some of the barriers to a fully digitized claims management process include multiple stakeholders,

TABLE 15.1 Steps toward developing a digitized claims process in a US context.

From →			To →	
	Steps			
Many system gaps	1	Customer receives claim from provider	Automated cloud-based claims process	↓ • Claim from provider automatically undergoes first check, is transferred to cloud
	2	Customer sends claim to insurer		
	3	Claim prepared		
Many manual tasks	4	Technical claims auditing	Fast, fully digital process with fewer steps	↓ • Fully integrated, real-time claims auditing by self-learning algorithms, in the cloud • Approval or decline sent to provider and customer from cloud via app or email
	5	Medical claims auditing		
	6	Claim approval or decline send to customer		
Slow and Cost-intensive	7	Payment to customer initiated	Improved customer experience	↓ • Automatic initiation of payment to provider or customer
	8	Customer receives payment		
	9	Customer transfers payment to provider		

Steps 1, 7, and 9 are mostly done manually; Steps 2-6 and 8 have gaps and discontinuities.
Source: *Adapted from Singhal S, Dash P, Schneider T, Chowdhary S, Aggarwal H. For better healthcare claims management, think "digital first". McKinsey & Company; 2019 [cited 2021 Dec 14]. Available from: https://www.mckinsey.com/industries/healthcare-systems-and-services/our-insights/for-better-healthcare-claims-management-think-digital-first.*

regulatory constraints, and also those related with data security and privacy concerns [10].

15.3.2 Europe

15.3.2.1 Claims processing in the Netherlands

In the Netherlands, around 100 million claims are processed from 40,000 healthcare providers. Paper claims were a huge administrative burden for payers, providers, and patients. The yearly cost of the Dutch claims process was estimated at around €460 million in 2002 [11]. To reduce costs, automation was required to reduce errors and claims processing times. Interoperability was a high priority to streamline the claims process between healthcare providers and the 20 payers (insurance companies) so standards and interfaces could "speak" the same language to interact with 500 different claims software packages [11].

To facilitate communication, an internet-based, national infrastructure was implemented, with a secure claims routing hub and registries for unique identification of healthcare providers, payers, and patients. The hub is essentially a large clearinghouse which allows practices and organizations to transmit electronic claims to insurance companies in a secure manner. This national data infrastructure can be viewed as an ecosystem of technology, processes, and organizations that are needed to collect, store, maintain, distribute, and use for different end users. For an analogy, the rail infrastructure is not only made of tracks and trains but also of resources, people, and material required to maintain it, ticketing, traffic control rules and regulations, and other passenger services. In 2010 approximately 90% of the claims produced in the Netherlands were exchanged and processed electronically after the establishment of the national infrastructure, standards (clinical terminologies), and interfaces [11]. This resulted in significant savings estimated between €100 and €300 million for the Dutch healthcare system annually [11].

15.4 Claims processing systems in Low-and-Middle Income Countries

15.4.1 Open-source Insurance Management Information System

The open-source Insurance Management Information System (openIMIS) [12] is an open-source platform developed as a collaborative effort between the Swiss [13,14] and German Development Cooperation [15,16] that fosters health financing processes for health and social protection. The software has enabled support of diverse insurance models including nationalized (Nepal), district-based (Tanzania), and community-based models such as Mutual Health Organizations (MHOs; Cameroon, Democratic Republic of Congo, and Chad). The web-based platform allows for exchange of information between beneficiaries, health service providers, and payers of the health financing scheme. The software is classified as a "global good" which is free to use, modify, and redistribute with support from a virtual community.

The web-based software allows the exchange of information between beneficiaries, health service providers, and the payers of the health financing scheme (Fig. 15.2). The highly customizable and modular software helps manage:

- Beneficiaries (the individuals enrolled in insurance who receive benefits)
- Benefit packages (services covered and negotiated prices)
- Providers
- Service claims generation, review, and processing
- Client feedback
- Monitoring and data analysis

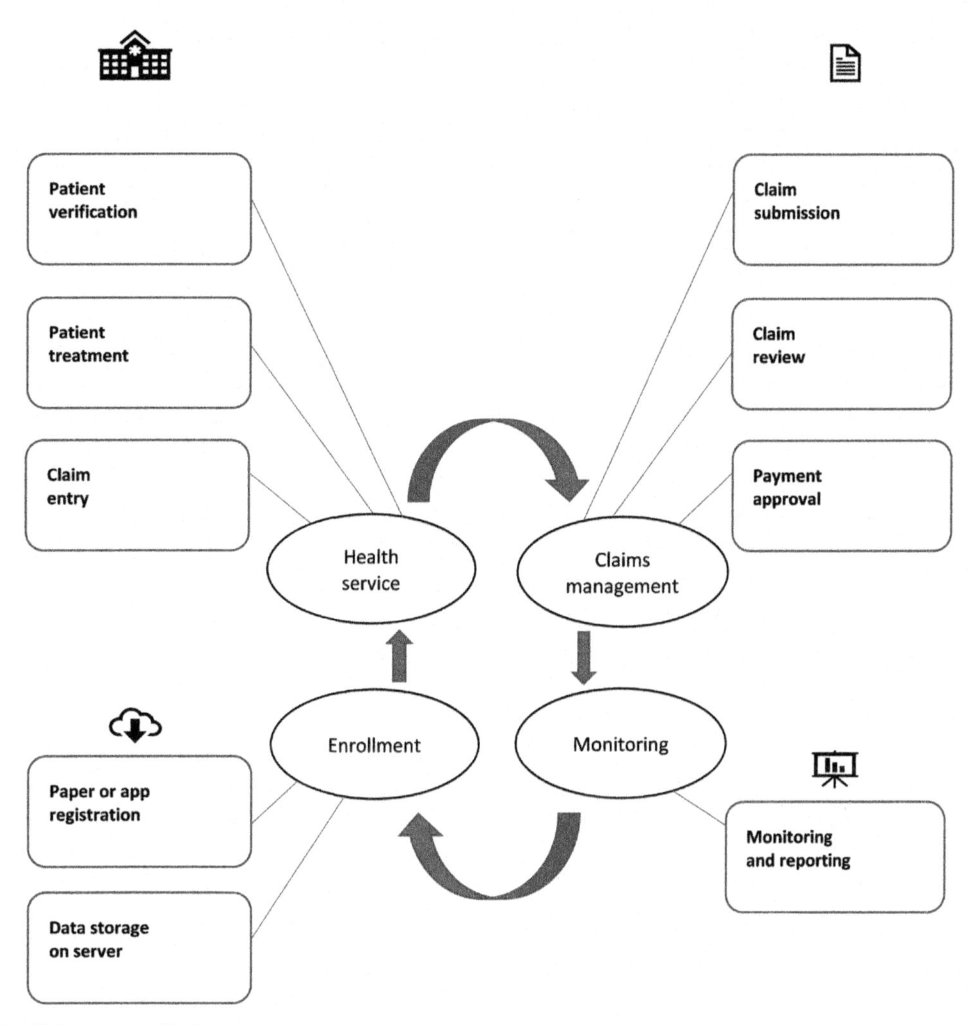

FIGURE 15.2 openIMIS claims integration workflow.

Since health financing schemes require an efficient implementation to undertake the complex business processes, scheme operators in LMICs struggle to achieve UHC, as they often lack robust technological infrastructures. openIMIS software allows scheme operators an "in-house" IT solution to manage health financing workflows and avoid expensive license fees from commercial software packages.

15.4.2 Implementation of openIMIS

15.4.2.1 Nepal

In 2016 the government of Nepal introduced the Social Health Insurance program with an initial roll-out to three of the country's 77 districts, focused mainly on the informal sector. The family scheme, with a family of up to five members contributing €30, receives a benefit package of €800 per family per year.

The openIMIS system for Nepal was adapted from the implementations in Tanzania and Cameroon. From the beginning, it was used to manage business processes of the insurance scheme; like beneficiary management and claim adjudication. In 2017 the Nepal Health Insurance Act was passed, which mandates that every Nepali citizen should be covered by health insurance. The law also enabled the formation of the Health Insurance Board (HIB) of Nepal. The scheme reached 65% of the country (41 out of 77 districts), with an aim to reach 100% by 2020.

The HIB transitioned to openIMIS. The tool has enabled enrollment and claims processing to support Nepal in implementing the scheme nationally. The system has also developed Android-based apps for enrollment which enable enrollment assistants to go door-to-door to add households to the national scheme. The web-based claims-entry and adjudication significantly reduces the effort needed for paper-based transactions and paperwork at the facility level. The scheme has enabled Nepal to insure approximately 4.8 million individuals, which is 16.2% of the total Nepali population [17]. The new features added in Nepal will help with interoperability, but would also provide valuable products for the global openIMIS users. The software has developed the Claim-Artificial Intelligence (AI) architecture that has helped reduce the workload for processing claims (Fig. 15.3).

The IT team at HIB and their engagement with the developers and implementers of the

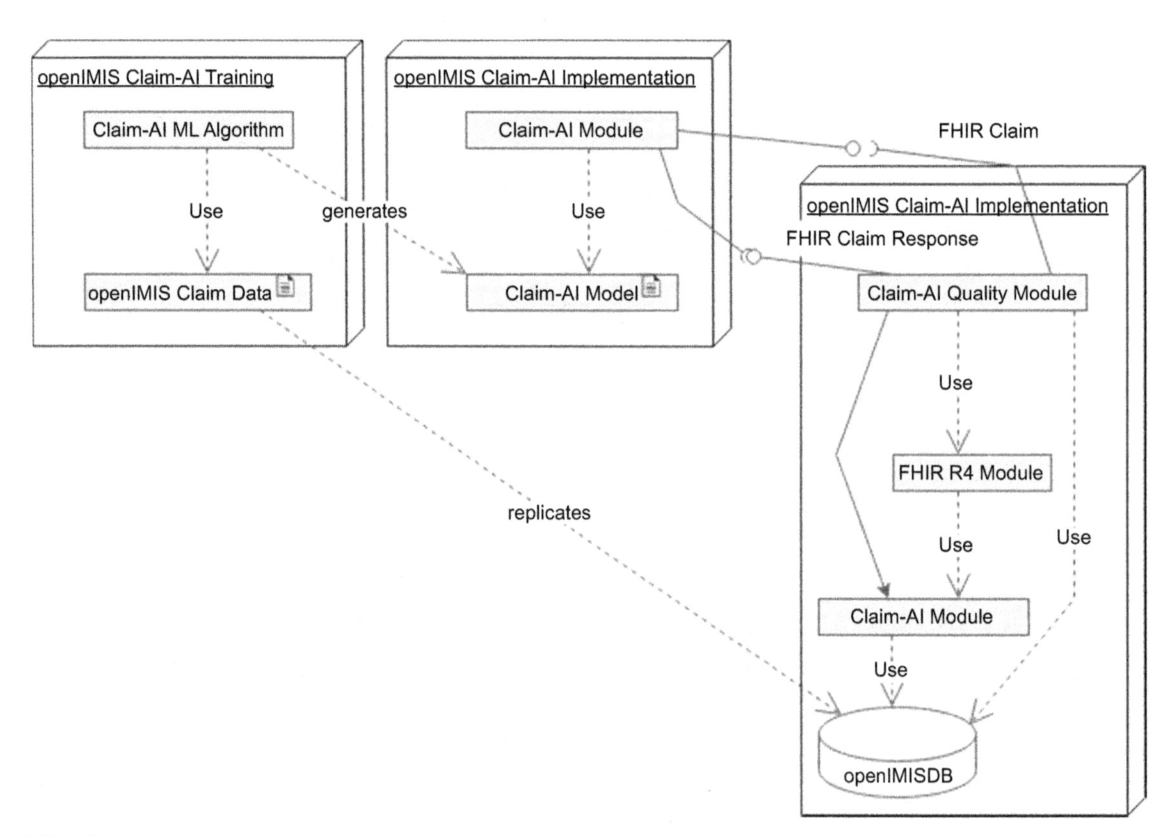

FIGURE 15.3 openIMIS Claims-AI architecture in Nepal. [18]

openIMIS community to introduce new features had developed the software further. These new features have helped with interoperability, but this will also add valuable products to global community of openIMIS users.

15.4.2.2 *Tanzania*

The implementation for openIMIS was originally developed in Tanzania (2012) and financed through the Swiss Development Corporation (SDC) with technical support from the Swiss Tropical and Public Health Institute (Swiss TPH); both the SDC and Swiss TPH are international aid organizations. The program initially started out as a pilot in one region and later expanded to three. The formal government roll-out of openIMIS was later expanded to the 26 regions in mainland Tanzania. The program is implementing the Improved Community Health Funds (iCHF) model, and the country is using the CHF IMIS as the main technology solution for running their operations. All of the components for IMIS are available either online, offline, and mobile phone format. The system is constantly developed in the country based on the inputs from stakeholder needs and integrates openIMIS in the overall IT landscape.

15.4.2.3 *Chad*

A similar program funded by the SDC was implemented in Chad known as the Support Project for the Health Districts (Programme d'Appui aux Districts Sanitaire au Tchad—PADS), a health development program. The implementation of openIMIS was launched as pilot in 2018 to digitize the operations at a district-based MHO in Danamadji. The PADS contributes to the National Strategy of Universal Health Coverage (Stratégie Nationale de Couverture Sanitaire Universelle—SN-CSU). However, PADS has been involved in supporting the implementation of openIMIS in the informal sector for a network of MHOs since 2010.

15.4.2.4 *Cameroon*

In 2013 the IMIS developed in Tanzania was customized to manage micro health insurance schemes in various dioceses with the Bamenda Ecclesiastical Provincial Health Assistance (BEPHA) Cameroon. The Swiss TPH supported the system's technical implementation with a bilateral agreement with the BEPHA Cameroon including a no-cost license to customize the source code. The web-based component of the system is in use; however, the pilot for mobile phone is expected to be rolled out shortly. The system from the five diocese level schemes mainly in the North West and South West regions use it for beneficiary enrollment and system management.

15.4.2.5 *Democratic Republic of Congo*

The Health System Support Program (Programme d'Appui au Systéme de Santé dans la Province du Sud Kivu—PASS) a social and health development program funded by the SDC operates through the financing, technical assistance, and capacity building to improve the technical platform for development. To revitalize the MHO, support was started in 2017 for the implementation of the management information system of the MHO activities (enrollment, premium collection, identification, and claims processing management). In order to professionalize the insurance business processes, the openIMIS software was used in nine MHOs and supported eight health zones to make healthcare accessible and improve the quality of the care.

15.5 OpenHIE and claims processing

OpenHIE is a global community whose mission is to improve the health of the underserved by having open and collaborative development and support for country driven large-scale health information sharing architectures. The community supports interoperability by building a reusable architectural framework that enables a service-oriented approach, which leverages information standards for the exchange of health information.

The architecture denotes logical components that make it possible for health data to be shared across information systems between facilities, across regions, or countries. The functions of the components are designed to be interoperable and support multiple solutions.

The OpenHIE [19] architecture (described more in Chapter 8) interacts in various contexts under the software components to ensure the events at a point-of-care (data) are gathered within the HIE. This is accomplished as the exchange normalizes the context of health information which is created across multiple dimensions which include:

- Who received health services
- Who provided the health services
- Where the services were received
- What particular care and services were received
- What treatments were received
- Who owns the financial responsibility

Designed to identify and address the healthcare financing data and data exchange needs, as well as respond to future needs, the OpenHIE Health Financing toward UHC working group [20] works synergistically with the OpenHIE community to ensure that data exchange processes and requirements meet the needs of the healthcare financing communities. The working group primarily focuses on the functions and data needed by the health purchaser, defined by OpenHIE as any institution that buys healthcare goods, services, and interventions on behalf of a covered population. Although its efforts are open to any health financing-related scenario, the working group prioritizes using national health insurance use cases as a basis for evaluating the health financing requirements.

Besides serving as a collaborative workspace for sharing best practices and proposing solutions to healthcare financing data exchange, some of the working group's goals include:

- Identify and prioritize foundational requirements needed to meet data elements and data exchange needs of healthcare financing;
- Identify and create alignment around standardized terminologies that will meet the data and data exchange needs of the international healthcare financing communities;
- Work to develop and/or identify solutions that meet these requirements;
- Develop documented data sharing use cases that describe the fundamental flow of information to support strategic purchasing;
- Build or refine OpenHIE workflows to incorporate health finance data sharing use cases;
- Represent country needs as they implement health purchasing schemas within the auspices of a national data sharing architecture;
- Collaborate with other stakeholder groups to identify data exchange needs; and
- Engage and collaborate with developers and implementers working with health insurance/finance solutions, such as openIMIS (open insurance management information system).

Issues around the financing of healthcare services are receiving strong recognition by international partners and national governments. Early development and adoption of integrated digital tools play a critical role in a successful implementation of UHC strategies. The goal is to ensure that solutions like openIMIS are able to use standards-based integrations that support data sharing between beneficiaries, health service providers, and payers. At the time of writing this chapter, the data exchanges to support these activities are being developed. It is expected that transactions supporting enrollment, coverage eligibility, and claims will be outlined in the OpenHIE Architecture Specification.

15.5.1 Proposed function of health financing in OpenHIE Architecture

The openIMIS community and others have been working with the OpenHIE community to ensure that data exchange processes and requirements meet the needs of healthcare financing communities and develop and adapt OpenHIE workflows to incorporate health finance data sharing use cases and country needs. Fig. 15.4 illustrates the anticipated role of health financing as it is integrated into the OpenHIE landscape, supporting *health financing and insurance* business domain services within an HIE.

15.5.2 Interoperability use cases

Countries and organizations that have adopted an eHealth strategy based on Health Level Seven (HL7) Fast Healthcare Interoperability Resources (FHIR) are able to implement more efficient digital workflows to strengthen their road to UHC. The standards-based approach also opens up opportunities for supporting a range of HIE workflows and interacting other HIE components and registries (e.g., Shared Health Record,

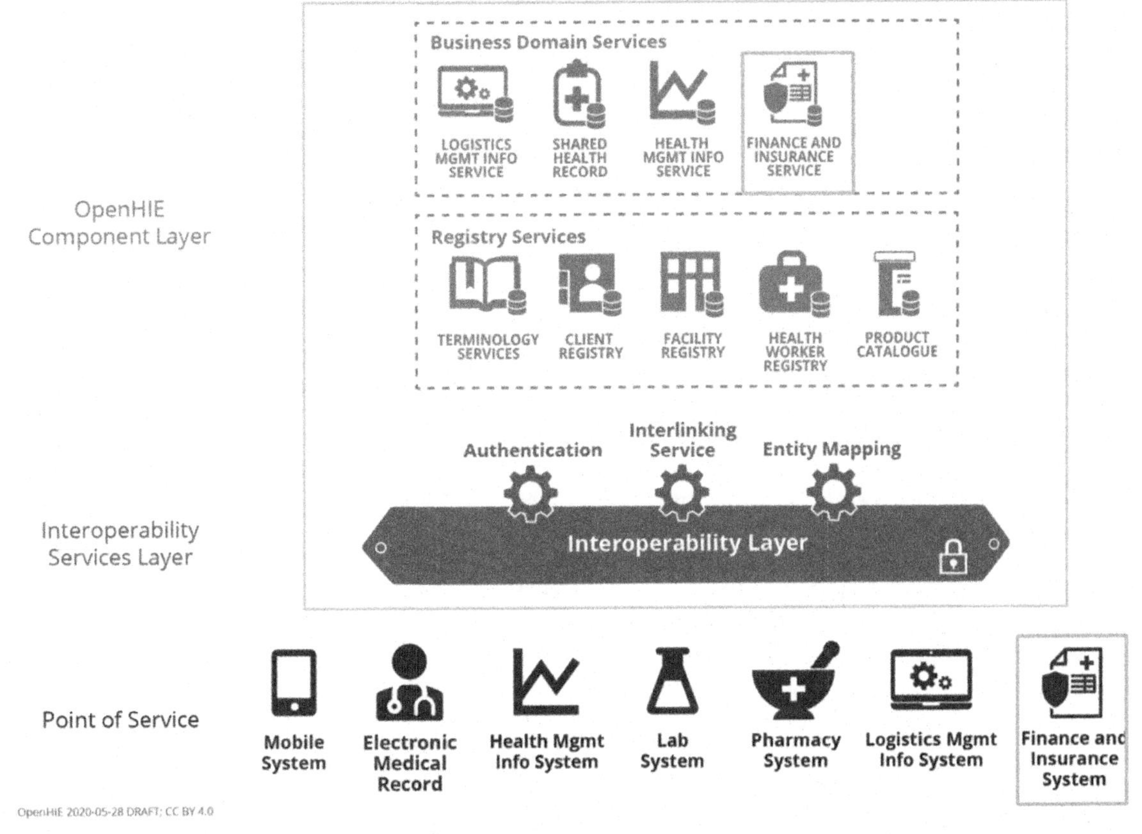

FIGURE 15.4 The OpenHIE architecture with the Finance and Insurance components highlighted.

Client Registry, Facility Registry, Product Registry, Terminology Services) as well as a move toward tools like openIMIS that can support the role of health financing as an OpenHIE reference technology.

One approach to supporting interoperability is to utilize FHIR. As an example, openIMIS now possesses a set of HL7 FHIR compatible Application Programming Interface (APIs) that allow the exchange of patient and claims data with other information systems in the health sector.

15.6 Summary

Achieving UHC for all individuals is an important endeavor and a focus of the WHO. One key to accomplishing this is creating a robust financing scheme that minimizes the administrative overhead by reducing delay and cost. Healthcare financing is a complex scheme that includes all activities related to the "mobilization, accumulation, and allocation of money to cover the health needs of the people" [1].

Processing claims is a large component of any healthcare finance scheme but can be expensive and time consuming. Processing each claim is a multistep endeavor, requiring submission, adjudication, payment, and settlement, which adds a high volume of data and administrative burden. These processes can be lengthy, time-consuming, and expensive detracting from the overall funding available in support of healthcare activities and becoming a barrier to achieving UHC.

HIE can provide efficiencies by digitizing this process. Additionally, the global community has developed solutions that are ready for implementation, thereby removing the requirement for a country to custom build systems to support these activities. openIMIS and OpenHIE have created reusable architecture frameworks that allow for the exchange of claims information, beneficiary enrollment and status, and monitoring and reporting. These frameworks are available under licenses that allow countries, particularly LMICs, to utilize them without fees to the developers, enabling more affordable solutions. Creating efficient, ready-to-implement systems and supporting automated claims processing allow more financial resources to be spent on healthcare rather than administration.

Questions for discussion

1. What benefits do HIE networks offer to healthcare financing schemes?
2. Currently US HIE networks are not clearinghouses for insurance claims processes. Why do you think this is the case?
3. Where is your nation in its pursuit of universal healthcare? Are claims processed using health information technologies? If so, are HIE networks leveraged to submit and/or process claims?

Acknowledgments

The authors thank the following Regenstrief Institute staff members who helped with the content and support the OpenHIE Community: Jennifer Shivers, Jamie Thomas, and Michelle Cox. We further recognize and appreciate the OpenHIE Health Care Financing Community [21], especially Uwe Wahser, Saurav Bhattarai, and Daniel Futerman who provide leadership in the working group.

References

[1] The Global Health Observatory. Health financing. Geneva: World Health Organization; [cited 2022 Mar 17]. Available from: https://www.who.int/data/gho/data/themes/topics/health-financing.
[2] World Health Organization. Universal Health Coverage. Geneva: WHO; 2022 [cited 2022 Mar 17]. Available from: https://www.who.int/news-room/fact-sheets/detail/universal-health-coverage-(uhc).

[3] World Health Organization. Universal Health Coverage Partnership annual report. Geneva: WHO; 2019.
[4] Patient Protection and Affordable Care Act of 2010. US public law 111-48.
[5] Oracle. Oracle health insurance: modernizing claims processing and adjudication. [cited 2021 Dec 14]. Available from: https://www.oracle.com/industries/financial-services/insurance/health-insurance-modernizing-claims-processing/#time.
[6] Burke J. Health analytics: gaining the insights to transform health care. John Wiley & Sons; 2013.
[7] McNeill D, Davenport TH. Analytics in healthcare and the life sciences: strategies, implementation methods, and best practices. Pearson Education;; 2014.
[8] O'Neil C. Weapons of math destruction: how big data increases inequality and threatens democracy. Broadway Books; 2016.
[9] Kordzadeh N, Ghasemaghaei M. Algorithmic bias: review, synthesis, and future research directions. Eur J Inf Syst 2021;31:388–409.
[10] Singhal S, Dash P, Schneider T, Chowdhary S, Aggarwal H. For better healthcare claims management, think "digital first". McKinsey & Company; 2019 [cited 2021 Dec 14]. Available from: https://www.mckinsey.com/industries/healthcare-systems-and-services/our-insights/for-better-healthcare-claims-management-think-digital-first.
[11] Ingun P, Streveler D, Brown K, Kanter A, Rietberg A, Hesp C. The World Health report: Health Systems Financing. The role of information systems in achieving universal health coverage. World Health Organization; 2010.
[12] openIMIS. Open-source Insurance Management Information System. [cited 2021 Dec 8]. Available from: https://openimis.org/.
[13] Schweizerische Eidgenossenschaft Confederation. Homepage. [cited 2021 Dec 8]. Available from: https://www.eda.admin.ch/deza/en/home.html.
[14] Institute STaPH. Universal health coverage: designing and implementing insurance management information systems. [cited 2021 Dec 8]. Available from: https://www.swisstph.ch/en/about/scih/sysu/imis/.
[15] Deutsche Gesellschaft fur Internationale Zusammenarbeit (GIZ). Homepage. [cited 2021 Dec 8]. Available from: https://www.giz.de/en/html/index.html.
[16] Federal Ministry for Economic Cooperation and Development. Homepage. [cited 2022 Apr 7]. Available from: https://www.bmz.de/en.
[17] Nepal Government. Health Insurance Board (Nepal). [cited 2022 Apr 7]. Available from: https://hib.gov.np/en/.
[18] Dobre D. Artificial Intelligence as a global good. AI supported claim adjudication with openIMIS. [Open Health Information Exchange, 2021], 2021; online.
[19] OpenHIE. Open Health Information Exchange. [cited 2022 Feb 21]. Available from: https://ohie.org.
[20] OpenHIE. Health financing towards UHC subcommunity. 2022 [updated Mar 14; cited 2022 Apr 14]. Available from: https://wiki.ohie.org/display/SUB/Health + Financing + towards + UHC + Subcommunity.
[21] OpenHIE. Health Financing Data Community. [cited 2022 Apr 7]. Available from: https://ohie.org/practice-area/health-financing-data/.

SECTION 4

Impacting health care delivery and outcomes

CHAPTER

16

Evidence base for health information exchange

Willi L. Tarver[1,2], *Pallavi Jonnalagadda*[1] *and Saurabh Rahurkar*[1,2]

[1]The Center for the Advancement of Team Science, Analytics, and Systems Thinking in Health Services and Implementation Science Research (CATALYST), The Ohio State University College of Medicine, Columbus, OH, USA [2]Richard M. Fairbanks School of Public Health, Indiana University-Purdue University Indianapolis, Indianapolis, IN, USA

LEARNING OBJECTIVES

By the end of this chapter, the readers should be able to:

- Summarize the available scientific evidence on the impact of health information exchange (HIE) on health outcomes.
- Discuss trends in scientific studies on the impact of HIE over time.
- Describe those factors associated with beneficial impact of HIE on clinical processes as well as patient outcomes.
- Discuss the gaps in available evidence on the impact of HIE.

16.1 Introduction

Health information exchange (HIE) is believed to boost efficiencies, reduce healthcare costs, and improve outcomes as a result of improved availability of health information in healthcare as well as public health. As such, many nations have dedicated policy efforts to promote electronic exchange of health information (see Chapter 3). In the United States, the Health Information Technology for Economic and Clinical Health (HITECH) Act was enacted in 2009 to expand the use of health information technology (HIT) in the healthcare system. As discussed in previous chapters, this act directed $19.2 billion toward HIT and infrastructure investments from the American Recovery and Reinvestment Act. Initial funds were used to not only incentivize eligible healthcare providers and hospitals to adopt the use of certified electronic health records (EHRs) that enabled electronic HIE, but also to support development of HIE infrastructure [1]. Moreover, innovative healthcare delivery models such as the hospital readmission reduction program [2], accountable care organizations [3], bundled payments [4], and patient-centered medical homes [5] that require HIE were also implemented.

DOI: https://doi.org/10.1016/B978-0-323-90802-3.00019-8

More recently, legislation such as the Medicare Access and CHIP Reauthorization Act of 2015 (MACRA) and the 21st Century Cures Act further fueled the continued adoption of interoperable HIE by providers [6].

Owing to many of these policies and programs, HIE in the United States is now ubiquitous. Outside of the United States, initiatives such as the Digital Healthcare Act (Germany) [7], Hospital Future Act (Germany) [7], and Quality and Outcomes Framework (United Kingdom) [8] have sought to promote interoperable HIE. While HIE in these regions is still evolving and far from universal, the motivations behind these policies and programs remains the same. Specifically, these initiatives are geared toward achieving theorized benefits to health outcomes from HIE to improve healthcare while lowering costs. However, is there really evidence for these benefits? What does the existing literature examining HIE say about its effects on health outcomes?

In this chapter, we examine the evidence for the effect of HIE on health outcomes by reviewing a broad body of peer-reviewed literature. We will identify outcomes that researchers have used to study how HIE affects healthcare as well as explore several other characteristics that influence this relationship. We also discuss how the evidence base for the healthcare effects of information exchange has evolved concurrent to the landscape of HIE. Additionally, we identify outcomes for which there is strong evidence of HIE as well as those where the evidence for HIE is weak. Finally, we examine the areas where there are knowledge gaps in what we know about how HIE affects healthcare.

16.2 Methods

This chapter provides an overview of the current evidence examining HIE's impact on health outcomes and builds on two previously published systematic reviews [9,10]. The first review, published in 2015, covered the timeframe from January 1980 to May 2014 (hereafter, referred to as Period 1) [10]. An updated review was published in 2018 and covered the timeframe from June 2014 to June 2017 (hereafter, referred to as Period 2) [9]. In this chapter, we examine newer evidence regarding how HIE affects health outcomes, comparing recent evidence to prior evidence while expanding on what is known based upon the newer findings.

Consistent with the previous reviews, we conducted a systematic review of the literature focused on HIE and health outcomes based on the Preferred Reporting Items for Systematic Reviews and *Meta*-Analyses (PRISMA) methodology [11]. We searched the PubMed and Scopus databases from July 2017 to December 2021 for articles using the following HIE-related search terms: "electronic health information exchange," "health information exchange," "health information interchange," "electronic document exchange," "information exchange," and "electronic data exchange"; along with terms related to effectiveness: "outcome evaluation," "impact," "effect," "association," "correlation," "assessment," "influence," "relationship," "examination," "evaluation," and "ramifications." For this review, we only included quantitative peer-reviewed empirical publications in the English language. Nonempirical articles such as letters to the editor, policy briefs, governmental reports, commentaries, and other nonpeer-reviewed publications were excluded. We also excluded qualitative studies and other reviews.

The keyword search identified 818 articles, to which we applied the two-stage process illustrated in Fig. 16.1. Based on article title and abstract, two reviewers (SR and WLT) identified those that evaluated HIE and health outcomes. In this first stage, we attempted to be as inclusive as possible (higher sensitivity) to not miss any relevant articles. For example, if we were unclear if a study met our inclusion or exclusion criteria after reviewing the abstract, we erred on the side of inclusion to review the full text of the article in stage 2. Articles for which an abstract could not be found were also included for full text review

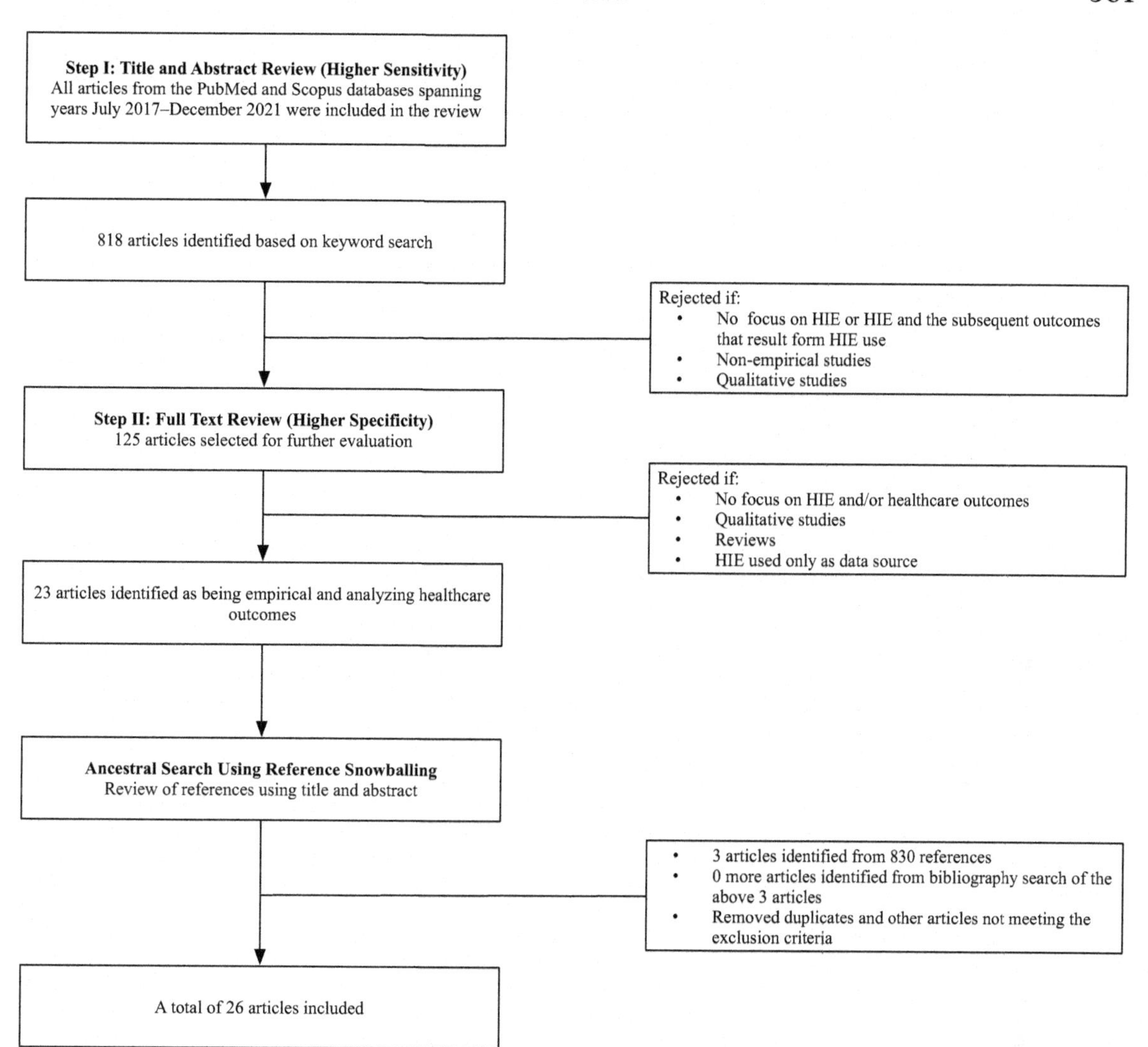

FIGURE 16.1 The systematic search strategy used in the current analysis.

in stage 2. Stage 1 resulted in the inclusion of 125 articles. In stage 2, we reviewed the full text of these 125 articles and selected those that evaluated the relationship between HIE and specific healthcare outcomes (e.g., healthcare utilization, healthcare costs, quality of care, disease surveillance). Outcomes like organizational outcomes and perceptions of HIE (e.g., provider perceptions of utility of HIE) were not included. Further, articles that used HIE networks only as a data source to create cohorts were also excluded. Stage 2 resulted in a list of 23 included articles.

Lastly, we performed an ancestral search of the references of the 23 articles from stage 2 using the snowball technique to recursively examine reference lists of these articles for any additional articles that may have been missed by the database search. This process yielded an additional three articles. Throughout the process (see Fig. 16.1), any disagreements were reconciled by consensus.

At the end of this process, we identified 26 articles consisting of 226 individual analyses published between July 2017 and December 2021 as many of the included studies examined more than one health outcome fitting the inclusion criteria. Analyses were considered discrete if they examined different outcomes, and/or different settings. For instance, in the study by Everson et al. [12], HIE was examined in relation to length of stay, likelihood of CT, likelihood of MRI, likelihood of X-ray, likelihood of admission, and total charges. Therefore this study analyzed a total of six outcomes. Similarly, in the study by Elysee et al. [13], 30-day readmission rates were examined in the inpatient and outpatient settings; therefore this study examined a total of two outcomes.

For each included article, we extracted various information including country of origin, study design (e.g., randomized control trial, quasi-experimental study, cohort study, cross-sectional study), as well as the setting and population studied [e.g., primary care physicians, hospital, emergency department (ED)]. We also extracted information on the health outcomes examined in the analysis which were grouped into the following categories: healthcare utilization (e.g., readmissions, redundant lab tests), public health (e.g., public health reporting, surveillance), healthcare costs (e.g., total care costs), quality-of-care measures (e.g., medication adherence, medication reconciliation), and patient satisfaction (e.g., communication with physicians, overall patient satisfaction, satisfaction with care received during visit). Additionally, we extracted information on several HIE-related characteristics such as the type of HIE being evaluated (e.g., community HIE, enterprise HIE, vendor-facilitated HIE). When possible, we also extracted information on whether a study assessed actual HIE usage (Yes/No), the patient consent model for data use in an HIE (Opt-in/Opt-out), and the mechanism used to access HIE information (Push/Pull). Since the landscape of HIE is now starting to focus more on interoperability, we identified if the article had a focus on interoperability (Yes/No). Studies were identified as using measures of actual usage if they used HIE log files or EHR audit data. We labeled the consent model to be "Opt-out" if all patients were enrolled for participation in HIE and "Opt-in" when any given patient explicitly objected to participation in HIE. An interoperability focus was determined based on whether the HIE resulted in integration of external data into the EHR.

Finally, we identified the relationship between HIE and health outcomes in individual analyses as "beneficial," "no effect," and "not beneficial." The relationship was considered "beneficial" if an analysis found a statistically significant positive association for positive outcomes or a negative association for negative outcomes. Conversely, if the analysis found a statistically significant positive association for negative outcomes or negative association for positive outcomes, the relationship was considered "not beneficial."

In order to examine the evolving nature of evidence over time, we aggregated data from our review with that from previous reviews that used an identical methodology [9,10]. The total sample had 77 studies (51 from the previous reviews, 26 from the current review) comprising a total of 383 analyses (157 from the previous reviews + 226 from the current review).

We summarized each of the extracted variables to examine the articles included in the current study. We then examined differences in study characteristics between studies that found a beneficial association with HIE and those that did not using a Chi-square analysis or Fisher's exact test as appropriate. We conducted all analyses in STATA/MP version 16. Statistical significance was set at $P < .05$.

16.3 Evidence base for the effect of Health Information Exchange on health outcomes

Findings are presented in relation to each of the three individual time periods. Then we present the findings from our comparison of the evidence base and evolution of evidence over time. A complete list of each article identified in each time period is provided at the end of this chapter in discrete bibliographies, stratified by time period.

16.3.1 Period 1 (January 1980–May 2014) overview

Importantly, each time period is characterized by policies and initiatives that supported the adoption of HIE. For example, Period 1 ranges from January 1980 to May 2014. While the majority of this period consists of isolated efforts in select locations to promote early versions of HIE, the latter studies—particularly those from the United States—should be viewed in light of landmark legislation. Namely, during this time period, the HITECH Act and the Patient Protection and Affordable Care Act were signed into law. The specifics of how these policies promoted adoption of EHRs while supporting HIE are discussed in Chapter 3. Financial incentives under HITECH's Meaningful Use (MU) program were offered starting 2011 through 2019. Stage 1 MU starting in 2011 focused on developing the capacity to exchange information electronically among providers and authorized entities, whereas stage 2 starting in 2014 required a minimum level of HIE. This review concluded that little evidence existed in the scientific literature that HIE impacted costs, use of health services, or quality of care. In addition, many of the early studies were limited in terms of study settings, outcomes examined, and the use of more rigorous study designs suited for establishing causation.

16.3.2 Period 2 (June 2014–June 2017) overview

Period 2 ranges from June 2014 to June 2017 and aligns with the transition from HITECH's MU program to the Merit-based Incentive Payment System introduced by MACRA. Another policy of interest in this period is the 21st Century Cures Act passed in 2016 which formally defined interoperability and included provisions to prohibit information blocking (see Chapter 6) to promote HIE. This review found that studies evaluating community HIEs were more likely to find benefits than studies that evaluated enterprise HIEs or vendor-facilitated exchanges. In addition, this review found that studies with more rigorous designs reported benefits of HIE among several outcomes such as reduction in duplicated procedures, reduced imaging, lower costs, and improved patient safety.

16.3.3 Period 3 (July 2017–December 2021) overview

Period 3 ranges from July 2017 to December 2021. During this period, the Office of the National Coordinator for Health Information Technology (ONC) published draft versions of the Trusted Exchange Framework and Common Agreement (TEFCA), that facilitates HIE by advancing interoperability (see Chapter 21). Concurrently, as part of its strategic goal to promote interoperability, the ONC established a core set of data elements that providers were required to share, called the United States Core Data for Interoperability. Additionally, the ONC encouraged use of standards such as Fast Healthcare Interoperability Resources (FHIR) to develop interoperable applications to improve healthcare.

To provide a consistent structure, the remainder of the chapter is organized as follows. Study characteristics are provided for the included studies for each review period. We then provide an overview of the findings for Period 3, while comparing and contrasting these findings to Periods 1 and 2. Lastly, we examine how various characteristics of existing studies and the analyses within relate to whether or not a study finds a benefit from the use of HIE and explore relevant trends over time.

16.3.4 Descriptive characteristics from contemporary literature

Table 16.1 describes the characteristics of all studies and periods individually as well as combined. Overall, from January 1980 to December 2021 (see Table 16.1, "Total" column), there were 77 articles examining HIE and its association with health outcomes. Nearly 80% of the included studies examining HIE were based in the United States. In terms of study design, a quarter of the studies used experimental study designs. The most common study setting was the ED, followed by the inpatient and outpatient settings respectively. Approximately 58% of the studies analyzed healthcare utilization, whereas 10% examined public health outcomes. The most common HIE type across the studies was the CHIE/RHIO (Community-based HIE/Regional Health Information Organization; see Chapter 1).

The 26 published articles from Period 3 included 226 analyses. In this most recent set of studies (see Table 16.2, "July 2017–December 2021" column), about 9.3% of the analyses focus on HIE outside the United States. HIE literature is dominated by observational study designs such as cohort studies (49.6%), while experimental study designs such as randomized controlled trials (9.7%) and quasi-experimental designs (19%) contributed to only about 1-in-3 analyses. Our review finds that a majority of the analyses were conducted in the outpatient setting (72.6%). By far, the most studied health outcomes in the HIE literature are those that focus on quality of care (36.3%) and patient satisfaction (34.1%). Together with healthcare utilization (23.0%), analyses focused on these three

TABLE 16.1 Descriptive characteristics of studies reviewed.

Variable	January 1980–May 2014 (N = 27 studies)	June 2014–June 2017 (N = 24 studies)	July 2018–December 2021 (N = 26 studies)	Total (N = 77 studies)
Study location				
United States	19 (70.4)	20 (83.3)	21 (80.8)	60 (77.9)
Others	8 (29.6)	4 (16.7)	5 (19.2)	17 (22.1)
Canada	1 (3.7)	1 (4.2)	–	2 (2.6)
Finland	1 (3.7)	–	–	1 (1.3)
Israel	4 (14.8)	2 (8.3)	–	6 (7.8)
Netherlands	1 (3.7)	–	–	1 (1.3)
Sweden	1 (3.7)	–	–	1 (1.3)
South Korea	–	1 (4.2)	–	1 (1.3)
Taiwan	–	–	5 (19.2)	5 (6.5)
Study design				
Randomized controlled trial	5 (18.5)	2 (8.3)	2 (7.7)	9 (11.7)
Quasi-experimental study	1 (3.7)	5 (20.8)	4 (15.4)	10 (13.0)

(*Continued*)

TABLE 16.1 (Continued)

Variable	January 1980–May 2014 (N = 27 studies)	June 2014–June 2017 (N = 24 studies)	July 2018–December 2021 (N = 26 studies)	Total (N = 77 studies)
Cross-sectional study	1 (3.7)	2 (8.3)	3 (11.5)	6 (7.8)
Cohort study	20 (74.1)	15 (62.5)	17 (65.4)	52 (67.5)
Study setting				
Emergency department	14 (51.9)	8 (33.3)	3 (11.5)	25 (32.5)
Inpatient	8 (29.6)	6 (25.0)	4 (15.4)	18 (23.4)
Community	–	3 (12.5)	1 (3.9)	4 (5.2)
Outpatient	1 (3.7)	3 (12.5)	13 (50.0)	17 (22.1)
Inpatient and outpatient	1 (3.7)	2 (8.3)	3 (11.5)	6 (7.8)
Other	3 (11.1)	2 (8.3)	2 (7.7)	7 (9.1)
Outcomes analyzed				
Healthcare utilization	21 (77.8)	12 (50.0)	12 (46.2)	45 (58.4)
Healthcare costs	9 (33.3)	11 (45.8)	3 (11.5)	23 (29.9)
Quality of care	7 (25.9)	5 (20.8)	11 (42.3)	23 (29.9)
Public health	1 (3.7)	4 (16.7)	3 (11.5)	8 (10.4)
Patient satisfaction	2 (7.4)	0 (0.0)	5 (19.2)	7 (9.1)
Year				
1987	1 (3.7)	–	–	1 (1.3)
1998	1 (3.7)	–	–	1 (1.3)
1999	1 (3.7)	–	–	1 (1.3)
2002	1 (3.7)	–	–	1 (1.3)
2006	1 (3.7)	–	–	1 (1.3)
2008	2 (7.4)	–	–	2 (2.6)
2009	1 (3.7)	–	–	1 (1.3)
2010	2 (7.4)	–	–	2 (2.6)
2011	3 (11.1)	–	–	3 (3.9)
2012	6 (22.2)	–	–	6 (7.8)
2013	4 (14.8)	–	–	4 (5.2)

(Continued)

TABLE 16.1 (Continued)

Variable	January 1980–May 2014 (*N* = 27 studies)	June 2014–June 2017 (*N* = 24 studies)	July 2018–December 2021 (*N* = 26 studies)	Total (*N* = 77 studies)
2014	4 (14.8)	4 (16.7)	–	8 (10.4)
2015	–	7 (29.2)	–	7 (9.1)
2016	–	5 (20.8)	–	5 (6.5)
2017	–	8 (33.3)	8 (30.8)	16 (20.8)
2018	–	–	6 (23.1)	6 (7.8)
2019	–	–	5 (19.2)	5 (6.5)
2020	–	–	4 (15.4)	4 (5.2)
2021	–	–	3 (11.5)	3 (3.9)
Measure of usage				
Actual usage measured	4 (14.8)	8 (33.3)	3 (11.5)	15 (19.5)
Not measured	23 (85.2)	16 (66.7)	23 (88.5)	62 (80.5)
HIE mechanism				
Pull	11 (40.7)	13 (54.2)	10 (38.5)	36 (46.8)
Push	10 (37.0)	6 (25.0)	5 (19.2)	21 (27.3)
Both	4 (14.8)	2 (8.3)		6 (7.8)
Multiple or unknown	2 (7.4)	3 (12.5)	11 (42.3)	14 (18.2)
HIE access				
Portal	0 (0.0)	9 (37.5)	5 (19.2)	14 (18.2)
Others	27 (100.0)	15 (62.5)	21 (80.8)	63 (81.8)
HIE type				
CHIE/RHIO	12 (44.4)	15 (62.5)	14 (53.9)	41 (53.3)
Vendor-facilitated	9 (33.3)	4 (16.7)	3 (11.5)	7 (9.1)
Enterprise	–	3 (12.5)	2 (7.7)	14 (18.2)
Other	6 (22.2)	2 (8.3)	7 (26.9)	15 (19.5)

The percentages in each cell represent the counts in that cell as a proportion of all studies in that column. For example, for variable "study design," under "January 1980–May 2014 (*N* = 27 studies)" the percentage for the category "cohort study" was calculated as a function of 20 divided by 27 (=74.1).
For the variable "outcomes analyzed," individual studies could assess multiple outcomes. Therefore, the total count for each category exceeds the total *N* of studies as multiple studies may have been evaluated within each category. Percentages for this variable are calculated as for other variables as a function of all studies in that column. *CHIE/RHIO*, Community-based HIE/Regional Health Information Organization; *HIE*, Health Information Exchange.

TABLE 16.2 Descriptive characteristics of analyses reviewed.

	January 1980–May 2014 (N = 94 analyses)	June 2014–June 2017 (N = 63 analyses)	July 2017–December 2021 (N = 226 analyses)	Total (N = 383)
Study location				
United States	59 (62.8)	48 (76.2)	205 (90.7)	312 (81.5)
Others	35 (37.3)	15 (23.8)	21 (9.3)	71 (18.5)
Study design				
Randomized controlled trial	17 (18.1)	4 (6.4)	22 (9.7)	43 (11.2)
Quasi-experimental study	12 (12.8)	9 (14.3)	43 (19.0)	64 (16.7)
Cross-sectional study	5 (5.3)	4 (6.4)	49 (21.7)	58 (15.1)
Cohort study	60 (63.8)	46 (73.0)	112 (49.6)	218 (56.9)
Study setting				
Emergency department	51 (54.3)	17 (27.0)	14 (6.2)	82 (21.4)
Inpatient	30 (31.9)	19 (30.2)	11 (4.9)	60 (15.7)
Community	–	7 (11.1)	2 (0.90)	9 (2.4)
Outpatient	1 (1.1)	13 (20.6)	164 (72.6)	178 (46.5)
Inpatient and outpatient	4 (4.3)	2 (3.2)	27 (12.0)	33 (8.6)
Other	8 (8.5)	5 (7.9)	8 (3.5)	21 (5.5)
Outcomes analyzed				
Healthcare utilization	67 (71.3)	25 (39.7)	52 (23.0)	144 (37.6)
Healthcare costs	11 (11.7)	18 (28.6)	4 (1.8)	33 (8.6)
Quality of care	12 (12.8)	10 (15.9)	82 (36.3)	104 (27.2)
Public health	2 (2.1)	10 (15.9)	11 (4.9)	23 (6.0)
Patient satisfaction	2 (2.1)	–	77 (34.1)	79 (20.6)
Years				
1987	2 (2.1)	–	–	2 (0.5)
1998	5 (5.3)	–	–	5 (1.3)
1999	2 (2.1)	–	–	2 (0.5)
2002	4 (4.3)	–	–	4 (1.0)

(Continued)

TABLE 16.2 (Continued)

	January 1980–May 2014 (*N* = 94 analyses)	June 2014–June 2017 (*N* = 63 analyses)	July 2017–December 2021 (*N* = 226 analyses)	Total (*N* = 383)
2006	4 (4.3)	–	–	4 (1.0)
2008	6 (6.4)	–	–	6 (1.6)
2009	3 (3.2)	–	–	3 (0.8)
2010	15 (16.0)	–	–	15 (3.9)
2011	13 (13.8)	–	–	13 (3.4)
2012	16 (17.0)	–	–	16 (4.2)
2013	13 (13.8)	–	–	13 (3.4)
2014	11 (11.7)	8 (12.7)	–	19 (5.0)
2015	–	18 (28.6)	–	18 (4.7)
2016	–	16 (25.4)	–	16 (4.2)
2017	–	21 (33.3)	46 (20.4)	67 (17.5)
2018	–	–	65 (28.8)	65 (17.0)
2019	–	–	23 (10.2)	23 (6.0)
2020	–	–	73 (32.3)	73 (19.1)
2021	–	–	19 (8.4)	19 (5.0)
Measure of usage				
Actual usage measured	20 (21.3)	21 (33.3)	12 (5.3)	53 (13.8)
Not measured	74 (78.7)	42 (66.7)	214 (94.7)	330 (86.2)
HIE mechanism				
Multiple or unknown	6 (6.4)	3 (4.8)	118 (52.2)	127 (33.2)
Pull	39 (41.5)	27 (42.9)	63 (27.9)	129 (33.7)
Push	34 (36.2)	23 (36.5)	42 (18.6)	99 (25.9)
Both	15 (16.0)	10 (15.9)	3 (1.3)	28 (7.3)
HIE access				
Portal	–	22 (34.9)	27 (12.0)	49 (12.8)
Other	94 (100)	41 (65.1)	199 (88.1)	334 (87.2)
Outcome effect				
Beneficial	54 (57.5)	43 (68.3)	64 (28.3)	161 (42.0)

(Continued)

TABLE 16.2 (Continued)

	January 1980–May 2014 (N = 94 analyses)	June 2014–June 2017 (N = 63 analyses)	July 2017–December 2021 (N = 226 analyses)	Total (N = 383)
No effect	30 (31.9)	15 (23.8)	152 (67.3)	197 (51.4)
Not beneficial	10 (10.6)	5 (7.9)	10 (4.4)	25 (6.5)
HIE type				
CHIE/RHIO	43 (45.7)	31 (49.2)	81 (35.8)	155 (40.5)
Vendor-facilitated HIE	–	11 (17.5)	73 (32.3)	84 (22.0)
Enterprise HIE	30 (31.9)	19 (30.2)	2 (0.9)	51 (13.3)
Other	21 (22.3)	2 (3.2)	70 (31.0)	93 (24.3)

CHIE/RHIO, Community-based HIE/Regional Health Information Organization; *HIE*, Health Information Exchange.

outcomes comprise 93% of all health outcomes studied in the 226 analyses. Over 94% of the analyses did not measure actual HIE usage and considered organizational adoption of HIE as being synonymous with use. Nearly 9-in-10 analyses focus on modes other than web-based portals (e.g., dashboards, event notifications, prepopulated forms) to engage in HIE. Only about 30% of analyses in this period report a beneficial effect to health outcomes from HIE.

16.3.5 Evolution of evidence of the effects of Health Information Exchange over time

It is helpful to examine these findings by comparing and contrasting them with those from Periods 1 and 2. As discussed above, and in previous chapters, the HIE landscape both in the United States and in other countries has evolved significantly and as a result of this, the nature of evidence has as well. As such, examining all periods together presents evidence for HIE over four decades, from 1980 to 2021. While each of the periods identified 23–27 studies that fit identical inclusion criteria, the number of outcomes analyzed more than doubled from 94 in Period 1 (see Table 16.2, "January 1980–May 2014" column) to 226 in Period 3 (see Table 16.2, "July 2017–December 2021" column). It is likely that the continued and growing support for HIE as well as the need to better understand how HIE affects health outcomes may be responsible for this increase. Further, as HIE becomes widespread, there is increased availability of data from mature HIEs. This may explain the steady increase in the number of studies from the United States over time. Similarly, since HIE in other countries is still in early stages, studies from outside the United States are few, representing a handful of nations. Over the 41-year period examined here, countries other than the United States represented in this literature include: Canada, Finland, Israel, Netherlands, South Korea, Sweden, and Taiwan. An important limitation of this review, however, is the exclusion of non-English articles. It may be the case that evidence on HIE exists in other nations during each time period, including the most recent period, even though it was not accessed by the authors.

Overall, studies from both the United States and other countries have relied mostly on observational designs while experimental designs such as randomized controlled trials or quasi-experimental approaches were used by less than

30% of studies in each period. Similar trends are also applicable at the analysis-level. However, almost 61% of analyses with experimental designs were in Period 3 as opposed to less than half of that (27.1%) in Period 1. This is critical since this implies that the newer studies are capable of generating stronger evidence due to more rigorous designs. This is especially seen in Period 2 (see Table 16.2, "June 2014–June 2017" column), when stronger evidence emerged linking HIE with reduced healthcare costs. HITECH was enacted under the premise that HITs would lower healthcare costs, yet less than 2% of all studies since 2017 examined healthcare costs as an outcome. It is likely that over the years, with HIE networks reaching maturity, benefits to healthcare costs and utilization became more evident. In Period 3, studies of quality of care and patient satisfaction constituted 70% of the studies. With the shift from volume-based to value-based healthcare after the introduction of MACRA, it appears there is a greater emphasis on quality of care and patient-centered outcomes like satisfaction.

Differences were also seen in the choice of study setting, the measurement of actual HIE usage, and the type of HIE studied. The type of study settings changed over time. During Period 1, the ED was the most common setting, whereas in Period 2, it was the inpatient setting. HIE is especially relevant in the ED setting because of the importance of timely intervention. Additional information about a patient obtained from an HIE can provide a more complete picture to the ED physician and thus aid in clinical decision making. This may be why early studies (represented in Period 1) mostly focused on this care setting. During Periods 1 and 2, EHR adoption steadily increased. By 2015 96% of all acute nonfederal hospitals had adopted EHRs [14]. With Centers for Medicare & Medicaid Services providing financial incentives for the MU of EHRs, it is likely that there was an increase in the use of HIE in the inpatient setting for Medicare and Medicaid populations that tend to have more complex medical needs [15]. Across the three time periods, there were steady gains in HIE among hospitals. While ambulatory settings have lagged in the adoption of EHRs, there was a steady rise in adoption in this setting with 72% of office-based physicians using certified EHRs by 2019 [16]. These changes were also reflected in the HIE literature with a dramatic increase in analyses examining the outpatient setting for benefits from HIE. The recent policy initiatives aimed at increasing interoperability may mitigate some of the barriers to HIE traditionally reported by ambulatory care providers, particularly difficulties in integrating external data with EHR systems [17].

Another difference across the three time periods was the emergence of vendor-facilitated HIE, which is represented in nearly a third of the studies in Period 3. Leading EHR vendors have established large HIE networks that compete with state-led efforts [18]. There is some concern among experts that the increasing popularity of vendor-initiated HIE will create "islands" of HIE, where HIE between systems using different EHR vendors may be impeded leading to negative effects on cost and quality of care. Indeed, there is evidence that there was a wide gap in HIE activity between hospitals using an EHR from a dominant vendor and hospitals using an EHR from a nondominant vendor in markets with the highest competition [19]. It is expected that provisions to address information blocking in the 21st Century Cures Act will discourage the creation of HIE "islands."

More articles assessed actual HIE usage in Periods 1 and 2, than in Period 3, when only about 5.3% of the studies measured actual usage of HIE. Despite the wealth of information available in HIE log and EHR audit files, these sources as objective measures of HIE remain underutilized for research purposes [20,21]. In a survey of HIEs across the United

States, less than a quarter supported research, and about 30% neither planned to support nor had future plans to support research [22]. HIEs that do support research share certain characteristics. They have the ability to create de-identified datasets and execute data use agreements with research universities. Further, they also require approvals from institutional review boards and approval of data sharing research by an oversight body (e.g., ethics committee) [22]. The main barrier to using HIE data for research is the law. Health Insurance Portability and Accountability Act created a floor for privacy and security of protected health information (PHI). However, individual state laws regarding health records may be more stringent thereby creating barriers [21]. Recent policy initiatives have been geared to encourage sharing of data and may therefore lead to more research that uses log file data from HIE networks in the coming years. For instance, the 21st Century Cures Act through TEFCA aims to create a network of networks to aid flow of information among authorized entities and has provisions to curtail information blocking. It also proposes that researchers can access PHI remotely with appropriate security and privacy safeguards. Moreover, the Cures Act also calls for the United States Department of Health and Human Services to convene a working group to study the use of PHI for research.

Lastly, even though MU emphasizes the use of HIE for public health activities, public health outcomes have not been commonly studied. Under MU stage 1, reporting immunizations, ED visits for syndromic surveillance, and laboratory results was optional. In 2014, MU stage 2 considered these three capabilities mandatory [23]. The less stringent MU requirements likely explain the dearth of studies in Period 1. However, the number of studies examining public health outcomes in Periods 2 and 3 are similar even though they represent nearly 16% and 5% of all the published articles in the two periods, respectively. One major barrier to electronic reporting of public health measures is the capacity of public health agencies to receive this data [23]. In 2014 21% of stage 2 hospitals reported that their local jurisdictions could not receive surveillance data, 15% reported their jurisdictions lacked the capacity to receive laboratory results, and 9% could not submit immunization results [23]. Even as recently as 2019, the top two challenges reported by 1-in-4 hospitals with respect to public health measures were capacity-related and interface-related. Surveys from 2017 and 2018 indicate that these challenges are enduring [24]. Recent initiatives like TEFCA and the Centers for Disease Control and Prevention's Data Modernization Initiative could potentially mitigate these reporting challenges and set the stage for more studies examining public health outcomes in relation to HIE.

We also examine how various characteristics of existing studies and the analyses within relate to whether a beneficial relationship is identified (see Table 16.3). Specifically, we analyzed the likelihood of finding a beneficial effect for a given category of a variable in comparison to all other categories within the same variable. As such, by geographic location, analyses from studies based in the United States were less likely to benefit from HIE (25.9% vs 91.7%) when compared to studies based in other countries. Healthcare utilization (45.1% vs 24.7%) and quality of care (40.8% vs 23.4%) were more likely to benefit from HIE compared to other outcomes. On the other hand, HIE was less likely to improve patient satisfaction (7.8% vs 41.4%) compared to other outcomes. Based on the most recent evidence, compared to other settings, HIE was less likely to produce benefits in the outpatient setting (23.9% vs 44.8%). Further, the mechanism as well as the mode of accessing HIE were also related to benefits to health outcomes from HIE. Specifically, benefits from HIE were more likely when HIE used the "pull" mechanism or was query-based

TABLE 16.3 Relationship between study characteristics and reporting a beneficial relationship.

	Beneficial relationship observed					
	January 1980–May 2014		June 2014–June 2017		July 2017–December 2021	
Variable	Variable, *n* (%) vs other, *n* (%)	*P*-value	Variable, *n* (%) vs other, *n* (%)	*P*-value	Variable, *n* (%) vs other, *n* (%)	*P*-value
Geographic location						
United States	39 (66.1) vs 15 (42.9)	.028	35 (72.9) vs 8 (53.3)	.155	53 (25.9) vs 11 (52.4)	.010
Outcomes analyzed						
Healthcare utilization	34 (50.7) v. 20 (74.1)	.038	12 (48.0) vs 31 (81.6)	.005	23 (44.2) vs 41 (23.6)	.004
Healthcare costs	7 (63.6) vs 47 (56.6)	.659	14 (77.8) vs 29 (64.4)	.304	1 (25.0) vs 63 (28.4)	.882
Quality of care	9 (75.0) vs 45 (54.9)	.188	9 (90.0) vs 34 (64.2)	.107	31 (37.8) vs 33 (23.0)	.017
Public health	2 (100.0) vs 52 (56.5)	.219	8 (80.0) vs 35 (66.0)	.354	3 (27.3) vs 61 (28.4)	.937
Patient satisfaction	2 (100.0) vs 52 (56.5)	.219	–	–	6 (7.8) vs 58 (39.0)	<.001
Setting						
Inpatient	15 (44.1) vs 39 (65.0)	.049	12 (57.1) vs 31 (73.8)	.18	13 (34.2) vs 51 (27.1)	.377
Outpatient	1 (100.0) vs 53 (57.0)	.387	10 (76.9) vs 33 (66.0)	.451	38 (22.6) vs 26 (44.8)	.001
Inpatient and outpatient	1 (25.0) vs 53 (58.9)	.18	1 (50.0) vs 42 (68.9)	.573	5 (18.5) vs 59 (29.7)	.228
Community	–	–	6 (85.7) vs 37 (66.1)	.293	1 (50.0) vs 63 (28.1)	.494
Emergency department	34 (66.7) vs 20 (46.5)	.049	10 (58.8) vs 33 (71.7)	.328	4 (28.6) vs 60 (28.3)	.983
HIE mechanism						
Push	23 (46.9) vs 31 (68.9)	.032	23 (69.7) vs 20 (66.7)	.796	13 (28.9) vs 51 (28.2)	.924
Pull	32 (59.3) vs 22 (55.0)	.68	24 (64.9) vs 19 (73.1)	.491	33 (50.0) vs 31 (19.4)	<.001
Both	6 (40.0) vs 48 (60.8)	.136	7 (70.0) vs 36 (67.9)	.897	0 (0.0) vs 64 (28.7)	.273
Study design						
Cohort study	45 (75.0) vs 9 (26.5)	<.001	29 (63.0) vs 14 (82.4)	.144	30 (26.8) vs 34 (29.8)	.612

(*Continued*)

TABLE 16.3 (Continued)

	Beneficial relationship observed					
	January 1980–May 2014		June 2014–June 2017		July 2017–December 2021	
Variable	Variable, n (%) vs other, n (%)	P-value	Variable, n (%) vs other, n (%)	P-value	Variable, n (%) vs other, n (%)	P-value
Randomized controlled trial	3 (17.7) vs 51 (66.2)	<.001	2 (50.0) vs 41 (69.5)	.418	6 (27.3) vs 58 (28.4)	.909
Quasiexperimental study	2 (16.7) vs 52 (63.4)	.002	8 (88.9) vs 35 (64.8)	.151	21 (48.8) vs 43 (23.5)	.001
Cross-sectional study	4 (80.0) vs 50 (56.2)	.295	4 (100.0) vs 39 (66.1)	.159	7 (14.3) vs 57 (32.2)	.014
Type of HIE measure						
Actual usage measured	10 (50.0) vs 44 (59.5)	.448	9 (42.9) vs 34 (81.0)	.002	5 (41.7) vs 59 (27.8)	.292
HIE access						
Portal	–	–	18 (81.8) vs 25 (61.0)	.09	17 (63.0) vs 47 (23.6)	<.001
HIE type						
CHIE/RHIO	29 (67.4) vs 25 (49.0)	.072	23 (74.2) vs 20 (62.5)	.319	25 (30.9) vs 39 (26.9)	.526
Vendor-facilitated HIE	–	–	5 (45.5) vs 38 (73.1)	.074	15 (20.6) vs 49 (32.0)	.073
Enterprise HIE	14 (46.7) vs 40 (62.5)	.148	13 (68.4) vs 30 (68.2)	.985	1 (50.0) vs 63 (28.1)	.494

Each row compares the specified variable with all other variables within that category. For example, let us consider the category "healthcare utilization" under the variable "outcomes analyzed." From Table 16.1, there are 52 analyses examining healthcare utilization, while 174 analyses examined other outcomes. Note in Table 16.2 the values for healthcare utilization under the column for Period 3 (July 2017–December 2021). Of the 52 analyses examining healthcare utilization, 23 analyses (or 44.2% of the 52 analyses) found a beneficial effect. Of the 174 analyses examining other outcomes, 41 analyses (or 23.6% of the 174 analyses) found a beneficial effect. *CHIE*, Community Health Information Exchange; *HIE*, Health Information Exchange; *RHIO*, Regional Health Information Organization.

(57.9% vs 19.4%). Web-based portals (94.4% vs 23.6%) also had a higher likelihood of producing benefits compared to other modes of accessing HIE. However, this may be because of a wide range of HIE approaches such as dashboards, event notifications, and prepopulated forms represented in the "other" category. Studies using a quasi-experimental design were found to be more likely to find a benefit from HIE (48.8% vs 24.7%). Lastly, when it comes to HIE type, vendor-facilitated HIE had a higher likelihood of producing benefits (20.6% vs 34.0%) compared to other types of HIE.

With respect to geographic location, the likelihood of studies published in the United States finding a benefit from HIE decreased over time. Specifically, studies based in the United States were more likely to benefit from HIE (66.1% vs 42.9%) during Period 1. However, there was no statistically significant difference found in Period 2, and Period 3 found that studies based in the United States were less likely to benefit from HIE. Importantly, each of the international studies identified during Period 3 were located in Taiwan which has a national health insurance that provides universal, mandatory coverage (see Chapter 30). Conversely, the United States continues to experience challenges for facilitating data exchange between disparate systems facing technical interoperability and network interoperability challenges.

When it comes to outcomes analyzed, healthcare utilization was consistently found to be less likely to benefit from HIE compared to other outcomes for Periods 1 (50.7% vs 74.1%) and 2 (48.0% vs 81.6%). However, this outcome was found to be more likely to benefit from HIE in Period 3. Again, we found during Period 2 that studies with stronger designs assessing healthcare utilization found HIE to be beneficial. Some of this finding may be a result of the stark increase in studies with stronger designs that we observed over the course of this period. This finding may also be a result of the maturation of HIE utilization. Early studies were focused on first generation systems and in healthcare systems where HIE usage was low. Given the growth of HIE, particularly among more advanced EHR systems, providers are able to more meaningfully utilize these systems and realize their benefits.

During Period 1, EDs were more likely than other settings to benefit from HIE (66.7% vs 46.5%), while inpatient settings were significantly less likely to benefit from HIE (44.1% vs 65.0%). While there was no difference in the likelihood to benefit from HIE across settings during Period 2, the outpatient setting was found to be less likely to benefit from HIE when compared to other settings in Period 3. During the earlier stages of HIE, ambulatory care providers lagged in the adoption of interoperable HIE when compared to other settings such as ED settings. Similarly, benefits from HIE were more likely when HIE used the "pull" mechanism or was query-based. This is a change from Period 1 where the "push" mechanism led to more benefits from HIE (46.9% vs 68.9%). This may be related to the increased usage of HIE in the outpatient setting, as "push" HIE or direct exchange is widely used in provider-to-provider electronic exchange of patient information, typically to improve care coordination. These trends can signify the increased reliance on HIE by reimbursement programs, such as the MU Program and Promoting Interoperability Program. These programs aim to shift patients from presenting to the ED for care to settings such as primary care and ambulatory care. As a result, research in these areas has become more of a priority which has a heavier reliance on "pull" HIE mechanisms.

While cohort studies were more likely than other study design to find a benefit from HIE (75% vs 26.5%) during Period 1, randomized controlled trials (17.7% vs 66.2%) and quasi-experimental studies (16.7% vs 63.4%) were less likely to find a benefit from HIEs when compared to other study designs. No differences were found in Period 2. Analyses using quasi-experimental study designs were more likely to find a benefit from HIE in Period 3, while cross-sectional study designs were less likely to find a benefit. With respect to quasi-experimental studies, these were difficult to conduct during the infancy of HIE. However, over time with the enactment of federal programs to support HIE, more opportunities arose to lend themselves to quasi-experimental research. When it comes to HIE type, vendor-facilitated HIE had a higher likelihood of producing benefits compared to other types of HIE. This may be due to the rise of certified EHR systems, with some EHR systems controlling more of the EHR market share. Many of these systems have HIE integrated within their EHRs, making it easier to exchange health information within, and between, networks that share the same EHR system.

16.3.6 Gaps in the current evidence

While researchers are finding evidence for more and more of the theorized benefits from

HIE over time, there remain some notable gaps remain in the literature. Most evidence on the benefits of HIE comes from studies that measure health outcomes as they relate to the presence or absence of the ability to engage in information exchange (e.g., adoption of HIE) as opposed to objective measures (e.g., observed usage of HIE functionality). In other words, studies rarely measure if healthcare delivery and practices where HIE is used differ in terms of health outcomes from those where no HIE is used. Over the last 40 years, less than 20% of all studies representing less than 14% of all outcomes analyzed used objective measures to examine the relationship between HIE use and health outcomes. Even though a provider may have the ability to engage in HIE, providers can choose not to use certain functions that are available within their EHR system which may limit the scope of HIE. Similarly, providers may not use certain functions due to being unaware that their EHR systems have those capabilities. The increasing availability of data from HIE log and EHR audit files presents promising opportunities to explore the benefits from HIE utilization.

As discussed in here as well as in Chapter 3, with the widespread adoption of HIE, there has been a push to promote interoperability. To identify if this shift in strategy was reflected in the literature, we extracted data on whether a given study had an interoperability focus. In our review, an exceedingly small number of studies examined interoperable HIE accounting for less than 3% of all studies (~4% of all analyses). One possible reason for this may be that interoperability continues to remain a challenge. While newer data sharing protocols are geared toward making integration of data into the EHR easier in theory, thus supporting interoperability; organizational barriers may persist. Concerns related to privacy and security may make organizations disinclined to share and/or integrate external data into their systems. Further, while newer protocols are supported by major vendors, implementation often requires building additional web services and/or application programming interfaces to support specific use cases. While some of these issues may be addressed by governance that oversees development of judicious data use agreements, others may require technologies supporting interoperability to mature and become more widespread.

Analyses of public health outcomes found benefits due to HIE, including from studies with more rigorous study designs. These benefits include increased public health reporting, improved immunization registries, and prompt event notifications—outcomes which support core public health functions. In 2019 the world experienced a global pandemic of coronavirus disease (COVID-19) caused by the severe acute respiratory syndrome coronavirus-2 (SARS-CoV-2). With over 495 million cases and 6 million deaths globally, the COVID-19 pandemic was one of the deadliest pandemics in recent history. Due to the theorized benefits as well as those public health benefits for which evidence exists, HIE had the potential to help manage several public health functions in light of the COVID-19 pandemic. Despite Period 3 coinciding with this pandemic, our review did not find any studies that focused on COVID-19-related use cases of HIE. Further, we only identified one published study which discussed the implementation of HIE tools in this context [25]. Although it is possible that studies examining HIE in this context may still be ongoing, presently this area remains understudied.

16.4 Conclusion

In this chapter, we reviewed the evidence base of HIE over the last four decades. The landscape of HIE has evolved significantly over this time period as technologies supporting HIE approached maturity concurrent with significant support from government agencies. While most studies continue to be from the

United States, the body of research examining HIE in global contexts is constantly growing with additional countries being represented. At the current point in time, high-quality studies suggest that HIE can improve outcomes such as healthcare utilization and quality of care. This translates to improvements in specific measures such as ED and inpatient readmissions, unplanned visits to the ED, hospitalization rates, duplicate lab and imaging tests, duplication of medications, and length of stay in the ED and inpatient setting. HIE may also improve care transitions, decrease rates of hospital acquired infections, increase cancer screening, ensure completeness of information, minimize rates of adverse drug events, allow shared decision making, and enhance patient satisfaction. Notwithstanding the benefits, it is important to note that the HIE literature suggests that these benefits may be more visible in some settings (e.g., inpatient, outpatient) compared to others (such as the ED). Further, benefits due to HIE may be differential based on HIE type, and with the changing HIE market, this evidence base continues to grow. HIE is at a critical juncture in its development with increasing focus on interoperability and integration of data into the EHR. Moreover, current policy and technological trends (discussed in Chapter 3 and Chapter 21) in the United States as well as globally present exciting opportunities for disruption in the HIE landscape. While HIE has come a long way, there is an abundance of room for progress. As such, the full scope of benefits to health outcomes is yet to be realized with the proliferation of HIE literature to incorporate more diversity in characteristics such as outcomes, study designs, technologies, HIE types, and settings.

Questions for discussion

1. How have the benefits to health outcomes from HIE use changed over time? Which health outcomes have received the most benefits from HIE? Which health outcomes are the benefits yet to be realized?
2. What are some barriers to studying the effect of HIE?
   a. Why is there a lack of quasiexperimental studies and randomized controlled trials in the field of HIE?
   b. What are the barriers to stronger study designs?
   c. How can the barriers to stronger study designs in this field be overcome?
3. With the expansion of interoperability initiatives, what kind of health outcomes would you expect to be impacted by HIE in the future?
4. If HIE conditions were completely interoperable, what kind of studies would you propose?
5. How do you anticipate the landscape of HIE will change with the proliferation of interoperability initiatives such as FHIR?

Acknowledgments

We note that each author contributed equally to the research and writing of this chapter.

References

[1] Blumenthal D. Launching HITECH. N Engl J Med 2010;362(5):382–5.
[2] Jackson CT, Trygstad TK, DeWalt DA, DuBard CA. Transitional care cut hospital readmissions for North Carolina Medicaid patients with complex chronic conditions. Health Aff (Millwood) 2013;32(8):1407–15.
[3] Adler-Milstein J, Jha AK. Sharing clinical data electronically: a critical challenge for fixing the health care system. JAMA 2012;307(16):1695–6.
[4] Williams C, Mostashari F, Mertz K, Hogin E, Atwal P. From the Office of the National Coordinator: the strategy for advancing the exchange of health information. Health Aff (Millwood) 2012;31(3):527–36.
[5] Leventhal T, Taliaferro JP, Wong K, Hughes C, Mun S. The patient-centered medical home and health information technology. Telemed J E Health 2012;18(2):145–9.
[6] H.R.2 – Medicare Access and CHIP Reauthorization Act of 2015, 2015–2016 Sess. (2015).

[7] Goldwasser Y, Gordon WJ, Brönneke JB, Stern AD. On the brink of a digital health care transformation: what Germany can learn from the United States: Health Affairs; 2021. Available from: https://www.healthaffairs.org/do/10.1377/forefront.20211018.865750/full/.

[8] Roland M. Linking physicians' pay to the quality of care—a major experiment in the United Kingdom. N Engl J Med 2004;351(14):1448–54.

[9] Menachemi N, Rahurkar S, Harle CA, Vest JR. The benefits of health information exchange: an updated systematic review. J Am Med Inform Assoc 2018;25 (9):1259–65.

[10] Rahurkar S, Vest JR, Menachemi N. Despite the spread of health information exchange, there is little evidence of its impact on cost, use, and quality of care. Health Aff (Millwood) 2015;34(3):477–83.

[11] Moher D, Liberati A, Tetzlaff J, Altman DG. Preferred reporting items for systematic reviews and *meta*-analyses: the PRISMA statement. Ann Intern Med 2009;151 (4):264–9.

[12] Everson J, Kocher KE, Adler-Milstein J. Health information exchange associated with improved emergency department care through faster accessing of patient information from outside organizations. J Am Med Inform Assoc 2017;24(e1):e103–10.

[13] Elysee G, Yu H, Herrin J, Horwitz LI. Association between 30-day readmission rates and health information technology capabilities in US hospitals. Medicine (Baltimore) 2021;100(8):e24755. Available from: https://doi.org/10.1097/MD.0000000000024755.

[14] Henry J, Pylypchuk Y, Searcy T, Patel V. Adoption of electronic health record systems among US non-federal acute care hospitals: 2008–2015: HealthIT.gov; 2016. Available from: https://www.healthit.gov/data/data-briefs/adoption-electronic-health-record-systems-among-us-non-federal-acute-care-1.

[15] Rahurkar S, Vest JR, Finnell JT, Dixon BE. Trends in user-initiated health information exchange in the inpatient, outpatient, and emergency settings. J Am Med Inform Assoc 2020;28(3):622–7.

[16] Office of the National Coordinator for Health Information Technology. National trends in hospital and physician adoption of electronic health records: HealthIT.gov; 2022. Available from: <https://www.healthit.gov/data/quickstats/national-trends-hospital-and-physician-adoption-electronic-health-records>.

[17] Patel V, Pylypchuk Y, Parasrampuria S, Kachay L. Interoperability among office-based physicians in 2015 and 2017: HealthIT.gov; 2019 [1–12]. Available from: <https://www.healthit.gov/data/data-briefs/interoperability-among-office-based-physicians-2015-and-2017>.

[18] Adler-Milstein J, Lin SC, Jha AK. The number of health information exchange efforts is declining, leaving the viability of broad clinical data exchange uncertain. Health Aff (Millwood) 2016;35(7):1278–85.

[19] Everson J, Adler-Milstein J. Engagement In hospital health information exchange is associated with vendor marketplace dominance. Health Aff (Millwood) 2016;35(7):1286–93.

[20] Adler-Milstein J, Adelman JS, Tai-Seale M, Patel VL, Dymek C. EHR audit logs: a new goldmine for health services research? J Biomed Inform 2020;101:103343.

[21] Saks MJ, Grando A, Millea C, Murcko A. Advancing the use of HIE data for research. Ariz State Law J 2020;52:145.

[22] Parker C, Reeves M, Weiner M, Adler-Milstein J. Health information exchange organizations and their support for research: current state and future outlook. Inquiry 2017;54 0046958017713709.

[23] Heisey-Grove D, Chaput D, Daniel J. Hospital reporting on meaningful use public health measures in 2014: HealthIT.gov; 2015. Available from: <https://www.healthit.gov/data/data-briefs/hospital-reporting-meaningful-use-public-health-measures-2014>.

[24] Richwine C, Marshall C, Johnson C, Patel V. Challenges to public health reporting experienced by non-federal acute care hospitals, 2019: HealthIT.gov; 2021. Available from: <https://www.healthit.gov/data/data-briefs/challenges-public-health-reporting-experienced-non-federal-acute-care-hospitals>.

[25] Wu DC, Lin HL, Cheng CG, Yu CP, Cheng CA. Improvement the healthcare quality of emergency department after the cloud-based system of medical information-exchange implementation. Healthcare (Basel) 2021;9(8).

CHAPTER

17

Measuring the value of health information exchange

Brian E. Dixon[1] *and Caitlin M. Cusack*[2]

[1]Center for Biomedical Informatics, Regenstrief Institute, Inc., Indianapolis, IN, USA [2]Insight Informatics, Washington, DC, United States

LEARNING OBJECTIVES

At the end of this chapter, the reader should be able to:

- Define evaluation in the context of health information exchange.
- Compare and contrast the various categories of evaluation.
- List and describe the domains of evaluation commonly examined in health information exchange.
- Identify the various roles recommended for inclusion as part of the evaluation team.
- Discuss the importance of developing an evaluation plan.
- Outline important considerations to the design of an evaluation plan.
- State the key sections or components of an evaluation plan.
- Prepare an evaluation plan to measure some aspect of health information exchange.
- Describe why dissemination is an important aspect of evaluation.

17.1 Introduction

Given limited evidence on the effective use of health information exchange (HIE) to improve outcomes for patients and populations as described in Chapter 16, there is a clear need to evaluate the implementation, use, and impact of HIE by those investing in it within a community, state, or nation. While literature reviews and journal articles argue for comparative studies and research agendas, the evidence base for HIE will not be developed by research scientists alone. Demonstrating HIE's effectiveness in reducing costs, improving outcomes, and creating more efficient care delivery systems comes from a combination of scientific research and practice-based evaluation. This chapter describes strategies and methods for evaluating HIE,

Health Information Exchange
DOI: https://doi.org/10.1016/B978-0-323-90802-3.00012-5

principally from the perspective of a health system or other entity engaged in the implementation or use of HIE within an enterprise or across a community, state, or nation.

The chapter begins with a review of the various types of evaluation, including research. Then the chapter outlines a strategy and the methods for the evaluation of HIE. Finally, the chapter provides guidance for how to disseminate outcomes from HIE development, implementation, adoption, and use. Only by evaluating HIE and sharing lessons will the evidence base for HIE be strengthened. It is incumbent upon all of us in both academia and practice to further develop the evidence base to ensure the sustainability of HIE networks.

17.2 The spectrum of evaluation

Evaluation seeks to examine the "worth, merit, or significance" [1] of an object (e.g., program, HIE, device). Many organizations routinely conduct evaluations to determine whether their business operations, internal initiatives, or external partnerships are effective. Efforts found to be effective are sustained or expanded, and ineffective efforts are either improved or terminated. These activities are often labeled as quality improvement projects, lean manufacturing, six sigma, or operations research. Research, therefore, is just one type of evaluation performed to determine whether an information system, program, or process is meritorious.

Despite the fact that many healthcare organizations routinely evaluate their clinical or administrative operations, healthcare leaders often equate evaluation of HIE with research and therefore entrust it to academics. In the mid-2000s the US Agency for Healthcare Research and Quality (AHRQ) awarded grants to over 100 health systems across America to implement health information technology (health IT) [2]. The list of grantees included a number of organizations seeking to deploy HIE in their local community or across their state [3,4]. Each grantee organization was asked to complete an evaluation as a component of their project. While projects led by academic research organizations submitted evaluation plans in a timely fashion, projects led by health systems and community organizations struggled to develop their evaluation plans [5]. In a series of meetings with grantees, AHRQ learned that practice-based organizations viewed evaluation as synonymous with scientific research and therefore struggled to come up with what they perceived as "rigorous research" of their HIE efforts.

Many in healthcare associate the term "research" with a randomized controlled trial (RCT) in which subjects are randomly assigned to either receive a new medication (drug) or a placebo (an inert substance also referred to as a sugar pill). While RCTs are considered the hallmark of scientific research for demonstrating the effectiveness of a new medication, therapy, or health delivery process, they are not the only form of scientific research performed in healthcare. Nor are they the only kind of evaluation that can support the implementation and adoption of new technologies in healthcare. In fact, RCTs are very challenging to do in the domain of health IT and HIE, because it is often either unethical to deny HIE benefits to some people in a community or impractical to partially implement HIE in a health system. Moreover, the use of RCTs to study HIE is time consuming and costly as they require significant human resources to coordinate the implementation of HIE into carefully selected, controlled environments. Therefore the health system must utilize an array of evaluation methods beyond RCTs to study HIE and other information technologies [5–7].

17.2.1 Evaluation categories

Evaluations of HIE can be grouped into the following categories: formative evaluation, summative evaluation, and scientific research.

17.2.1.1 Formative evaluation

Formative evaluation takes place before or during implementation with the aim of improving the design and performance of the technology being implemented [6]. Evaluations of this type are sometimes referred to as "playing smallball," a baseball analogy that suggests the goal of a formative evaluation is not to hit a Grand Slam but to simply make a base hit [8]. For HIE, formative evaluations tend to be focused on a singular aspect of the exchange and thus can be carried out by a relatively small team overseen by a project manager or program director. For example, the project director may wish to ensure that healthcare organization leaders are on board with the formation of an HIE effort in the community, or the creation of a new HIE service. A stakeholder analysis would facilitate systematic collection of feedback from the healthcare leaders useful to decision-making at the local HIE while simultaneously providing insights useful to other HIEs that could be shared in the form of a whitepaper or professional conference presentation.

Formative evaluation can occur during multiple phases of HIE development as summarized in Table 17.1. Several existing HIE efforts have used formative evaluation to assess readiness for HIE adoption [9–12], the design of HIE services [13,14], or the early adoption of HIE in an organization or geographic region [15–17]. Qualitative methods, those that focus on open ended questions and emergent discovery of knowledge, lend themselves well to this form of evaluation.

Although formative evaluations occur most often before or during implementation of HIE services, they can be performed after implementation. Postimplementation formative evaluations typically enable networks to ensure that HIE services continue to perform well months or years after implementation. Periodic review of HIE network utilization data as well as focus groups with users can ensure services are meeting organizational goals. Data collected from

TABLE 17.1 The stages of HIE in which formative evaluation can be used to gather insight, lessons, and evidence.

	Formation	Development	Implementation	Operations
Purpose of the evaluation	To understand or clarify the need for HIE.	To understand user needs or rationale for design decisions.	To understand how recently introduced HIE services are impacting health system structures and processes.	To ensure that HIE services are being delivered efficiently and effectively.
Examples	Review of available literature to convince stakeholders of the need for HIE. Analyze the readiness of organizations in the community to engage in HIE. Observe clinicians' request and use of information from outside providers or organizations to identify potential workflow improvements given HIE.	Conduct a focus group to gather ideas on the design of services offered by the HIE. Interview IT staff at HIE member organizations to gather input on the design of the HIE architecture. Survey healthcare organizations to assess market interest and customer price points. Scan market.	Review project team materials to assess whether the implementation is on schedule and within budget. Observe clinical users to assess access to and early adoption of HIE services and applications. Assess the quality of data transmitted from source systems (e.g., laboratory information system).	Review user requests or issues (e.g., helpdesk tickets) to assess performance of HIE services. Observe clinical users to assess the use of HIE services in routine clinical care delivery. Periodic assessment of data quality from existing and new source systems. Interview users about their satisfaction with HIE services and requests for new functions or services.

This table includes examples of formative evaluation methods for assessing specific aspects of HIE. *HIE*, Health information exchange.

formative evaluations postimplementation can generate ideas for new functionality or services for development. These evaluations focus on organizational and work processes postimplementation, not outcomes (e.g., reduced costs).

17.2.1.2 *Summative evaluation*

Summative evaluation, which can be referred to as ex-postevaluation (meaning after the event), typically occurs after implementation, and focuses on the impact of a given technology. Most often this form of evaluation is used to measure whether or not a technology such as HIE achieved its desired aims or goals. Summative evaluations focus on outcomes, and not process.

For example, a summative evaluation might measure the impact of HIE on specialty care referrals from primary care clinicians. The emphasis in an e-referral project might be on care coordination, including timeliness of follow-up by specialists and primary care physicians' satisfaction with the service, instead of simply counting the number of e-referrals sent by primary care doctors.

In other words, summative evaluation measures the value of HIE with respect to financial, clinical decision-making, healthcare delivery, and patient as well as population outcomes. This kind of evaluation can also be used to measure HIE usage, such as measuring how many patients' records in the HIE are accessed or under what conditions emergency department (ED) clinicians access the HIE. The results of summative evaluations can be shared in the form of reports or peer-reviewed journal articles in addition to conference presentations. Most often, these evaluations are used to demonstrate to executive leadership or the Board of Directors that HIE network participation or an HIE service is paying dividends for the organization. Summative evaluations often use quantitative methods, although qualitative methods are used in some cases.

Real-world examples of summative evaluations performed in HIE include the following:

- Measuring the impact of HIE on repeated diagnostic imaging and related costs in emergency back pain evaluation [18];
- Quantifying a reduction in ED admissions following the implementation of HIE-based alerts [19];
- Synthesis of interviews with providers across six states to evaluate the impact of statewide HIE programs [20];
- Assessment of the association between HIE system usage and 30-day same-cause hospital readmissions [21];
- Interviewing clinicians about their use and perceptions of an HIE-based intervention after its implementation in two US Department of Veterans Affairs (VA) facilities [22]; and
- Measuring unique users who viewed a publicly available dashboard built on top of an HIE network designed to track COVID-19 infections and hospitalizations in a state or region [23].

17.2.1.3 *Scientific research*

Scientific research aims at producing generalizable knowledge using replicable methods to measure the impact of HIE on some outcome. While summative evaluation also measures outcomes, scientific research attempts to control for various extraneous factors such as organizational, behavioral, or policy factors. By controlling for these extraneous factors, scientists seek to find out whether and how much HIE influenced the outcome beyond policy changes (e.g., Meaningful Use, 21st Century Cures Act) or a charismatic HIE champion. Furthermore, scientific research can examine patterns and trends beyond a single HIE implementation. For example, a cross-sectional study might survey hospitals about their adoption and usage of HIE to infer trends across a state, region, or nation. Scientific research also includes RCTs as well as large observational studies of patient populations, provider organizations that participate in HIE, and HIE initiatives themselves. Quantitative, qualitative, and mixed-methods studies are all used in scientific research.

Real-world examples of scientific research performed on HIE include the following:

- A randomized trial that examined whether HIE among specialists and general practitioners in rural Japan impacted outcomes among patients at low-to-moderate risk of cardiovascular disease, kidney disease, and stroke [24];
- A national examination of US ambulatory, office-based, provider volume of HIE use during referrals from primary care to specialty care along with the factors (e.g., practice, market, population) associated with higher use [25];
- A study of length of stay among hospital readmissions to a different hospital with and without the presence of HIE across a network of Israeli hospitals managed by the same integrated healthcare provider and payer [26];
- A cluster randomized trial among primary care providers in the VA to study the impact of an HIE-based event notification service on time to follow-up after an acute care event and rehospitalizations [27];
- A survey of providers that used an HIE-based event notification service to explore the organizational capabilities associated with and perceptions of HIE service use [28];
- A controlled before-after study that examined the impact of an HIE-based service on provider reporting of communicable disease cases to public health authorities [29];
- A statewide survey of ambulatory clinics to examine the inhibitors, including technological, organizational, and environmental contexts, to HIE with external clinics and external hospitals [30]; and
- A mixed-methods study of HIE users to understand HIE adoption and acceptance between users groups and care settings across England that utilized the Unified Theory of Acceptance and Use of Technology [31].

17.2.2 Domains of evaluation

No matter the type, evaluation examines one or more aspects of HIE. Prior work developed a framework [32] that defines five broad domains in which evaluation of HIE can occur (see Table 17.2). Each domain is broad, encompassing a range of possible questions that a health system, HIE initiative, policymaker, or research scientist might wish to ask. While the Value domain focuses on the impact of HIE on outcomes, the other domains support evaluation questions that address the impact of HIE or its components (e.g., technical aspects, a certain type of data) on patients, providers, organizations, usage, or adoption. This framework is useful for thinking about the kinds of questions certain stakeholders might ask about the development, implementation, or use of HIE.

17.3 Developing an evaluation plan

To effectively evaluate an aspect of an operational HIE initiative or the development of HIE for a specific use case, one must have a plan. The plan outlines the goals of both the HIE project as well as the evaluation; it specifies what is to be measured, how it is to be measured, and by whom; it considers costs, personnel, and timelines; and serves as a blueprint for the team conducting the evaluation. Although aspects of the evaluation will likely evolve and change during execution, it is critical to the success of an evaluation to begin with a well-constructed plan.

The following sections outline the various components of an evaluation plan. One can think of the section headers as a checklist of elements that could be embodied in a

TABLE 17.2 Domains of evaluation for HIE.

Domain	Description	Evaluation question examples
Technology	Evaluations in this domain focus on the technical aspects of HIE, including performance of the software, hardware, and architectural choices made by the HIE. This domain also allows for comparison of technical designs, maintenance costs, and system usability.	What is the accuracy of the master person index? Which text mining methods can best identify active medications in a hospital discharge summary? Which data encryption tools perform well in a federated HIE network of mental health clinics?
Data	Evaluations in this domain focus on the data captured, stored, and managed by the HIE. This can include the quality of the data from various sources as well as which data are accessed under what conditions by certain types of user groups.	Which sources of data are most accessed by primary care clinicians? How complete and timely are immunization records sent by emergency departments? Under what conditions do clinicians click on discharge summaries that are more than 5 years old?
Implementation	Evaluations in this domain focus on the facets of design, use, and implementation of HIE in a health system or community. They can range from measuring adoption by certain providers to the cost of interface development to the challenges of mapping local terminologies to a reference terminology.	What is the average total cost associated with implementing an interface to emergency department information systems for syndromic surveillance? Which providers tend to use the HIE and under what conditions? How many full-time equivalents are needed to staff the helpdesk at HIEs of various sizes and maturity levels?
Policy	Evaluations in this domain focus on the influence of local, state, and national policies on the adoption and use of HIE. Evaluations can examine stakeholder engagement as well as aspects of privacy. They can also include measuring the degree to which use is mandated by hospital administration.	What is the impact of the "Promoting Interoperability" program from the Centers for Medicare & Medicaid Services on the adoption and use of HIE among physician practices with less than five providers? What impact did the Information Blocking final rule have on expanding HIE access to nonaffiliated hospitals? Would a change in privacy policy impact the adoption and use of HIE among patients in a given state or region?
Value	Evaluations in this domain focus on the impact of HIE on clinical and population outcomes. They can further measure the effect of HIE on healthcare costs, utilization, and access.	Does HIE between VA and non-VA providers improve access to care or outcomes for Veterans? Can HIE between primary care and specialty providers improve the coordination of care? Does the use of HIE improve the ability to correlate vaccine status with severe disease, hospitalizations, and death?

This table includes evaluation questions representative of each domain. *HIE*, Health information exchange; *VA*, Veterans Affairs.
Source: *Adapted from Dixon BE, Zafar A, Overhage JM. A framework for evaluating the costs, effort, and value of nationwide health information exchange. J Am Med Inform Assoc. 2010;17(3):295–301.*

document shared amongst a team as well as stakeholders, such as the people or organization funding the evaluation. The content in these sections is derived from the authors' many years of evaluating HIE as well as from their work with AHRQ grantees seeking to do the same. A corollary document that those interested in HIE evaluation might find valuable is the "Guide to Evaluating Health Information Exchange Projects" published by AHRQ [33].

17.3.1 The evaluation team

One of the first tasks to evaluating HIE is putting together the right team. Just as HIE development and implementation teams involve multiple individuals with different expertise, so does the evaluation team. The evaluation team can be led by someone from the implementation team, or it could be a consultant hired to conduct the evaluation. While the exact composition of the evaluation team will vary depending on the goals of the evaluation, one should consider including experts in the following areas: evaluation methodology, healthcare operations, technical implementation, clinical care, and project management. In addition, having someone who represents the patient or consumer viewpoint could be helpful. Each of these areas is considered below.

17.3.1.1 Evaluation methodology

The benefits of working with an expert in evaluation methodology when conducting an evaluation are obvious. For HIE evaluation it is best to identify someone who is experienced in health services or public health evaluations. These individuals can be recruited from academic organizations, or they may be employed by a consulting firm. Experts in evaluation methodology may advise on what to measure, how to measure the outcomes of interest, and the process for conducting the evaluation. Furthermore, they may assist in the analysis and interpretation of results. Experts can further provide oversight of evaluation activities, human subjects' protection, and confidentiality of evaluation data including compliance with the Health Insurance Portability and Accountability Act of 1996.

17.3.1.2 Health care operations

Experts in this area are individuals with detailed understanding of the administrative and business side of healthcare organizations. They can be particularly helpful when measuring impact of HIE on healthcare workflows. Such an expert can communicate with organizational staff and administrators before and during the evaluation, represent their needs to the evaluation team, and help determine what healthcare organizations and stakeholders need to collect or extract from administrative systems as part of the evaluation. In addition, healthcare operations expertise can help determine the validity of measures for financial assessments of HIE costs and savings, such as reduced utilization of services.

17.3.1.3 Technical implementation

Experts in this area are individuals who are familiar with health IT systems and HIE transactions. They can help the evaluation team determine what is feasible to extract from electronic health record (EHR) systems, clinical data warehouses, or other components of the HIE in order to measure system performance, HIE usage, volume of transactions, or impact on patient and population outcomes. Technical experts are often familiar with health IT data standards as well as how data are entered and stored in systems. They can further assist the evaluation team in managing the data it will ultimately collect for analysis.

17.3.1.4 Clinical care

Experts in clinical care are current or former practicing clinicians who understand clinical decision-making processes as well as workflow. They can inform study designs that aim at measuring the impact of HIE on patient outcomes as well as diagnosis, treatment plans, or care coordination. Clinical expertise is especially important to evaluation efforts that seek to measure adherence to clinical guidelines, clinical performance, patient safety, or quality of care. Sometimes it is possible to recruit a senior clinician with administrative experience who can inform both clinical and operations aspects of an evaluation. In other instances, this role may be filled by a clinician champion involved in the implementation of HIE within a health system or community.

17.3.1.5 *Project management*

Experts in project management are important not only for implementation of HIE but also its evaluation. Evaluations can involve complex data collection from multiple EHR systems or organizations, and efforts to obtain consent from study participants, as well as schedule observations of workflow, require coordination. An experienced project manager can support execution of the evaluation plan by coordinating team activities while helping to ensure the evaluation is completed on time and within budget.

17.3.1.6 *Patient (consumer) representation*

Patients and their caregivers can provide useful insights into the type of metrics or study questions that would be most beneficial to other patients and caregivers. If the evaluation seeks to measure patient satisfaction, quality of life, or patient reported outcomes, consider adding one or more patient representatives to the evaluation team. Ideally, patient representatives should be familiar with the healthcare consumer experience and able to share first-hand experiences of being a patient or caregiver.

17.3.2 Defining goals, objectives, and stakeholders

To measure the impact of HIE, one must first define the impact(s) to be measured. Planning an evaluation therefore begins by defining the goals and objectives of the HIE, and it requires defining the stakeholders who care about whether the HIE is successful or fails.

First, identify key stakeholders who care about the success of HIE. These stakeholders might be those who are funding the implementation of HIE, or they may be the participants in HIE. Health systems are often stakeholders in HIE as are clinicians. However, there may be other groups that stand to benefit if HIE is successful, or lose if HIE fails. It is these stakeholders who will be interested in the results of the evaluation, and their perspective matters to the evaluation plan.

Next, enumerate the goals and objectives of HIE, usually within a particular use case. For example, a community may wish to improve the exchange of immunization records to enhance the ability of the health system to both measure vaccine coverage and forecast vaccines for a particular patient population (e.g., children, the elderly). Such goals and objectives would likely suggest an evaluation plan that would seek to measure a change in documented vaccine administration records, as well as accurate vaccine forecasts generated for the patient population of interest. The objectives of an evaluation plan (e.g., what it seeks to measure) stem from the goals and objectives of HIE mediated by stakeholders. Table 17.3 provides an example showing the alignment between the goals and objectives of a project to electronically report laboratory results to public health authorities mediated by the interests of stakeholder groups.

17.3.3 Identifying potential measures

Once the stakeholders, goals, and objectives are known, the evaluation team can then identify potential measures. Eventually the evaluation project will measure some change resulting from the HIE. This might be a change in patient attitudes or knowledge, provider attitudes or knowledge, efficiency of care processes, or clinical or population outcomes.

TABLE 17.3 Example alignment of health information exchange goals and objectives mediated by stakeholder groups for the use case of electronic laboratory reporting.

Goal and objective of the health information exchange	Stakeholder groups and their interests	Evaluation plan objectives (measures)
Goal: To improve the completeness and timeliness of disease reporting by successfully transmitting laboratory results electronically to public health authorities in a given state or region. **Objective**: To exchange at least 80% of laboratory results from private hospitals and independent laboratories electronically within 18 months.	Public health department—receiving complete lists of cases faster. Health systems—cutting costs for paper and time to fax results to health department. Providers—reducing costs and time for faxing lab results to health authorities.	Measure change at the health department in the number and percent of fax-based laboratory reports to electronically delivered laboratory reports. Measure change in time (# days) between when the laboratory test was performed and when it was reported to a public health department. Measure change in time (# minutes) clinic and laboratory staff spend handling laboratory reports. Measure change in number of laboratory reports received from stakeholders per unique disease case (redundant reporting).

Although measurement is an action (verb), evaluations use measures (nouns) or variables to indicate whether a change has occurred. Measures can be clinical or process indicators such as blood pressure versus the number of days to schedule an appointment. A successful evaluation is one that selects feasible measures, or measures that are readily available and can be objectively collected for analysis.

The first step in selecting measures for a given evaluation is to generate a list of candidate measures. There are two methods for generating the list: (1) perform a literature review and (2) brainstorm possible measures. While either method can generate a list of candidate measures, they complement one another and thus both methods should be used to ensure that a comprehensive list of candidate measures is generated.

A literature review is a process to identify relevant material from both peer-reviewed and gray literature (i.e., information that falls outside the mainstream of published journals and monographs), reading through the material, and analyzing the information in the material. Librarians in hospitals, academic medical centers, or the public library are excellent resources to consult when conducting a literature review. They can assist in designing a broad but specific search. Furthermore, they can help identify relevant sources of gray literature that may not appear in an online search.

The second method involves gathering the evaluation team plus key stakeholders to brainstorm measures of interest. Brainstorming is a group exercise designed to generate ideas through open and constructive discussion. Healthcare executives and clinical leaders are familiar with a wide range of indicators they review on a regular basis: indicators they might want to see affected by HIE. Evaluation experts will also be familiar with commonly used indicators in prior evaluations. Discussion should center on the goals and objectives of the HIE use case as well as the evaluation. Candidate measures should be related to the evaluation target.

The group should solicit ideas from all attendees and emphasize that "no idea is a bad idea." Keep in mind that this list will be further reviewed, discussed, and paired down. Therefore it is best to start with a large list since many measures will be eliminated when the evaluation plan is finalized.

17.3.4 Designing the evaluation

Now that the team has a list of possible measures, it is time to design the evaluation. The evaluation team must decide upon the study design and methods. The study design, whether formative, summative, or scientific research, should be informed by the stage of HIE development and purpose of the evaluation, as discussed at the beginning of the chapter. The study methods should be informed by the study design.

Study methods produce the data and are grouped into three categories: quantitative, qualitative, and mixed. In general, quantitative methods produce numbers that describe what has changed, while qualitative methods produce information that describes why or how a change occurred. Mixed-methods use a combination of quantitative and qualitative methods to produce a more comprehensive understanding of an outcome. Table 17.4 summarizes and compares study methods as well as example data they produce.

TABLE 17.4 Comparison of study methods and the data they produce.

Study methods	Examples of methods	Examples of data produced
Quantitative	Surveys/questionnaires	• Likert scale values 1 to 5 based on respondents' answer selection. • Demographics of the subjects. • Ordinal data based on respondents' multiple-choice answers.
	Analysis of administrative datasets such as diagnosis codes or user access logs.	• Count of each International Classification of Diseases-10 code recorded for patients in the emergency department. • List of clinical users and the date/time they accessed the health information exchange portal or viewer.
	Analysis of clinical datasets such as laboratory results or postsurgical outcomes.	• Count of HbA1c tests performed for patients with diabetes. • Average value of HbA1c test results. • List of patients with a 30-day readmission following a surgical procedure.
Qualitative	Observations	• Lists of activities performed by clinicians during the observation period. • After synthesis, patterns of activities or decision-making processes during a shift.
	Interviews	• Pages of transcribed questions and answers from the people interviewed. • Video or audio of the interviews; notes taken by the study team.
	Focus groups	• Pages of transcribed discussion among small groups of people. • Video or audio of the sessions. • Notes from the focus group leader and observers.
	Document review	• Copies of notices of privacy practice from clinics. • Notes taken during implementation team meetings over an 18-month period.

An example of a mixed-methods study evaluating HIE is "Exploring the Utilization of and Outcomes from Health Information Exchange in Emergency Settings" funded by AHRQ [34]. This project examined use of HIE by ED providers as well as the impact of HIE use on patient outcomes through three evaluation studies:

1. Using data across six years from the Indiana Network for Patient Care, an HIE network that spans the State of Indiana described in Chapter 22, the study quantified the use of HIE over time in over 90 EDs throughout the state.
2. Based on qualitative interviews with ED physicians, nurses, and administrators sampled across urban, suburban, and rural EDs connected to the Indiana HIE network, the study examined the antecedents, motivations for use, and other factors that influence use of HIE among ED providers.
3. Using quantitative, patient-level data from the Indiana HIE network linked with usage logs from the HIE, the study examined the association between HIE use and ED utilization and the decision to admit a patient to hospital following an ED visit.

The study employed a concurrent mixed-methods design, meaning that the three aims were conducted in parallel. However, data and findings from one aim could influence the conduct of research in the other aims. For example, quantitative data from Aim 1 were used to influence the sampling and questions used in the interviews. Specifically, the researchers used data on whether certain EDs were "high utilizers," "moderate utilizers," or "low utilizers" of the HIE network to ensure interviews were conducted with users from each group. Low utilizers were not necessarily in rural areas or smaller (EDs) As the research progressed, results from one aim also supported interpretation of results from another aim. Specifically, findings from Aim 2 helped to explain potential reasons why patient outcomes in Aim 3 were not always consistent across (EDs)

A good example to illustrate how the various methods worked together can be illustrated in the team's analysis of HIE usage patterns over time. Usage was generally consistent across settings, which is expected years after implementation. However, in 2015, use increased significantly before leveling off again at a new, higher level of steady utilization [35]. These quantitative data were interesting, but the data alone could not explain the sudden increase in usage or why it remained high thereafter. Interviews with ED providers found that several large volume providers implemented single sign on (SSO) functionality in 2015, enabling providers to login to the HIE portal with a single click from their EHR system. This facilitated easier access to "outside information" on patients. Instead of opening a web browser, navigating to the HIE site, logging into the HIE network (using a separate username and password), and looking up the patient using information such as a name and birthdate, the SSO functionality allowed providers to click on a button within their EHR system and automatically login to the HIE network to view medical records for the patient whose record was opened locally. When asked what features make the HIE easy to use, providers overwhelmingly commented that SSO facilitates their use because it makes their job easier. The qualitative data helped the research team interpret their earlier finding, enabling them to synthesize results in a way that explains changes in HIE use over time.

Another AHRQ-funded study [36] of interest also used mixed methods to examine the impact of a new HIE service that prepopulated forms for reporting positive cases of notifiable conditions (e.g., COVID-19, chlamydia, HIV, measles) to public health authorities. This is often described in the public health informatics literature as electronic case reporting [37,38]. Interviews with providers allowed the team to understand how the HIE service was perceived by frontline clinicians [39], which helped the team interpret mixed quantitative results. The HIE-based intervention was significantly effective at improving the reporting of notifiable conditions [29], although effectiveness varied across conditions. Clinician feedback helped explain that automation of routine processes in high volume clinics works well, but in clinics with low volumes clinicians still felt bothered by reporting processes regardless of whether they were paper-based or automated. Based on these two HIE studies, mixed methods are strongly recommended for HIE-based studies as they enable interpretation of heterogeneous patterns in outcomes, work processes, organizational policies, and use of HIE by various types of providers.

A final AHRQ-funded study to keep an eye on in the future is Health Dart [40], which uses Fast Healthcare Interoperability Resources along with other technical standards to directly integrate HIE into clinicians' EHR systems. The project aims to improve the efficiency and effectiveness of HIE by better aligning HIE use into providers' workflow making it easier for them to access the information and knowledge in HIE networks. The project will be implemented in waves across providers, and it will focus on a selected set of conditions including chest pain, abdominal pain, dizziness, back pain, pregnancy, arrhythmia, and dyspnea. Researchers will use multiple methods, including surveys, focus groups, HIE usage log files, and data from the EHR, to measure acceptance by clinicians, observe the rates of data utilization, and assess the impact of HIE on clinical outcomes. The project, funded in 2020, is likely to produce several findings of interest to the HIE community and expand the HIE evidence base.

17.3.5 Data sources

The next step in the process is identifying the sources of the data to support evaluation of the potential measures for the target study design. Data are everywhere in the health system as well as in health information systems. The challenge is defining how the data are to be captured or extracted so they can be used in the evaluation. Furthermore, the team needs to consider where the extracted data will be stored for use during the analysis phase. There are likely to be many data of interest, but only a limited set of data that can be feasibly captured from health services or extracted from existing systems.

Given the proposed study design and list of candidate measures, the team should systematically identify the sources and extraction methods for the data that will be used for each proposed measure. Potential sources include laboratory information system, radiology information system, ED information system, billing system, registration system, disease registry, pharmacy orders, medication administration systems, audit logs of an EHR, personal health record system, and nursing documentation. Other systems to consider include enterprise clinical data warehouse, interface engines that move data between information systems, edge servers that queue incoming or outgoing messages or documents, or the client registry. Some of these systems will be readily available to the HIE or health system, while others (e.g., disease registry, immunization information system) might be available through a partner, such as the public health authority, insurance company, or independent laboratory.

Each system will likely have a different process by which the team can extract, transform, and load (ETL) data into a study database that will enable analysis. This is where having technical expertise on the evaluation team will be vital. Moreover, extracting data from information systems managed by partners may require coordination and discussions with their technical staff. External data sources may also require executing a data use agreement or business associate agreement, a task that can be handled by the project manager with review and input from legal counsel and project director. Keep in mind that legal agreements can take weeks to months to negotiate and finalize.

A final consideration is how the data captured by the evaluation team (e.g., interview data) or extracted from an information system (e.g., laboratory results) will be analyzed. Qualitative data usually require multiple iterations in which the raw notes or documents are synthesized into themes and patterns. Quantitative data often need manipulation prior to their use in an analysis. For example, laboratory test result data are often quite complex—especially microbiology results. Some results might have a numeric value and a reference range, allowing the team to easily assess whether the value falls inside or out of the range and is therefore indicative of disease or a given health status. Yet many results are reported as cryptic values of "present" or "suspected. Sent to public health lab for confirmation" leaving the final result determination up to the evaluation team when analyzing the data, often in consultation with the clinical expert on the team. Moreover, many patients with a given disease, such as diabetes, may not have a formal, documented diagnostic code for the disease. Therefore the team may need to derive a formula for determining, based on available data, whether a given patient has a particular disease or outcome. The need to transform data prior to analysis should be considered when discussing how best to capture data for a given measure.

17.3.6 Assessing feasibility of evaluation measures

Reaching this step in the planning process is not an easy task. However, by systematically thinking through the study design, evaluation methods, potential measures, data sources, and data extraction methods, the team will be well aware of the challenges, complexities, and effort that may be required to complete each candidate evaluation measure. This awareness will be useful in assessing feasibility of the candidate evaluation measures.

For this phase, the team discusses the candidate measures, the sources of the data for those measures, and the relevant ETL methods, in the context of the study design and evaluation methods. To guide the discussion, we suggest asking the team to collectively place each candidate measure in one of the quadrants within a 3×3 Decision Matrix (Fig. 17.1) [41]. The measures should be considered with respect to two aspects: (1) their importance to stakeholders and (2) their feasibility to capture. Measures that are both important to stakeholders and feasible to obtain for analysis should be prioritized in the evaluation plan. Quadrants 1-to-3 are

		Feasibility		
		1: Feasible	2: Feasible with Moderate Effort	3: Not Feasible
Importance	1: Very Important	(1)	(2)	
	2: Moderately Important	(3)	(4)	
	3: Not Important	(5)		

FIGURE 17.1 A decision matrix to guide the selection of important and feasible measures for use in the final evaluation plan. Source: *Adapted from Cusack CM, Byrne CM, Hook JM, McGowan J, Poon E, Zafar A. Health information technology evaluation toolkit: 2009 Update (Prepared for the AHRQ National Resource Center for Health Information Technology under Contract No 290-04-0016). AHRQ Publication No 09-0083-EF. Rockville, MD: Agency for Healthcare Research and Quality; 2009.*

marked in green to suggest that, after discussion, the measures placed in them should be retained for the final evaluation plan. The measures in quadrants 4 and 5 should be further discussed and kept in the plan as time and resources permit. Measures that are not feasible, meaning that their capture or extraction would come at a large expense or significant time, should be eliminated. The goal is to help the team prioritize the measures that will best meet stakeholder needs given the budget, time, and people available to perform the evaluation.

17.3.7 Finalizing the plan

With a completed decision matrix, the team is ready to finalize the evaluation plan. At this stage, the output from each section above can be combined into a single document. The document should be drafted by the team, internally reviewed, and potentially reviewed by external experts or advisors. Once fully drafted, the plan can be presented to a funder for review, or it can be shared with a Board for advice and consent. Once approved by stakeholders, the team will be ready to execute the plan.

The information in Box 17.1 is a sample outline for the various sections to be included in the evaluation plan document. Each final measure should be fully described, although the exact elements and sections included in the plan may vary depending on the study design.

BOX 17.1

Sample evaluation plan outline.

- **I.** Overview of the HIE Project or Organization
- **II.** Goals and Objectives of the HIE Project or Use Case for Evaluation
- **III.** Questions or Objectives of the Evaluation
- **IV.** Evaluation Measures
  - **a.** First Measure—Quantitative or Qualitative?
    - **i.** Description of Measure
    - **ii.** Timeframe for Measurement
    - **iii.** Study Design/Method
    - **iv.** Data Collection Plan
      - **1.** Data Source and Description
      - **2.** Data Extraction Methods, including the name of any specific database field name where the data are stored
    - **v.** Analysis Plan
      - **1.** Data Coding Methods
        - **a.** Quantitative Data: How should the data be calculated or transformed prior to analysis?
        - **b.** Qualitative Data: Which themes is the team trying to find in the unstructured notes/documents?
      - **2.** Data Analysis Methods
      - **3.** Power Calculations or Sample Size Considerations
      - **4.** Tools or Software to Support the Analysis
  - **b.** Repeat the above for each subsequent measure.
- **V.** Budget Considerations

Conclusion

17.4 Dissemination of findings

Evaluating the impact of an HIE project or intervention remains incomplete until the results or lessons from the evaluation are shared. Disseminating findings is what builds the evidence base for HIE and provides closure to the evaluation. Stakeholders interested in the evaluation, including funders, will want to see a report or presentation. There are benefits to disseminating the findings more broadly to peers (e.g., other organizations that may be HIE initiatives or health systems) as well as the biomedical science community. Showcasing findings may encourage others to invest in HIEs, provide evidence of the value and sustainability of an HIE, and promote the need for interoperability of healthcare data to improve outcomes and quality of care. In addition, presentations at professional or scientific conferences can improve the reputation of the evaluation team members as well as the organization for which they work. Publication of the results in a peer-reviewed journal also enhances stature of individuals and organizations. These dissemination methods enable others in the HIE and health IT communities to learn from the experiences of implementing or using HIE.

17.4.1 Strategies for success

Although dissemination beyond the local environment may be challenging, it is feasible as many audiences are interested in the outcomes from and barriers to HIE. Results from the evaluation plus a well-documented evaluation plan provide sufficient inputs into developing an abstract, article, or manuscript for submission to a professional conference or journal. The resources in Table 17.5 provide

TABLE 17.5 Resources to help health information exchange (HIE) networks disseminate results from evaluations with multiple stakeholder groups.

Resource	Description	Features	Source	Citation
Communicating with scientific audiences				
Writing Evaluation Reports	This site features several resources that outline key considerations for effectively reporting evaluation findings and essential elements of evaluation reporting. There are report checklists and suggestions for data visualizations that will make your reports interesting and informative for readers.	Report Checklists Visualizations	National Science Foundation Collaborators	[42]
Statement on Reporting of Evaluation Studies in Health Informatics (STARE-HI)	Guidelines created to help individuals structure a document that reports the findings from an evaluation. The advice in STARE-HI can guide the evaluation team in drafting an article for submission to a peer-reviewed journal.	Guidance for Peer-Reviewed Journals	International Medical Informatics Association (IMIA)	[43,44]
STARE-HI mini	Based on STARE-HI but focused on helping individuals prepare informatics conference papers.	Guidance for Informatics Conference Papers	IMIA	[45]

(Continued)

TABLE 17.5 (Continued)

Resource	Description	Features	Source	Citation
How to Write a Paper or Conference Abstract	This is a blog post by an academic on how to craft a successful abstract. The guidance in this post provides a blueprint for evaluation teams to succinctly state their findings useful in many contexts, including peer-reviewed article submissions, professional conference abstract submissions, and communicating with stakeholders.	Guidance for Conference Abstracts		[46]
Purdue Online Writing Lab	This university website offers a lot of helpful tips for how to write abstracts as well as full reports and research papers. The site is especially helpful with grammar and style as well as references, including APA and MLA. The site offers help in specific subjects, like engineering and technical writing, making more practical than other sites geared toward academic writing.	Guidance for Abstracts, Full Reports, Research Papers Grammar and Style References Engineering, Technical, as well as Academic Writing	Purdue University	[47]
Communicating with broader audiences				
Just Plain Data Analysis	This resource offers suggestions for how to present numerical evidence from evaluations for use in policymaking contexts. The advice can guide evaluation team members in presenting their findings to conference attendees, board members, and the general public.	Guidance for Policymaking Contexts		[48]
Communicating with Your Community	This site features multiple resources on how to "raise awareness about ... your organization's accomplishments." There are guides on creating press releases, brochures, websites, and direct mail campaigns. These guides help organizations focus their message and get out the word about the work they are doing in the community. HIE networks could use the tools to disseminate evaluation findings or create awareness about how the HIE network is impacting care delivery and population outcomes in a community.	Press Releases Brochures Websites Direct Mail	Center for Community Health and Development at the University of Kansas	[49]

further advice and guidance on disseminating findings from HIE evaluations.

17.5 Emerging trends

17.5.1 A growing evidence base

There has been significant growth in HIE evaluation studies over time. As depicted below in Fig. 17.2, the number of HIE-related research articles published each year increased to around 250 starting in 2015. Growth of HIE-related research appears to coincide with the growth of early HIE efforts globally in the late 2000s as well as policies like the Health Information Technology for Economic and Clinical Health Act that encouraged the adoption and use of HIE (see Chapter 3 for details on these policies). The year 2021 saw a decrease in HIE-related evaluation studies, which may be due to the global COVID-19 pandemic or a backlog of articles to be indexed in PubMed.

Recently the United States shifted its "Meaningful Use" program into the current "Promoting Interoperability" program [50]. Whereas prior policy focused primarily on the adoption and use of EHR systems with some HIE requirements, newer policies focus on promoting greater use of interoperability within enterprises and HIE across health delivery systems. Current and future policy creates an environment that encourages the conduct of HIE evaluations. Health services and informatics researchers will likely capitalize on favorable policy conditions to examine the implementation of current and future HIE-related policies. Furthermore, evaluation studies will be encouraged to help guide decisions about which policies are working, which ones should be sunset, and what new polices are needed to optimize HIE across the health system in the United States and globally.

17.5.2 Return on investment

Despite a growing evidence base, there is continued need for evaluation. This is especially true for results of return-on-investment (ROI) analysis, which continues to represent a minority of the available evidence. Health systems, accountable care organizations, and policymakers are all keen to understand whether HIE can result in reduced healthcare costs either by improving the efficiency of health services or through savings afforded by better outcomes that coincide with lower utilization.

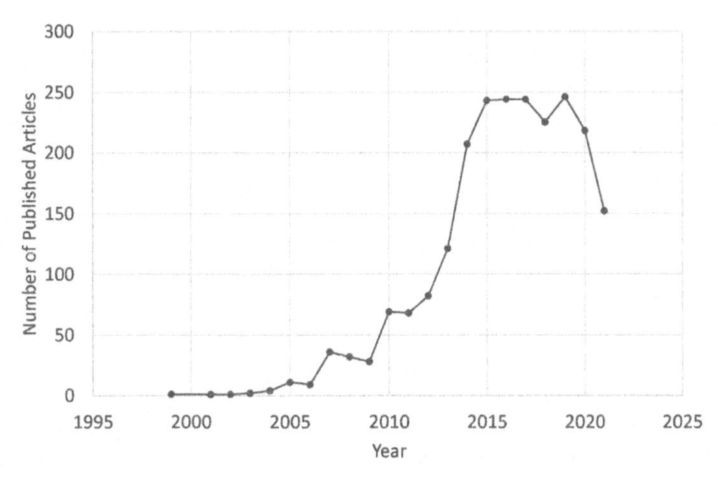

FIGURE 17.2 Number of health information exchange-related articles indexed in PubMed since 1995.

Where possible, evaluation teams should consider adding economic expertise to facilitate conduct of ROI as a component of HIE evaluation. Funders of HIE evaluations are encouraged to support ROI analyses to advance this segment of the evidence base.

17.6 Summary

The evaluation of HIE remains a need for a health system in the middle of reform. Despite growth in the adoption and use of HIE, the evidence base supporting its business case, as well as best practices, is limited. More work is necessary to measure the impact of HIE on clinical as well as population outcomes, in addition to the business of healthcare delivery. Readers are encouraged to not only contribute to the development and implementation of HIE but also the evaluation of it.

Questions for discussion

1. Under what circumstances might summative evaluation be considered research? How about vice versa? Is one better than the other?
2. Which study designs and methods lend themselves best to evaluations on a "shoestring budget?"
3. What are the ethical implications of conducting an evaluation of HIE in a community setting?
4. How might the evaluation plan for a low-to-middle income country differ from an evaluation plan in the United States?
5. Who are potential funders of HIE evaluation in the United States? Internationally?
6. Why should health systems or accountable care organizations fund evaluation of HIE? Isn't research funding best left to government?

References

[1] Scriven M. Minimalist theory: the least theory that practice requires. Am J Evaluation 1998;19(1):57–70.
[2] Mosquera M. HHS awards $139 million to drive adoption of health care IT. Washington: Washington Technology; 2004 [cited 2022 Jan 13]. Available from: <https://washingtontechnology.com/2004/10/hhs-awards-139-million-to-drive-adoption-of-health-care-it/340623/>.
[3] Nocella KC, Horowitz KJ, Young JJ. Against all odds: designing and implementing a grassroots, community-designed RHIO in a rural region. J Healthc Inf Manag 2008;22(2):34–41.
[4] Agency for Healthcare Research and Quality. State and regional demonstration projects. Rockville, MD: Agency for Healthcare Research and Quality; 2009 [updated Dec 2014; cited 2021 Dec 27]. Available from: <http://healthit.ahrq.gov/ahrq-funded-projects/state-and-regional-demonstration-projects>.
[5] Poon EG, Cusack CM, McGowan JJ. Evaluating healthcare information technology outside of academia: observations from the national resource center for healthcare information technology at the Agency for Healthcare Research and Quality. J Am Med Inform Assoc 2009;16(5):631–6.
[6] McGowan JJ, Cusack CM, Poon EG. Formative evaluation: a critical component in EHR implementation. J Am Med Inform Assoc 2008;15(3):297–301.
[7] Cresswell K, Sheikh A, Franklin BD, Krasuska M, Nguyen HT, Hinder S, et al. Theoretical and methodological considerations in evaluating large-scale health information technology change programmes. BMC Health Serv Res 2020;20(1):477.
[8] Johnson KB, Gadd C. Playing smallball: approaches to evaluating pilot health information exchange systems. J Biomed Inform 2007;40(6 Suppl):S21–6.
[9] Dixon BE, Miller T, Overhage JM. Assessing HIE stakeholder readiness for consumer access: lessons learned from the NHIN trial implementations. J Healthc Inf Manag 2009;23(3):20–5.
[10] Overhage JM, Evans L, Marchibroda J. Communities' readiness for health information exchange: the National Landscape in 2004. J Am Med Inform Assoc 2005;12(2):107–12.
[11] Martin TR, Gasoyan H, Pirrotta G, Mathew R. A national survey assessing health information exchange: readiness for changes to Veterans Affairs access standards. Perspect Health Inf Manag 2021;18(3):1i.
[12] Alexander GL, Rantz M, Galambos C, Vogelsmeier A, Flesner M, Popejoy L, et al. Preparing nursing homes for the future of health information exchange. Appl Clin Inform 2015;6(2):248–66.

[13] Revere D, Dixon BE, Hills R, Williams JL, Grannis SJ. Leveraging health information exchange to improve population health reporting processes: lessons in using a collaborative-participatory design process EGEMS (Wash DC) 2014;2(3)[cited 2022 Jan 13] [Article 12 p.] Available from. Available from: https://www.ncbi.nlm.nih.gov/pmc/articles/PMC4371487/.
[14] Reeder B, Revere D, Hills RA, Baseman JG, Lober WB. Public health practice within a health information exchange: information needs and barriers to disease surveillance. Online J Public Health Inform 2012;4(3).
[15] Abramson EL, McGinnis S, Edwards A, Maniccia DM, Moore J, Kaushal R. Electronic health record adoption and health information exchange among hospitals in New York State. J Eval Clin Pract 2012;18(6):1156–62.
[16] Vest J. Health information exchange: the determinants of usage and the impact on utilization [3397326]. Bryan, TX: The Texas A&M University System Health Science Center; 2010.
[17] Byrne CM, Mercincavage LM, Bouhaddou O, Bennett JR, Pan EC, Botts NE, et al. The Department of Veterans Affairs' (VA) implementation of the Virtual Lifetime Electronic Record (VLER): findings and lessons learned from Health Information Exchange at 12 sites. Int J Med Inform 2014;83(8):537–47.
[18] Bailey JE, Pope RA, Elliott EC, Wan JY, Waters TM, Frisse ME. Health information exchange reduces repeated diagnostic imaging for back pain. Ann Emerg Med 2013;62(1):16–24.
[19] Indiana Health Information Exchange. ADT alerts for reducing ED admissions: a case study. Indianapolis, IN: Indiana Health Information Exchange; 2013 [cited 2022 Jan 3]. Available from: <https://mpcms.blob.core.windows.net/bd985247-f489-435f-a7b4-49df92ec868e/docs/4f798bc8-4c8f-4dce-b145-cab48f3d8787/ihie-adtalerts-case-study.pdf>.
[20] Dullabh P, Hovey L, Ubri P. Provider experiences with HIE: key findings from a six-state review. Bethesda, MD: NORC at the University of Chicago; 2015 [cited 2022 Jan 13]. Available from: <https://web.archive.org/web/20180412053126id_/https:/http://www.healthit.gov/sites/default/files/reports/provider_experiences_with_hie_june_2015.pdf>.
[21] Vest JR, Kern LM, Silver MD, Kaushal R. The potential for community-based health information exchange systems to reduce hospital readmissions. J Am Med Inform Assoc 2014;22:435–42.
[22] Franzosa E, Traylor M, Judon KM, Guerrero Aquino V, Schwartzkopf AL, Boockvar KS, et al. Perceptions of event notification following discharge to improve geriatric care: qualitative interviews of care team members from a 2-site cluster randomized trial. J Am Med Inform Assoc 2021;28(8):1728–35.
[23] Dixon BE, Grannis SJ, McAndrews C, Broyles AA, Mikels-Carrasco W, Wiensch A, et al. Leveraging data visualization and a statewide health information exchange to support COVID-19 surveillance and response: application of public health informatics. J Am Med Inform Assoc 2021;28(7):1363–73.
[24] Nakayama M, Inoue R, Miyata S, Shimizu H. Health information exchange between specialists and general practitioners benefits rural patients. Appl Clin Inform 2021;12(3):564–72.
[25] Apathy NC, Vest JR, Adler-Milstein J, Blackburn J, Dixon BE, Harle CA. Practice and market factors associated with provider volume of health information exchange. J Am Med Inform Assoc 2021;28(7):1451–60.
[26] Flaks-Manov N, Shadmi E, Hoshen M, Balicer RD. Health information exchange systems and length of stay in readmissions to a different hospital. J Hosp Med 2016;11(6):401–6.
[27] Dixon BE, Judon KM, Schwartzkopf AL, Guerrero VM, Koufacos NS, May J, et al. Impact of event notification services on timely follow-up and rehospitalization among primary care patients at two Veterans Affairs Medical Centers. J Am Med Inform Assoc 2021;28(12):2593–600.
[28] Wiley KK, Hilts KE, Ancker JS, Unruh MA, Jung HY, Vest JR. Organizational characteristics and perceptions of clinical event notification services in healthcare settings: a study of health information exchange. JAMIA Open 2020;3(4):611–18.
[29] Dixon BE, Zhang Z, Arno JN, Revere D, Joseph Gibson P, Grannis SJ. Improving notifiable disease case reporting through electronic information exchange-facilitated decision support: a controlled before-and-after trial. Public Health Rep 2020;135(3):401–10.
[30] Chandrasekaran R, Sankaranarayanan B, Pendergrass J. Unfulfilled promises of health information exchange: What inhibits ambulatory clinics from electronically sharing health information? Int J Med Inform 2021;149:104418.
[31] Watkinson F, Dharmayat KI, Mastellos N. A mixed-method service evaluation of health information exchange in England: technology acceptance and barriers and facilitators to adoption. BMC Health Serv Res 2021;21(1):737.
[32] Dixon BE, Zafar A, Overhage JM. A framework for evaluating the costs, effort, and value of nationwide health information exchange. J Am Med Inform Assoc 2010;17(3):295–301.
[33] Pan E, Byrne CM, Damico D, Crimmins M. Guide to evaluating health information exchange projects (Prepared for the Agency for Healthcare Research and Quality under Contract No. 290200900023-I).

Rockville, MD: Agency for Healthcare Research and Quality; 2014 [cited 2021 Dec 27]. Available from: <http://healthit.ahrq.gov/health-it-tools-and-resources/guide-evaluating-health-information-exchange-projects>.
[34] Exploring the utilization of and outcomes from health information exchange in emergency settings. Rockville, MD: Agency for Healthcare Research and Quality; 2017. Available from: <https://digital.ahrq.gov/ahrq-funded-projects/exploring-utilization-and-outcomes-health-information-exchange-emergency>.
[35] Rahurkar S, Vest JR, Finnell JT, Dixon BE. Trends in user-initiated health information exchange in the inpatient, outpatient, and emergency settings. J Am Med Inform Assoc 2021;28(3):622–7.
[36] Dixon BE, Grannis SJ, Revere D. Measuring the impact of a health information exchange intervention on provider-based notifiable disease reporting using mixed methods: a study protocol. BMC Med Inf Decis Mak 2013;13(1):121.
[37] Public Health Informatics Institute. Advancing electronic case reporting (eCR) of sexually transmitted infections (STIs). Decatur, GA: Public Health Informatics Institute; 2016. Available from: <https://phii.org/ecr-sti>.
[38] Haque SN, Dixon BE, Grannis SJ, Pina J. Public health informatics. In: Finnell JT, Dixon BE, editors. Clinical informatics study guide: text and review. 2nd ed. Zurich: Springer International; 2022. in press.
[39] Revere D, Hills RH, Dixon BE, Gibson PJ, Grannis SJ. Notifiable condition reporting practices: implications for public health agency participation in a health information exchange. BMC Public Health 2017;17(1):247.
[40] Agency for Healthcare Research and Quality. Improving healthcare processes and outcomes by directly integrating health information exchange data in the clinical workflow. Rockville, MD: Agency for Healthcare Research and Quality; 2021 [cited 2022 Jan 13]. Available from: <https://digital.ahrq.gov/ahrq-funded-projects/improving-healthcare-processes-and-outcomes-directly-integrating-health>.
[41] Cusack CM, Byrne CM, Hook JM, McGowan J, Poon E, Zafar A. Health information technology evaluation toolkit: 2009 Update (Prepared for the AHRQ National Resource Center for Health Information Technology under Contract No 290-04-0016). AHRQ Publication No 09-0083-EF. Rockville, MD: Agency for Healthcare Research and Quality; 2009.
[42] Center for Advancement of Informal Science Education. Evaluation reporting and dissemination. 2021 [cited 2022 Jan 13]. Available from: <https://www.informalscience.org/evaluation/reporting-dissemination>.
[43] Brender J, Talmon J, de Keizer N, Nykanen P, Rigby M, Ammenwerth E. STARE-HI – statement on reporting of evaluation studies in health informatics: explanation and elaboration. Appl Clin Inform 2013;4(3):331–58.
[44] Talmon J, Ammenwerth E, Brender J, de Keizer N, Nykanen P, Rigby M. STARE-HI – Statement on reporting of evaluation studies in Health Informatics. Int J Med Inform 2009;78(1):1–9.
[45] de Keizer NF, Talmon J, Ammenwerth E, Brender J, Nykanen P, Rigby M. Mini Stare-HI: guidelines for reporting health informatics evaluations in conference papers. Stud Health Technol Inform 2010;160(Pt 2):1206–10.
[46] Kelsky K. How to write a paper or conference proposal abstract. 2011 [cited 2021 Dec 27]. Available from: <http://theprofessorisin.com/2011/07/12/how-tosday-how-to-write-a-paper-abstract/>.
[47] Purdue Online Writing Lab. West Lafayette, IN: Purdue University; 2021 [cited 2022 Jan 13]. Available from: <https://owl.purdue.edu/owl/purdue_owl.html>.
[48] Klass G. Just plain data analysis: finding, presenting, and interpreting social science data.. 2nd ed. New York: Rowman and Littlefield Publishers; 2012.
[49] Center for Community Health and Development. Chapter 6. Communications to promote interest. The University of Kansas; [cited 2022 Jan 13]. Available from: <https://ctb.ku.edu/en/table-of-contents/participation/promoting-interest>.
[50] Centers for Medicare and Medicaid Services. Promoting interoperability programs. Baltimore, MD: Centers for Medicare & Medicaid Services; 2020 [updated 2021 Feb 11]. Available from: <https://www.cms.gov/Regulations-and-Guidance/Legislation/EHRIncentivePrograms>.

CHAPTER

18

Leveraging HIE to facilitate large-scale data analytics

Eileen F. Tallman[1], *Drew Richardson*[2], *Todd M. Rogow*[3], *David C. Kendrick*[4,5] *and Brian E. Dixon*[1,6]

[1]Department of Epidemiology, Richard M. Indiana University Fairbanks School of Public Health, Indiana University, Indianapolis, IN, USA [2]Indiana Health Information Exchange, Indianapolis, IN, USA [3]Healthix, New York, NY, USA [4]MyHealth Access Network, Tulsa, OK, USA [5]Department of Medical Informatics, University of Oklahoma, Norman, OK, USA [6]Center for Biomedical Informatics, Regenstrief Institute, Inc., Indianapolis, IN, USA

LEARNING OBJECTIVES

At the end of the chapter, the reader should be able to:

- Define analytics and discuss how it supports achieving the goals outlined in many nations' digital health strategy.
- Describe the data, information, knowledge, wisdom pyramid.
- Describe how health information organizations can provide real-time analytics to health systems to improve population health outcomes.
- List ways in which analytics can provide value for HIEs and participants in public health and healthcare organizations.
- Explain how analytics are supported in an HIE.
- Identify barriers to implementing analytics in an HIE.
- Understand how HIE architecture models can impact analytics.
- List and describe three types of analytics that can be used at an HIE.

18.1 Introduction

Electronic health data are abundant in much of the globe. Mobile phone applications, wearable technologies like heart rate monitors and smart watches, social media services, and healthcare information systems all collect health-related data leading to the accumulation of massive amounts data. Once a nation has

Health Information Exchange
DOI: https://doi.org/10.1016/B978-0-323-90802-3.00017-4

established a robust infrastructure for amassing data, it next seeks to leverage those data to infer insights and drive outcomes, such as reductions in healthcare costs or improvements in population health outcomes. However, generating meaningful population health insights remains a major challenge for health systems around the world. The key to leveraging abundant data resources is health analytics, a term that has become synonymous with artificial intelligence (AI) and other innovations in digital health that garner headlines and drive innovation in the health sector.

In this chapter, we discuss how the methods of health analytics can be used by health information exchange (HIE) networks and health information organizations (HIOs) to derive value for health systems and populations. We examine some of the important ways in which HIOs can incorporate analytics into their services and some of the barriers they may face. We also discuss the common analytical approaches HIE networks can use to improve population health outcomes. First, we begin with the basics of analytics and analytical approaches, establishing a foundation upon which we can discuss the integration of an analytic platform into an HIE network.

18.2 Foundations for analytics

Analytics is the "discovery, interpretation, and communication of meaningful patterns found in data, as well as the application of data patterns for effective decision-making" [1]. *Population health management* is made up of strategies, processes, and tools that gather demographic and clinical data and use them to carry out population health practices [2]. Population health management relies on *population health analytics,* which applies quantitative methods to the gathered data to generate insights. Population health analytics is increasingly used in health systems, and there is a high demand for ways to incorporate these tools into existing information systems. Population health analytics is key to meeting the goals of the Triple Aim as a framework for optimizing health system performance, and when used analytics can improve value-based care, reduce costs, and generate population health insights such as identifying health behavior patterns and establishing risk groups [3].

Analytics often leverages large amounts of data, also known as *big data*. Big data are characterized by four V's: volume, velocity, variety, and veracity. Data volumes in healthcare can be enormous, with vital signs gathered on intensive care patients every hour or even minute. The data in healthcare come from a wide variety of locations (clinics, hospitals, pharmacies, etc.), and from each location, a variety of data types are gathered (e.g., health interviews, patient registration, sensors). The combination of high data volumes and real-time data flows makes healthcare data some of the potentially highest velocity forms of Big Data. Finally, before they can be used for analytics, raw data need to be cleaned, linked, stored, and managed, and derived information needs to reach the right people at the right time and in the right form for immediate consumption and comprehension.

The processes of data organization, normalization, and validation are necessary to assure the veracity of the data and may occur at many points. For example, clinic staff may have quality control procedures for data entry before sending information to a HIE to be sorted, normalized, and exchanged so that data analysis can occur (see Fig. 18.1B). Furthermore, raw data consist of multiple, unorganized observations that need to become something more meaningful, and at its peak, generate wisdom. The progression of raw data to wisdom is best illustrated by the Data Information Knowledge Wisdom (DIKW) pyramid, which can be seen in Fig. 18.1A.

The DIKW pyramid is a hierarchy that starts with raw data, which is then transformed into information when it has been organized or structured in a way that it can be used for a

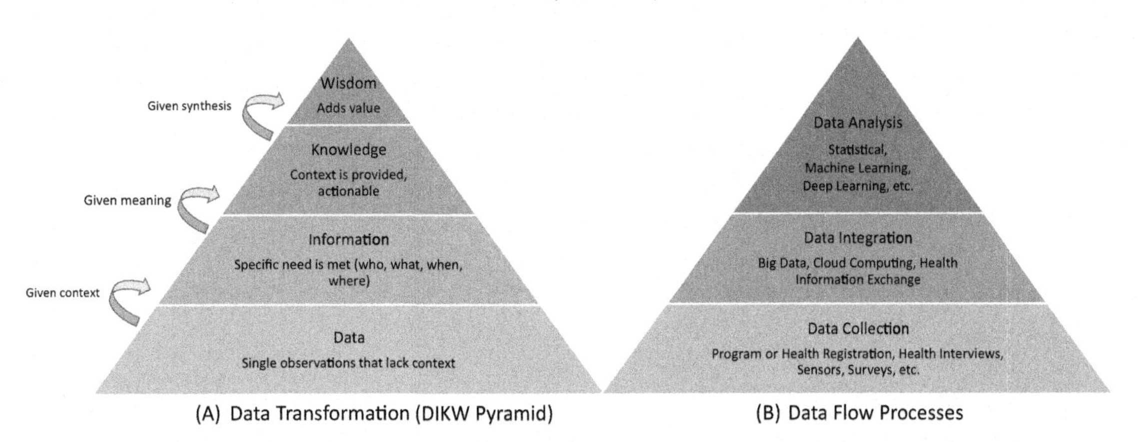

FIGURE 18.1 Putting the DIKW pyramid and data flow processes together. (A) The DKIW pyramid; (B) data flow processes [4]. Source: *Models are derived from Kristoffersenristoffersen E, Blomsm(Kristoffersen E, Blomsma F, Mikalef P, Li J. The smart circular economy: a digital-enabled circular strategies framework for manufacturing companies. J Bus Res 2020;120:241–61).*

specific need [1]. It can provide the who, what, when, and where for an observation [4]. For example, a percentage shown next to a label for "Giardia lamblia" becomes meaningful when we know it represents the percentage of individuals with giardiasis in a specific zip code in the same month. Next, information becomes knowledge when it can be examined with context beyond the dataset. In the giardia example, the information can be combined with expertise from a health department to identify an outbreak and locate the water source. Finally, at the top of the pyramid, raw data yield information that has generated knowledge, which over time and with experience, becomes wisdom. Wisdom enables judgment, increases effectiveness, and adds value after knowledge has been acquired [1]. The health department could use wisdom to eliminate the cause of giardia and generate prevention strategies.

There are three analytical approaches that facilitate the movement of raw data from the base level of the DIKW pyramid to the information, knowledge, and wisdom levels of the pyramid. These analytical approaches, which are called "descriptive," "predictive," and "prescriptive," are discussed later in the chapter, but their relationship to the DIKW pyramid can be seen in Fig. 18.2.

18.3 Analytical maturity

Analytical maturity is evaluated through *analytical maturity models* that describe milestones and provide guidance, measurement, and evaluation at advancing stages of analytical capacity. Different fields, such as business, software development, and healthcare, have discipline-specific analytic models. The models can help improve the business of analytics by establishing milestones an HIE can achieve to accomplish different levels of analytic capacity. They are also useful to help an organization objectively assess baseline analytics capabilities to identify resources they might need to progress toward more advanced stages in the model. One such example is the Healthcare Information and Management Systems Society (HIMSS) Adoption Model for Analytics Maturity (AMAM), which is made up of eight stages [5] that can be seen in greater detail in Table 18.1.

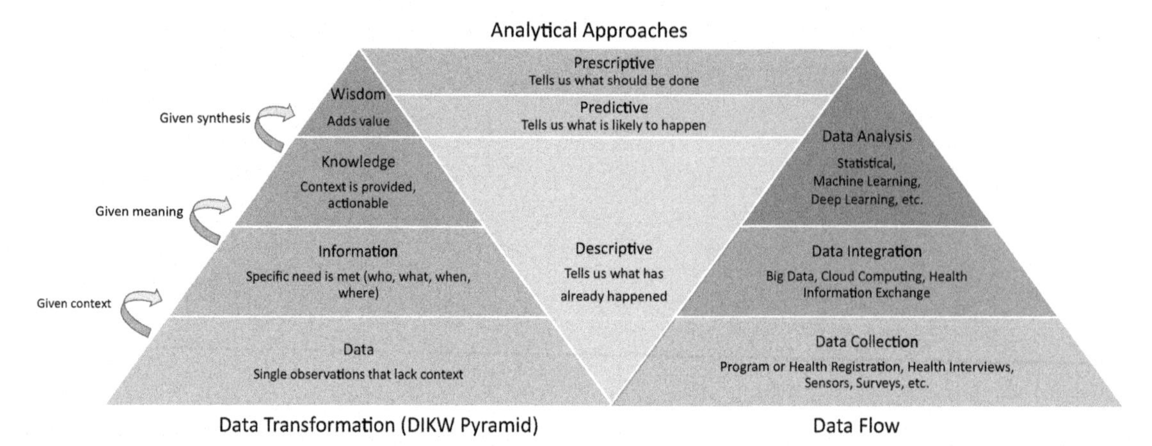

FIGURE 18.2 The DKIW pyramid (left), three analytical approaches (middle), and data flow processes (right)[4] . Source: *Models are derived from Kristoffersen's Smart CE framework (Kristoffersen E, Blomsma F, Mikalef P, Li J. The smart circular economy: a digital-enabled circular strategies framework for manufacturing companies. J Bus Res 2020;120:241–61).*

18.4 Analytical approaches

There are three primary analytical approaches that are widely used across industries and can be implemented for HIE: descriptive, predictive, and prescriptive. In the next sections, we explore these analytical approaches in detail.

18.4.1 Descriptive analytics

Descriptive analytics are used to describe populations, events, and behaviors, or to summarize datasets to make them more interpretable [1]. They explain what has already happened in a dataset. They help bridge the gap between our understanding of past population health behaviors and how they influence future population health outcomes [1]. Descriptive analytics are typically displayed in the form of percentages and frequencies and use basic statistics like mean, median, and standard deviation to describe a dataset. Most population health analyses use descriptive analytics. They are useful for generating reports or adding context to more advanced analyses. In the context of analytical maturity, descriptive analytics can be used at lower-level stages. For example, the HIMSS AMAM places descriptive analytics capacity in Stage 3 [5]. Some examples of descriptive analytics include prevalence and incidence of disease, conditions, or events. In terms of population health, descriptive analytics can tell us if individuals with an age-related risk for breast cancer are being screened in the community or what portion of the state has Type I and Type II diabetes mellitus.

18.4.2 Predictive analytics

Predictive analytics *forecasts* the likelihood of future health events or outcomes by using population- and individual-level data [1]. In other words, they tell us what might happen; they do not have complete accuracy. Predictive analytics are generated through modeling and simulations and they work by identifying patterns in a dataset that can be used to forecast future behavior [6]. Of note, predictive analytics are not a priori, or hypothesis-driven, but are instead a posteriori, or based on observations from the data. Therefore it can be challenging to determine what questions to ask a

TABLE 18.1 Summary of HIMSS Adoption Model for Analytics Maturity (AMAM) [5].

Maturity level	Analytical capabilities
0: Fragmented Point Solutions	• Desire to learn about adding analytics • Has need for insights • Wants to improve decision-making • No governance
1: Foundation Building: Data Aggregation and Initial Data Governance	• Actively accumulating data • Has centralized data storage that supports historical and consolidated access • Developing analytics strategy • Brings basic data together from appropriate systems
2: Core Data Warehouse Workout: Centralized Database With an Analytics Competency Center	• Enterprise data warehouse exists, is accessible, and contains data. • Data warehouse can be used for ad hoc queries and descriptive reporting. • Analytics competency center manages analytic skills, standards, and education. • Activities are aligned with the organization's overall strategic goals. • Data governance is maturing; basic clinical and operational tasks are supported (e.g., patient registries).
3: Efficient, Consistent, Internal and External Report Production and Agility	• Mastery of enterprise descriptive reporting • Varying parts of the organization can corral data, work with it, and easily generate historical and current reports. • Data quality is stable and predictable. • Tools are standardized and broadly available. • Data warehouse access is managed and reliable.
4: Measuring and Managing Evidence-Based Care, Care Visibility and Waste Reduction	• Direct analytical data assets, skills, and infrastructure focused on improving clinical, financial, and operational programs. • Makes effort to understand and optimize clinical care through analytics resources that support evidence-based care, tracks and reports care and operational variability, and uses analytics to identify and minimize clinical and operational waste.
5: Enhancing Quality of Care and Population Health, and Understanding the Economics of Care	• Demonstrate expanded point-of-care oriented analytics and support of population health. • Align data governance to support quality-based performance reporting and economics of care.
6: Clinical Risk Intervention and Predictive Analytics	• Demonstrate maturity of predictive analytics. • Demonstrate expanded focus on advanced data content and clinical support.
7: Personalized Medicine and Prescriptive Analytics	• Can leverage advanced datasets (e.g., genomics, biometrics) to support personalized medicine. • Deliver mass customization of care combined with prescriptive analytics.

predictive model ahead of time. Because predictive analytics use patterns, their predictions are only as useful as long as the patterns in the dataset are true and accurate representations of reality. Some of these challenges can be mitigated by using more data, because, as long as all other elements are the same, analytics using larger volumes of data are more likely to be truly representative of the truth (e.g., have narrower confidence intervals). Therefore algorithms trained with larger datasets are more likely to account for more complexities and features in the dataset—and yield more accurate predictions. Only organizations with a high level of analytical maturity can reliably use predictive analytics—the HIMSS AMAM does not include predictive analytics until Stage 6.

Predictive analytics are not just needed in day-to-day clinical decision-making. They are used heavily to support the business operations of an organization, especially to help optimize the performance of a healthcare system within its existing business models, which range from fee-for-service to value-based contracts to full risk contracts. Population health-focused predictive models can be used to reduce costs and improve quality metrics for value-based payment models and quality programs [such as Merit-based Incentive Payment System (MIPS) and meaningful use], as well as optimize the management of a population's health. For example, emergency room readmissions could be reduced by improving care coordination for those most at risk of the readmission events [7]. First, the patients who are most at risk need to be identified. Predictive models can be used to identify these patients by applying machine learning techniques or statistical methods to the available data to help identify electronic phenotypes that match the characteristics of at-risk patients. An example of predictive analytics can be found in Box 18.1, which features Healthix, a community-based HIE network in New York City, and its analytics platform, which is used to identify population risk scores for the purpose of risk management [8].

18.4.3 Prescriptive analytics

Prescriptive analytics also uses simulations, usually through machine learning, to create suggestions with the aim of improving decision-making [6]. It is the most-impactful, but least-used out of the three types of analytics because it requires advanced analytical maturity. According to HIMSS AMAM, prescriptive analytics takes place in organizations who have reached Stage 7 [5]. Prescriptive analytics attempts to quantify the impacts of future decisions [1], enabling organizations enabling them to make better choices and avoid negative consequences. Prescriptive analytics can be used for clinical decision-making in a healthcare setting, which relies on real-time data and workflow automation. Predictive and prescriptive analytics can be used in combination as described in Box 18.2. In this example, 30-day readmission rates are predicted, and then prescriptive methods are used to determine the best interventions for prevention of readmissions in high-risk patients.

18.5 Drivers of analytics in health systems

Recent national policies in health information technology in the United States emphasize interoperability over analytics. This could suggest that the United States is, by and large, still stuck at low levels of analytical maturity. However, analytics are increasingly championed at the national level. In its national roadmap for interoperability, the Office of the National Coordinator for Health Information Technology (ONC) sets a goal that real-time

BOX 18.1

Healthix Population Risk Scores.

Leveraging analytical technology to make real change

Healthix is one of the largest public, community-based HIE networks in the nation, bringing together over 9000 healthcare facilities across Southern New York State. Healthix provides secure access to clinical data of more than 20 million patients for treatment, care coordination, and quality improvement. Data available through Healthix include a broad range of clinical information electronically delivered, in real time, 24/7 with each patient encounter from across New York State.

Among many service offerings Healthix provides Healthix Analytics, which provides dashboards and reports to support population health management, patient outreach, and readmission management. The analytics service, powered through a partnership with HBI Solutions, Inc. (HBI), provides predictive risk scores, early identification of serious health conditions, and helps prevent avoidable emergency department (ED) visits and hospitalizations. Risk scores are calculated daily using clinical information, medical encounters, and social determinants of health (SDOH) data from across a broad spectrum of HIE data contributors. Although many providers were using Healthix's real-time alerts triggered by acute care events, increasingly providers seek ways to close gaps in care, identify high-risk patients who are "lost to care," or understand why patients are frequently utilizing emergency room services. This requires large-scale analytics leveraging multiple HIE data sources.

Healthix chose to partner with HBI, a vendor that understands the merit of integrating predictive analytics with HIE services, especially in Healthix's case, where New York State privacy and policy considerations must be built into the offering. The predictive risk insights show what is likely to happen to a patient or member in the future, allowing care teams to proactively intervene before the untoward event occurs and helps organizations allocate resources where they are needed most. The predictions include estimated costs, utilization (ED visit, inpatient admissions), mortality, chronic disease development (diabetes, heart failure, etc.), and high-cost/high-morbidity events like stroke, heart attack, and suicide.

HBI approaches machine learning by tuning and calibrating the models on each customer's dataset, which provides the highest accuracy for each customer, as each customer's population and datasets vary widely. During the calibration process, HBI utilizes longitudinal data over multiple years to thoroughly derive and test each model before placing the model into production. HBI uses Hadoop Spark, a combination of open-source architectures for big data management and processing, for the model feature selection process, and the R statistical programming language for model development and calibration. Once the algorithm is finalized, it is layered into a PMML (Predictive Model Markup Language) engine, which works with Healthix's core HIE system powered by InterSystems HealthShare.

Overall, partnership with HBI helps Healthix fulfill its mission of mobilizing health information across the communities they serve to advance patient care. Healthix Analytics is just one example of this, supporting the patient, not just by bringing together their digital health records, but in leveraging data and making data actionable for those providing direct care or management services. This service builds upon

BOX 18.1 (*cont'd*)

the robust base of clinical records available through Healthix. Using risk scores targets specific conditions, enabling those treating the patient to become proactive in their practices. Highlighting a patient's risk score gives providers the foresight to enroll the individual into preventive care programs or provide a needed office visit to avoid an undesirable outcome, whether that is being readmitted to a hospital or developing a chronic condition.

Putting Actions into Practice

In the summer of 2020, at the height of the COVID-19 pandemic, Healthix began working with New York City's health agencies, which includes the agency that oversees health for the city's school children. The school health agency is charged with the supervision of >1 million children's health between the ages of 6–18 throughout the five boroughs. Specifically, their goal was to use Healthix data to support patient outreach and care coordination, and to help young patients and their families better manage their COVID-19 susceptibility, especially in the context of clinical conditions such as asthma, and mental health diagnoses. This was especially critical as youngsters were learning remotely under the most trying of circumstances. Healthix's goal was to provide the program with access to real-time clinical data, which would supplement available claims and clinical data, as well as share risk scores for those students in these specified health areas. Recognizing that working with a large, complex health agency, with its many specialized bureaus and subdivisions and little-to-no technical or systems integration would pose a challenge, Healthix began with a step-by-step approach to gain some initial traction. Their hope was that over time, the agency would be able to cross-pollinate ideas across various departments and divisions, enabling them to leverage more and more of the available data and technology that Healthix offers over time—thus adding the HIE as a core component of their public health infrastructure.

Healthix analysts began the public schools project by properly matching the identities between Healthix and the school health agency roster. Their initial match rate of 97% helped validate that Healthix had substantial overlap. Once data started flowing, they began to see benefits—within the first few months additional diagnoses uncovered potential findings for 13,000 children with asthma, 9000 for depression, and 11,000 for anxiety. Preliminary results showed 10,000 students had a change in diagnosis within the first few months. The real-time nature of Healthix's data provided the agency with timely understanding of the health risks of the students they were serving. It became clear that there is widespread potential benefit of the use of HIE data and analytics services across bureaus caring for family and child health, disease control, mental hygiene, and health equity and community wellness (see Table 18.2).

TABLE 18.2 COVID-19 susceptibility in children (6–18 years) in New York City's five boroughs.

Risk class	Number	Percentage
Low	999,659	99.9
Moderate	654	0.065
High	108	0.11
Very high	4	0.0004
Total	1,000,425	100

Healthix, New York State's largest public HIE, was engaged to provide COVID-19 risk scores for all children with one or more chronic conditions to help New York City's health department prioritize outreach and care coordination. The table represents overall risk class as identified for New York City's school population and their respective number and percentage for reference.

BOX 18.1 (*cont'd*)

Based upon its mature Enterprise Master Patient Index (eMPI) as well as over a decade of aggregated clinical data, Healthix Analytics provides information to target, personalize, and manage care for patients at-risk. An example of the analytics report can be seen in Fig. 18.3. It identifies patient risk before a diagnosis is made to aid in prevention and wellness initiatives. Most compelling is the fact that empowering the city program with risk scores on asthma, mental hygiene, and COVID susceptibility has helped officials become more proactive in reaching out to school nurses and care managers to intervene with students currently at-risk in these areas.

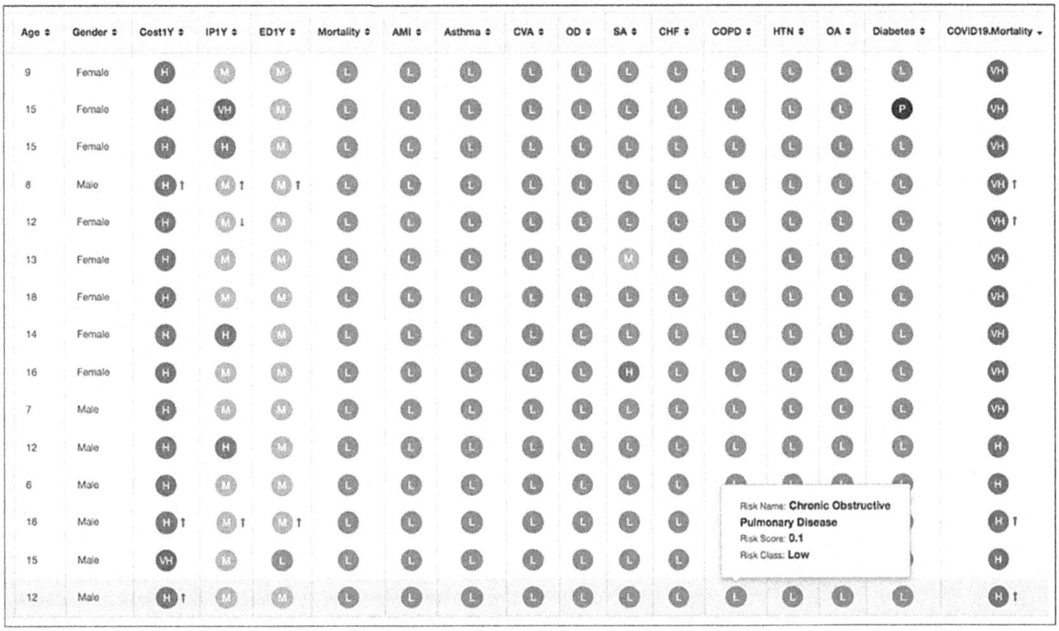

Age	Gender	Cost1Y	IP1Y	ED1Y	Mortality	AMI	Asthma	CVA	OD	SA	CHF	COPD	HTN	OA	Diabetes	COVID19.Mortality
9	Female	H	M	M	L	L	L	L	L	L	L	L	L	L	L	VH
15	Female	H	VH	M	L	L	L	L	L	L	L	L	L	L	P	VH
15	Female	H	H	M	L	L	L	L	L	L	L	L	L	L	L	VH
8	Male	H ↑	M ↑	M ↑	L	L	L	L	L	L	L	L	L	L	L	VH ↑
12	Female	H	M ↓	M	L	L	L	L	L	L	L	L	L	L	L	VH ↑
13	Female	H	M	M	L	L	L	L	L	M	L	L	L	L	L	VH
18	Female	H	M	M	L	L	L	L	L	L	L	L	L	L	L	VH
14	Female	H	H	M	L	L	L	L	L	L	L	L	L	L	L	VH
16	Female	H	M	M	L	L	L	L	L	H	L	L	L	L	L	VH
7	Male	H	M	M	L	L	L	L	L	L	L	L	L	L	L	VH
12	Male	H	H	M	L	L	L	L	L	L	L	L	L	L	L	H
6	Male	H	M	M	L	L	L	L	L	L	L	[illegible]	[illegible]	[illegible]	[illegible]	H
16	Male	H ↑	M ↑	M ↑	L	L	L	L	L	L	L	[illegible]	[illegible]	[illegible]	[illegible]	H ↑
15	Male	VH	M	L	L	L	L	L	L	L	L	[illegible]	[illegible]	[illegible]	[illegible]	H
12	Male	H ↑	M	M	L	L	L	L	L	L	L	L	L	L	L	H ↑

Risk Name: **Chronic Obstructive Pulmonary Disease**
Risk Score: **0.1**
Risk Class: **Low**

FIGURE 18.3 Diagram of Healthix predictive risk report.

analytics will be used to improve health delivery by 2030 [10]. HIE networks and HIOs are uniquely positioned to support the progression from data to wisdom and support the advancement of analytical maturity for health systems and other healthcare stakeholders who are ready to take the next step. However, according to a 2018 national survey of 89 HIOs, only 39% reported offering analytics as a value-added service [11].

Globally, multiple nations are driving their health systems toward greater use of analytics. Israel, for example, desires to be a global leader in digital health technologies, including AI. Already boasting over 500 digital health start-ups, Israel created a $1 million shekel ($276 million) investment fund focused on commercializing its "gold mine" of health data [12]. These companies are banking on the nations existing interoperable systems that make large healthcare datasets ripe for analytics. Many other developed nations similarly seek to employ advanced computational approaches to healthcare delivery, all of which have a mature national electronic health record (EHR) deployment whose data can be examined using analytical approaches. Nations with centralized national healthcare models have an advantage. However, in the United States, trends toward value-based payment models and risk sharing with providers also drive interest in health analytics. The advanced payment models drive the desire of health systems to leverage analytics in support of population health.

18.6 How does analytics support promoting interoperability and reporting goals?

As mentioned in previous chapters, the US Promoting Interoperability Programs (formerly called EHR Incentive Programs/Meaningful Use) are made up of three stages [13], summarized below:

- Stage 1 established requirements for electronic health records and data capture.
- Stage 2 encouraged the use of EHR to meet continuous quality improvement goals defined by the National Quality Strategy (NQS).
- Stage 3 focused on advanced usage of EHR to improve health outcomes.

Analytic approaches are needed to meet the goals of Stage 3 while Stages 1 and 2 establish the technical foundations required to access data across health systems to be integrated into those approaches. The shift in focus to population health management, clinical care coordination, and standardized data for widespread HIE requires the ability to contextually analyze the current and steady progress of a health system within a community [14].

In addition, Stage 3 of Promoting Interoperability requires Medicaid providers to report annually on quality and performance measures. Value-based programs, like the MIPS, require reports for six measures (e.g., poor diabetes control and depression screening) while some Accountable Care Organizations (ACO's) report on an additional 10 measures (e.g., breast cancer screening, statin use) [15]. Providers need access to quality data to generate value-based reports, but they also need access to real-time, robust data to know whether they are on track to meet required standards and to actually improve population health. Population health management requires the iterative use of analytics to keep a health system informed about its progress and improve care for the population that they serve. Providers face challenges because many technology tools in the health space were developed to capture information about billing and volume, but not quality and outcomes [16]. An example of how HIE can support population health management goals is illustrated in Box 18.3, which describes how MyHealth, Oklahoma's statewide HIE, employs analytics to help its members achieve the quality reporting goals for the Promoting Interoperability programs (formerly Meaningful Use).

Furthermore, health systems rely on intra- and intersystem health data from multiple sources to gain population insights or to generate reports [17]. This is especially true for smaller providers or rural clinics, whose patients may need to visit multiple facilities. Rural patients may visit facilities outside of town or county boundaries. In all of these scenarios, real-time data can be difficult to obtain. In

BOX 18.2

Combining predictive and prescriptive methods.

Predictive and prescriptive methods are often used in combination. It can sometimes be a bit confusing to differentiate them because they both use simulations and machine learning. Predictive analytics answers the question "What will happen?" while prescriptive analytics answers "Based on predictions of all possible outcomes, what should I do?" [6].

A study by Bertsimas et al. [9] applied machine learning methods to a dataset with over 300 variables collected between 2011 and 2014. The first aim of the study was to use predictive methods to determine whether preoperative or a combination of pre- and postoperative data could best predict the 30-day readmission events of patients who have undergone surgery. They evaluated the quality of their prediction using the false positive rate and the sensitivity of the test. The results of their predictive tests showed that 30-day readmission predictions were more accurate with both pre- and postoperative variables.

The predictive methods were useful in trying to describe what will likely happen to surgical patients after they are discharged. The application of prescriptive methods would build upon this to inform a decision, action, or program to address the problem. Thus the next step in the process is to try to prevent 30-day readmissions ("what should I do?"). In the study, prescriptive methods were applied to enable clinical decision support based on the preoperative predictive models [9]. For these prescriptive methods, the investigators simulated altering preoperative hematocrit values before surgery to prevent postsurgery 30-day readmissions. The results predicted that presurgical blood transfusions to a target hematocrit would reduce postoperative 30-day hospital readmissions by 5%–20% for one model and 4%–19% for a second model.

response, providers may collect claims data from external sources in lieu of EHR access, but they often contain a shallow supply [16] and the process is often time consuming and inaccurate, and exchange is usually delayed [18]. HIOs are well positioned to meet challenges faced by health systems because of their ability to enhance interoperability, data sharing, and data quality. They can leverage aggregate data from repositories and act as a data steward to support analytics in real time. In addition, HIOs can normalize or add structure to unstructured data prior to use [21].

In the next section, we discuss how the introduction of analytics in an HIE network can help health systems meet local and national population health goals.

18.7 How can HIOs provide real-time analytics to meet population health goals?

An *analytic platform* is an enterprise technology solution that contextualizes data [22] and usually exists in the form of a user-friendly web application or a dashboard. The platform is an important component of facilitating analytic capacity and makes analytics accessible for both an HIE network and its members. If you are familiar with software like Tableau, Microsoft PowerBI, or Oracle Analytics Cloud, you are already acquainted with an analytic platform. These platforms often include visualization tools, cross-platform functionality, and ad hoc query capabilities.

Many analytic platforms are used to build customized modules and they may be used for forecasting, creating predictive risk models, generating dashboards, or geospatial analysis. Overall, having an analytic platform can increase the value of available aggregate data by using it to generate insights and actionable knowledge.

For example, if an emergency department is overextended and lacks staffing resources, an analytic platform could be used to create a

BOX 18.3

MyHealth makes meaningful use easy.

MyHealth Access Network is Oklahoma's statewide HIE network, connecting more than 80% of all healthcare activity on 4 million patients as they visit more than 1400 sites of care using more than 40 different electronic health record (EHR) systems across Oklahoma and thousands of hospitals and clinics nationwide. MyHealth receives real-time data on more than 110,000 clinical encounters each day, complete with diagnoses, procedures, medications, allergies, lab results, vital signs, radiology, immunization, and more. For most people, medical histories go back more than 10 years, providing a rich historical record as well as a current health status as it evolves in real time. Participants include hospitals, clinics, federally qualified health centers, behavioral health, tribal health systems, health plans, state agencies, pharmacies, social services agencies, and early childhood education programs.

MyHealth's primary mission is to ensure that every patient has their complete health record available wherever and whenever it is needed for decisions about their care. In addition, MyHealth participants agreed to expanded data uses for public health and research use cases. Regarding public health, MyHealth has played a key role in Oklahoma's response to the COVID-19 pandemic by providing data and analysis to the Oklahoma State Department of Health, the Governor's Response Team, private sector providers, and the general public. The company has a mature, structured process for evaluating research requests to ensure the protection of patient, provider, and participant privacy while enabling innovation and the derivation of new knowledge. MyHealth has supported research studies and innovations submitted to numerous local, state, and federal agencies, including the National Institutes of Health and Agency for Healthcare Research and Quality.

As an HIE, MyHealth fields data request routinely from network participants, researchers, and even patients, and since 2012, MyHealth has used a formalized process for participants (and their partners) to request data for specific purposes. Each of the proposed use cases is carefully vetted through MyHealth's committee and board processes and if approved, become a formal part of the library of approved use cases. Over time, custom data product requests evolve into standard "shrink-wrapped" product offerings.

MyHealth analytics stack

There are several components to MyHealth's analytics technology stack, which is composed of the tools used to complete data processing from the point at which data gathered all the way through to the knowledge and wisdom that are generated. Each component of the technology plays an important role, and over time every component has been changed or replaced as better performing or lower cost solutions have become available. Most recently, the shift to cloud-native technologies has enabled new approaches to analytics and has removed

BOX 18.3 (*cont'd*)

dependencies on localized hardware and single vendor technology stack. The full analytics stack can be seen in Table 18.3.

It is important to understand that HIE technologies are always evolving, making continual evaluation of the performance and cost of current vendors a key activity. In a recent landmark agreement with the State of Oklahoma, MyHealth has agreed to serve as the Statewide HIE and the State Designated Entity, and MyHealth will be overseeing the deployment of core HIE technologies from Orion Health Solutions, which is the chosen software platform of the state Medicaid agency. This transition is currently in process.

MyHealth analytics products and services

Analytics services are the most important and most significant growth area of the HIO's business and services, and its major drivers have been the COVID-19 pandemic and the shift to value-based payment models. The COVID-19 pandemic increased recognition by public health agencies that the HIE has the most complete real-time dataset available to provide disease surveillance, vaccine administration information, hospital bed utilization, and many other analytics related to the response. Meanwhile, the shift to value-based payment models and increased need to accept risk have seen many large provider organizations recognize the need for complete real-time information on which to manage the care and utilization of their attributed patients, as well as a complete historical record to support risk prediction and patient identification for population health management.

MyHealth offers analytics products and services of two types—those that are standardized for specific customers and broadly approved data use cases, and those that are produced as custom work for specific approved use cases resulting from unique data requests.

MyHealth broadly approved analytics

MyHealth provides many broadly approved analytics products and services. Governance-approved models for Patient Attribution form the foundation of all analytics services at MyHealth, enabling the sharing of populations of patients' data. These are based on previously approved algorithms for healthcare (e.g., primary care, oncologic medical home, behavioral health, etc.) with attribution relationships.

MyHealth has a web-based provider portal that shows complete medical records for >4 million people. They also provide a Fast Healthcare Interoperability Resource (FHIR) format via application programming interface (API) that enables capable EHRs to pull specific data elements. MyHealth helps organizations make use of Electronic Clinical Quality Measures (eCQMs), which were created to support Value-Based Payment Models such as the Comprehensive Primary Care (CPC) initiative, a 4-year multipayer initiative created to improve primary care, and its successor, CPC+ [19]. The company also offers Claims Data Analytics. Originally part of the CPC initiative, MyHealth receives monthly claims data from more than 2.5 million lives in Oklahoma and provides measures such as all-cause 30-day readmissions, ER and inpatient utilization, and total cost of care. Legislation under consideration at the time of this writing would also make MyHealth the All Payer Claims Database for Oklahoma, further enhancing the data density and expanding the use cases that can be supported for healthcare stakeholders in Oklahoma.

As a part of their standard analytics services, MyHealth generates regular reports that can help organizations achieve Meaningful Use, perform

BOX 18.3 (*cont'd*)

well on MIPS, meet the interoperability requirements of the Medicare Condition of Participation rules, and comply with ONC's new Data Blocking rules. The Care Fragmentation Alerting system, which is an advanced version of admission, discharge, and transfer (ADT), provides a daily digest of all clinical activity on attributed patients and includes visits of all types (inpatient, ER, and outpatient), procedures, and providers involved, from all locations within Oklahoma as well as all other locations participating in the Patient Centered Data Home nationally. It also provides visit data from Consolidated Clinical Document Architecture (CCDA) documents, making the CFA reports much more useful than simple ADT alerting. Numerous provider organizations have significantly increased revenues by achieving more timely follow-up with patients after ER or inpatient discharge, reductions in 30-day readmissions, and avoided duplicate testing. MyHealth also supplies a Care Gap Alerting system, which generates reports on events (breast and colon cancer screening, blood pressure, etc.) relevant for quality programs such as Healthcare Effectiveness Data and Information Set (HEDIS), MIPS, and others. The Care Gap reports are made available to subscribing providers or payers at least monthly, enabling the payer or provider to close gaps throughout the year, rather than just at the end of the measurement window. One large payer reported that a large EHR vendor delivered them ~45,000 care gaps across five states. By comparison, MyHealth, as an HIE, provides more than 360,000 potential care gap closing events monthly, just on the Oklahoma population.

MyHealth also delivers a national award-winning Social Needs Screening and Alerting program. Created as part of Center for Medicare and Medicaid Innovation (CMMI) Accountable Health Communities (AHC) program, which aims to address gaps between clinical care and community services [20], MyHealth created a novel method for leveraging real-time clinical data to trigger social needs screenings to the patients' phones while they are waiting to be roomed in the clinic or ED. Patients who report a social need are immediately referred to relevant social services nearby and near where they live. All screening and referral results are provided back to clinical practices so that each patient's social needs can be accounted for in their clinical plans. This program has served more than 2.6 million patients in Oklahoma since 2018 and has had a massive impact on health and services in Oklahoma. The program thrived during COVID-19, because even though visits were shifting to telemedicine, patients still have their mobile phones to receive and respond to the screenings. This type of program represents an area where HIE networks are uniquely able to deliver services and improve outcomes, and when combined with clinical and claims data, the social needs data offer perhaps the most important substrate for an advanced, impactful community health analytics program.

MyHealth Custom Analytics

MyHealth Custom Analytics can be just about anything including:

- Research study support
- Public health COVID-19 analytics and consultation services
- Market share analytics

The custom services have been applied in many ways. For example, MyHealth has provided lifetime medical and healthcare utilization history for subjects enrolled in an NIH-funded study of the impact of early childhood education. They also supported a $15 million AHRQ study in the Evidence Now program, in which dozens of small primary care practices were enrolled in a program to improve care quality by receiving regular updates on their performance on four quality measures. For this program, MyHealth calculated

BOX 18.3 *(cont'd)*

the metrics utilizing data from more than 20 different EHR vendors and hundreds of sites of care across Oklahoma. Furthermore, since the beginning of the pandemic, MyHealth has provided COVID-19 consultation to the Oklahoma State Department of Health, the Governor's Response team, and to several Tribal Health Departments. MyHealth COVID-19 analytics are reviewed in weekly press and public briefings as well.

predictive risk model that can identify superusers of emergency department services based on discharge method (e.g., to home, to a facility, to a family member 's home, with home healthcare). Maybe they would learn that patients who are discharged to their homes where there is no support return to the emergency department more frequently. The emergency department could then strategize to improve the discharge plan and evaluate outcomes from that intervention.

Prior to implementing an analytic platform, or participating in organizational analytics, an HIE network must have organizational governance and policies supporting and enabling the use of data for analytics. Once these things are in place, the technology requirements include (1) an interoperable HIE transaction system, (2) a centralized transaction data store, (3) clinical terminology management software (e.g., Terminology Services), and (4) an enterprise master person index software [23]. In other words, the HIO or network must possess the core technologies described in Chapters 8–12. These technologies provide a foundation upon which an analytic platform can be developed as a core HIE service or point of service application.

There are two roles that HIOs can play with respect to achieving the nationwide goal of real-time analytics for population health. First,

TABLE 18.3 MyHealth analytics stack.

Function	Tool(s)
Data Acquisition	• HL7 Data: Postgres database in Amazon Web Services (AWS) o Receives all HL-7 data for each domain in near real time from the Central Data Repository. • Claims Data: SQL-Server o Hosts the claims data, provides a working repository for claims data analytics, and also supports several analytics products.
Development	• Programming Language: C# • Query Language: SQL • Markup Language: HTML5 • Visualization: Tableau • Development Planning and Tracking: JIRA stack
Extract, Transform, and Load (ETL)/ Extract, Load, Transform (ELT):	• SQL • Tableau Prep
Data Visualization	• Tableau Server with the Data Management Add On

HIOs can enable analytics within health systems, which involves the use of analytic platforms. Under this scenario, the analytic platform becomes a local point of service application that leverages data from the HIE network. Second, HIOs can provide analytics as a core HIE service within the network—that is, the HIE serves as the analytic platform. We discuss these roles in the following sections.

18.7.1 HIOs as enablers of analytics

Many health systems have existing analytic platforms that are used to generate intra-system insights through an Enterprise HIE or an EHR vendor-based exchange. However, the use of a proprietary vendor can limit data acquisition, transformation, and utilization if the vendor will only allow exchange with matched-vendor health systems. As a result, these platforms may be insufficient to meet national population health goals, which rely on a variety of data from public health departments, pharmacies, and ancillary/wraparound services. As a result, HIE members may request additional analytical assistance from HIE network resources.

HIOs have an advantage as independent, third-party organizations that have the capacity to work with multiple health system participants. They can reduce some of the existing gaps between intra- and intersystem data sharing through technical infrastructure and governance and, in turn, enhance population health analytics. Their focus is on community-wide sharing, which discourages information blocking, and they can extract, transform, and load (ETL) data from intersystem electronic medical records based on an entire geographic region [21].

Customer demands are likely to drive an HIO to perform as an enabler of analytics. One common request is that an HIO make data available in file formats digestible by the customer's existing platform or data warehouse. This often requires flat files, like comma-separated values or American Standard Code for Information Exchange (ASCII), that hold data for one record in each line. It is usually requested that these files have uniform formatting and data rules so that the data can be batched overnight without errors. Some HIO data requests are for CCDA documents that summarize a patient's record into a single file. These can be requested in batch for many patients or, more often, via IHE queries that request the CCDA's one at a time per patient as activity occurs. Most recently, data are being requested in HL7's FHIR APIs that can enable cross-platform data transfer of the data. A particular strength of the FHIR API approach is the ability to provide specific data elements, such as an individual lab test or vital sign, on demand, and without human intervention or effort.

18.7.2 HIOs as a provider of analytics-as-a-service

Analytics-as-a-service (AaaS) is a cloud-based service that supports the process of using data to generate insights that are incorporated into a general use analytical platform [24]. AaaS differs from a standard analytical platform in three important ways. First, it requires a use fee for services as they are requested. Unlike in the case of a standard subscription, which requires a fixed recurring payment for an entire package, an HIO participant would not have to pay for services that they are not using. As a result, AaaS benefits HIE networks that support smaller ACOs and rural health systems and participants who are in need of affordable services [25]. It distributes HIO workload because analytics services are developed as needed, and it also creates space for new services to be developed and deployed over time [24]. Furthermore, HIO participants can share and use data from multiple health systems and other unique data sources, unlike a typical EHR vendor-mediated subscription service, which requires matched-vendor platform exchange [18]. Second, AaaS is cost-effective because through it, reusable components are developed. This allows for rapid development and deployment of services, less engineering time, and more consistency across services. AaaS increases interoperability because it creates incentive for all organizations to provide high-quality data on a timely basis, and the data, insights, resources, and expertise are more easily shared between HIO participants [24]. Finally, AaaS reduces capacity constraints because it is flexible, scalable, and easily upgradable. These benefits reduce both maintenance needs at the HIO and the number of skilled staff needed by HIO participants.

18.7.3 HIO use of a vendor-supplied analytics platform

While some HIOs have the consumer demands, staffing and funding capacity, to build an analytics platform on top of their HIE, some do not. Some reasons for these limitations were mentioned in Chapter 5. For example, HIOs may have limited opportunities to increase a customer base if they are operating within a region that has a small population a small geographic size. Therefore they may cater to very specific needs. In larger regions, HIOs may need to grow quickly or advance their capacity to better serve a region. In these cases, HIE leadership may choose to partner with a third-party vendor who can supply an analytics platform. For example, CyncHealth, formerly Nebraska Health Information Initiative (NEHII), partnered with a vendor that specializes in population health analytics to improve real-time data monitoring [26]. During the COVID-19 pandemic, CyncHealth further expanded their partnerships to include a company specializing in a cloud-based eMPI and another specializing in data quality and interoperability to rapidly expand their capacities [27]. As mentioned in Box 18.2, Healthix, an HIE in New York, partnered with HBI Solutions to improve their predictive analytic capacities across communities in their region.

18.7.4 Conveying value

Regardless of whether an HIO acts as an enabler of analytics or provides analytics for a region, it is critical that they are able to convey their value to participants. This can be done through careful messaging. HIOs/HIEs should determine what services are needed by the region or health system it serves ahead of time.

18.8 Barriers to analytics

18.8.1 Low-to-middle-income countries

Although there is an abundance of data around the world, access and the ability to harness insights are not evenly distributed. Low-to-middle-income countries (LMICs) face many barriers to data access and the adoption of widespread analytics. LMICs have a high burden from communicable and noncommunicable disease, and population in these countries may be widely spread out, as almost a third of the populations in these countries live hours away from available healthcare services [28] and other resources. The COVID-19 pandemic underscored the importance of digital solutions implemented at scale and the need for HIE in LMICs, and it also encouraged its growth. However, large-scale digital solutions are often implemented in partnership with governments, and many LMIC governments possess limited resources [28].

Open-source solutions can be used to mitigate some barriers to data acquisition, analytics, and HIE in LMICs. Open-source solutions have the capacity to allow experts such as software engineers, health information professionals, and analysts to contribute to advancing HIE efforts while maintaining independence from proprietary technology stacks.

One example is OpenHIE, which is community of practice that provides open and collaborative development and support for country-driven, large-scale health information–sharing architectures. It is driven by a community of volunteers and partnering organizations to improve global health. DHIS2 is an open-source software that provides a web-based platform with some analytic and data visualization capabilities, and it has been used to improve population health in Africa.

Barriers can also be overcome through collaborations between tech innovators and government and public health ministries. These partners can make use of existing open-source solutions to expand the scale of the digital solutions they develop. For example, Nigeria uses DHIS2 as its national health management information system. The Surveillance Outbreak Response Management and Analysis System (SORMAS), an open-source, scalable eHealth platform, was developed as a collaboration between the Nigeria Centre for Disease Control and the Helmholtz Center for Infection Research in Germany during the Ebola crisis in 2014 to help manage the disease through early detection [29]. The user-friendly platform can be used by surveillance, laboratory staff, hospital staff, and more to collect and report communicable disease data [30]. The platform was scaled during the COVID-19 pandemic and is now used in several countries in Africa, Asia, and Europe [30].

18.8.2 Barriers to HIE analytics

18.8.2.1 Financial

One major barrier to HIE analytics is the upfront expense of adding or building an analytics layer to an existing HIO. Costs include hiring engineering staff and data scientists to develop analytics platforms or applications or the cost of working with a vendor. However, these upfront costs can be recouped after the infrastructure has been developed and maintenance costs can be mitigated over time if an HIO can continue to create demand for analytics services and convey their value to participants.

18.8.2.2 Data collection

A core function of an HIE is to continuously measure and refine data quality with its participating data sources. This is no different than in other HIE areas, but it is important that stakeholders be aware that analytics will likely result in the need for data quality measurement and a program for continuous data quality improvement.

18.8.2.3 Methodology selection

Organizations choosing to implement analytics may have difficulties selecting methodologies. Often, it is difficult to know what to look for, what to measure, or what tools to use, and thus it can be difficult to know where to start. It is therefore important to have strong leadership in the HIE with at least some understanding of the value and limitations of analytics. This leadership could come from analytics leaders across the HIE, from an analytics working group, or from a designated analytics leader within the HIE.

18.8.2.4 Organizational

HIE analytics may be heavily impacted by a number of issues unique to the participants involved. According to experts at Deloitte [31], barriers to analytics may be organizational in nature, related to data ownership, the result of unclear roles and responsibilities, or caused by resource competition.

- Organizational—HIE participants may rely on their IT or financial departments as the owner of analytics responsibilities due to the general understanding that they are responsible for enterprise data or business insights. Similar competing needs may exist where clinical analytics or genomics and translational research are performed within an organization.

- Data ownership issues—Participants may have staff that have contributed a lot of effort to work around data inefficiencies to generate insights and be effective in their environment. Some of those techniques become the informal status quo and as a result, data ownership can become personal and politicized. These issues can transfer into collaboration with an HIE.
- Unclear roles and responsibilities—Staff involved in analytics may have competing priorities (e.g., projects, resources, department demands, etc.) and limited guidance (could be leadership, protocols, or standard operating procedures) or formal decisions about how to proceed. Leadership in this area may span across multiple departments, which can be difficult to coordinate.
- Resource competition—Many organizations suffer from limited access to managers and analysts with a combination of knowledge about public and population health and healthcare and technical and communication skills. HIEs should hire their own managers and analysts, but this can be challenging because they are high in demand.

To address organizational barriers, experts at Deloitte [31] suggest that HIO staff can:

- identify organization leaders that will serve as champions for the analytics program;
- align analytics resources with enterprise priorities;
- establish clear roles and responsibilities to help enable effectiveness; and
- promote a culture of analytics.

In addition, the HIE architecture model may contribute both strengths and weaknesses when incorporating analytics, which will be discussed in the next section.

18.9 Impact of HIE architecture models on analytics

Common HIE data architecture models, which can be centralized, federated, and hybrid, can impact HIE analytics. As mentioned in Chapter 8, a centralized HIE model is advantageous when it comes to pulling data from multiple sources. HIEs are positioned well to perform analytics using the data from the centralized storage locations that are created in this model. Centralized models require the HIE to scale data, computing, and analytics resources. This requires stricter governance policies around data use, as well as technical processes including the use of an eMPI (Chapter 12) to assure individual identity resolution is accurate, and code normalization capabilities to ensure that data are not duplicated either from within or between sources sending in the same information [32].

A federated model can have fewer requirements for policy and governance, and it may assuage participant concerns about allowing a separate organization to permanently hold and store their data, creating real or perceived protections against privacy breaches and data ownership issues. This has the potential to speed up the acquisition of data sources for analytics. Unfortunately, a strictly federated approach to data acquisition also creates a significant barrier to analytics, because calculations and algorithms can only be applied to data collocated on a single compute instance—that is, it is not possible to calculate HbA1c control for lab results stored in electronic health record systems of dozens of provider organizations without querying it and bringing it all together. Federated interoperability is not designed to support this kind of broad, shallow query, which can result in transaction counts on the order of 10^{10}. This approach is usually not acceptable given that transaction counts of 10^7 are considered a denial-of-service attack on the internet. In addition, setup and maintenance of federated data feeds can be difficult, and the assurances of data completeness and quality are more difficult to achieve [32].

Hybrid models use both a centralized data repository and a record locator service to ensure stronger data tracking. These models are better suited for analytics than federated alone, in that they can make use of healthcare and population health management tools, like ADT alerts that require a master patient index, or clinical decision support tools can facilitate clinical analytics, risk stratification, and medical research, and also allow participants to use their own data to improve care and monitor patient outcomes [32]. The hybrid model has the potential to provide governance flexibility and potentially lowers barriers to data acquisition, but retains some limitations of the federated models, such as unknown amounts of missing data and limitations on the amount and timing of data available due to dependencies on targeted queries. The ideal approach to data infrastructure for health analytics is to have a middle data tier to which most, if not all data, are shared across the maximum number of organizations possible in real time. One of the best-known examples of a middle tier enabling analytics is the Google search engine, which continuously crawls, gathers, and stores web content in servers owned by Google so that Google's powerful and proprietary search engine can be used to organize and search the data. As a healthcare middle tier, an HIE can store the data and apply identity resolution, code normalization, standardization, and data structure optimization to the data, enabling the maximal number of use cases and assures performance while minimizing impact on live clinical systems. An important goal of an HIE-mediated middle tier would be to cover all geographies and develop data exchange to ensure that for each patient living in an HIE's service area, 100% of all health record data are available. CIVITAS Networks for Health, the trade association of HIEs and regional health improvement organizations, supports such a network, called the Patient Centered Data Home, which achieves this level of connectivity for more than 40 HIE networks, which together exchange billions of healthcare transactions annually to enable the largest network of middle tiers in the United States.

18.10 Emerging trends

The field of analytics as it applies to HIE is growing and rapidly changing. Increasingly, machine learning and AI are being used to improve healthcare decision-making and population health outcomes and as a result they are being integrated into analytics platforms that are used by HIEs. Machine learning is increasingly used to generate better predictive models and when combined with AI may improve clinical decision support by resolving the complexities of data elements documenting patient care into conclusions about the impact of interventions on outcomes. One such example is the potential for applying machine learning techniques to extract SDOH data that are typically collected by administrative staff, clinicians, or public health workers [33]. As SDOH data become a focus in public health and healthcare, more information may need to be collected. Machine learning may enable derivation of the social needs of patients from other sources and eliminate some of the manual effort to ensure that the information is present, further enhancing data completeness and quality.

Furthermore, the National Committee for Quality Assurance (NCQA) continues to evolve the HEDIS, which is used by more than 90% of health plans in the United States to measure care and service performance. The NCQA recently added a Data Aggregator Validation certification program process, which helps to ensure the accuracy of aggregate health data used in reporting [34]. Increasingly, data certification is being touted as an option for ensuring that data quality reaches certain standards and the NCQA is no exception, as they will now designate certified partner status for those data streams that are validated by them. This may eliminate some of the barriers to use of data from HIEs, because previously only data taken directly from EHRs were considered standard supplemental data for HEDIS measurement. Many community-based HIEs are becoming certified partners, bringing revenue streams to HIE networks that allow HIEs to focus on analytics services as well as projects that ensure better quality of the data used to study population health.

18.11 Summary

Analytics can be used within health systems to achieve population health goals and meet reporting requirements. The incorporation of analytics into health information systems is a challenge, but there are many ways in which HIEs can help. Lower levels of analytical maturity can be achieved when HIEs are able to enhance interoperability and data quality for a health system. HIEs can help to increase analytical capacity by enabling analytics or by providing analytics as a service through the HIE or in partnership with a proprietary vendor. There are many barriers that exist to adding analytics to a health system, including financial, data collection, methodological, and organizational. LMICs face additional challenges due to government challenges and a lack of resources but can rely on open-source innovations and partnerships to create digital solutions. Last, when HIEs implement analytics, it is important to consider their HIE model and how that will impact their analytical capabilities.

Questions for discussion

1. How is the role of HIE as an Enabler of Analytics different than an HIE who provides Analytics-as-a-Service?
2. What are two types of organizational barriers an HIE may face when trying to implement analytics?
3. When should an HIE consider the analytical maturity of their organization?
4. What are three types of Analytical Approaches? Provide an example of each.

Acknowledgments

The authors greatly appreciate the efforts of Joseph Walker, CISSP, Julie Ladehoff, MBA, Jennifer Faries, MBA, Dewey Molenda, Charlie Clegg, Lance Butler, Kari Adams, Greg Conover, Stacie Kaze, Matthew Weeden, Clint Ryan, Jennifer Brock, Mena Weigant, Tim Cooper, and Robert Cobianchi all of MyHealth Access Network, Oklahoma, Eric Widen, MHA, Thomas Moore, MPA, Naitik Patel, MBA, and Vivienne DeStefano who contributed the work described in the Healthix case study.

References

[1] Kasthurirathne SN, Ho YA, Dixon BE. Public health analytics and big data. In: Magnuson JA, Dixon BE, editors. Public health informatics and information systems. 3rd ed. Switzerland AG: Springer Nature; 2020.

[2] McNemar E. What is the role of data analytics in population health [Internet]. XTelligent Healthcare Media; 2021. Available from: https://healthitanalytics.com/features/whatistherole-ofdataanalytics-inpopulationhealthmanagement.

[3] Institute for Healthcare Improvement. The IHI Triple Aim. [Internet]. n.d. Available from: http://www.ihi.org/Engage/Initiatives/TripleAim/Pages/default.aspx.

[4] Kristoffersen E, Blomsma F, Mikalef P, Li J. The smart circular economy: a digital-enabled circular strategies framework for manufacturing companies. J Bus Res 2020;120:241–61.

[5] Healthcare Information and Management Systems Society. Adoption Model for Analytics Maturity (AMAM) [Internet]. n.d. Available from: https://www.himss.org/what-we-do-solutions/digital-health-transformation/maturity-models/adoption-model-analytics-maturity-amam.

[6] Król K, Zdonek D. Analytics maturity models: an overview. Information 2020;11(3):142.

[7] David G, Smith-Mclallen A, Ukert B. The effect of predictive analytics-driven interventions on healthcare utilization. J Health Econ 2019;64:68–79.
[8] Healthix. Healthix Analytics [Internet]. New York, NY. n.d. Available from: https://healthix.org/what-we-do/healthix-services/healthix-analytics-2/.
[9] Bertsimas D, Li ML, Paschalidis IC, Wang T. Prescriptive analytics for reducing 30-day hospital readmissions after general surgery. PLoS One 2020;15(9):e0238118.
[10] Office of the National Coordinator for Health Information Technology. Interoperability roadmap: a shared, nationwide interoperability roadmap version 1.0.: U.S. Department of Health and Human Services; 2021 [updated May 5, 2021]. Available from: https://www.healthit.gov/topic/interoperability/interoperability-roadmap.
[11] Adler-Milstein J, Garg A, Zhao W, Patel V. A survey of health information exchange organizations in advance of a nationwide connectivity framework. Health Aff (Millwood) 2021;40(5):736–44.
[12] Comstock J. A 'gold mine' of data is driving Israel's billion-shekel bet on digital health [Internet]. EMEA: HIMSS Media; 2019. Available from: https://www.mobihealthnews.com/news/emea/gold-mine-data-driving-israels-billion-shekel-bet-digital-health.
[13] U.S. Centers for Medicare & Medicaid Services. Promoting interoperability programs. Baltimore, MD: U.S. Centers for Medicare & Medicaid Services; 2021 [updated August 5, 2021]. Available from: https://www.cms.gov/Regulations-and-Guidance/Legislation/EHRIncentivePrograms.
[14] Bresnick J. What does the stage 3 meaningful use rule mean for analytics?: XTelligent Healthcare Media; 2015. Available from: https://healthitanalytics.com/news/what-does-the-stage-3-meaningful-use-rule-mean-for-analytics.
[15] U.S. Centers for Medicare & Medicaid Services. Quality measures: APP requirements [Internet]. Baltimore, MD: U.S. Centers for Medicare & Medicaid Services; 2021. Available from: https://qpp.cms.gov/mips/app-quality-requirements.
[16] Fields RW, Gandhi N. Tools for population health management. Prim Care 2019;46(4):529–38.
[17] U.S. Centers for Medicare & Medicaid Services. Value-based programs. Baltimore, MD: U.S. Centers for Medicare & Medicaid Services; 2020. Available from: https://www.cms.gov/Medicare/Quality-Initiatives-Patient-Assessment-Instruments/Value-Based-Programs/Value-Based-Programs.
[18] Bell A, Owen C, Soule D, Crawford E. Pairing HIE data with an analytics platform: four key improvement categories: HealthCatalyst; 2019. Available from: https://www.healthcatalyst.com/insights/HIE-data-analytics-platform-key-phm-goals/.
[19] U.S. Centers for Medicare & Medicaid Services. Comprehensive primary care initiative [Internet]. Baltimore, MD: U.S. Centers for Medicare & Medicaid Services; 2021. Available from: https://innovation.cms.gov/innovation-models/comprehensive-primary-care-initiative.
[20] U.S. Centers for Medicare & Medicaid Services. Accountable health communities model [Internet]. Baltimore, MD: U.S. Centers for Medicare & Medicaid Services; 2022. Available from: https://innovation.cms.gov/innovation-models/ahcm.
[21] Indiana Health Information Exchange. Population health from an HIE perspective. Indianapolis, In: Indiana Health Information Exchange; 2017. Available from: https://www.ihie.org/population-health-hie-perspective/
[22] Techopedia. Analytics platform: Janalta Interactive; 2017. Available from: https://www.techopedia.com/definition/29493/analytics-platform
[23] Widen EC. Improve patient and member health using data science to predict health risks and reduce practice variation [Internet]. HBI Solutions; 2017. Available from: https://hbisolutions.com/wp-content/uploads/2017/11/HBI-White-Paper.pdf
[24] Lismont J, Tine Van C, Óskarsdóttir M, Seppe vanden B, Baesens B, Lemahieu W, et al. Closing the gap between experts and novices using analytics-as-a-service: an experimental study. Bus Inf Syst Eng 2019;61(6):679–93.
[25] Monica K. Enabling targeted health data exchange for efficient patient care: EHR intelligence; 2019. Available from: https://ehrintelligence.com/news/enabling-targeted-health-data-exchange-for-efficient-patient-care
[26] CyncHealth. NEHII and KPI Ninja to present on population health infrastructure as the definitive solution to sustainability and value-based care at HIMSS20 [Internet]. Omaha, NE2020. Available from: https://cynchealth.org/nehii-and-kpi-ninja-to-present-on-population-health-infrastructure-as-the-definitive-solution-to-sustainability-and-value-based-care-at-himss20/
[27] BusinessWire. Nebraska Health Information Initiative (NEHII), NextGate, InterSystems and KPI Ninja Partner to Support Statewide COVID-19 Data Collection and Reporting [Internet]. 2020. Available from: https://www.businesswire.com/news/home/20200504005033/en/Nebraska-Health-Information-Initiative-NEHII-NextGate-InterSystems
[28] Bode M, Goodrich T, Kimeu M, Okebukola P, Wilson M. Unlocking digital healthcare in lower- and middle-income countries [Internet] McKinsey & Company; 2021Available from. Available from: https://www.

mckinsey.com/industries/healthcare-systems-and-services/our-insights/unlocking-digital-healthcare-in-lower-and-middle-income-countries.

[29] Exemplars in Global Health. SORMAS in Nigeria: adapting a fully integrated surveillance system to track COVID-19 [Internet]. n.d. Available from: https://www.exemplars.health/emerging-topics/epidemic-preparedness-and-response/digital-health-tools/sormas-nigeria

[30] SORMAS. How it works [Internet]. SORMAS; n.d. Available from: https://sormas.org/how-it

[31] Morris M, Radin J, Brooks M. Organizing for analytics in health care: Deloitte; 2013. Available from: https://www2.deloitte.com/content/dam/Deloitte/us/Documents/life-sciences-health-care/us-lshc-analytics-in-health-care.pdf

[32] Bresnick J. How health information exchange models impact data analytics: Xtelligent Healthcare Media; 2015. Available from: https://healthitanalytics.com/news/how-health-information-exchange-models-impact-data-analytics

[33] Nelson H. Using machine learning to extract SDOH data, EHR clinical notes [Internet]. EHR Intelligence: Xtelligent Healthcare Media; 2021. Available from: https://ehrintelligence.com/news/using-machine-learning-to-extract-sdoh-data-ehr-clinical-notes

[34] National Committee for Quality Assurance. Data aggregator validation [Internet]. Washington, DC. Available from: https://www.ncqa.org/programs/data-and-information-technology/hit-and-data-certification/hedis-compliance-audit-certification/data-aggregator-validation/

CHAPTER

19

Health information exchange: incorporating social and environmental determinants of health into health information exchange

Katie S. Allen[1], Nora J. Gilliam[2], Hadi Kharrazi[3], Melissa McPheeters[4] and Brian E. Dixon[1,2]

[1]Center for Biomedical Informatics, Regenstrief Institute, Inc., Indianapolis, IN, USA [2]Department of Epidemiology, Richard M. Fairbanks School of Public Health, Indiana University, Indianapolis, IN, USA [3]Biomedical Informatics and Data Science Section, Johns Hopkins School of Medicine, Baltimore, MD, USA [4]RTI International, Research Triangle Park, NC, USA

LEARNING OBJECTIVES

By the end of the chapter, the reader should be able to:

- Accurately define and differentiate between various social determinants of health (SDOH) (Section 19.1).
- Understand the importance of including SDOH data within an HIE network (Section 19.2).
- Explore case examples of utilizing various SDOH types in a clinical setting (Section 19.2).
- Describe how different SDOH data types are collected and documented (Section 19.3).

19.1 Introduction

Health factors [1] are the characteristics or attributes that change the likelihood of a person developing a medical condition. Health systems often capture care related factors such as clinical factors (e.g., labs, blood pressure, treatments) or the quality of care delivered. Health systems also capture a limited number of behavioral factors such as tobacco or alcohol use. However, a much broader range of determinants exist beyond care factors that have a large influence on overall health. This chapter focuses on social and environmental factors, typically referred to as the social determinants of health (SDOH). Including SDOH in health information exchange (HIE) networks enables clinicians to see a more holistic view of their patients, allows healthcare

Health Information Exchange
DOI: https://doi.org/10.1016/B978-0-323-90802-3.00023-X

providers to depict their population more accurately, and empowers healthcare systems to identify potential health disparities. However, their implementation and actual use within the healthcare setting is still gaining momentum. This is due, in part, to the wide variety and format or SDOH factors, as well as the complexity involved in implementing them, including changes in clinician workflows and an evidence base to support their use.

This chapter defines SDOH factors, including examples of sources and formats. This chapter further explores how SDOH factors present unique opportunities and challenges related to HIE and details how these data are collected and stored. Additionally, we discuss the overall value of incorporating SDOH in HIE, both for patients and health systems.

19.2 Section 1. Defining social determinants of health

The importance and desire to incorporate SDOH into healthcare have been gaining momentum due to increased understanding of how social factors influence health [2,3]. Additionally, healthcare providers are recognizing that the growing health disparities and healthcare problems cannot be addressed by medical care alone [4]. SDOH factors can be individual level (i.e., those specific to the patient) or aggregate/neighborhood level (i.e., those specific to the community where the patient resides). Thus SDOH is a term collectively assigned to nonclinical individual factors (e.g., income, food insecurity, housing challenges) or conditions within a person's environment (e.g., neighborhood deprivation) [5]. The environment includes all geographies where a person is born, currently lives, works, plays, and socializes.

SDOH include a broad range of factors (Fig. 19.1) which are grouped into five major domains: (1) economic stability, (2) education access and quality, (3) healthcare access and quality, (4) neighborhood and built environment, and (5) social and community context [6]. Many factors are interconnected. SDOH factors may affect health outcomes either through supportive/positive or detrimental mechanisms.

19.2.1 Economic stability

This SDOH domain is related to financial well-being and can include the ability to build wealth, manage debt, and more importantly, as it relates to healthcare expenses, recover from unexpected financial shocks [7]. For example, diabetic patients who need both proper nutrition and medication to prevent negative outcomes such as hospitalization may experience different outcomes based on their economic stability. A diabetic patient with financial means to afford prescribed insulin and select high-quality foods at the grocery store will often have different outcomes than diabetic individuals who have trouble affording their medication or nutritious food. Ample evidence ties economic stability to positive health outcomes [8,9], including among individuals with the same medical underlying health conditions.

19.2.2 Education access and quality

Educational factors (e.g., amount of schooling, quality of that schooling) have been associated with higher levels of morbidity (e.g., having multiple conditions/diseases), higher prevalence of chronic disease, and shorter life expectancy [10]. Education is highly interconnected with work and economic conditions, and can support health, while at the same time, poor health can affect educational pursuit. In a simple example, hunger affects the ability of a child to learn and focus on their schoolwork. Higher levels of education may also provide individuals with greater ability

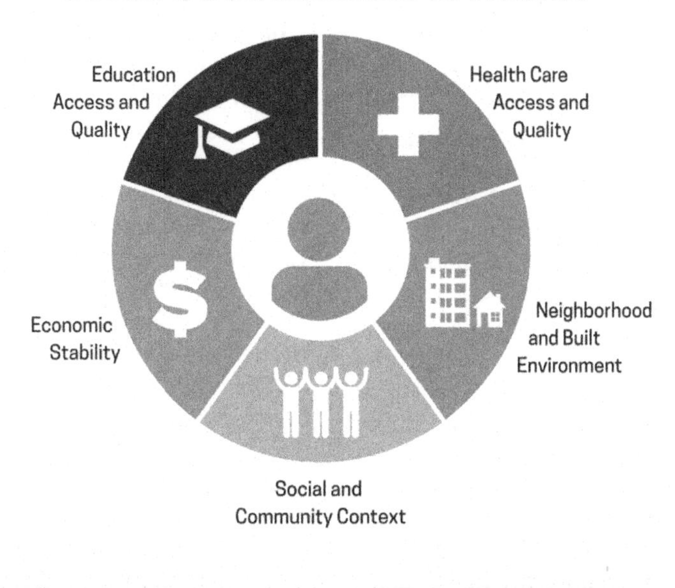

FIGURE 19.1 The social determinants of health or conditions in the environments where people are born, live, learn, work, play, worship, and age that affect a wide range of health, functioning, and quality-of-life outcomes and risks. *Image courtesy: Office of Disease Prevention and Health Promotion, US Department of Health and Human Sciences. What influences health: Healthy People 2030 [Internet]. [cited 2022 Apr 10]. Available from: https://health.gov/healthypeople/objectives-and-data/social-determinants-health.*

to parse and respond to scientific materials related to their health. This is referred to as health literacy and affects decisions individuals make related to their health.

19.2.3 Healthcare access and quality

This SDOH domain covers a range of areas related to access to care including insurance coverage, distance to care facilities (e.g., hospital, specialty care), or the quality of care received. In the United States, insurance has a large effect on the ability to access care and receive routine screenings. Evidence from the Affordable Care Act suggest that expansion of insurance coverage improved access to routine care [11], which can reduce preventable hospitalizations [12].

19.2.4 Neighborhood and built environment

The "built environment" refers to the human-made characteristics within the areas we work and live. This includes all aspects of the neighborhood including walkability, land use, distance from traffic or waste sites, and access to recreational areas [13]. Built environment considers factors such as physical structures (e.g., buildings, sidewalks) and pollutants (e.g., smoke, drinkable water). However, it also encompasses neighborhood elements such as safety (e.g., walkability, traffic patterns, violence rates). Built environment SDOH can play important, but different, roles in overall health. For example, access to sidewalks and playgrounds has been associated with reduced weight and better outcomes in conditions such as cardiovascular disease and depression/anxiety [14].

19.2.5 Social and community context

This domain encompasses relationships and interactions with all those in a community (e.g., family, friends, neighbors, coworkers). Social-connectedness has been associated with reduced depression/anxiety, substance abuse, and lowering risky behaviors in adolescents [15]. Additionally, loneliness and social isolation have been linked to negative cardiovascular outcomes such as higher blood pressure [16]. There is an abundance of evidence showing community-dwelling older adults suffer from increased negative health outcomes, including higher risk for mortality and issues related to cognitive function, when they are socially isolated [17,18].

SDOH cover a very broad array of characteristics that pertain to a person's everyday life. Many of them are interconnected (e.g., education and economic stability, economics and neighborhood). Each SDOH can influence health, positively or negatively [4,19], and most are not within the direct control of the healthcare community. Achieving positive health outcomes is influenced by these factors, so understanding what factors may be playing a role in the life of their patient is important for clinical decision making. Collecting and utilizing data about SDOH are an important piece in treating patients and managing the population within a healthcare system. HIE could play a valuable role in improving health by ensuring these data elements are available to clinicians and health system administrators when it is needed. The next section will explore how SDOH data can be utilized to enhance care management and potentially create cost efficiency for the healthcare system (Box 19.1).

19.3 Section 2. The role of health information exchange in social determinants of health

There have been national [23] and international [24] calls made to enhance health information technology to incorporate data beyond

BOX 19.1

Other key terms and definitions.

Several terms are often utilized interchangeably with SDOH, but they do not mean precisely the same concept. This chapter defines SDOH, but it is important to know and understand the other terminology utilized and how and when to apply it [20].

Social risk factors. Social risk factors include SDOH, but these factors are considered to always have a negative effect. For example, housing is a SDOH characteristic. Housing can be stable (e.g., able to make payments/rent on home) or unstable (e.g., recently evicted). When housing is unstable, it is considered to be a social risk factor [21].

Social needs. Social needs are social risk factors with the patient's preference and priorities considered. For example, a patient may have multiple risk factors but the current need is housing because they have a pressing need for a safe place [21]. Identifying social needs of highest importance to the patient can be a challenge. However, social needs screening tools have increased in availability and use and are a good method for identifying social needs from the patient's perspective [22].

clinical factors using HIE networks. This is largely due to the value HIE can bring in combining multiple sources of data and delivering it through multiple mechanisms. This is valuable at the patient level, such as for predicting risk or delivering patient-specific services, as well as the population level for more rapidly identifying community-level risk factors.

At the individual level, an initial priority focuses on identifying social needs and addressing those to improve health outcomes. However, once social needs are collected, it is the role of the HIE network to deliver these data in a way that can be viewed by the clinician or made actionable. Systems such as FindHelp (formerly Aunt Bertha) are social care networks designed to connect patients to social resources. Health systems utilize screening tools to identify SDOH influencing the health outcomes of the patient. These data are entered into the electronic health records (EHR/HIE) and leveraged for referrals for services, such as food pantries or social workers. Referral networks are increasingly available within the EHR [25] and HIE to allow clinicians to identify local services patients may benefit from (e.g., housing assistance). In the case of CyncHealth [26], a HIE in Nebraska & Iowa, the technology includes the ability to order those services to address patient needs. CyncHealth's system sends the order to the service (e.g., food pantry) which can message the clinician or otherwise mark the service as delivered. Clinicians can follow up on the orders to ensure they were met. However, many of these initiatives are in the early stages and it is not yet known whether clinicians will successfully integrate them into their practice or whether the initiatives will have a demonstrable effect on patient outcomes.

Beyond identifying needs and addressing them, clinical data can be combined with social data to predict need and healthcare utilization. The research community has been focused on designing and implementing systems that incorporate SDOH data and assessing the impact on health outcomes. For example, studies found that combining all available information—current and historical clinical data and social variables—allowed for predicting whether a patient was likely to revisit an emergency department [27–29]. However, another study focused on predicting whether patients would need social services did not find benefit from including SDOH factors [30]. Another study examined the influence of social variables on 30-day hospital readmission risk for pediatric patients. They found that utilizing SDOH variables would enhance the hospital's ability to predict readmission and provide nonclinical interventions to avoid the hospitalization [31]. However, it is important to note that many of these interventions have not been deployed widely as the evidence base is still growing.

This area of research focuses on which type and level of SDOH factor influence health outcomes and for what conditions. Additionally, researchers seek to implement these interventions for larger populations, attempting to determine whether health outcomes will be improved when they are put into a real-world setting.

Predictive models can be utilized to target population level interventions as well. In Maine, an algorithm was deployed to predict hypertension diagnosis within 12 months [32]. The results of this algorithm classify groups of people most at risk for hypertension and related cardiovascular issues. This allows public health and healthcare systems to target and enhance hypertension-related initiatives in areas of the community most likely to benefit. Use of SDOH-enhanced HIE can also allow health systems to identify disparities in health, monitor the overall health of their population [33], and appropriately target underserved populations for intervention. Nationwide efforts, such as *All In: Data for Community Health* [34], consist of multisector partnerships working to share data and combine clinical and public health datasets with data from housing, education, and social services. There are numerous active projects, covering a variety of SDOH areas.

Two examples include connecting communities to diabetes screening and prevention tools to care coordination for homeless individuals. The overall goal of this partnership is to improve community health outcomes by connecting data sources to identify gaps and needs in the community.

The Centers for Medicare and Medicaid Services (CMS) have moved toward value-based payment models, which incentivize maintaining a healthy population [35] versus the more traditional model of paying for specific instances of clinical care. Value-based programs reward providers with incentives for the quality of care they give as it relates to both patients and population [36]. Examples of CMS value-based programs include the Medicare Access and CHIP Reauthorization Act of 2015 and the Merit-based Incentive System's Promoting Interoperability. Learning to access and make use of SDOH to improve population health thus could be beneficial to populations and to the health systems that serve them.

In addition to payment initiatives, technology-based initiatives have increased awareness around, and incentivize use of, SDOH. HITECH, and specifically the Meaningful Use provisions, established criteria for healthcare providers for the collection of social and behavioral history [23,37]. Meaningful Use included provisions for standardizing the collection of SDOH via logical observation identifiers names and codes (LOINC) and other existing terminologies. (See Chapter 10 for more details on HIE standards.)

The incorporation of SDOH into HIE has the potential to provide value to individual patients, communities, and healthcare systems. This is accomplished with targeted interventions, like identifying needs and addressing them, and through aggregating and viewing SDOH at the population level. The United States has incentivized these activities through both payment reimbursement models as well as technology legislation. However, SDOH covers a broad range of characteristics and complexity as to how they are identified and stored. The next sections will examine how SDOH data are collected and how they can be incorporated into HIE.

19.4 Section 3. Incorporation of social determinants of health into health information exchange

19.4.1 Data collection and storage

There are several challenges to incorporation of SDOH into HIE. First, SDOH data have a wide variety of person- or population-level factors that must be handled separately. Second, SDOH collection does not fit neatly into the existing clinical data workflows. Finally, while the availability of data standards to support the collection, storage, or exchange of SDOH is increasing, they do not yet cover all aspects of SDOH and widespread adoption is limited.

In addition to covering several domains, each SDOH domain may be multifaceted and include both individual- and community-level measures. For example, a person has an income level specific to them but resides in an area with a median income level. These two income levels may be disparate. To further illustrate, a person may reside in a US Census Tract (neighborhood designation) that has a low median income or a high percentage of poverty. There may be environmental effects on the individual based on the level of poverty around them. However, the individual may have a high income and not be personally affected by poverty (e.g., affords food and housing). Collecting and understanding the impact of both individual- and community-level factors are thus important.

Practically, an HIE would need to know the person's address to associate it with census tract data and a method for linking the address geocode with the applicable community-level variables and know the individual's metrics as well and have a way of combining them.

Different SDOH variable types need to be stored within the HIE in a way that associates them with the patient. This requires data collection processes, semantic standards for identifying the different variables, and syntactic standards for exchanging the data. This has been a focus of the HIE and SDOH communities since approximately 2013, when the National Academy of Medicine formed a committee to improve clinical management of SDOH data. This culminated in the publication of recommended social and behavioral domains for inclusion in EHRs. These SDOH factors included race and ethnicity, education, financial-resource strain, stress, depression, physical activity, tobacco use, alcohol use, social connection or isolation, intimate-partner violence, residential address, and census-tract median income [38].

Furthermore, since 2013, there has been active work to identify the proper screening tools and methods for incorporating SDOH data into clinical workflows. Relevant to HIE, however, is the critical piece of semantic and syntactic standards. In conjunction with the focus on which SDOH should be collected, there have been efforts to create standard vocabulary to enable data sharing. This has sparked large initiatives as it relates to standards, such as the Gravity Project [39], which is identifying SDOH for collection and actively coordinating with standards development organizations in the creation of proper structured vocabularies. Additionally, the Gravity Project is supported by HL7 International, ensuring these efforts will meet standards for storing, exchanging, and retrieving SDOH data. (More detail on standards is available in Chapter 10.)

19.4.1.1 Data management

As with all data elements included within HIE, governance rules should be considered when deciding how to collect, store, and utilize SDOH. (See Chapter 4 for more details on governance.) Additionally, the various levels of data offer unique strengths and weaknesses to consider.

19.4.2 Aggregate/population data

Typically, aggregate/population-level data have limited governance associated with them and are often publicly available. This allows for easier linkage to the HIE. However, such flexibility comes with weaknesses. Due to their aggregated nature, population-level SDOH may be too broad to be useful at the person-level, and thus lack specificity or be inaccurate/not applicable for the individual patient. Also, community-level SDOH data may be complex. For example, the American Community Survey (US Census Bureau) offers thousands of variables across different strata [40]. Selecting and managing these variables can be difficult for a large population. Finally, integration within the existing EHR/HIE data models may be challenging. EHR/HIE data are primarily designed for individual data variables gathered at the point of care. SDOH data that are aggregate may not fit neatly into one of the existing clinical categories. Efforts are underway within several collaborative communities to align these types of data to common data models such as observational medical outcomes partnership (OMOP) [41] and patient centered outcomes research institute (PCORI) [42], which will require substantial updates to the syntactic and semantic standards needed to transmit and store SDOH data

19.4.3 Person-level data

Individual-level data often have increased governance that may preclude their access when they are not provided directly by the patient. For example, connecting to other registries or datasets, such as state-managed education and workforce data, requires navigating the rules and legislation that governs those datasets. Each country and state set their own rules for how these datasets are governed, which may dictate how they can be shared, whether they can be stored, who can utilize them, and for what purpose. However, person-level SDOH are often easier to code using standards and incorporate into the existing data model, because they more closely align with standard clinical variables and demographics. There is still work required to incorporate these data types into common data models such as OMOP and PCORnet.

19.4.4 Metadata/hierarchies

An additional challenge related to data management of SDOH is the limited metadata, hierarchies, and definitions that exist. For example, does unemployment include those voluntarily out of the workforce (e.g., retired, stay-at-home parent) or only those who wish to be employed but are not currently? Understanding what each variable means is key to maximizing its potential for improving health outcomes. More importantly for HIE, as partners exchange SDOH data, it is imperative to ensure that SDOH data elements mean the same concept to both partners, just as we would for clinical data exchange (e.g., laboratory results). Much of this is still under development [39,43], with a growing literature base to clarify and specify definitions and support the development of standards and metadata.

Several other challenges exist related to SDOH data that are worth noting. First, storage of SDOH data is not without costs. SDOH can amount to a considerable size of variables to be stored and this may not be cost-effective for smaller organizations. Second, temporality concerns are raised with respect to SDOH data. The frequency of updates may vary depending on the type of variable (i.e., American Community Survey is updated annually but Census variables are not). This may also have implications on the usefulness of the data, which needs to be considered when integrating the data into predictive models [44], dashboards, or clinical care.

19.5 Emerging trends

The collection and use of SDOH in the context of HIE is relatively new. Efforts have been made, with varying degrees of success, to incorporate social factors into HIE in support of predicting use, supporting population, and connecting patients to needed social services. Even these activities are relatively recent compared to the evolution of HIE networks. Accordingly, future efforts related to evaluation of operational SDOH/HIE integrations will be important.

As the efforts in this space advance, there are movements to fully integrate HIE with community resources, such as the Population Health OutcomEs aNd Information EXchage (PHOENIX), which combines HIE clinical data with SDOH to support population health [45]. Additionally, innovators are envisioning Social HIE (S-HIE), which fully connect social services and the delivery of healthcare [46] and community health records. S-HIE will combine geographic, neighborhood, and patient characteristics to enable population health management [47].

19.6 Summary

SDOH are critical pieces of the overall health of an individual and of the community. Incorporating these data into HIE networks has the potential to provide value by improving the ability of clinicians to deliver patient-centered care, the ability of healthcare systems to effectively manage their populations, and for improvement of community health outcomes. This is incentivized by value-based payment structures as well as an increased focus on identifying and addressing disparities in health. However, including SDOH within HIE is not without challenges. SDOH data do not always fit neatly into the existing data model or syntactic and semantic coding systems. Aggregate data may not have a significant effect on patient-level health outcomes. However, SDOH has shown potential for improving prediction models to prevent adverse health outcomes, like readmission, and to facilitate access to needed social services. The incorporation of SDOH into clinical care, and the use of HIE networks to facilitate these activities, will continue to be an important topic in the years to come.

Questions for discussion

1. What are SDOH and how might they influence the health outcomes of an individual? Of a population?
2. What are the differences between individual-level and population-level SDOH? How might these differences influence management of these data in an HIE network?
3. How might a community-based HIE network incorporate SDOH to support healthcare systems in population health management?
4. What are the facilitators and barriers to capturing SDOH data in the clinical setting? How might HIE be deployed to address these?

References

[1] County Health Rankings. Health factors [Internet]. County Health Rankings & Roadmaps. [cited 2022 Apr 2]. Available from: <https://www.countyhealthrankings.org/explore-health-rankings/measures-data-sources/county-health-rankings-model/health-factors>.

[2] Woolf SH, Braveman P. Where health disparities begin: the role of social and economic determinants – and why current policies may make matters worse. Health Aff (Millwood) 2011;30(10):1852–9.

[3] Adler NE, Newman K. Socioeconomic disparities in health: pathways and policies. Health Aff (Millwood) 2002;21(2):60–76.

[4] Braveman P, Egerter S, Williams DR. The social determinants of health: coming of age. Annu Rev Public Health 2011;32:381–98.

[5] Office of Disease Prevention and Health Promotion, US Department of Health and Human Services. What influences health: Healthy People 2030 [Internet]. [cited 2022 Apr 10]. Available from: <https://health.gov/healthypeople/objectives-and-data/social-determinants-health>.

[6] Centers for Disease Control. Social determinants of health: know what affects health [Internet]. [cited 2022 Feb 15]. Available from: <https://www.cdc.gov/socialdeterminants/index.htm>.

[7] Weida EB, Phojanakong P, Patel F, Chilton M. Financial health as a measurable social determinant of health. PLoS One 2020;15(5):e0233359.

[8] Walker RJ, Strom Williams J, Egede LE. Influence of race, ethnicity and social determinants of health on diabetes outcomes. Am J Med Sci 2016;351(4):366–73.

[9] Walker RJ, Smalls BL, Campbell JA, Strom Williams JL, Egede LE. Impact of social determinants of health on outcomes for type 2 diabetes: a systematic review. Endocrine. 2014;47(1):29–48.

[10] Ross CE, Wu C. The links between education and health. Am Sociol Rev 1995;60(5):719.

[11] Lau JS, Adams SH, Park MJ, Boscardin WJ, Irwin CE. Improvement in preventive care of young adults after the Affordable Care Act: the Affordable Care Act is helping. JAMA Pediatr 2014;168(12):1101–6.

[12] Wen H, Johnston KJ, Allen L, Waters TM. Medicaid expansion associated with reductions in preventable hospitalizations. Health Aff (Millwood) 2019;38(11):1845–9.

[13] Healthy People 2020 [Internet]. US Department of Health and Human Services. Available from: <http://www.healthypeople.gov/2020/topicsobjectives2020/objectiveslist.aspx?topicId = 8>.

[14] McCormack GR, Cabaj J, Orpana H, Lukic R, Blackstaffe A, Goopy S, et al. A scoping review on the relations between urban form and health: a focus on Canadian quantitative evidence. Health Promot Chronic Dis Prev Can 2019;39(5):187–200.

[15] Steiner RJ, Sheremenko G, Lesesne C, Dittus PJ, Sieving RE, Ethier KA. Adolescent connectedness and adult health outcomes. Pediatrics 2019;144(1):e20183766.

[16] Xia N, Li H. Loneliness, social isolation, and cardiovascular health. Antioxid Redox Signal 2018;28(9):837–51.
[17] Nicholson NR. A review of social isolation: an important but underassessed condition in older adults. J Prim Prev 2012;33(2–3):137–52.
[18] DiNapoli EA, Wu B, Scogin F. Social isolation and cognitive function in Appalachian older adults. Res Aging 2014;36(2):161–79.
[19] Braveman P, Gottlieb L. The social determinants of health: it's time to consider the causes of the causes. Public Health Rep 2014;129(Suppl 2):19–31.
[20] Green K, Zook M. When talking about social determinants, precision matters [Internet]. Health Affairs Blog. Available from: <https://www.healthaffairs.org/do/10.1377/hblog20191025.776011/full/>.
[21] Alderwick H, Gottlieb LM. Meanings and misunderstandings: a social determinants of health lexicon for health care systems. Milbank Q 2019;97(2):407–19.
[22] Kreuter MW, Thompson T, McQueen A, Garg R. Addressing social needs in health care settings: evidence, challenges, and opportunities for public health. Annu Rev Public Health 2021;42(1):329–44.
[23] Hripcsak G, Forrest CB, Brennan PF, Stead WW. Informatics to support the IOM social and behavioral domains and measures. J Am Med Inform Assoc 2015;22(4):921–4.
[24] Cresswell KM, Sheikh A. Health information technology in hospitals: current issues and future trends. Future Hosp J 2015;2(1):50–6.
[25] Pennic J. Aunt Bertha taps Innovaccer to boost its SDOH program [Internet]. HIT Consultant; 2019 [cited 2021 Apr 1]. Available from: https://hitconsultant.net/2019/10/14/aunt-bertha-taps-innovaccer-to-boost-its-sdoh-program/#.YHWpQi2ca-4.
[26] CyncHealth [Internet]. CyncHealth. [cited 2021 Dec 30]. Available from: <https://cynchealth.org>.
[27] Vest JR, Ben-Assuli O. Prediction of emergency department revisits using area-level social determinants of health measures and health information exchange information. Int J Med Inform 2019;129:205–10.
[28] Chang H-Y, Hatef E, Ma X, Weiner JP, Kharrazi H. Impact of area deprivation index on the performance of claims-based risk-adjustment models in predicting health care costs and utilization. Popul Health Manag 2021;24(3):403–11.
[29] Hatef E, Ma X, Rouhizadeh M, Singh G, Weiner JP, Kharrazi H. Assessing the impact of social needs and social determinants of health on health care utilization: using patient- and community-level data. Popul Health Manag 2021;24(2):222–30.
[30] Kasthurirathne SN, Vest JR, Menachemi N, Halverson PK, Grannis SJ. Assessing the capacity of social determinants of health data to augment predictive models identifying patients in need of wraparound social services. J Am Med Inform Assoc 2018;25(1):47–53.
[31] Symum H, Zayas-Castro J. Identifying children at readmission risk: at-admission vs traditional at-discharge readmission prediction model. Healthcare (Basel) 2021;9(10).
[32] Ye C, Fu T, Hao S, Zhang Y, Wang O, Jin B, et al. Prediction of incident hypertension within the next year: prospective study using statewide electronic health records and machine learning. J Med Internet Res 2018;20(1):e22.
[33] Gamache R, Kharrazi H, Weiner JP. Public and population health informatics: the bridging of big data to benefit communities. Yearb Med Inform 2018;27(1):199–206.
[34] All In: Data for Community Health [Internet]. [cited 2022 Apr 2]. Available from: <https://www.allindata.org/about-us/>.
[35] Brewster AL, Fraze TK, Gottlieb LM, Frehn J, Murray GF, Lewis VA. The role of value-based payment in promoting innovation to address social risks: a cross-sectional study of social risk screening by US physicians. Milbank Q 2020;98(4):1114–33.
[36] Centers for Medicare and Medicaid Services. What are value-based programs? [Internet]. 2020 [cited 2020 Dec 1]. Available from: <https://www.cms.gov/Medicare/Quality-Initiatives-Patient-Assessment-Instruments/Value-Based-Programs/Value-Based-Programs>.
[37] Blumenthal D, Tavenner M. The "Meaningful Use" regulation for electronic health records. N Engl J Med 2010;363(6):501–4.
[38] Adler NE, Stead WW. Patients in context – EHR capture of social and behavioral determinants of health. N Engl J Med 2015;372(8):698–701.
[39] HL7 International. Gravity Project [Internet]. [cited 2020 Dec 1]. Available from: <https://www.hl7.org/gravity/>.
[40] United States Census Bureau. American Community Survey (ACS) [Internet]. [cited 2021 Jan 15]. Available from: <https://www.census.gov/programs-surveys/acs>.
[41] Phuong J, Zampino E, Dobbins N, Espinoza J, Meeker D, Spratt H, et al. Extracting patient-level social determinants of health into the OMOP common data model. AMIA Annu Symp Proc 2021;2021:989–98.
[42] PCORnet. ADVANCE – Expanding SDOH across PCORnet [Internet]. [cited 2022 Apr 2]. Available from: <https://pcornet.org/news/category/network-partner/advance/>.
[43] Freij M, Dullabh P, Lewis S, Smith SR, Hovey L, Dhopeshwarkar R. Incorporating social determinants of health in electronic health records: qualitative study

of current practices among top vendors. JMIR Med Inform 2019;7(2):e13849.

[44] Tan M, Hatef E, Taghipour D, Vyas K, Kharrazi H, Gottlieb L, et al. Including social and behavioral determinants in predictive models: trends, challenges, and opportunities. JMIR Med Inform 2020;8 (9):e18084.

[45] Korzeniewski SJ, Bezold C, Carbone JT, Danagoulian S, Foster B, Misra D, et al. The Population Health OutcomEs aNd Information EXchange (PHOENIX) program – a transformative approach to reduce the burden of chronic disease. Online J Public Health Inform 2020;12(1):e3.

[46] Nguyen OK, Chan CV, Makam A, Stieglitz H, Amarasingham R. Envisioning a social-health information exchange as a platform to support a patient-centered medical neighborhood: a feasibility study. J Gen Intern Med 2015;30(1):60–7.

[47] Hatef E, Weiner JP, Kharrazi H. A public health perspective on using electronic health records to address social determinants of health: the potential for a national system of local community health records in the United States. Int J Med Inform 2019;124:86–9.

[48] Hahn RA, Truman BI. Education improves public health and promotes health equity. Int J Health Serv 2015;45(4):657–78.

CHAPTER

20

Cross-border Health Information Exchange to Achieve World Health Outcomes

Nimish Valvi[1], *Jennifer Shivers*[1,2] *and Paul G. Biondich*[2]
[1]Center for Biomedical Informatics, Regenstrief Institute, Inc., Indianapolis, IN, USA
[2]Global Health Informatics, Regenstrief Institute, Inc., Indianapolis, IN, USA

LEARNING OBJECTIVES

By the end of the chapter, the reader should be able to:

- Understand the background of interstate health exchange in the United States.
- Understand benefits of Patient Summary and eDispensing in cross-border health data exchange in the European context.
- Understand the role of Towards the European Health Data Space in cross-border health data exchange in the European context.

20.1 Introduction

Before we can effectively talk about cross-border health information exchange (HIE) networks, we must first address what we think of as borders. Hagen defines borders as *"the lines dividing distinct political, social, or legal territories, are arguably the most ubiquitous features within the field of political geography."* [1] In certain areas of the world, these borders can be between states or districts that may operate under differing legal frameworks within the same nation. For the purposes of this chapter, we will focus on examples where the HIE network is *operating across local, regional, state, and national boundaries.* The nature of crossing different legal, social, and political boundaries is challenging, and one must ascertain the tough job to align entities operating within a specific legal, political, and social context. The challenge for cross-border HIE networks is magnified because of the potential differences in each of the aforementioned contexts. Therefore, the challenges of cross-border HIE are less about technology, which has been in place to effectively do HIE for years. The challenges for cross-border HIE are more human in nature. One must consider the differences in context and the impact of creating a system that may be operating across nations with different

Health Information Exchange
DOI: https://doi.org/10.1016/B978-0-323-90802-3.00029-0

levels of information literacy, legal frameworks, and mind-sets.

In this chapter, we examine cross-border exchange efforts in multiple parts of the world. We explore examples to highlight the complexities and demonstrate effective strategies for managing cross-border situations.

20.2 Cross-border Health Information Exchange

20.2.1 United States

In 2009, Healthbridge, an HIE network in Cincinnati, Ohio and the Indiana Health Information Exchange (IHIE) in Indianapolis, IN developed an 'electronic postman' approach to exchange clinical health data between Ohio and Indiana to reduce the use of fax for exchange of clinical information. Patient-centered care seeks to strengthen patient-clinician interactions, promotes communication, and increases patient involvement in management of their health. To increase patient-centered care, access to accurate and timely health data is essential for informed health-decision making. In addition to the lack of health information at the first visit, studies have shown patients receiving care in emergency departments do not receive timely follow-up after discharge [2–4]. Patients who do not receive timely follow-up care are more likely to return to the emergency department with worsening conditions [2–4]. Moreover, because all health care is not local, there are gaps in patient health information with inadequate patient-centered care. The widespread adoption of electronic health record (EHR) systems now improves the decision-making with the availability of patient health information during a patient visit. Despite considerable progress with improved patient consent and governance leading to exchange of EHR data, much of the information about a patient remains siloed within hospitals and health systems.

These challenges have seen relief with the onset of HIE networks that serve as a secure, comprehensive storage and exchange centers that receive patient information from various community and health organizations. In 2009, Congress decided to modernize the HIE process after the passage of the HITECH Act, which offered incentives to states and local governments to develop initiatives for regional HIE networks [5]. The HIE networks have adopted various technologies to improve provider access to patient health information which is both collected and maintained by other organizations. Exchange of health information by HIE networks have addressed the issues of quality, safety, and efficiency, and they have been timely and comprehensive. HIE has improved patient safety, reduced duplicate procedures, and lowered costs. These regional HIE networks have widened the scope exchanging health information electronically, but networks still remain largely at the regional and state level.

In 2012, the Sequoia Project began the management of the Nationwide Health Information Network (NwHIN), now referred to as eHealth Exchange, which focused on exchange of health information among government agencies. The Sequoia Project also directed an interoperability framework 'Carequality' which expanded to non-governmental agencies, including private care providers, hospitals, and clinics. In addition, EHR vendor companies like EPIC and Cerner, have expanded their scope of health data exchange beyond their systems.

20.2.1.1 Patient-Centered Data Home

HIE networks need to expand their regions and states to increase their utility and impact. To leverage the positions of the regional HIEs, the Strategic Health Information Exchange Collaborative (SHIEC) initiated the Patient-Centered Data Home (PCDH) in order to share data among HIE networks across the United States. The PCDH creates an opportunity for a comprehensive medical history of a patient irrespective of where they seek care.

In 2016, the PCDH initiative was piloted in the Central, Western, and Heartland regions of the United States. At the end of 2018, the PCDH connected 26 HIE networks from across the regions which accounted for half of the population of the United States. The Heartland region included seven HIE networks in five states: East Tennessee Health Information Network in Knoxville, Tennessee; Great Lakes Health Connect in Grand Rapids, Michigan; HealthLINC in Bloomington, Indiana (now part of IHIE); Indiana Health Information Exchange in Indianapolis, Indiana; Kentucky Health Information Exchange in Frankfort, Kentucky; Michiana Health Information Network in South Bend, Indiana (now part of IHIE); and The Health Collaborative in Cincinnati, Ohio. In the pilot year, within the Heartland HIE networks, approximately 8.5 million admission, discharge, and transfer (ADT) messages were exchanged. This initiative has offered a pragmatic grass-roots level approach to achieve national interoperability.

20.2.2 Africa

Mitigation of disease spread is critically important in cross-border areas, other corridor hotspots, and water-ways. These environments are dynamic, with frequent interaction between transport and other migrant workers and vulnerable resident populations, including economically disadvantaged women and youth. Health services in these areas for human immunodeficiency virus (HIV), tuberculosis (TB), and sexual and reproductive health (SRH) are often limited, inaccessible, or unaffordable. Key challenges include lack of coordination, leading to duplication of effort and poor targeting of resources, and a policy environment that inhibits access to affordable services for key and vulnerable populations, including mobile populations and difficulties sustaining service delivery.

The need for sharing of health information developed from the Cross-Border Health Integrated Partnership Project (CB-HIPP), a regional project funded through the United States Agency for International Development (USAID) and the East Africa Mission (EAM). The program was implemented to address the need to integrate health services in the strategic cross-border areas and other transport sites in sub-Saharan East, Central, and Southern Africa. The project developed a cross-border health unit (CBHU) that revealed the need for a robust health database for the cross-border population in Busia, Kenya and Tororo district, Uganda.

The target population in the cross-border region mainly serves female sex workers (FSW), men having sex with men (MSM), people who inject drugs (PWID), transport workers (truck drivers and assistants), miners, border agency staff, fishermen, vulnerable young girls and women, individuals diagnosed with HIV, and tuberculosis. The HIE is enabling a real-time and secure exchange of patient and service delivery data across the cross-border health facilities. By tracking the number of patients through a screening tool built into the Point of Care (POC) systems, records are stored in the Client Registry (**Chapter 12**) and Shared Health Record (**Chapter 11**) for the purpose of policy decision making at the local and country level and to customize packages of care at the facility level.

The cross-border digital health solution is built on open standards and open software to facilitate monitoring health of mobile populations with access to HIV and other services at different health facilities across the Kenya-Uganda border. It uses the Open Health Information Exchange (OpenHIE) architecture (**Chapter 8**) to facilitate the transfer of information between various POC systems. The participating POC systems include KenyaEMR, AMPATH MRS, and UgandaEMR, all distributions of the Open Medical Record System (OpenMRS) customized to support continuum of care across several programs like HIV, TB, and maternal and child health (MCH).

The interoperability layer is Open Health Information Mediator (OpenHIM), which is customized to facilitate the exchange of data between participating systems. The client registry is based on the Open Extensible Master Patient Index (OpenEMPI) used to aggregate and manage clinical data to maintain a master list of patients that can be accessed by participating systems to uniquely identify patients. The Shared Health Record (SHR) is the Open Shared Health Record (OpenSHR), an OpenMRS-based data repository that leverages Integrating the Healthcare Enterprise (IHE) profiles to store and query information.

20.2.3 Europe

In Europe, citizens are increasingly crossing borders for reasons such as travel for business, leisure, or for visiting family and friends; visits unrelated to healthcare. However, some of the travel can produce demands to access health services in another member state. Europeans have always been able to access healthcare for free in other member states; however, access is subject to their local and national legislations on social protection. With the increase in this movement of goods, services, and people across the European Union (EU), it became a priority for member states to organize their national healthcare systems. This situation has a created a need for patient health information to be available securely at hospitals, clinics, and pharmacies for citizens to access health services in member states.

The exchange of patient health data among organizations is a significant challenge due to security and privacy concerns. In the European context, cross-border healthcare is defined in Directive 2011/24/EU of the European Parliament and the Council of 9 March 2011 [6]. In practical terms, cross-border healthcare is complex, since each European country has a National Healthcare System governed by its own sovereign regulatory framework which creates a barrier for efficient health data exchange [7]. The strategy that the European Union (EU) has adopted was commenced in 2008 to develop a framework for an interoperable exchange of electronic health (eHealth) information within the EU Member States, which would address Patient Summary (PS) and the ePrescription services, using Smart Open Services for European Patients (epSOS) [8].

In 2008, after the launch of epSOS, the initiative gradually expanded the number of participating countries to create a large-scale pilot of 25 countries and 50 beneficiaries. The epSOS enabled the development of a practical eHealth framework and an Information & Communication Technology Infrastructure for aiding interoperable access to patient health information, namely to provide PS and ePrescription (ePS) between different EU healthcare systems. This facilitates the sharing of information needed for healthcare coordination and the continuity of care across member states.

Some of the standardized elements of patient data included in the PS are the following:

- Patient demographics (e.g., name, date of birth, gender).
- Relevant medical summary (e.g., current medical illness, major surgeries, allergies).
- A list of current medications the patient is currently taking, which includes all prescribed medication.
- Information regarding the summary itself, mainly addressing when and by whom was the summary created or updated.

The ePS serves two main functions:

- Enable electronic transmission of the drug prescription from EU country A to a pharmacy in EU country B where it is being retrieved.
- eDispensing (eD), as it suggests is the dispensing of the drug to the patient (country of treatment) after the retrieval of an ePS, and the submission of a report for the dispensed medications to the country of origin.

As a result, access to personal health information across the EU will provide immense benefits to the citizens such as:

- If someone has an accident in another EU member state, clinicians will have immediate access to health information about the individual (e.g., allergies or intolerance to certain medications, presence of chronic health conditions). This will greatly improve the time to provide effective treatment.
- Increase in quality of care across all EU member states and provide continuity of care for citizens all across EU member states.
- The sharing of health information will prevent the need to repeat similar laboratory or radiology tests reducing the costs and saving time for the hospital.

The epSOS initiative dictates a vision for each country to deploy a National Contact Point (NCP) for eHealth, this serves as a bidirectional interface between the national health IT infrastructure and the one provided by the European infrastructures that support eHealth functions. The successes of the epSOS project have now been utilized for other European projects which aim to define a minimal data set and the related business rubrics to regulate the exchange.

To enable the adoption of a common format for the PS, the European Commission advised the European Committee for standardization group of Health Informatics (CEN/TC 251) to create a standard for PS based on the International Patient Summary (IPS) project and also develop an implementation guide. The standards were developed in partnership with Health Level-7 (HL7) using the European Guidelines on cross-border care (i.e., eHN EU PS Guidelines) as a preliminary step which emerged from the epSOS large-scale pilot. The IPS standard was published in 2019 entitled "prEN 17269 – The Patient Summary for Unplanned, Cross-border Care" [9]. Following the standard, a guidance document for European implementation, the technical specification "prTS 17288-The International Patient Summary: Guidance for European Implementation Technical Specification" [9], described how the standard PS can be deployed in the European context.

These features will be tested in the frame of the Trillium II project, which is an EU/US Cooperation for Global Interoperability in Digital Health initiative. Trillium II is enabling the IPS standard that will allow access and sharing of health information for unplanned and emergency care as and when needed, which will include information on allergies, immunizations, relevant medical and surgical history, implants, and medications.

Since 2019, citizens of Finland were able to buy medicines using e-prescriptions in Estonia and Luxembourg; while doctors will be able to access patient summaries of citizens from the Czech Republic. The roll out of the two services in 25 EU countries is expected to be implemented by 2025. The current status as of March 2022 is listed in Table 20.1.

20.2.3.1 Legal and financial aspects

In the legal context, healthcare providers for cross-border eHealth must comply with the Directive 2011/24/EU regarding patient's rights. The Directive addresses the rights (i.e., right to access data, right to erase and correct data, and the right to know who accessed the data) and the rules which govern access to healthcare in another EU country and assure European eHealth systems achieve a high level of trust and security. The Directive provides a key provision for the creation of NCPs that should have facilities to provide patients practical assistance who need to make informed decisions. In addition, the NCPs should make it easier for patients to understand the structure of cross-border prescriptions. The exchange of health data is governed by the European and national legislation regarding the protection of personal information. This domain is currently governed by the General Data Protection Regulation (2016/679/EC) [10].

TABLE 20.1 Implementations of Patient Summary and eDispensing solutions in Europe.

Health data of citizens from the countries below:	**Can be consulted by doctors from the countries below, using the Patient Summary:**
Czech Republic	Luxembourg, Croatia, Portugal, France
Malta	Czech Republic, Luxembourg, Croatia, Portugal, France
Portugal	Malta, Luxembourg, Croatia, Czech Republic, Spain
Croatia	Malta, Portugal, Czech Republic, Luxembourg, France
Spain	Portugal
Doctors from the countries below:	**Can access health data of citizens coming from:**
Croatia	Czech Republic, Malta, Portugal
Luxembourg	Croatia, Czech Republic, Malta, Portugal
Malta	Portugal, Croatia
Portugal	Malta, Croatia, Czech Republic, Spain
Czech Republic	Croatia, Malta, Portugal
France	Czech Republic, Croatia, Malta, Portugal,
ePrescriptions of citizens from countries below:	**Can be retrieved in pharmacies in:**
Croatia	Finland, Estonia, Portugal
Estonia	Finland, Croatia
Finland	Estonia, Croatia, Portugal
Portugal	Estonia, Finland, Croatia
Pharmacists of countries below:	**Can dispense ePrescriptions presented by citizens from:**
Croatia	Finland, Estonia, Portugal
Estonia	Finland, Croatia, Portugal
Finland	Estonia, Portugal, Croatia
Portugal	Finland, Croatia

In order for cross-border exchange of electronic health records, the most important aspect is the secure identification of patients and healthcare providers. This step is addressed within the legal instrument in the EU regarding cross-border electronic identification is Regulation (EU) 2014/910, known as the electronic Identification, Authentication, and trust Services (eIDAS) [11].

For the development of a generic cross-border eHealth services, the Connecting Europe Facility (CEF), a key EU funding instrument of the Innovation and Networks Executive Agency (INEA) provided financial support for 16 Member States [12]. The INEA is responsible to promote job growth through investment in infrastructure and supports a trans-European network in the fields of transport, energy, and digital services.

20.2.3.2 Towards the European Health Data Space (TEHDAS)

The TEHDAS project is a joint collaboration of 25 European countries (21 EU members and four other European countries) which develops principles for the secondary use of health data. The program is coordinated by the Finnish Innovation Fund, Sitra and has been active since February 2021. The goal of the project is *"that in the future European citizens, communities and companies will benefit from secure and seamless access to health data regardless of where it is stored"* [13]. The system aims to build on protecting individual data and support the portability of their health data, with guidelines as stated from Article 20 of the General Data Protection Regulation (GDPR). The project will promote the access and exchange of different types of health data (e.g., electronic health records, genomics data, patient registries), to support health care delivery (primary use) but also for data to be available for public health, research and making health policy decisions (secondary use). The project has its focus on the following:

- Engage dialogue between other European projects and policymakers about European Health Data Space
- Ensure sustainable secondary use of data in Europe
- Develop governance towards cross-border co-operation between European countries in the secondary use of health data
- Promote reliable and compatible access to secondary use of health data
- Clarify the role of individuals in secondary use of health data and encourage dialogue to include them on the use of health data for research and policymaking

In the past, cross-border sharing of health was limited and project-based, with little or no legal bases or common practices for the use of secondary health data in Europe. With a lack of clarity on the GDPR and varying interpretations led to the underuse of secondary data for research and decision-making. The project has gained further impetus due to the COVID-19 pandemic, which highlighted the urgent need for European-wide sharing and coordination of health data. (Box 20.1) The project has been divided into eight work packages that are led by different organizations across the countries. Work-packages 1–3 are directly linked with the execution of the project, and 4–8 are thematic, which are linked to the secondary use of health data (Table 20.2).

BOX 20.1

COVID-19 passports.

While this may not be the typical health information exchange, the need to reliably share COVID-19 vaccination status while traveling has become a large issue regarding sharing health data across borders. Latin American countries such as Panama are aligning with the European COVID Passport processes and status. The key features of the certificate are that it is available in digital and/or paper format with a QR code, it is safe and secure, valid in all EU countries; and is available in the national language and English.

The digital certificate is a digital proof that a person has either been vaccinated against COVID-19, received a negative test result, or recovered from COVID-19. The vaccine certificates were deemed equivalent to the EU Digital COVID Certificate.

TABLE 20.2 Work-package steps under the TEHDAS project in Europe.

Work-package	Activity
Execution linked work-packages	
1. Coordination	• Implementation managed and coordinated by the Finnish Innovation Fund Sitra
2. Dissemination	• Communication of project deliverables and results managed by Finnish Innovation Fund Sitra
3. Evaluation	• Assessment of project objectives managed by Shared Services of the Ministry of Health, EPE, Portugal
Thematic work-packages	
4. Outreach engagement and sustainability	• Engage with national health authorities of participating countries and international stakeholders to incorporate their views. • Ensure project results are incorporated in future EU legislation
5. Sharing data for health	• Develop options for governance for the exchange of secondary data between European countries based on transparency, citizen engagement, and common good • Recommend European countries on national legislation to enable cross-border exchange and secondary use of health data
6. Data quality	• Develop guidance on data anonymization and reconcile disparate data • Promote digital transformation of European health systems
7. Connecting the dots	• Provide options for technical interoperability • Encourage participation of future users (e.g., researchers, policymakers, technical implementers, companies, and institutions) in designing services
8. Citizens	• Gain understanding on citizens' attitude towards sharing their health data • Raise awareness and inform people of the benefits of using secondary data

20.2.4 Latin America

In Latin America, there appear to be two emerging use cases for health information exchange across borders. The first is the need to provide healthcare for people migrating across the region and more recently to support safe travel during the COVID-19 pandemic.

20.2.4.1 *Brazil & French Guiana*

The borders between Brazil and French Guiana is an endemic region for malaria. [14] This led to a Franco-Brazilian cooperation agreement in 1996 to create a Joint Commission for Cross-Border cooperation between French Guiana and Brazil. [15] Moreover, a sub-working group has been working on health-related issues since 2009, which resulted in a regular exchange of information on malaria between the Guianese and Brazilian surveillance authorities. However, there are notable differences in data formats, update frequencies, spatial and temporal aggregation; lack of contextual information (i.e., metadata); as well as limited recipients for the information on both sides of the border. Due to these inconsistencies, there was a need to have a unified vision to address the malaria situation in the cross-border area.

In this context, there was a need to build a cross-border malaria information system (CBMIS). This system needed to specify reproducible methods based on data harmonization rules, the use of free technological solutions, as well as good practices for information representation and dissemination. In order to facilitate data and knowledge dissemination to public health stakeholders, managers, health officers, and the general public data visualization tools would be needed.

20.2.4.1.1 Study area

The cross-border area was defined as the area between the municipalities of both the countries French Guiana and Brazil, as a coherent territory with a continuous living population. For French Guiana, this included Ouanary, Saint-Georges, and Camopi with an approximate population of 201, 4,220, and 1,828 inhabitants as of 2017, [16] respectively; while for Brazil it includes Oiapoque with an estimated population of 27,270 inhabitants in 2019. [17]

20.2.4.1.2 Data sources & Definition of Cross-Border Malaria Cases

Information regarding individual malaria cases is collected monthly in French Guiana through the delocalized surveillance system Centers for Prevention and Care (Centers Délocalisés de Prévention et de Soins [CDPSs]) operated by Cayenne Hospital, in operation since 2007. In the cross-border area of French Guiana, currently there are four CDPSs: Ouanary, Saint-Georges, Camopi, and Trois-Sauts (Camopi municipality). A malaria case is defined as any positive rapid diagnostic test (RDT) (SD BIOLINE Malaria Ag Pf/Pan in French Guiana). [15] These tests only distinguish *P falciparum* and non-*P falciparum* species. The system is unable to explicitly identify *new attacks* of malaria (i.e., new infection due to a new mosquito bite), notifications based on follow-up of malaria cases, treatment failures, or *P vivax* relapses within the database.

For Brazil, information on individual malaria cases is provided by the Malaria Epidemiological Surveillance Information System (Sistema de Informações de Vigilância Epidemiólogica de Malaria [SIVEP-Malária]) is managed by the information technology department of the unified health system (Departamento de Informática do Sistema Único de Saúde) of the Brazilian Ministry of Health. [15] Brazil uses a thick smear of microscopy, which allows the identification of all *Plasmodium* species in addition to the use of RDT (SD BIOLOINE Ag Pf/Pv). [15] Malaria cases related follow-up consultations, treatment failures, and relapses are referred to as the treatment verification slides (lâminas de verificacão de cura [LVCs]). A repeat case of malaria is considered as an LVC for *P vivax* (or for *P falciparum*) if treatment was received against P vivax (or for *P falciparum*) within the last 60 days (40 days for *P falciparum*). A *new case* is defined if it is a non-LVC case. [15] Monthly anonymized cases are sent by the SIVEP-Malária to the CBIMS through a partnership with the Oswaldo Cruz Foundation (Fundação Owaldo Cruz [Fiocruz]).

A *cross-border* malaria case is defined as per the definitions of the national surveillance systems and that was associated with (1) a notification center, (2) patient's residential address, or (3) a possible transmission location, located in the previously defined cross-border area. [15]

20.2.4.1.3 Data Harmonization System

Data harmonization was achieved by transforming the data from the two national information systems to develop a common, harmonized data model. The steps for the data flow and the harmonization process for the transfer protocols are illustrated in Fig. 20.1.

The common, harmonized model relied as much as possible on the existing international standards, for those not available national or normative representations based on the knowledge areas and consensual use of the study. The data harmonization consisted of changes in data type (e.g., conversion of string type to integer and unit conversion for patient age from months to years). An extract, transform, and load (ETL) process was implemented using the free software Talend Open Studio for Big Data for all transformation rules.

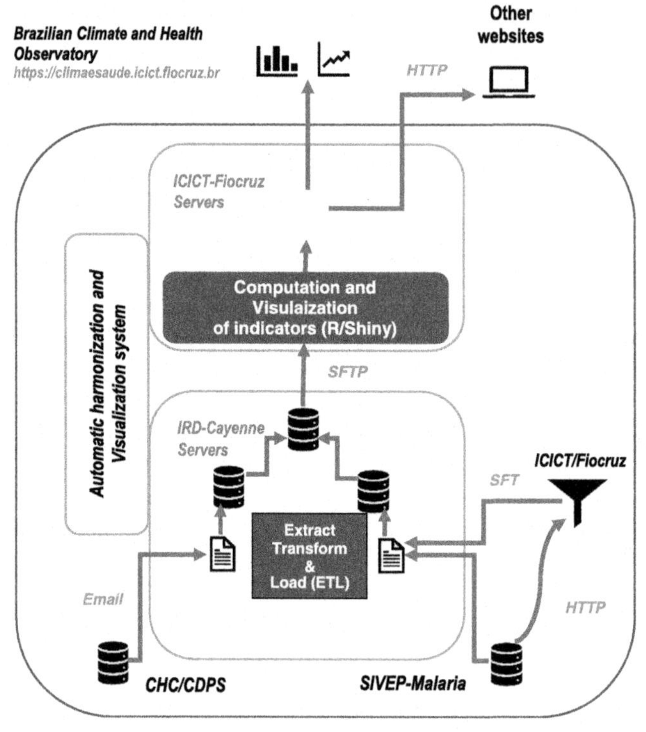

FIGURE 20.1 System architecture and data information flow of Cross-border Malaria Epidemiological Surveillance Information System in Brazil and French Guiana.[15]

20.3 Summary

Exchanging health data across state and national borders is a challenge due to issues related to personal information privacy laws and policies. Varying degrees of complexities arise, be it at the state level in a US context or different EU Member States, having different national regulatory frameworks or managing coordinated infectious disease mitigation across national borders. Various efforts have been undertaken to overcome challenges like interoperability, record linking, governance, and inadequate infrastructure. These challenges differ based on regions that need greater importance due to the spread of vector-borne illnesses or recently with the COVID-19 pandemic. Technology exists for health information to move across borders, but most of these barriers exist due to a lack of resources, trust, and legal clarity.

Policymakers have noticed an urgent need for timely, transparent, and secure sharing of health information during the on-going pandemic. This led to an impetus in sharing of health information in the United States and also in the European Union. More collaboration is needed on international classifications and terminologies to facilitate compatibility in the future. This will certainly help in lowering the costs and barriers to carry out the business needs of health; moreover, it will be important in supporting citizens for their fundamental right to health information.

Questions for Discussion

1. Describe some of the projects in the United States that have led to the growth of cross-border health information exchange?
2. What was the role of the Cross-Border Health Integrated Partnership Project (CB-HIPP) to address the needs of mobile populations in Africa? Which of the open software and technologies have helped to address cross-border health issues?
3. How is Europe addressing the challenges of cross-border health exchange? What regulation and project are driving forward an EU collaboration towards cross-border health information exchange?
4. What steps did Brazil and French Guiana take to address the need for malaria surveillance for their mobile populations in their cross-border region?

Acknowledgements

The authors appreciate Dr. Karmen Williams, Steven Wanyee, Daniel Otzoy, and James Kariuki for sharing their valuable insights and expertise in cross-border health data exchange.

References

[1] Diener A, Hagen J. Borderlines and borderlands: political oddities at the edge of the nation-state. Rowman & Littlefield Publishers, Inc.; 2010.
[2] Gavish R, Levy A, Dekel OK, Karp E, Maimon N. The association between hospital readmission and pulmonologist follow-up visits in patients with COPD. Chest. 2015;148(2):375–81.
[3] Naderi S, Barnett B, Hoffman RS, et al. Factors associated with failure to follow-up at a medical clinic after an ED visit. Am J Emerg Med 2012;30(2):347–51.
[4] Newton AS, Rosychuk RJ, Dong K, Curran J, Slomp M, McGrath PJ. Emergency health care use and follow-up among sociodemographic groups of children who visit emergency departments for mental health crises. Cmaj. 2012;184(12):E665–74.
[5] Hochman M, Garger J, Robinson E. Health Information Exchange after 10 years: Time for a More Assertive Approach. Health Aff 2022; Accessed February 1.
[6] 2011/24/EU Directive on the application of patients' rights in cross-border healthcare (Cross-border Directive). 2011.
[7] Nalin M, Baroni I, Faiella G, et al. The European cross-border health data exchange roadmap: Case study in the Italian setting. J Biomed Inf Jun 2019;94:103183. Available from: https://doi.org/10.1016/j.jbi.2019.103183.
[8] epSOS project. Accessed December 1, 2021. https://ec.europa.eu/digital-single-market/en/news/cross-border-health-project-epsos-what-has-it-achieved.
[9] Health Informatics - The Patient Summary for Unscheduled, Cross-border Care. In: Standardization ECf, editor. 2019.
[10] Regulation (EU) 2016/679 of the European Parliament and of the Council of 27 April 2016 on the protection of natural persons with regard to the processing of personal data and on the free movement of such data, and repealing Directive 95/46/EC (General Data Protection Regulation) (Text with EEA relevance) ELI: http://data.europa.eu/eli/reg/2016/679/2016-05-04.
[11] eIDAS website. Accessed December 3, 2021. https://www.eid.as.
[12] Accessed December 3, 2021. https://ec.europa.eu/inea/en/connecting-europe-facility.
[13] Towards the European Health Data Space (TEHDAS). Accessed March 25, 2022.
[14] da Cruz F, Peiter P, Carvajal-Cortes J, Dos Santos Pereira R, do Socorro Mendonca Gomes M, Suarez-Mutis M. Complex malaria epidemiology in an international border area between Brazil and French Guiana: challenges for elimination. Tropical Medicine and Health 2019;24. Available from: https://doi.org/10.1186/s41182-019-0150-0.
[15] Saldanha R, Mosnier E, Barcellos C, Carbunar A, Charron C, Desconnets J-C, et al. Contributing to elimination of cross-border malaria through a standardized solution for case surveillance, and data interpretation: development of a cross-border monitoring system. Journal of Medical Internet Research Public Health and Surveillance 2020;10.2196/15409. Available from: https://doi.org/10.2196/15409.
[16] Available from: Institut National de la Statistique et des Études Économiques (INSEE). [accessed 01.02.22].
[17] Available from: Instituto Brasileiro de Geografia e Estatística (IBGE). [accessed 01.02.22].

CHAPTER

21

Future directions for health information exchange

Julia Adler-Milstein[1], *Chantal Worzala*[2] *and Brian E. Dixon*[3,4]

[1]Center for Clinical Informatics and Improvement Research, University of California, San Francisco, CA, USA [2]Alazro Consulting LLC, Takoma Park, MD, USA [3]Department of Epidemiology, Richard M. Fairbanks School of Public Health, Indiana University, Indianapolis, IN, USA [4]Center for Biomedical Informatics, Regenstrief Institute, Inc., Indianapolis, IN, USA

LEARNING OBJECTIVES

- To describe current and near-future topics that will shape the evolution of health information exchange.
- To describe large-scale policy frameworks that seek to streamline approaches to HIE nationally and internationally.
- To describe how the COVID-19 pandemic has shifted thinking about the role of HIE networks.

21.1 Introduction

As health information exchange (HIE) continues to evolve, its future appears likely to be particularly shaped by two factors: policy and the pandemic. While these factors target addressing unmet needs—particularly in building toward large-scale HIE infrastructure—overall it does not appear that we are heading toward "one right way" to approach HIE. In this chapter, we address a set of topics that reflect core areas of ongoing change where policy, the pandemic, and other forces are actively at play.

We begin by describing a major policy effort underway in the United States to create a national framework to facilitate nationwide exchange—the Trusted Exchange Framework and Common Agreement (TEFCA). Under TEFCA, Americans should expect to see greater exchange of data, particularly across different types of HIE networks (e.g., community-based, vendor, enterprise). While this will reflect important progress, it could also exacerbate a current challenge in which we lack solutions to integrate multiple sources of health information and present that information in a way that is easy for patients, clinicians, and other key stakeholders to use. We therefore turn to a discussion of challenges related to interoperability

Health Information Exchange
DOI: https://doi.org/10.1016/B978-0-323-90802-3.00005-8

usability—characterizing the current pain points, describing emerging solutions, and discussing how standards are lacking to support better data integration that would facilitate improved usability.

Outside of the United States, we examine the Joint Action Towards the European Health Data Space (TEHDAS), a recent initiative of the European Union (EU). Through a series of policies enacted at both continental and individual nation levels, Europe hopes to make routinely captured health data available across borders to support public health and research. These policies are likely to shape how data are used globally beyond their original intent for treatment, payment, and healthcare operations.

Current and future policies, including TEFCA and TEHDAS, were influenced by the COVID-19 pandemic that occurred during the early phases of their implementation. Therefore we conclude the chapter by exploring the impact of the pandemic on HIE for the future. Several efforts are underway in the United States to move HIE networks toward public health data utilities. We examine this concept and consider the benefits and challenges of treating HIE networks as public utilities.

21.2 A unified approach to nationwide exchange

Summary. The development of nationwide infrastructure to support sharing of health information has been discussed for decades and may be on the verge of being realized through the TEFCA called for under the 21st Century Cures Act [1]. The foundational governance rules for TEFCA were released in January 2022 and the network-of-networks approach to nationwide exchange will be operationalized in the coming months and years. The success of TEFCA is not guaranteed as participation is voluntary. However, growing expectations that health information will be shared and will available when and where it is needed could encourage participation.

21.2.1 Federal support for health information exchange

The first federal program to offer significant funding for HIE, The Health Information Technology for Economic and Clinical Health (HITECH) Act, provided short-term funding to states to facilitate the exchange of health information among stakeholders in local, regional, and statewide efforts. Beginning in 2010, the Office of the National Coordinator for Health Information Technology (ONC) provided almost $550 million in grants through the State HIE Cooperative Agreement Program [2]. Evaluations of that program noted considerable variation across states "based on state context and program factors" [3]. Arguably, state and regional efforts to create HIE networks reflect the local nature of much healthcare and the importance of trust relationships in creating the conditions for exchange. However, they also lead to a fragmented approach to exchange with regard to the technical approaches adopted and governance approaches implemented, including who has access to information for what purposes and under what policies to keep information private and secure.

21.2.2 The health information exchange landscape

Today, there are an estimated 89 operational health information organizations (HIOs), down from 106 in 2014 [4]. During the COVID pandemic, a number of state and regional HIE networks developed tools to support both healthcare providers and public health officials in collecting, analyzing and sharing clinical data, test results, alerts, and healthcare capacity information needed to coordinate the response to the pandemic [5]. While some of these HIEs connect with each other, most notably through the Patient Centered Data Home, they are not yet all connected through a single, nationwide approach for exchange [6]. Efforts to expand exchange can be hampered by the significant effort it takes to create data sharing agreements that are acceptable to all parties, including possible competitors and actors that have competing interests, such as providers and payers. State and regional exchanges also face challenges overcoming competitive concerns (including from health IT vendors offering HIE networks), ensuring financial sustainability, and addressing federal regulations [4].

21.2.3 Nationwide exchange

Under HITECH, ONC launched efforts to support nationwide exchange under the Nationwide Health Information Network (NwHIN). In 2012 the NwHIN transitioned out of the federal government to become a nonprofit public–private collaboration, the eHealth Exchange. Today, eHealth Exchange connects federal agencies and nonfederal healthcare organizations across the country [7]. Other approaches to support national exchange have also developed over time, notably Carequality, which is a nonprofit, private sector interoperability framework to connect health information networks and other implementers (such as electronic health record vendors) with each other [8]; and the CommonWell Health Alliance, a vendor-neutral network [9]. In addition, several major electronic health record (EHR) vendors have also developed the capability to connect their customers with one another, as well as through the other national exchanges like the eHealth Exchange.

However, none of these approaches connect all actors across the healthcare system to support a full range of exchange purposes or to meet all of the exchange needs of participants. Notably, the national exchanges primarily support the sharing of patient-level data for treatment purposes. According to an ONC analysis of data from the American Hospital Association, hospitals used three different electronic methods for sending and receiving summary of care records in 2019, suggesting that no single connection could fulfill all their information sharing needs [10]. In addition, 7 in 10 hospitals face at least one challenge in reporting to public health using electronic means [11].

21.2.4 Trusted Exchange Framework and Common Agreement basics

The 21st Century Cures Act (2016) called on the ONC to "convene appropriate public and private stakeholders to develop or support a trusted exchange framework for trust policies and practices and for a common agreement for exchange between health information networks" [12]. The statute called out the need for common rules for trusted exchange, including organizational and operational policies and methods to authenticate participants in exchange, as well as a process for filing and adjudicating noncompliance. ONC named The Sequoia Project to be the Recognized Coordinating Entity (RCE) that would work with ONC to develop and operationalize TEFCA through a public–private collaborative funded under a Cooperative Agreement. The RCE is also tasked with providing governance and oversight for the TEFCA and creating a sustainability plan.

The stated goals of TEFCA are to:

- establish a universal policy and technical floor for nationwide interoperability;
- simplify connectivity for organizations to securely exchange information to improve patient care, enhance the welfare of populations, and generate healthcare value; and
- enable individuals to gather their health information [13].

The TEFCA does not create a new health information network. Rather, it creates a governance and legal structure (Fig. 21.1) to allow existing, and possibly new, HIE networks and HIOs to exchange information and sets common expectations, obligations and technical approaches for those that choose to join. By setting a single set of rules that are embedded in legal contracts, TEFCA allows those participating in TEFCA exchange to share information across networks without having to develop one-off agreements. It also creates a single set of technical requirements to support TEFCA exchange. The vision is to allow participants such as healthcare providers, payers, public health agencies, and individuals to be able to share and gather information nationwide through a single connection of their choosing.

At the center of TEFCA connectivity will be a small set of Qualified Health Information Networks (QHINs) that will be designated by the RCE to have met specific eligibility requirements to demonstrate that they can reliably manage high volumes of exchange in accordance with specific technical requirements. The RCE has stated that the QHINs will be expected to handle hundreds of millions of transactions per day, support nationwide exchange, and be subject to specific performance metrics. Thus they will serve as central nodes for efficient exchange of health information at a national scale. This infrastructure will facilitate automated exchange across other health information networks that participate in TEFCA. Many of the state and regional HIEs that exist today would not necessarily have the technical infrastructure to become a QHIN. However, they could establish connectivity with a QHIN to connect their own participants into nationwide exchange, while also providing additional local and value-add services.

The key instrument underlying TEFCA exchange is a Common Agreement that sets forward legally binding requirements addressing

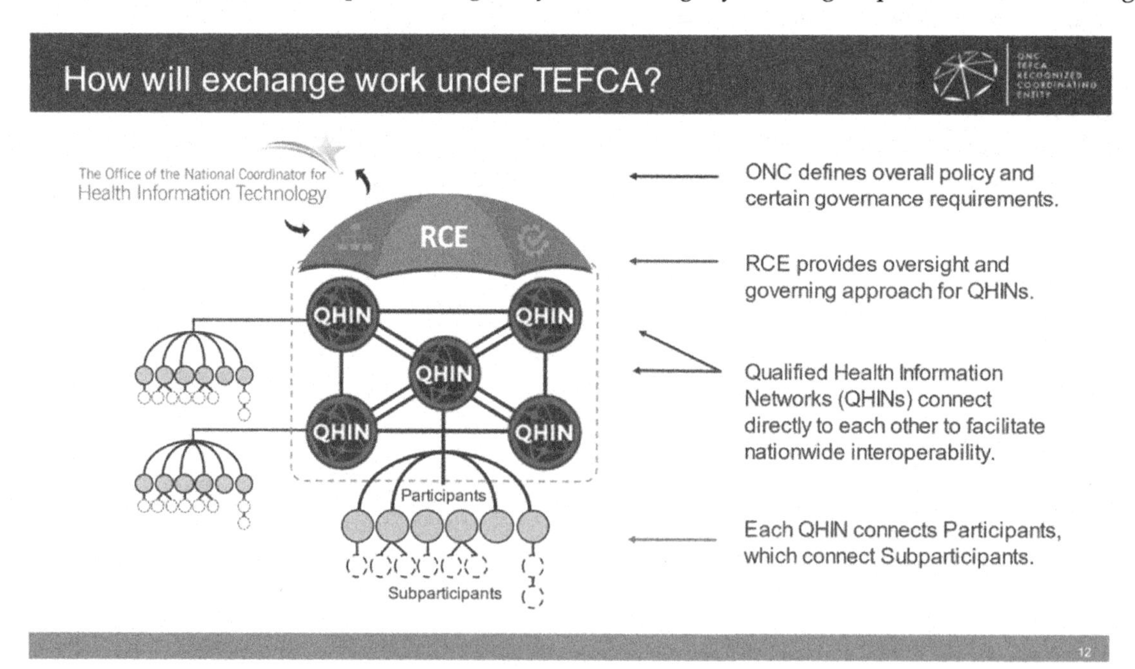

FIGURE 21.1 Organizational roles and responsibilities under TEFCA. *TEFCA*, Trusted Exchange Framework and Common Agreement. Source: *Published with permission of the ONC Recognized Coordinating Entity (http://www.rce.sequoiaproject.org).*

the parties to and purposes of exchange, expectations for collaboration and nondiscrimination in exchange, privacy and security requirements, and the technical approach to exchange. The Common Agreement will be signed by each QHIN and the RCE. Each QHIN will also be required to flow down key elements of these data sharing requirements in the legal agreements they have with health information networks and other actors that they support and that want to be part of TEFCA exchange (QHIN Participants and Subparticipants).

One key element of trusted exchange is standard approaches for privacy and security. In recognition of that, the Common Agreement provides specific requirements for QHINs and other participants in TEFCA exchange. Most connected entities will likely be Covered Entities under the Health Insurance Portability and Accountability Act (HIPAA; which generally covers healthcare providers, payers and clearing houses) or Business Associates of Covered Entities, and thus already be required to comply with the HIPAA privacy and security requirements. However, some parties to TEFCA exchange may not covered by HIPAA. Therefore, to create a common standard, the Common Agreement requires entities not covered by HIPAA to protect individually identifiable information that they reasonably believe is part of TEFCA exchange in substantially the same manner as HIPAA Covered Entities protect Protected Health Information, including most provisions of the HIPAA Privacy and Security Rules.

21.2.5 Trusted Exchange Framework and Common Agreement launch

In January 2022, both ONC and the RCE released foundational documents to launch TEFCA. These include:

- The Trusted Exchange Framework, which sets forth principals that embody the federal approach to guide nationwide exchange over time [14].
- The Common Agreement Version 1, which is the legal agreement outlining the expectations and requirements for participation in TEFCA exchange, key elements of which will also flow down to other entities participating in exchange [15].
- The QHIN Technical Framework that specifies the technical requirements for exchange among QHINs, which is built on approaches that are in widespread, production use today, including Integrating the Healthcare Enterprise (IHE) Profiles to support queries, responses, and message delivery. The QHIN Technical Framework also provides details on how QHINs will interact with the RCE Directory, which will play a key role in routing queries, responses, and messages across entities sharing information via TEFCA exchange (see Box 21.1) [16].
- A Fast Healthcare Interoperability Resource (FHIR) Roadmap that establishes a process to leverage the FHIR standard to support exchange in TEFCA. Stakeholders and policymakers have emphasized the need for TEFCA to align with the tremendous growth in and support for FHIR (see Box 21.2) [17].

The timeline put forward by the RCE and ONC suggests that the process of vetting organizations and designating them as QHINs will begin in the first half of 2022, with the first group of QHINs designated before the end of the year. The QHINs will then need to work with the health information networks, EHR vendors, and other entities that want to connect with them for TEFCA exchange to ensure that their contracts include the appropriate flow-down provisions [13].

The Common Agreement puts forth a set of six Exchange Purposes:

- Treatment (as defined in HIPAA)

BOX 21.1

QHIN technical framework (QTF).

The QTF describes the functional and technical requirements that a QHIN must meet and specifies the technical underpinnings for QHIN-to-QHIN exchange, including the specific standards to be implemented. The QTF enables two information exchange modalities for QHINs:

- QHIN Query, including Patient Discovery (IHE XCPD), Document Query (IHE XCA), and Document Retrieve (IHE XCA)
- QHIN Message Delivery (IHE XCDR)

To ensure secure communications and support privacy, the QTF also addresses: certificate policy, secure channel, authentication, and authorization.

The RCE Directory Service will support exchange by including information on all of the end points connected through QHIN-to-QHIN exchange. It is an HL7 FHIR-based service. QHINs will be responsible for updating information about their Participants and Subparticipants on an ongoing basis.

BOX 21.2

Fast Healthcare Interoperability Resource (FHIR) Roadmap.

The federal government has prioritized adoption of the HL7 FHIR standard to support data-level exchange of information. Today, most FHIR-based exchange is point-to-point, and the standard is not yet widely used in network-based exchange. However, ONC and the RCE have published an FHIR Roadmap to support FHIR-based exchange within the TEFCA framework by 2025 in three stages:

- Stage 1—FHIR Content Support: FHIR-based exchange is possible within QHINs' own networks and IHE-based exchange can support sharing content formatted to the FHIR standard (or payloads), with additional coordination among the parties to exchange.
- Stage 2—Network-Facilitated FHIR Exchange: QHINs provide network infrastructure to facilitate Participants and Subparticipants from different QHINs independently engaging in FHIR-based exchange.
- Stage 3—Network-Brokered FHIR Exchange: In addition to Stage 2 functions, QHINs may broker FHIR payloads by routing FHIR application programming interface (API) transactions between Participants and Subparticipants from different QHINs.

- Payment (as defined in HIPAA)
- Healthcare operations (as defined in HIPAA),
- Public health,
- Government benefits determination (such as the Social Security Administration assessing eligibility for disability benefits), and

- Individual access services, which supports people in gathering their health information from across various providers and other entities.

In an effort to build on existing capabilities used by HIE networks today, the RCE has stated that responses will only be required for treatment and individual access services in the beginning. However, as detailed guidance for the other exchange purposes is provided, they will also become standard purposes for exchange.

21.2.6 Considerations for the future

The RCE and ONC have followed an open process to gather stakeholder feedback and incorporate it into the foundational documents for TEFCA. However, there are still key questions to be answered as it is operationalized. For example, some stakeholders have questioned whether TEFCA is needed, given the other national networks and interoperability frameworks that exist in the private sector. Observers have also questioned whether entities will engage in TEFCA, given that participation is voluntary and participants in TEFCA will need to modify existing data use agreements. A related issue is funding and sustainability. The federal government has not made any funding available to QHINs, which will need to develop a clear business case for their services that offer sufficient value for any fees that are charged. Moreover, HIE networks and other participants will need to evaluate both how to participate in TEFCA exchange and the business case for doing so.

A unified approach to nationwide exchange could create significant efficiencies by decreasing the complexity of connecting to others and increasing the number of entities that participate in exchange. The engagement of the federal government in TEFCA also could encourage participation by reassuring entities that this particular exchange effort will be enduring.

Federal engagement in a multipurpose nationwide exchange model also creates a forum for collaboration for all stakeholders to pursue advances in interoperability. For example, the COVID pandemic highlighted the need to collaboratively address information sharing to support public health activities, including case and lab results reporting, case investigation, and sharing of information on health system capacity. Additional use cases, such as research, could also be addressed through TEFCA over time. The development of a single source of connectivity to accomplish multiple exchange purposes would create efficiencies by reducing the need for multiple connections and collaborations to accomplish different goals.

In addition, the launch of TEFCA comes at a time when demands for health information to be shared are growing. The growing ubiquity of information technology solutions in retail, banking, and other areas has created consumer expectations that health information will also be available electronically [18]. In addition, the Centers for Medicare & Medicaid Services (CMS) has established expectations for providers and payers to share data electronically [19,20].

To that end, the Common Agreement establishes a broader set of Exchange Purposes than any of the existing health information networks—such as payment, public health, and individual access services—which could draw new participants into nationwide HIE and create demand from end-users, even when participants may have competitive positions. For example, consumers generally do not like to manage multiple provider portals and could see significant value in being able to gather all their health information through a consumer-facing app or portal. Payers may want to leverage TEFCA to query providers for the patient information they need to close care gaps (such as missing immunizations or preventive screenings), complete quality measures, or submit data to Medicare and other payers for risk-adjustment purposes. And, to the extent TEFCA delivers on the promise of more efficient and simplified exchange, providers with limited connectivity today, such as small physician offices and postacute care providers, may choose to engage.

Observers have also asked whether and how TEFCA could interact with other regulatory requirements, including the prohibition on information blocking that was included in the 21st Century Cures Act. In its final rule defining what is not information blocking, ONC stated: "it would be premature to establish special treatment for entities that join the TEFCA. We may reconsider this suggestion at a later date" [12]. It is also possible that other federal agencies, such as the CMS, point to TEFCA in future regulations, similar to the ways in which CMS requires the use of certified health IT by healthcare providers in the Promoting Interoperability Program or references specific ONC standards for use by payers in the Patient Access and Interoperability rules.

The success of TEFCA is not a foregone conclusion. However, the recent launch suggests that the effort has momentum to deliver on its promise of more efficient and simplified nationwide exchange. Key factors determining its success will include the engagement of the federal government and the growing expectations by consumers and stakeholders that health information will be available electronically to support a variety of uses.

Looking forward, QHINs will be asked to report metrics that will help to gauge how widely it is used. Initial metrics in the QTF include, for example, the number of organizations and facilities that have been connected, by type (e.g., hospital, public health entity, payer); the number of clinicians connected; the number of transactions processed; and average response types. Public reporting of these data, as well as more systematic evaluation of the program would be valuable in measuring success of the initiative.

21.3 An emerging challenge: usability of interoperability

Summary. Substantial effort over the past decade has resulted in greater levels of HIE [21] and this will only expand as TEFCA moves forward. Greater availability of electronic health information can help support a number of different use cases, which span from individual patient and clinician use to population and public health applications. When individual patients (or their caregivers) or clinicians have greater access to electronic health data, it is not uncommon that those data come from multiple sources and are not integrated to offer a single, comprehensive picture of health information. For example, a patient may have their records from multiple health systems connected to their smartphone, but those records still exist and have to be reviewed by the patient independently. Similarly, for clinicians, they may be able to access outside records from within their EHR system, but those records are not integrated into the EHR, such that clinicians have to review separate lists of encounters, problems, medications, etc. In both examples, electronic exchange has occurred but we have not integrated data in a way that facilitates its use and creates a holistic view of patient information. Moving forward, we will need to think about both the technical approaches and policy drivers that can help address these issues. Deriving value from increased electronic information sharing depends on this crucial but largely unrecognized issue.

21.3.1 The emerging challenge of interoperability usability

A growing number of studies have found that, even when information is available electronically, it is often not used. This is true both for patients and for clinicians. On the patient side, several studies have found a large gap between the percent of patients with electronic health data available to them, and the percent who ever or repeatedly access that data [22]. Today, patients can access their health data electronically in a number of different ways [23]. The most common method is via a patient portal offered by their healthcare provider or payer where the patient can register to view, download, or transmit their health information [24]. With increases in smartphone adoption and implementation of APIs, patients now may also have the option of viewing and downloading their health information to their smartphone [25]. However, even with new options for access, patient uptake remains low.

A contributor to low patient use is data fragmentation. For example, in a recent Medsphere blog post, the author described having "... portal access to 6 different providers, including two hospitals. Each portal holds information about me that the others don't have. Ironically, even though the two hospitals both use Cerner EHRs, their portals not only don't speak to each other, but were configured so differently that navigating each is a different experience" [26]. Research on designing more effective patient portals in the context of fragmented health systems suggests that "under such a fragmented setup, in order to see all of his or her information and interact with all of his or her providers, the patient must access multiple portals, each with a distinct interface, password, and username. Especially for patients with complex conditions who see multiple providers, this multiplicity of portals and access requirements may complicate their navigation of the system and limit their ability to manage their care" [27]. Taken together, these findings point to the challenge of designing approaches to patient-facing HIE that not only make data available but ensure that the data are usable by integrating fragmented patient records into a unified patient chart.

On the clinician-facing side, the issues are similar. A systematic review of clinician HIE usage and impact found overall low levels of use, concluding that studies "generally showed usage in less than 10% of patient encounters" [28]. Even more recent assessments of clinician HIE use have continued to find low levels [29,30]. Similarly, a national hospital survey revealed that 37% of hospitals report rarely or never using outside data available electronically, and when asked why, top reasons cited were (1) information is available but not integrated into EHR (cited by 52% of hospitals) and (2) information not presented in a useful format (e.g., too much information, redundant, or unnecessary information) (cited by 34% of hospitals) [31]. These findings reflect the reality that most approaches to HIE require clinicians to go outside of their local EHR (e.g., by logging in to a community longitudinal record) or to go to a separate tab in their local EHR that houses outside records [32]. A recent blog describing this issue characterized multiple consequences for clinicians, stating that "when data are viewable but not combined, clinicians are less likely to use data from outside sources; cognitive effort is spent marrying local EHR data with outside data (for example, moving between two or more problem lists, medication lists, or encounter lists); and time is consumed manually reconciling outside data with local data. Furthermore, unreconciled outside data typically cannot be included in clinical notes or used to drive decision support" [33].

21.3.2 Potential solutions

There is little disagreement that, in concept, the optimal solution would be a single, harmonized patient record that patients, clinicians, and other appropriate stakeholders could use. However, in practice, concerns have been raised about the importance of data provenance, and in particular reflecting the source-data entity. For example, if an imaging study was performed and interpreted by a radiologist at a small community hospital, that report may be used differently than had it been done at a flagship academic medical center. Indeed, prior work has cited lack of trust in outside records as a barrier to information use [10], and early interoperability solutions kept outside records data separate based on the assumption that clinicians in particular would find this approach more acceptable.

As real-world experience has accumulated, it has become clear that the downsides of such separation are substantial, and we have therefore started to pursue approaches that integrate and harmonize data sources. For example, the Indiana Health Information Exchange (IHIE) is developing an application called Health Dart that allows clinicians to query specific data directly from their EHR [34]. This FHIR application has specific query and response capabilities to allow a physician to retrieve patient information from outside sources without leaving their EHR. Moreover, what is presented to the clinician is not a list of outside documents, but precise data tailored to facilitate decision-making in a specific context (e.g., patient presents with chest pain). Research on its use and impact are underway and will serve as important evidence of the benefits of more integrated approaches to data retrieval.

In terms of more integrated approaches to data presentation, current research is limited. One recent study used a natural experiment with Epic System's HIE network—Care Everywhere—to assess the impact of a user interface design change that integrated one particular type of information—encounters [35]. As part of upgrading to the 2017 version, a new feature created a single, integrated, sequential list of local health system and external (from other Epic-based health systems) encounters presented in the Chart Review (CR) tab. Prior to this switch, outside records were only available through the Care Everywhere (CE) tab, a section of the EHR exclusive to outside record [36]. The new feature was supplementary, such that there was no change to user ability to view outside records via the CE tab. Using an interrupted time series analysis, within the health system, this encounter integration display change had a large impact on how often outside records were viewed. Specifically, the level of outside record views increased by 22,920 per week. There were increases in the level of views for all provider and encounter types: attendings (3675), residents (3277), and nurses (914); inpatient (1676), emergency (487), and outpatient (7228). While only a single-site study, this evidence suggests the large-scale effects, at least on HIE use, that can come from better data integration. It will be important to extend this evidence base to study the impact across different types of data and in different settings.

21.3.3 Key challenges to data integration

While it may seem the remaining work to achieve data integration across core clinical data domains is minor, there are major barriers that stem from the current scope and implementation of data standards. Even for data types that seem uniform, data standards have not been designed and implemented to address the challenges of data harmonization posed by trying to interoperate fragmented EHR systems.

Consider, for example, the case of lab results. There is a mature and widely accepted data standard (Logical Observation Identifiers, Names and Code (LOINC)) that is a clinical terminology to represent lab test orders and results [37]. However, in practice, LOINC has not been fully implemented, such that many lab tests and lab results found in a given EHR do not include the associated LOINC identifier, particularly in EHRs and other information systems that predate the development of LOINC (or have inherited data from older systems). This is problematic for many use cases, especially public health reporting [38]. Even if we were to solve this large-scale, costly issue by fully implementing LOINC across all EHRs, LOINC is insufficiently specific to achieve full standardization. Tests with identical LOINC identifiers often differ across other dimensions, such as machine calibration or reference ranges.

Manual efforts to translate across all possible combinations of dimensions—mapping lab equipment manufacturer, units of measurement, and reference range, across the thousands of different lab tests, and variations within each test—are a nonstarter. There are efforts, however, to map common tests that account for >90% of laboratory volume. High-volume tests like white blood cell count, glycosylated hemoglobin (HbA1c), etc. enumerate to around 2000 commonly performed tests across hospitals, commercial laboratories, and point-of-care testing locations [39]. Automated approaches exist in the Regenstrief LOINC Mapping tool (RELMA) to map common tests to local codes for a hospital or clinic [40,41]. Furthermore, the Association of Public Health Laboratories in coordination with the Centers for Disease Control and Prevention (CDC) is using automated and semiautomated approaches to support mapping efforts in support of COVID-19 reporting [42]. Although automated efforts have yielded results, these efforts do not scale efficiently as many local codes can map to more than one potential LOINC code necessitating human review. Even mapping to just the high-volume tests could be challenging for the nation across small-to-medium hospitals. Moreover, mapping to just high-volume tests may focus too much on clinical care, excluding secondary uses like quality measurement and public health [39]. These examples make clear why it has been difficult to achieve lab result integration, and many of the same issues apply to other core types of clinical data (e.g., medications). A single harmonized medical record would require an enormous breadth of standards that are less mature or nonexistent.

Looking ahead, it may be decades or longer before the needed standards are available and implemented. This leaves the question of whether we should be pursuing more pragmatic approaches to integrate data and create more user-friendly interoperability solutions. The key to success in the pragmatic approach is differentiating two scenarios. Again, using the lab result example, it relies on differentiating when the same test from different laboratories is sufficiently, clinically different that the results cannot be safely treated as equivalent versus when the distinctions, while genuine, are not clinically meaningful. Here, specialty societies may be a key actor to define the guidelines for their commonly used lab tests, describing when different data sources can be integrated and when they should be kept separate, which EHR vendors can then implement.

While a more pragmatic approach would help speed improved interoperability usability, there are potential risks. For example, integrating more, but not all, types of lab results could create inconsistency in what clinicians and patients see and experience, risking confusion and missed information. In addition, perspectives on which differences are clinically meaningful may differ by specialty for the same lab test. We lack a framework for how to balance the risks, benefits, and financial costs of integrating data at varying levels of customization. Instead, we default to the most conservative approach that largely keeps different data sources separate, likely overweighing these risks and undervaluing the tremendous potential gains from even modest increases in data integration. In addition, standards harmonization is only one part of the framework. Designing better approaches to data integration also requires consideration of where data are stored, at what level of granularity, and how we bring data sources together for different HIE use cases.

Ideally, new approaches will emerge that avoid the need for tradeoffs and can achieve user-friendly approaches to data integration that do not rely on perfect data standards. For example, machine learning and artificial intelligence approaches could identify the information needed given the patient context, including reconciling unstructured text notes, to present an easy-to-interpret clinical summary from multiple sources. This still may not include a single reconciled set of lab results but could perhaps produce a summary of whether a given result is trending up or down. In many clinical scenarios, and likely for patient use, this may be sufficient for decision-making. On the patient-facing side, some third-party applications are attempting to reconcile patient information across disparate sources [43] and could be buoyed by better data availability enabled by TEFCA. However, consumer demand for these solutions is not yet clear.

21.3.4 Considerations for the future

Looking ahead, there are no easy solutions to achieve a single, harmonized patient record that draws on the increasingly available set of electronic data that can be exchanged. What is clear is that the gap between what is available and what can be effectively used by clinicians and by patients will grow. For clinicians, we should continue to seek to comingle local EHR data with data from outside records, such that clinicians stay within their workflow and are presented with an integrated and logically organized (e.g., chronological) list of core data: encounters, lab results, problems, medications, etc. For patients, we will need something similar that solves the "many portals" issue in ways that create value. Given the substantial work required to achieve this final step of integrating data from disparate records, it is critical to pursue approaches that scale, potentially using artificial intelligence (AI)-based approaches, and can be supported by federal policy efforts.

21.4 International policies impacting health information exchange

Summary. There exist two major continent-wide initiatives that seek to expand HIE in Europe and Africa that are likely to impact the adoption and use of HIE globally in the next decade. Although each effort is nascent, both seek to enable cross-border data sharing while enhancing the capacity of each nation to facilitate HIE within its borders and with its geographical neighbors "in an effective, efficient, ethical, and lawful manner" [44].

21.4.1 Joint Action Towards the European Health Data Space

In Europe, the EU launched the Joint Action Towards the European Health Data Space or TEHDAS initiative in February 2021 to increase the secondary use of health data beyond treatment, payment, and healthcare operations [45]. As discussed in Chapter 6, these existing three use cases for HIE are the most common in the United States and globally. Through TEHDAS, the EU seeks to leverage routinely collected health data for public health and research, including innovations in health IT as well as pharmaceuticals and other clinical interventions. The initiative was heavily influenced by the COVID-19 pandemic, which made it challenging for EU nations to share data on SARS-CoV-2 infections, hospitalizations, and vaccinations.

Currently TEHDAS is in its initial phases. To date, the initiative held several workshops and discussion forms across Europe to inform its early discovery processes. The initiative published a report in early 2022 that detailed the results of these workshops [46]. The report identified a number of international, semantic standards and common data models, including LOINC, SNOMED-CT and Observational Medical Outcomes Partnership

(OMOP) [47], that are in use within Europe. The report did not make a definitive recommendation on the framework for TEHDAS. Over the next two years, TEHDAS plans to continue exploring available standards and frameworks to develop a final set of recommendations for implementation across the EU.

The final framework will be translated into a European Health Data Space (EHDS) [48], which will serve as a Web-based platform for accessing, standardizing, analyzing, and using health data from multiple countries for population health and research. It will likely be a federated network that leverages multiple data sources, including EHR systems, national patient registries, and genomics databases.

The EHDS and TEHDAS initiatives are heavily influenced by the General Data Protection Regulation (GDPR) (discussed in Chapter 3), which is an overarching policy framework for the privacy and security of data collected and managed by EU nations [49]. Moving forward, TEHDAS will define specific policy and governance recommendations that will enable each nation to pass legislation enabling cross-border health data sharing in support of the EHDS. Furthermore, TEHDAS will define governance of the EHDS, which will require representation from across the EU and stakeholder groups, including patients. In the initial reports from TEHDAS, a strong emphasis is given to consumer participation in governance of the EHDS as well as attitudes toward citizens sharing their information to support public health and innovation in the EU [50].

In many ways, TEHDAS appears to be consistent with the TEFCA efforts in the United States. In the coming decade, TEHDAS will likely develop a common framework and policy regulations for EU that will guide HIE efforts within nations and cross-border. Furthermore, the EHDS will be a platform through which nations can leverage population data to guide health policy, public health surveillance, and innovation in the biomedical sciences. As the initiative moves forward, evaluation of its impact and comparisons with TEFCA are in order to measure its progress and examine the challenges it will likely face given disparate approaches to HIE within nations and the landscape of policy regulations that will need to be harmonized.

21.4.2 African Union health information exchange efforts in support of public health

Summary. In 2020 the Africa Centers for Disease Control and Prevention (Africa CDC) formed a working group to make policy and technical recommendations for the adoption and use of HIE across the continent. Because of the COVID-19 pandemic, the working group was heavily influenced to focus on cross-border data sharing for public health use purposes. However, broadly the initiative seeks to establish a firm foundation for HIE in the future within nations and across the African Union (AU).

21.4.2.1 A framework for health information exchange in Africa

The report from the working group, released to AU Member States in 2021 [44], outlines policy and technical recommendations for the development of HIE across the continent, recognizing that most eHealth systems in AU states "use technologies that are functionally suboptimal, have limited capabilities to exchange and use data from other disparate systems, and some are unsustainable due to their proprietary nature."

The policy section outlines directions for future AU and Member States policies, including:

- A governance framework and oversight mechanisms that promote partnership and collaboration among AU Member States to address emerging and endemic diseases as well as public health emergencies.

- A legal framework that ensures each Member State complies with all the HIE policies and standards.
- Data privacy and security policies that ensure security, confidentiality, and controlled access to health information.
- Data use agreements that conform to national and continental privacy provisions.

The technical section recommends a set of common technical standards for HIE, including:

- eHealth system standards and development principles to ensure interoperability of digital health tools as they are introduced and managed by Member States;
- Communication protocols to enable device to device communication;
- Messaging and vocabulary standards to facilitate electronic data collection, exchange and retrieval of relevant data, metadata, information, and knowledge; and
- Security standards to enable the secure exchange of health information.

Initial recommendations and efforts are expected to focus on data exchange within and across borders for COVID-19 and HIV. Over time, the foundation established for HIE in these use cases could expand to enable better public health cooperation across other diseases, including chronic disease and injury prevention. The work will be supported by a range of stakeholders, including international donor organizations and the Africa CDC. Furthermore, it is anticipated that progress will be evaluated by Africa CDC and other groups engaged in strengthening public health infrastructure across the AU.

21.5 Models of health information exchange postpandemic

Summary. The challenges faced by many public health authorities in the United States is stimulating conversations about a new role for HIE networks postpandemic. Namely, HIE networks are beginning to be conceived of as public health data utilities. As a public utility, use of HIE networks would be required by the state, and public funding (state and/or federal) would be invested in the development and expansion of HIE infrastructure in all states and territories. This evolution would impact governance, funding models, and alter the marketplace for HIE. It is unclear whether this notion will catch on and disrupt the HIE landscape, but it has strong potential to change HIE in the United States.

21.5.1 Why evolve health information exchange into a public utility?

In Chapter 1, we examined the dominant types of HIE networks found around the world: enterprise, community-based, government-facilitated, vendor-facilitated, and health record banking. The various forms for HIE networks have evolved over the past two decades as infrastructures matured and new functions developed to meet clinical workflow as well as regulatory needs. A disruptor to these traditional HIE forms was the COVID-19 pandemic, suggesting that models of HIE might differ in the future.

The COVID-19 pandemic challenged the health system as well as governmental public health agencies [21]. Healthcare facilities, especially hospitals, asked the HIE networks in which they participated to support their efforts at tracking patients and populations impacted by COVID-19. Public health agencies also requested that HIE networks provide them with data and information on individuals tested for SARS-CoV-2, individuals hospitalized with COVID-19, and bed availability to inform surveillance efforts as well as response efforts such as routing patients to facilities with open beds. Information needs were significant, and the needs required timely response with data from HIE networks.

Existing, mature HIE networks stepped up to support their health systems and public health agencies. Enterprise HIE networks developed dashboards to inform health system leaders guiding triage and management of COVID-19 operations on patient volumes, bed availability, and staffing [51]. Networks within health systems also tracked inventory, such as personal protective equipment, to support the safety of healthcare workers.

At the community level, HIE networks tracked patient volumes, disease burden, and population characteristics for cities and regions [52,53]. An example is the IHIE working with the Regenstrief Institute to create a community-level dashboard of COVID-19 burden for the State of Indiana in United States (Fig. 21.2). The dashboard allowed health system leaders, as well as the public, to view data on admissions and comorbid conditions during the early phases of the pandemic. Later this dashboard tracked new epidemic waves due to the Delta and Omicron variants.

Similar efforts happened in New York, Texas, Oklahoma, and across the globe. In Israel, the national (government-facilitated) HIE network implemented new functionality that displayed a patient's COVID-19 status (e.g., infected, recovered) as well as their vaccination status to clinicians within the EHR system as they navigated patients' records (see Chapter 31). Within the US Veterans Health Administration (VHA), a community-based HIE in New York City was utilized to identify Veterans hospitalized with COVID-19 outside the VHA network [54], prompting primary care teams to follow up with vulnerable patients postinfection.

Another federal program that stimulated exchange with public health is the Strengthening the Technical Advancement & Readiness of Public Health via Health Information Exchange Program (STAR HIE Program) [55]. This program sought to build innovative HIE services that benefit public health agencies as well as improve HIE services available to support communities disproportionately affected by COVID-19. A few examples from this program include:

- Georgia Health Information Network: Connected correctional facilities as well as hospitals not previously sending COVID-19 results to the state health department.
- Kansas Health Information Network: Developed a method to automate reporting of key clinical information to the state health department following a COVID-19 positive test. This approach helped public health develop a robust registry of key data on vaccines, reinfections, immunity, and other information.
- More than 10 HIE networks around the nation received supplemental funding in 2021 from the STAR HIE Program to connect state immunization registries to HIE networks in support of sending and querying COVID-19 vaccination records. These efforts helped public health streamline data collection while supporting efforts by providers to verify vaccination status and generate community reporting on vaccinated populations.

All of these examples, along with many others, elevated the profile of HIE networks in their respective communities. Clinicians realized the value of HIE as did public health agencies. In many communities, the public also realized the benefits of HIE infrastructures for the first time. For example, the Regenstrief Institute dashboard with IHIE data was cited by the Indiana Department of Health and news media daily as the information source on hospitalizations and resource utilization.

21.5.2 What is a public health data utility?

As nations begin to recover from the multiple waves of COVID-19 infection, hospitalization,

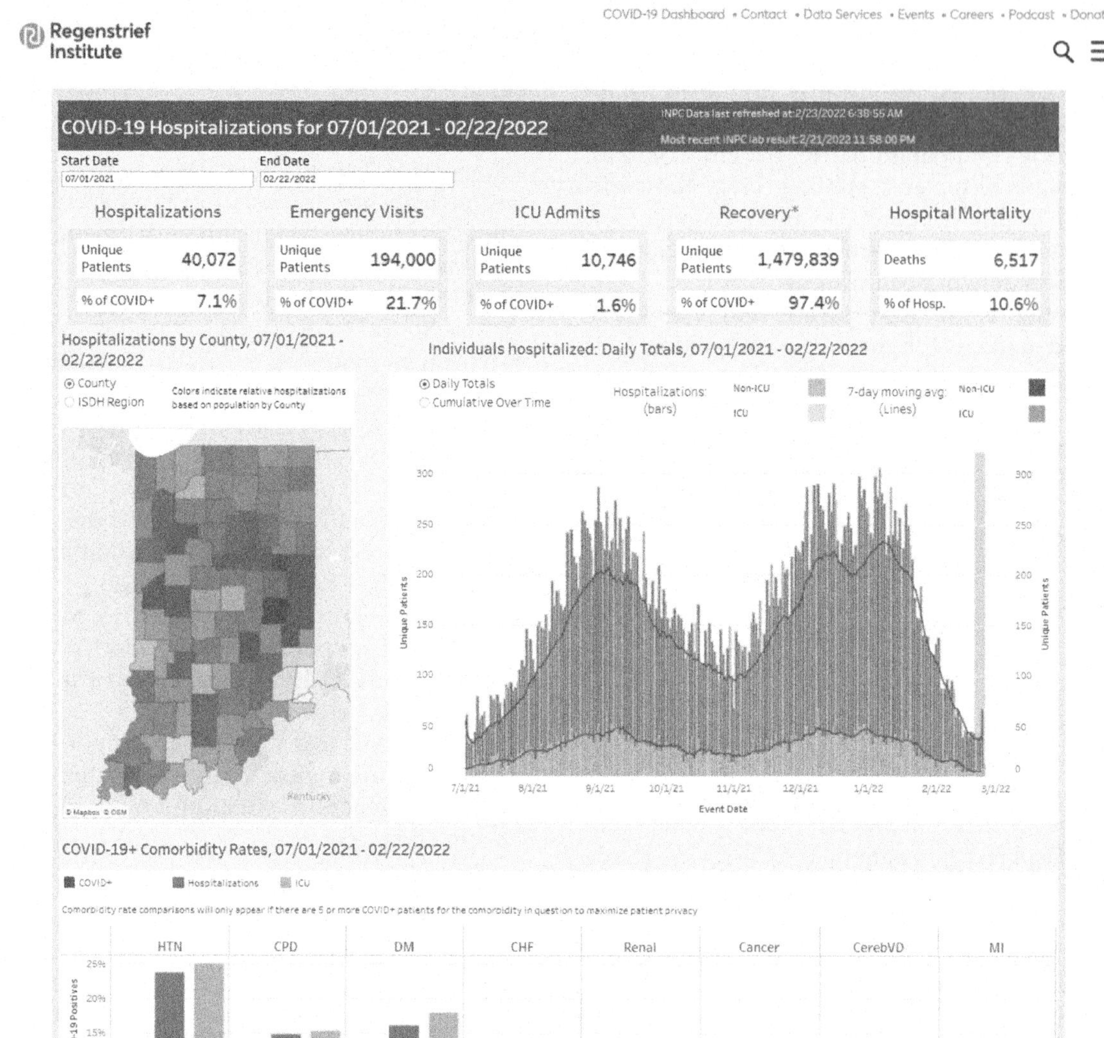

FIGURE 21.2 The Regenstrief Institute COVID-19 dashboard, powered by the Indiana Network for Patient Care that is managed by the Indiana Health Information Exchange. *CerebVD*, Cerebral vascular disease; *CHF*, chronic heart failure; *CPD*, chronic pulmonary disease; *DM*, diabetes mellitus; *HTN*, hypertension; *ICU*, intensive care unit; MI = Myocardial infarction.

and death, conversation now focuses on how best to strengthen the health system in preparation for the next pandemic as well as routine public health surveillance. One idea being discussed in the United States is a shift toward greater use of HIE networks for public and population health. The concept is that HIE networks would become a *public health data utility* in which the government would fund or underwrite the HIE infrastructure in exchange for greater utilization of the data and functions within the HIE network. Hospitals, clinics, and health systems would continue to participate in these HIE networks and asked to contribute toward the sustainability and maintenance of the infrastructure. Yet, HIE networks would no longer rely solely on private-sector funding, and governmental public health agencies would increasingly guide the evolution of HIE data and services. These networks could become QHINs under TEFCA, and collectively they could connect through an entity like the eHealth Exchange to create a national HIE network that would either supplement or replace existing quasinational networks like Carequality.

The concept of a public health data utility is a hybrid between the community-based and government-facilitated HIE models. On the one hand, state governments would compel adoption and use of the HIE through policy, making broader data and information available to users of the HIE network. State agencies would also benefit from those data and information, leveraging them to inform its activities such as surveillance and health policy. On the other hand, HIE networks would be managed by nongovernmental organizations that sit at the intersection of public health authorities and private healthcare institutions. Instead of investments in HIE infrastructure within a public health agency that might mirror that of what community-based networks provide today, investment would be made in a common infrastructure shared by government, nongovernmental, and private organizations. These infrastructures might use centralized or de-centralized architectures, but there would be a single designated HIE network for a given state or region. Much like the national HIE networks in Denmark (Chapter 28), Israel (Chapter 32), or the UAE (Chapter 33). However, if such networks exist at the state level, it remains unclear how such utilities would approach exchange of data across state lines.

21.5.3 A disruptive model for health information exchange

Some states in the United States, including Maryland (Chapter 25), were moving in this direction prepandemic. However, most community-based HIE networks remain independent of government, and not all HIEs have public health agencies as participants. The shift toward a public health data utility would be novel and potentially disruptive. Historically HIE networks grew out of private managed care organizations, so a greater role for government in HIE networks will be new for most of the United States. Second, governmental designation of an HIE network with requirement for participation by public and private health systems will likely challenge the sustainability of vendor-facilitated HIE networks. Health systems may no longer see value in paying for vendor-based networks if they can access the data they need from a statewide or regional HIE that will presumably connect them to nearly all of the providers in their region. Third, larger HIE infrastructures with significant participation by providers and governmental health agencies will likely prevent the establishment of sustainable independent, patient-mediated HIE networks. Networks developed in the private sector for patient directed exchange may struggle to garner financial support from healthcare providers when larger, more robust HIE networks exist that meet their needs. Any form of patient-mediated exchange will likely need to be wholly funded by patients subscribing to services, and patient-driven HIE networks would likely need to interoperate with the public health data utilities.

21.5.4 Advantages for public health data utilities

Public health data utilities in each state or across regions would have a number of advantages. First, participation by all providers in a state or region would enhance the value of the HIE network for all participants. Comprehensive information would be perceived as valuable to all parties, and providers would have more confidence in using the data to drive clinical decisions. Second, economies of scale would make operations and maintenance easier to manage. It would also lower costs for providers as the core infrastructure would have financial support from the government. Governmental agencies would benefit greatly from timely, more complete data on populations. Population health activities, including accountable care, learning health systems, and addressing social determinants of health would all likely benefit from more comprehensive data available on populations in a state or region. Finally, a larger, sustainable HIE network with broader stakeholder input would likely enable coordination of HIE-based services for public and population health. Providers may not need to rely as much on third parties for services if the HIE could provide a similar service for participants. Moreover, there would be less need for multiple interfaces and/or APIs for the same function across different platforms. Strategic planning could result in shared services and approaches much like those seen in Denmark and Israel as well as the planned strategies for UAE.

21.5.5 Challenges to public health data utilities and the future

Public health data utilities would not be challenge-free, however. There are potential drawbacks to this model of HIE. First, coordination of HIE services and operations across a larger set of stakeholders would likely mean slower timelines for consensus-building and implementation of new functions and services. National HIE networks in Israel and Denmark are both plagued by inertia challenges in transitioning platforms as well as development of new functions. COVID-19 functionality, however, was rapid, so urgent needs can spur quick action. Second, a stronger role for government may make providers uncomfortable and lead to greater regulation of healthcare delivery. Most HIE networks today are principally designed for providers and health systems, meeting their needs and supporting primarily individual patient care. A shift toward governmental influence, even if equal to private providers at the beginning, may result in HIE services and priorities that challenge providers. Greater measurement of performance as well as safety and quality indicators could result in government desire for additional regulations on providers. Moreover, requirements from governmental authorities over provider participation and interfaces might result in greater burden on provider-based IT support teams. Ideally overreach of governmental authority and/or requirements on provider-based IT systems would be controlled for by open, transparent governance processes and consensus-building. The key would be for the nongovernmental entity managing the HIE network to adequately facilitate dialog and decision-making processes such that all parties are comfortable with requirements, fee structures, etc. So concerns would need to be actively managed by the HIE network on an ongoing basis.

It is unclear whether any state, multiple states, or the entire United States might move toward a public health data utility model of HIE. At the time of writing, this idea was being actively debated and discussed among public and private organizations, including many community-based HIE networks. While there are concerns and challenges, they could be addressed through active and robust governance. There are clear advantages, but these networks challenge powerful actors in the US health system, and their success is not guaranteed. Therefore public health data utilities are an emerging trend that could impact the HIE landscape if the concept gathers support and at least some states or regions adopt this model over the next few years.

21.6 Conclusion

To date, HIE development in the United States has been characterized by the philosophy of "let a thousand flowers bloom." This was driven by an understanding that there is no single best way to approach HIE and that local conditions and considerations in a given community, state, or region need to be taken into account to determine the approach to HIE that would be adopted and sustained. As those flowers have bloomed, the limitations of such a philosophy have come into focus. For example, with many different HIE networks in place, provider organizations are bearing the cost and complexity of connecting to multiple different networks (or choosing not to participate at all because no single network meets their needs). Similarly, patient care is fragmented such that their data ends up within different HIE networks. And, as we move around data from many different source systems and HIE networks, there are challenges in integrating that data to create a single, harmonized patient record. These limitations magnify in the context of a public health pandemic where complete, timely data are essential. As the COVID-19 pandemic unfolded in the United States, it became rapidly apparently that our diverse HIE ecosystem was not built to meet public health information needs.

Current efforts to advance HIE are guided by the need to address these limitations. Under TEFCA, TEHDAS, and public health utility models, we are layering new data sharing frameworks and governance on top of diverse HIE approaches in order to help them function more like a seamless whole. Success is not a forgone conclusion. While there are clear benefits of pursuing these efforts, the benefits do not always align with who will bear the costs. As a result, there are many questions about whether these new models will gain traction by attracting participation and achieving implementation in ways that realize the intended benefits.

Questions for discussion

1. What are the primary challenges that emerging efforts to improve HIE are tackling?
2. What are the key ways in which emerging efforts are addressing these challenges?
3. Are there key challenges that emerging efforts are not addressing? How might these challenges be addressed?
4. Are there ways in which the future directions described in this chapter complement each other? Are there ways in which they may come into conflict with each other?
5. If there is a new pandemic in the future, based on initiatives described in this chapter, in what ways should our HIE infrastructure be more prepared to respond and meet information sharing needs?

References

[1] Medicare Payment Advisory Commission. REPORT TO THE CONGRESS - Medicare Payment Policy. MedPAC; 2005. <https://www.medpac.gov/wp-content/uploads/import_data/scrape_files/docs/default-source/reports/Mar05_EntireReport.pdf>.

[2] State Health Information Exchange. HealthIT.gov. Last reviewed April 29, 2019. <https://www.healthit.gov/topic/onc-hitech-programs/state-health-information-exchange> [accessed 01.04.22].

[3] Gold M, McLaughlin C. Assessing HITECH implementation and lessons: 5 years later. Milbank Q 2016;94(3):654–87. Available from: https://doi.org/10.1111/1468-0009.12214.

[4] Adler-Milstein J, Garg A, Zhao W, Patel V. A survey of health information exchange organizations in advance of a nationwide connectivity framework. Health Aff (Millwood) 2021;40(5):736–44. Available from: https://doi.org/10.1377/hlthaff.2020.01497.

[5] Reavis T. Prepared and ready: America's HIEs and the response to COVID-19. Journal of AHIMA. <https://journal.ahima.org/Article-Details/prepared-and-ready-americas-hies-and-the-response-to-covid-19>; 2020 [accessed 04.04.22].

[6] Patient Centered Data Home. Strategic Health Information Exchange Collaborative (SHIEC). Published 2022. <https://strategichie.com/patient-centered-data-home/> [accessed 01.04.22].

[7] eHealth Exchange. Home, Available from: <https://ehealthexchange.org/>; 2022 [accessed 01.04.22].

[8] Members and supporters. Carequality, Available from: <https://carequality.org/members-and-supporters/>; 2022 [accessed 01.04.22].

[9] CommonWell Health Alliance. Home, Available from: <https://www.commonwellalliance.org/>; 2022 [accessed 01.04.22].

[10] Johnson C, Pylypchuk Y. Use of certified health it and methods to enable interoperability by U.S. non-federal acute care hospitals, 2019. ONC Data Brief 2021;(54):20.

[11] Richwine C, Marshall C, Johnson C, Patel V. Challenges to public health reporting experienced by non-federal acute care hospitals, 2019. ONC Data Brief 2021;(56):17.

[12] Office of the National Coordinator for Health Information Technology, Department of Health and Human Services. 21st Century Cures Act: Interoperability, Information Blocking, and the ONC Health IT Certification Program. Federal Register. <https://www.federalregister.gov/documents/2020/05/01/2020-07419/21st-century-cures-act-interoperability-information-blocking-and-the-onc-health-it-certification>; 2020 [accessed 04.04.22].

[13] The Sequoia Project. *User's Guide to the Trusted Exchange Framework and Common Agreement* – TEFCA. 2022;63 <https://rce.sequoiaproject.org/wp-content/uploads/2022/01/Common-Agreement-Users-Guide.pdf>.

[14] Office of the National Coordinator for Health Information Technology, Department of Health and Human Services. The Trusted Exchange Framework (TEF): Principles for Trusted Exchange 2022;13 <https://www.healthit.gov/sites/default/files/page/2022-01/Trusted_Exchange_Framework_0122.pdf>.

[15] Office of the National Coordinator for Health Information Technology, Department of Health and Human Services, 64. Common Agreement for Nationwide Health Information Interoperability; 2022. <https://rce.sequoiaproject.org/wp-content/uploads/2022/01/Common-Agreement-for-Nationwide-Health-Information-Interoperability-Version-1.pdf>.

[16] Office of the. Qualified Health Information Network (QHIN) Technical Framework. National Coordinator for Health Information Technology, Department of Health and Human Services, 36. QTF; 2022. https://rce.sequoiaproject.org/wp-content/uploads/2022/01/QTF_0122.pdf.

[17] Office of the National Coordinator for Health Information Technology, Department of Health and Human Services. FHIR Roadmap for TEFCA Exchange 2022;10 <https://rce.sequoiaproject.org/wp-content/uploads/2022/01/FHIR-Roadmap-v1.0_updated.pdf>.

[18] Harnessing electronic health data in the palm of your hand: new survey data shows increasing availability of patient-facing APIs and early uptake by patients. Health IT Buzz. <https://www.healthit.gov/buzz-blog/consumer/harnessing-electronic-health-data-in-the-palm-of-your-hand-new-survey-data-shows-increasing-availability-of-patient-facing-apis-and-early-uptake-by-patients>; 2021 [accessed 01.04.22].

[19] Policies and technology for interoperability and burden reduction. CMS. Available from: <https://www.cms.gov/Regulations-and-Guidance/Guidance/Interoperability/index#CMS-Interoperability-and-Patient-Access-Final-Rule>; 2021 [accessed 01.04.22].

[20] Promoting interoperability programs. CMS, <https://www.cms.gov/Regulations-and-Guidance/Legislation/EHRIncentivePrograms>; 2022 [accessed 01.04.22].

[21] Dixon BE, Caine VA, Halverson PK. Deficient response to COVID-19 makes the case for evolving the public health system. Am J Prev Med 2020;59(6):887–91. Available from: https://doi.org/10.1016/j.amepre.2020.07.024.

[22] Lin SC, Lyles CR, Sarkar U, Adler-Milstein J. Are patients electronically accessing their medical records? Evidence from national hospital data. Health Aff (Millwood) 2019;38(11):1850–7. Available from: https://doi.org/10.1377/hlthaff.2018.05437.

[23] Johnson C, Richwine C, Patel V. Individuals' access and use of patient portals and smartphone health apps, 2020. ONC Data Brief 2021;(57):14.

[24] Irizarry T, DeVito Dabbs A, Curran CR. Patient portals and patient engagement: a state of the science review. J Med Internet Res 2015;17(6):e148. Available from: https://doi.org/10.2196/jmir.4255.

[25] Adler-Milstein J, Longhurst C. Assessment of patient use of a new approach to access health record data among 12 US health systems. JAMA Netw Open 2019;2(8):e199544. Available from: https://doi.org/10.1001/jamanetworkopen.2019.9544.

[26] How patient portals are failing healthcare – and our patients. Medsphere. <https://www.medsphere.com/blog/how-patient-portals-are-failing-healthcare-and-our-patients/>; 2019 [accessed 01.04.22].

[27] Otte-Trojel T, de Bont A, Aspria M, et al. Developing patient portals in a fragmented healthcare system. Int J Med Inform 2015;84(10):835–46. Available from: https://doi.org/10.1016/j.ijmedinf.2015.07.001.

[28] Rudin RS, Motala A, Goldzweig CL, Shekelle PG. Usage and effect of health information exchange: a systematic review. Ann Intern Med 2014;161(11):803–11. Available from: https://doi.org/10.7326/M14-0877.

[29] Rahurkar S, Vest JR, Finnell JT, Dixon BE. Trends in user-initiated health information exchange in the inpatient, outpatient, and emergency settings. J Am Med Inform Assoc 2021;28(3):622–7. Available from: https://doi.org/10.1093/jamia/ocaa226.

[30] Apathy NC. Health Information Exchange Use in Primary Care (Ph.D. thesis). Indianapolis, IN: Indiana University – Purdue University Indianapolis; 2020 [accessed 01.04.22]. <https://www.proquest.com/docview/2437187770/abstract/96BB3448BCD44D07PQ/1>.

[31] Sharing Health Information for Treatment. American Hospital Association; 2018:5. <https://www.aha.org/system/files/2018-03/sharing-health-information.pdf> [accessed 01.04.22].

[32] Everson J. The implications and impact of 3 approaches to health information exchange: community, enterprise, and vendor-mediated health information exchange. Learn Health Syst 2017;1:e10021.

[33] Adler-Milstein J, Neinstein AB, Cucina RJ. Improving interoperability by moving from perfection to pragmatism. Health Affairs. Health Affairs Blog. Available from: <https://www.healthaffairs.org/do/10.1377/forefront.20210105.661344>; 2021 [accessed 01.04.22].

[34] Product spotlight: Health Dart. Indiana Health Information Exchange. <https://www.ihie.org/product-spotlight-fhir-chest-pain-app/>; 2020 [accessed 01.04.22].

[35] Adler-Milstein J, Wang MD. The impact of transitioning from availability of outside records within electronic health records to integration of local and outside records within electronic health records. J Am Med Inf Assoc 2020;27(4):606–12. Available from: https://doi.org/10.1093/jamia/ocaa006.

[36] Winden TJ, Boland LL, Frey NG, Satterlee PA, Hokanson JS. Care everywhere, a point-to-point HIE tool. Utilization and impact on patient care in the (ED.). Appl Clin Inform 2014;5(2):388–401. Available from: https://doi.org/10.4338/aci-2013-12-ra-0100.

[37] McDonald CJ, Huff SM, Suico JG, et al. LOINC, a universal standard for identifying laboratory observations: a 5-year update. Clin Chem 2003;49(4):624–33. Available from: https://doi.org/10.1373/49.4.624.

[38] Dixon BE, Siegel JA, Oemig TV, Grannis SJ. Electronic health information quality challenges and interventions to improve public health surveillance data and practice. Public Health Rep 2013;128(6):546–53. Available from: https://doi.org/10.1177/003335491312800614.

[39] Wu J, Finnell JT, Vreeman DJ. Evaluating congruence between laboratory LOINC value sets for quality measures, public health reporting, and mapping common tests. AMIA Annu Symp Proc 2013;2013:1525–32.

[40] Zunner C, Bürkle T, Prokosch HU, Ganslandt T. Mapping local laboratory interface terms to LOINC at a German university hospital using RELMA V.5: a semi-automated approach. J Am Med Inform Assoc 2013;20(2):293–7. Available from: https://doi.org/10.1136/amiajnl-2012-001063.

[41] Vreeman DJ, Hook J, Dixon BE. Learning from the crowd while mapping to LOINC. J Am Med Inform Assoc 2015;22(6):1205–11. Available from: https://doi.org/10.1093/jamia/ocv098.

[42] LOINC in vitro diagnostic (LIVD) test code mapping for SARS-CoV-2 tests. CDC. <https://www.cdc.gov/csels/dls/sars-cov-2-livd-codes.html>; 2022 [accessed 01.04.22].

[43] Digital health platform that combines all your medical records into one place. OneRecord. <https://onerecord.com>; 2022 [accessed 01.04.22].

[44] Africa Centers for Disease Control and Prevention. AU health information exchange: policy and standards for health information system. Addis Ababa: African Union; 2021.

[45] Joint Action Towards the European Health Data Space – TEHDAS. TEHDAS. <https://tehdas.eu/> [accessed 01.04.22].

[46] Identification of relevant standards and data models for semantic harmonization. TEHDAS. <https://tehdas.eu/app/uploads/2022/02/tehdas-identification-of-relevant-standards-and-data-models-for-semantic-harmonization-2022-02-03.pdf>; 2022 [accessed 01.04.22].

[47] Overhage JM, Ryan PB, Reich CG, Hartzema AG, Stang PE. Validation of a common data model for active safety surveillance research. J Am Med Inform Assoc 2012;19(1):54–60. Available from: https://doi.org/10.1136/amiajnl-2011-000376.

[48] European Health Data Space. European Commission. Published 2022. <https://ec.europa.eu/health/ehealth-digital-health-and-care/european-health-data-space_en> [accessed 01.04.22].

[49] TEHDAS suggests options to overcome data barriers. TEHDAS. <https://tehdas.eu/results/tehdas-suggests-options-to-overcome-data-barriers/>; February 28, 2022 [accessed 01.04.22].

[50] Package 8: citizens. TEHDAS, <https://tehdas.eu/packages/package-8-citizens/> [accessed 04.04.22].

[51] Reeves JJ, Hollandsworth HM, Torriani FJ, et al. Rapid response to COVID-19: health informatics support for outbreak management in an academic health system. J Am Med Inform Assoc 2020;27(6):853–9. Available from: https://doi.org/10.1093/jamia/ocaa037.

[52] Dixon BE, Grannis SJ, McAndrews C, et al. Leveraging data visualization and a statewide health information exchange to support COVID-19 surveillance and response: application of public health informatics. J Am Med Inform Assoc 2021;28(7):1363–73. Available from: https://doi.org/10.1093/jamia/ocab004.

[53] Tortolero GA, Brown MR, Sharma SV, et al. Leveraging a health information exchange for analyses of COVID-19 outcomes including an example application using smoking history and mortality. PLoS One 2021;16(6):e0247235. Available from: https://doi.org/10.1371/journal.pone.0247235.

[54] Sherman RL, Judon KM, Koufacos NS, et al. Utilizing a health information exchange to facilitate COVID-19 VA primary care follow-up for Veterans diagnosed in the community. JAMIA Open 2021;4(1):ooab020. Available from: https://doi.org/10.1093/jamiaopen/ooab020.

[55] STAR HIE Program. HealthIT.gov. <https://www.healthit.gov/topic/star-hie-program>; 2021 [accessed 01.04.22].

SECTION 5

Case studies in health information exchange

CHAPTER

22

The Indiana Health Information Exchange

J. Marc Overhage[1] *and John P. Kansky*[2]

[1]Enterprise Analytics Core, Elevance Health, Indianapolis, IN, USA [2]Indiana Health Information Exchange, Indianapolis, IN, USA

LEARNING OBJECTIVES

- Understand the pivotal role of data reuse in creating value through health information exchange.
- Appreciate why the highest value use cases have to be carefully prioritized to successfully grow health information exchange.
- Understand the approach that IHIE has successfully utilized to create mutual value to health information exchange participants.

Major themes

Significant themes that should be evident in this case study include the ongoing goal of sustaining value by improving the quality and efficiency of health and care. This goal was achieved through persistence, systematically building on successes and pragmatism.

22.1 Introduction

When we began to create what would become the Indiana Network for Patient Care (INPC), efforts to develop Community Health Information Networks had, with very few exceptions, failed. Initially, these efforts focused primarily on administrative transactions and depended on relatively expensive and difficult to implement technologies. Regenstrief Institute investigators created an enterprise medical record (EMR) system that integrated the disparate "best of breed" information systems common in health systems during the 1970s and 1980s. By the mid-1990s, Regenstrief started to extend the EMR to meet the needs of physicians of the Indiana University (IU) School of Medicine who routinely practiced across the county hospital system (then known as Wishard Memorial Hospital), the Veterans Health Administration (VHA) hospital, and University Hospital, as well as the patients they cared for across these facilities. They focused on clinical, rather than

Health Information Exchange
DOI: https://doi.org/10.1016/B978-0-323-90802-3.00022-8

administrative, functions in this work. The rapid evolution of Internet technologies combined with Regenstrief Institute investigators' leadership and experience with healthcare IT standards stimulated a technological development creating an opportunity to develop a low-cost scalable approach to what is now called health information exchange (HIE).

While the Indiana HIE (IHIE) grew out of a research initiative, an early emphasis on sustainability and practicality has ensured that broad adoption, long-term growth, and economic viability would be critical drivers for the network. These guiding principles served as the foundation for the 2004 incorporation of IHIE as a not-for-profit supporting organization [a community-based health information organization (HIO) based on definitions in Chapter 1] with the initial goals of:

- making Central Indiana a national leader in the use of electronic health information to deliver superior healthcare and to lower the cost of that care;
- developing and implementing an HIE network that enables hospitals, physicians, laboratories, pharmacies, and other health services providers to deliver faster, more accurate, safer, higher quality, and less redundant medical care to patients in Central Indiana;
- benefiting the work of medical and public health researchers by making available the unique databases that will be developed through the HIE network, which will, in turn, benefit hospitals, payers, pharmacy benefits managers, employers, public health agencies, drug companies, and ultimately patients; and
- facilitating the development and adoption of new health-related technologies which is likely to result in new job opportunities in the Central Indiana economy.

22.2 Context

Indiana, whose motto is "The Crossroads of America," reasonably represents the United States overall. It has a population of approximately 6.8 million that is 85% white, 10% black, and 7% Hispanic, with an age distribution similar to the rest of the United States. Slightly more than 20% of the population lives in rural areas. Indianapolis is the largest metropolitan statistical area with almost 30% of the population. Over half (56%) of the State's citizens are covered by employer-sponsored plans, 4.5% by individual plans, 16.8% by Medicaid, 14.6% by Medicare, and 6.1% are uninsured. Almost 1 in 5 Hoosiers (17.1%) rate their health as poor or fair, and over half (51.9%) rate it as very good or excellent.

As with many states, Indiana healthcare referral patterns cross state boundaries. Ft. Wayne in the northeastern corner and Evansville in the southwestern corners anchor care in their regions spanning adjacent states. Care in the state's southeastern corner is anchored by the Louisville, KY, and Cincinnati, OH markets. There are several large health systems in the State, including Indiana University Health, Franciscan Alliance, and Community Health Network. Indianapolis is home to one of the nation's largest essential healthcare systems in the nation, Eskenazi Health, which has a 333-bed hospital and 12 community health centers across the metro area. National systems, including Ascension Health and HCA, also have facilities in Indiana. There are 130 acute care hospital facilities in the state. Approximately 17,400 physicians practice in Indiana, with 8300 practicing in a primary care specialty. The majority of physicians are employed either directly or indirectly by hospitals.

In the mid-1990s, investigators at the Regenstrief Institute, an international leader in developing and evaluating health information technology, with funding from the Agency for Healthcare Research and Quality (AHRQ) and the National Library of Medicine (NLM), engaged central Indiana stakeholders, including health systems, public health departments, physicians, businesses, payers, and philanthropies to build on previous work to create the INPC [1]. The INPC is a contractual basis for the HIE network in the state that was initially managed and operated by the Regenstrief Institute but is now managed and operated by the not-for-profit IHIE.

Since 1994, Regenstrief investigators and IHIE have evolved the capabilities and expanded the scope of the INPC while maintaining its original focus and priorities. While developing the INPC, we focused on solving the problems of clinicians trying to care for patients with incomplete data. Patients were often seen by physicians in an emergency care setting, for example, without critical data about their condition and treatment being made available to the medical staff. The INPC was initially established with 27 data-sharing partners, including representation from hospitals, practices, community health clinics, and homeless care sites. Initial features included a secure wide-area network, a clinical data repository, and software to enable a cross-institutional combined view of an individual's medical results.

Over the next two decades, a series of grants from federal agencies (including the AHRQ, NLM, National Cancer Institute, and Office of the National Coordinator for Health Information Technology) and private foundations (Regenstrief Foundation, Markle Foundation, and Fairbanks Foundation) were used to capitalize the creation of the core technology infrastructure and operate the exchange [2–6]. During this time, Regenstrief investigators studied the core problems, including patient identity management, privacy and confidentiality, data normalization, and assessing the value created through HIE [7–10]. These are the subjects in Sections **1 and 2** of this book.

In 2003 a report commissioned by Indianapolis business community leaders identified life sciences as a priority for business development. In response, a new organization named BioCrossroads (http://www.biocrossroads.com) convened workgroups that determined that the community should foster the development of health information technology in Indiana. BioCrossroads commissioned the Boston Consulting Group to explore the most effective way to create and implement health IT in the community based on these recommendations.

Three significant, early challenges could have scuttled the development of IHIE. First, hospital Chief Information Officers asked whether IHIE (community-based HIE) competes with the individual hospital IT strategies to link physician offices (e.g., enterprise HIE). The community resolved this challenge by recognizing that the EHR systems in the hospitals addressed internal, institutional workflows and that participation in the city-wide network could globally reduce operating costs for the health systems.

Second, hospital Chief Financial Officers asserted, "I do not see any significant ROI (return on investment) and recommend to their Chief Executive Officers (CEOs) not to proceed." Fortunately, a ROI analysis showed that large-scale delivery of clinical results to ambulatory provider practices appreciably lowered costs resulting in measurable returns, in addition to likely intangible returns. Based on these results, the health system CEOs' vision that INPC is the infrastructure for future healthcare initiatives and cost savings carried the day.

The inevitable question of who would capitalize the project came to the fore. The Regenstrief Institute's development of the INPC coincided with overcoming the other challenges.

So, in 2004, Indianapolis civic leaders created IHIE to provide technical support and help develop a sustainable business model for the INPC. Major hospital systems agreed to provide startup capital for IHIE clinical results delivery service as prepaid fees. This blending of research and commercial perspectives proved a successful formula for the community-based HIE network.

The HIE landscape has changed in many ways over the last 18 years. By the time the HITECH Act passed in 2009, INPC leaders and stakeholders had over a decade of experience building community trust, assessing needs, and responding to issues such as privacy and security. HITECH, the 21st Century Cures Act, the emergence of EHR vendor-facilitated HIE networks, and other market dynamics dramatically changed the landscape. Current efforts to foster interoperability will not have the luxury of developing at this pace and must demonstrate value early in the implementation process. The high costs of building infrastructure may make it difficult for HIE networks to demonstrate their value to stakeholders at inception. Delaying value creation can slow the momentum of an HIE network. Emerging interoperability efforts do, however, have the advantage of existing data nomenclature standards such as Logical Observation Identifiers and Name Codes (LOINC) and RxNorm (see Chapter 10), technical solutions for patient matching (see Chapter 12), and commercial products for HIE, as well as greater visibility and acceptance of the value of HIE by healthcare leadership (see Chapter 16).

22.3 The Indiana Health Information Exchange

22.3.1 Organization

Initially, the Regenstrief Institute was responsible for the INPC's technical direction, implementation, and operations, including application and technical support. Over time, IHIE has completely assumed the responsibility for growing the technology and technical operations and expanded the technology partners. Today, IHIE is a statewide not-for-profit health data business and the organization that provides focus and infrastructure to expand the reach of currently available services, provide customer support, business development, technical resources, and physician liaisons. IHIE is also responsible for identifying potential sources of capital and assessing the feasibility of potential use cases, emphasizing the value of participation for different stakeholders.

The stakeholders in IHIE were aligned across several categories, including external environment, organizational environment, consensus about goals, consensus about means, unique local aspects of the market, consensus about roles, the potential value that IHIE could bring, and consensus around behavioral expectations [11].

IHIE is a nonprofit 501(c)3 supporting organization and is HITRUST certified. It operates through various governance structures that facilitate efficient consultation with diverse stakeholders. The primary stakeholder structure is a Board of Directors consisting of 16 organizations representing the hospital networks, public agencies, medical societies, physicians, consumers, and researchers. The most challenging work was establishing trusted organizational models, consensus on goals and requirements, and crafting participation agreements that met each party's legal, clinical, and ownership requirements. IHIE maintains active relationships with clinical and organizational leaders within INPC member organizations that provide guidance and expertise to assist future development. These relationships are multidisciplinary, encompassing technical, clinical, customer service, and users.

The INPC Management Committee, which operates separately from IHIE's Board of Directors, evaluates each new proposed INPC use case, such as adding a data type to the exchange, for its appropriateness. They assess aspects of the proposed change, including how many patients are affected, what organizations need to involve, and how to implement the new service. This approach has been in place since IHIE's inception. By understanding the stakeholders' objectives and developing the exchange to support those objectives, the Management Committee achieved a degree of social alignment primarily through a complex and somewhat organic communication process.

22.3.2 Community engagement

IHIE engages clinicians, health plans, and other organizations across the health ecosystem through direct outreach. Because of the community's emphasis on supporting healthcare, the life sciences, and health IT, many potential participants have existing collegial relationships that facilitate willingness to participate. Other factors that stimulate interest in participation are IHIE's cost-effective solution for results delivery and increasing interest and investment in health IT across Indiana. IHIE notes that its relationships and INPC participation have been built over a long time. They also benefit from an ongoing relationship with BioCrossroads to help facilitate discussions among stakeholders—particularly in the life sciences segment. Providers were often unaware of HIE (as a verb) early on, and a long period of education and communication was required to engage them. More recently, awareness is higher, though deep engagement still requires considerable time and effort. For example, members of the nursing home industry were in discussions with INPC for five years before the first long-term care facility signed a participation agreement in spring 2010.

As of December 2021, the INPC includes data from over 117 hospitals, two long-term care groups, local and national laboratories, including Labcorp and Quest, imaging centers, and pharmacies connected to INPC, with approximately 15 billion structured observations on over 15 million unique patients. Over 50,000 providers in 18,000 practices use the HIE. Indiana Medicaid shares administrative data, including prescription records. Nearly all Indiana emergency departments (EDs) are connected to capture real-time chief complaint data for biosurveillance and outbreak detection. The Indiana Department of Health (IDOH) and the Marion County Public Health Department share immunization information, public health laboratory results, and tumor (cancer) registry data. Images (PDF) of electrocardiograms from 47 health systems are available as well.

In 2009 five organizations were facilitating HIE in the State of Indiana. Over time, all five organizations have been subsumed or merged with IHIE so that, as of 2021, IHIE is the singular HIO connecting providers across the state. Driven in part by the critical need to share data during the COVID-19 pandemic, nearly all the remaining health systems that were not participating before 2020 have begun sharing data, leading to a genuinely statewide HIE network.

A critical factor in engaging participants is to offer relevant, valuable services. IHIE must be cautious in choosing what services to implement and in what order since each service needs to be financially self-sufficient; sources of participant engagement, sources of capital to create the service, technological capabilities, and business models have to be aligned. By alignment, we mean creating an architectural, operational, and business approach that distributes value across all stakeholders rather than funding. According to a 2006 Deloitte Center for Health Solutions report [12], while "financing and ROI issues often receive a disproportionate share of stakeholder attention, successful HIE [network]s keep their purpose and mission at the forefront." IHIE has focused on value and facilitating the business need to share patient data to improve quality, safety, and efficiency [12].

HIE networks are expected to improve efficiency and reduce healthcare costs. However, if their primary purpose becomes cost control, they will likely fail. IHIE has explored several value-added services that rely on normalized data. These include syndromic surveillance, emergency medical technician access, and INPC access at mass sporting events.

Not all services proved successful. For example, early on, IHIE had discussions with pharmacy benefit managers and payers about an incremental approach to e-prescribing. The initial step for this approach was to support the delivery of a printed medication history synthesizing data from multiple medication sources. A combination of factors resulted in IHIE's choice not to pursue this service. By the time IHIE had overcome the technical challenges and a business model evolved, e-prescribing had begun to expand rapidly. IHIE was essentially too late in fielding this service.

22.3.3 Use

Even when there is potential to improve the value of the care, providers find changing behaviors difficult given the extreme time pressure and many demands on their attention. IHIE created services to reduce barriers and simplify access. For example, the earliest service delivered a summary of each patient's data to the physician caring for them in the ED. The INPC used admission discharge transfer (ADT) messages generated when a patient was registered to trigger the system to print a summary on distinctively colored green paper, which clerical personnel placed with the paper documents used to manage the patients in the department. This approach ensured that, while the providers could log in and review or query data in detail, they always had ready access to crucial patient data without any effort other than to glance at the page.

Physicians have always sought additional detail in more complicated cases that represent a minority of patients. Many anecdotes exist of care improved by the data available through the INPC. Over the years, there were many efforts to increase the proportion of patients for which physicians took advantage of the INPC data through lookup using the CareWeb service. Still, it was not until single sign-on integration with the EMR physicians were using to care for their patients that were implemented late in 2014 that the proportion of patients for which INPC data were accessed materially increased [13]. Subsequently developed services like HealthDart (see Section 22.3.7) take this concept further by providing access to context-specific patient data by clicking a primary complaint-specific button in the EHR interface.

Other services such as DOCS4DOCS, the IHIE service that delivers results and reports to providers, are also built around providers' preferences for how they want results integrated into their practice's workflow.

22.3.4 Financial model

The operation of the exchange has been self-sustaining since 2011. Its operational costs are covered through its "bundled" subscription fees (including clinical messaging and clinical repository services). Initially, IHIE charged per transaction (clinical message delivered). However, growing aggregated transaction fees discouraged utilization among large providers, and IHIE transitioned to an "all you can eat" membership fee model based upon adjusted patient days. IHIE continually works to identify ways to leverage data, such as electronic lab reporting, event-triggered care management data and access, automated transmission of reportable condition data to the public health authority, and supporting disability eligibility determination by the Social Security Administration.

Organizations providing HIE face the challenge of any multiparty network service [14]. To survive, they must reach a critical mass of users. Expanding the number of users and uses allows IHIE to distribute the core costs of data capture, normalization, and storage. Cost distribution supports sustainability. Some value-added services become less expensive and more technologically feasible as more organizations share the costs of an HIE infrastructure. The cost of standardizing a given kind of data source is relatively independent of the volume of data produced; any organization supporting interoperability must focus its resources on the high-volume data producers to reach critical mass. In most communities, these will be the large health systems. Of course, integrating lower volume providers such as federally qualified health centers, public schools, and long-term care providers is essential, and costs may have to be subsidized through revenues from services, philanthropy, or other sources.

IHIE creates value primarily by extracting data out of silos within participant organizations and establishing trust in the community allowing the data to be aggregated and accessible by providers and other stakeholders who need the information to improve patient and population health. The INPC's architecture supports and facilitates data use and reuse. The term reuse, or secondary use, has a negative connotation. However, the reality is that in healthcare, nearly every use is reuse beyond the primary reason for collecting the data (e.g., documentation or billing). Therefore some prefer to use the term "continuous use" of data rather than "reuse." Regardless of what term is used, real-world data and information are valuable for a range of healthcare purposes. Therefore HIE networks create value when they can make data and information available in a wide range of contexts for use—in as many different ways as possible that produce value, support the HIEs mission, and contribute to sustainability.

HIE operations, like most service businesses, are labor-intensive. Building and maintaining interfaces to and from data sources and the initial and ongoing semantic normalization of data from different sources (i.e., "mapping") make up roughly half of the ongoing expenses. The training and support of new and existing customers make up another quarter. The remaining quarter is divided, in decreasing portions, among software, database setup and maintenance, project management, data center and hardware, and professional services. The business model created for access to the INPC clinical data repository relies on health systems paying a fee scaled by their size. This access will, in return, improve the quality, safety, and efficiency of care they provide. IHIE's sustainability strategy is based on principles key to HIE being a self-sustaining endeavor:

- HIE is a business
- Leverage high-cost, high-value assets
- No loss leaders
- Independent, local sustainability
- HIEs are natural monopolies
- There is an optimal size for an HIE—the need for scale
- Avoid grants for operational cost—HIE services must be able to generate revenue equal to or above expenses

Refer to Chapter 5 for more principles on sustaining HIE operations.

22.3.5 Technical approach

IHIE strives to keep its technical architecture simple to facilitate participation and engagement. The INPC system stores data in a federated model, with all data physically residing in a central location [6]. However, the source institution logically separates data, even though they operate in the same software system. Messages from source systems flow into one centralized process. The INPC standardizes HL7 message formats and maps local observation and report codes to standard codes (e.g., reference terminology described in Chapter 10). It also links multiple patient and physician identifiers for one individual to a global identifier (e.g., client registry as described in Chapter 12).

The INPC system matches patients within and across institutions, creating a longitudinal patient-centric record (e.g., shared health records described in Chapter 11). The current patient-matching infrastructure requires a patient identifier or medical record number assigned by a known registration authority to be associated with results or observations about the patient. A deterministic matching algorithm links multiple records for one patient, enabling a view of the patient's data, no matter its source.

Various data services require different standardization efforts. On the one hand, report delivery services such as DOCS4DOCS require relatively small (a few person-weeks) amounts of effort per data source, most of which is consumed by standardizing the local provider codes used to identify report recipients. INPC maps local laboratory, radiology, and drug codes to national terminology standards for other use cases.

Mapping to a standard code system, or reference terminology, allows the INPC to consolidate patient data in decision support, public health, and research. The INPC's perspective is that data can only be leveraged for use and reuse if represented in a standard format. Therefore supporting the use of LOINC and RxNorm were central to INPC's early work. Regenstrief developed, maintains, and supports LOINC for laboratory and other clinical observations. The INPC maps all institution laboratory codes to LOINC.

The use of CCDs, or continuity of care documents, has increased gradually as an alternative or additional format for exchanging data. More than 100,000 CCDs per month are currently received from 55 hospitals, yet this still represents a minority of all data exchanged. IHIE delivers CCDs to providers as part of certain services it offers, including through the DOCS4DOCS system. CCDs are retained, and specific data types are extracted and analyzed, when necessary, to support services or specific data needs. IHIE can also deliver CCDs in response to queries such as those originated by EPIC's Care Everywhere system. In addition, as part of the VHA's HIE efforts, IHIE exchanges CCDs with VHA facilities across the country. Unfortunately, providers are still dissatisfied with the content and workflow associated with CCDs as a medium for HIE [15].

Over the last decade, IHIE made several significant enhancements to the underlying technical infrastructure of the INPC. First, they completely redeveloped the software, moving from a locally developed hierarchical database to a commercial relational database (Oracle), and reimplemented the code in JAVA to create a contemporary, service-oriented architecture. Second, they fully virtualized the system and migrated it from the public hospital's data center, where the exchange had been hosted since its inception, to a contemporary hardware and storage environment in a commercial data center. This move increased reliability, performance, and security. One of the most critical technical infrastructure efforts IHIE undertook was creating and refining an improved process for interfacing participants. The process for "onboarding" new organizations had proven to be a rate-limiting step in the network's growth. It is also a challenge for other HIE networks and public health departments seeking to onboard providers.

IHIE's approach to onboarding included establishing a project management office, monthly status tracking, dedicated interface engineers, and detailed process maps. While this approach improved the process, IHIE was still unsatisfied with the progress rate and continued exploring enhancing its interfacing capability. They also established a master provider index (e.g., health worker registry as described in Chapter 14) with matching during the project. This functionality allows IHIE to link all data for a provider even though different provider identifiers might be used. For example, a drug enforcement admistration identification number might identify a prescription record from Surescripts (a national network for pharmacy claims data). In contrast, the local laboratory ID identifies a laboratory result for that provider. This linking capability facilitated access to the clinical data repository across provider organizations to aggregate data related to the provider for clinical data reporting and other similar functions.

A related technological improvement was creating a provider attribution system: a method for associating a patient with a specific provider accountable for their care. This system utilizes a predictive model (see Chapter 18) that uses data about the transactions passing through the exchange to identify providers who can be considered accountable or responsible for the patient's care. Analyzing which provider received laboratory results, wrote prescriptions, had encounters with them, and wrote notes about a patient over a specific period can inform which provider is providing the patient's care. This attribution is used, for example, to select the patients used for provider quality reporting. While in some quality programs, a member may specifically identify an accountable provider (e.g., a Primary Care Physician), the payor has to decide which patients quality a provider gets credit for in other programs. Because HIEs typically capture data for the entire population, they are uniquely positioned to measure quality since they can include all patients and not just those from a single payor. This unique capability was part of the rationale for IHIE developing its Quality Health First (QHF) program described below.

22.3.6 Privacy and confidentiality

The INPC contains, and IHIE's services disclose, highly confidential information protected by federal and state law. As a result, the governing agreements contain stringent confidentiality provisions. All information stored on and received through the INPC network must be kept confidential under all applicable laws, as well as each participant's own internal rules and regulations relating to the confidentiality of patient health information. The terms and conditions agreement that govern INPC members' participation in the INPC incorporate recent changes to the Health Insurance Portability and Accountability Act (HIPAA) under HITECH, a reporting process for severe breaches of confidentiality, and changes to support the 21st Century Cures Act implementation (see Chapter 6). The agreement allows the use of the repository data for prescribed treatment, public health and research, and purposes with oversight by the INPC Management Committee. Only authorized INPC member users associated with a given institution are given INPC access to the records of patients according to the agreed-upon "trigger and access window rules" based on the approved uses. It permits research on de-identified data extracts but prohibits analysis that compares institutions or providers, even if de-identified unless authorized explicitly by the involved parties.

Because the pool of patients is so large and inclusive, the INPC adopted more stringent rules than HIPAA requirements and constrains clinicians' access to a narrow subset of data necessary to meet the users' specific needs under a given set of circumstances. A few principles or rules are applied to limit the information that is made accessible.

IHIE based its first rule on "proximity" between patient and provider. The INPC knows when a patient has checked into a given facility because it receives all check-in ADT messages. It uses the information from the ADT messages to provide clinicians working within a given facility access to the INPC records for patients who are concurrently in that facility receiving care. IHIE has been using this proximity-based approach in Indianapolis EDs for years. They now employ the same method for clinicians and patients in each hospital.

The HIE network based its second rule on institutional privileges. This rule allows providers who have staff privileges at two or more INPC institutions to access the INPC data from all their institutions at once, so they can look at a patient's data as one record. In the combined view, individual results are footnoted with their institutional source to clarify the data's origin. Physicians already have the right to look at the medical record data in each hospital by virtue of their staff privileges; the INPC makes access more straightforward and the data more digestible.

Finally, the system can enable access to a patient's clinical data based on a patient-provider relationship as evidenced by a formally scheduled appointment. Access is enabled for a period around an appointment (the duration depends on the encounter setting), clinical allowing the provider to prepare for and follow up on the patient's care.

22.3.7 Services

IHIE offers three suites of services targeted at different customer groups: OneCare, PopCare, and GovCare.

22.3.7.1 OneCare

An important turning point in the evolution of HIE in Indiana was developing the DOCS4DOCS report delivery system (now part of IHIE's OneCare suite of services). When INPC first began exchanging data, they used a "pull" model offering a comprehensive view of patients' records at the point of care. In 2003 INPC learned that clinicians would not always look up data and wanted a "push" model. Regenstrief responded by developing DOCS4DOCS, a clinical messaging service that sends text reports such as laboratory, radiology, transcriptions, and cardiology from hospital source systems and delivers the information to affiliated providers. DOCS4DOCS provides three methods for physicians to receive or access clinical data from participating organizations:

- *Secure inbox*—the DOCS4DOCS portal is a secure, web-based "inbox." See Fig. 22.1.
- *Direct EHR Integration*—clinical messages can be delivered directly to an ambulatory

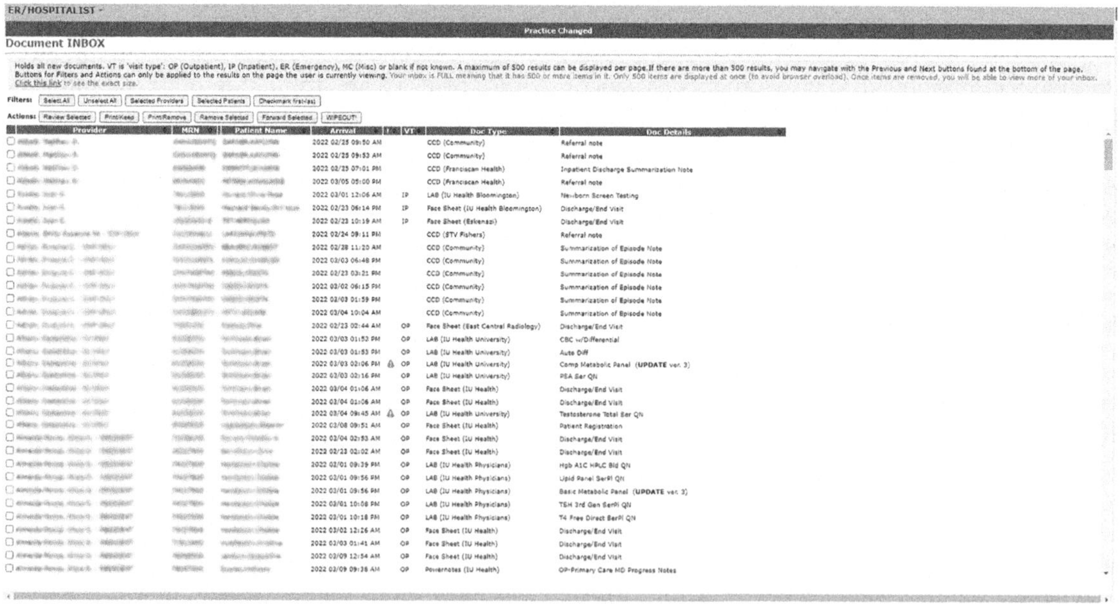

ER/HOSPITALIST -

Practice Changed

Document INBOX

Holds all new documents. VT is 'visit type': OP (Outpatient), IP (Inpatient), ER (Emergency), MC (Misc) or blank if not known. A maximum of 500 results can be displayed per page.If there are more than 500 results, you may navigate with the Previous and Next buttons found at the bottom of the page. Buttons for Filters and Actions can only be applied to the results on the page the user is currently viewing. Your inbox is FULL meaning that it has 500 or more items in it. Only 500 items are displayed at once (to avoid browser overload). Once items are removed, you will be able to view more of your inbox. Click this link to see the exact size.

Filters: Select All | Unselect All | Selected Providers | Selected Patients | Checkmark first-last

Actions: Review Selected | Print/Keep | Print/Remove | Remove Selected | Forward Selected | WIPEOUT!

Provider	MRN	Patient Name	Arrival	!	VT	Doc Type	Doc Details
[illegible]	[illegible]	[illegible]	2022 02/25 09:50 AM			CCD (Community)	Referral note
[illegible]	[illegible]	[illegible]	2022 02/25 09:53 AM			CCD (Community)	Referral note
[illegible]	[illegible]	[illegible]	2022 02/25 07:01 PM			CCD (Franciscan Health)	Inpatient Discharge Summarization Note
[illegible]	[illegible]	[illegible]	2022 03/05 05:00 PM			CCD (Franciscan Health)	Referral note
[illegible]	[illegible]	[illegible]	2022 03/01 12:06 AM		IP	LAB (IU Health Bloomington)	Newborn Screen Testing
[illegible]	[illegible]	[illegible]	2022 02/23 06:14 PM		IP	Face Sheet (IU Health Bloomington)	Discharge/End Visit
[illegible]	[illegible]	[illegible]	2022 02/23 10:19 AM		IP	Face Sheet (Eskenazi)	Discharge/End Visit
[illegible]	[illegible]	[illegible]	2022 02/24 09:11 PM			CCD (STV Fishers)	Referral note
[illegible]	[illegible]	[illegible]	2022 02/28 11:20 AM			CCD (Community)	Summarization of Episode Note
[illegible]	[illegible]	[illegible]	2022 03/03 06:48 PM			CCD (Community)	Summarization of Episode Note
[illegible]	[illegible]	[illegible]	2022 02/23 03:21 PM			CCD (Community)	Summarization of Episode Note
[illegible]	[illegible]	[illegible]	2022 03/02 06:15 PM			CCD (Community)	Summarization of Episode Note
[illegible]	[illegible]	[illegible]	2022 02/03 01:59 PM			CCD (Community)	Summarization of Episode Note
[illegible]	[illegible]	[illegible]	2022 03/04 10:04 AM			CCD (Community)	Summarization of Episode Note
[illegible]	[illegible]	[illegible]	2022 02/23 02:44 AM		OP	Face Sheet (East Central Radiology)	Discharge/End Visit
[illegible]	[illegible]	[illegible]	2022 03/03 01:52 PM		OP	LAB (IU Health University)	CBC w/Differential
[illegible]	[illegible]	[illegible]	2022 03/03 01:53 PM		OP	LAB (IU Health University)	Auto Diff
[illegible]	[illegible]	[illegible]	2022 03/03 02:06 PM	⚠	OP	LAB (IU Health University)	Comp Metabolic Panel (**UPDATE** ver. 3)
[illegible]	[illegible]	[illegible]	2022 03/03 02:16 PM		OP	LAB (IU Health University)	PSA Ser QN
[illegible]	[illegible]	[illegible]	2022 03/04 01:06 AM		OP	Face Sheet (IU Health)	Discharge/End Visit
[illegible]	[illegible]	[illegible]	2022 03/04 01:06 AM		OP	Face Sheet (IU Health)	Discharge/End Visit
[illegible]	[illegible]	[illegible]	2022 03/04 09:45 AM	⚠	OP	LAB (IU Health University)	Testosterone Total Ser QN
[illegible]	[illegible]	[illegible]	2022 03/08 09:51 AM		OP	Face Sheet (IU Health)	Patient Registration
[illegible]	[illegible]	[illegible]	2022 02/04 02:53 AM		OP	Face Sheet (IU Health)	Discharge/End Visit
[illegible]	[illegible]	[illegible]	2022 02/23 02:02 AM		OP	Face Sheet (IU Health)	Discharge/End Visit
[illegible]	[illegible]	[illegible]	2022 02/01 09:39 PM		OP	LAB (IU Health Physicians)	Hgb A1C HPLC Bld QN
[illegible]	[illegible]	[illegible]	2022 02/01 09:56 PM		OP	LAB (IU Health Physicians)	Lipid Panel SerPl QN
[illegible]	[illegible]	[illegible]	2022 03/01 09:56 PM		OP	LAB (IU Health Physicians)	Basic Metabolic Panel (**UPDATE** ver. 3)
[illegible]	[illegible]	[illegible]	2022 03/01 10:08 PM		OP	LAB (IU Health Physicians)	TSH 3rd Gen SerPl QN
[illegible]	[illegible]	[illegible]	2022 03/01 10:18 PM		OP	LAB (IU Health Physicians)	T4 Free Direct SerPl QN
[illegible]	[illegible]	[illegible]	2022 03/02 12:26 AM		OP	Face Sheet (IU Health)	Discharge/End Visit
[illegible]	[illegible]	[illegible]	2022 03/03 01:41 AM		OP	Face Sheet (IU Health)	Discharge/End Visit
[illegible]	[illegible]	[illegible]	2022 03/09 12:54 AM		OP	Face Sheet (IU Health)	Discharge/End Visit
[illegible]	[illegible]	[illegible]	2022 03/09 09:38 AM		OP	Powernotes (IU Health)	OP-Primary Care MD Progress Notes

FIGURE 22.1 The DOCS4DOCS user interface, a secure web-based inbox, allows users to manage clinical documents from all participants in Indiana Health Information Exchange.

provider's EHR via standards-based interfaces to dozens of different vendors' EHR systems.

- *Fax*—messages can be delivered to physician practices via facsimile if that is the providers' preferred clinical communication mode.

DOCS4DOCS uses HL7 interfaces to receive laboratory/transcription/radiology results, discharge summaries, operative notes, electrocardiograms, and other clinical messages from participating data sources. Users can choose which reports are delivered to their inbox, for example, inpatient versus outpatient, preliminary versus final, and report forwarding to other physicians involved in the patient's care. Data sources can "override" these options when delivery to specific providers is dictated by regulation. Data senders, such as hospitals and laboratories, pay a fee for the service of delivering their results to clinicians. DOCS4DOCS offers data delivery at a lower cost than alternatives, providing a value proposition to data senders. As a result, they are invested in the system at a business level. This approach to getting data to users consistently and reliably has driven growth and was the early basis of IHIE's sustainability planning. Over time, most providers have moved from receiving faxed reports to the inbox solution (Fig. 22.1). Today, larger providers use the direct EHR integration option, while most smaller practices use the Internet-based inbox option. Only a handful of practices continue to receive reports via facsimile.

Other services in the OneCare bundle include retrieving and viewing data from the INPC repository within a provider's EHR, transferring the data either as a CCD with the CCD Connect service or as fast healthcare interoperability resrouces (FHIR) bundles with the HealthDart service. OneCare also provides services to allow the provider to review data in INPC either using the CareWeb interface (Fig. 22.2), which offers sophisticated results review, searching, and graphing capabilities, or the Clinical Data Search services that offer streamlined search capability.

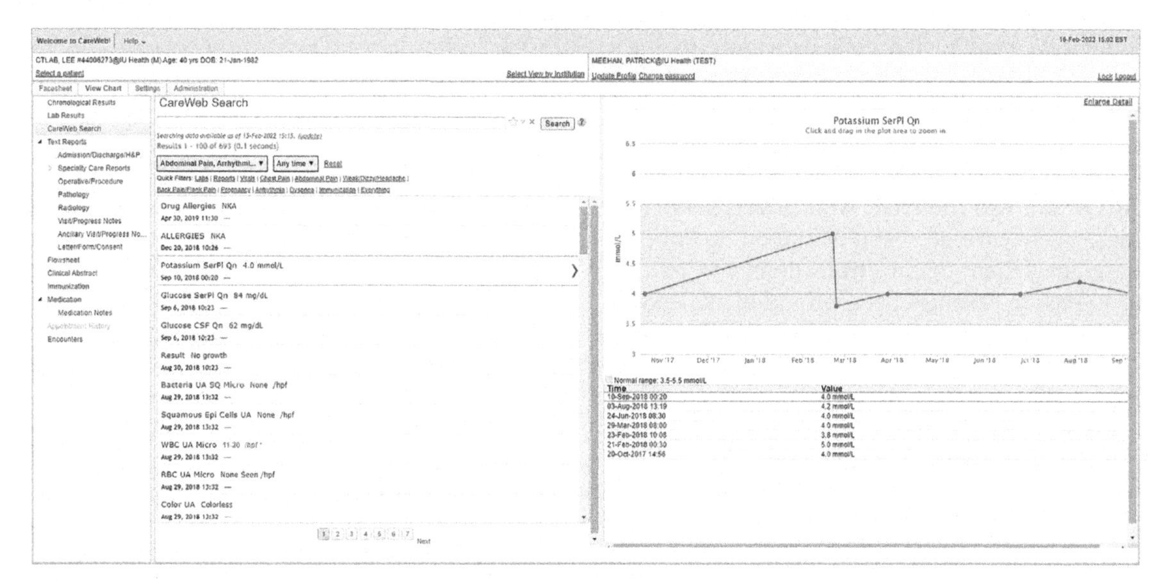

FIGURE 22.2 The CareWeb user interface provides a collection of capabilities to search and display structured and unstructured data across all Indiana Network for Patient Care participants.

The INPC and its Clinical Repository and Results Viewer provide a statewide health repository system that securely aggregates individual patient health information from multiple sources into a single virtual patient medical record (Fig. 22.2). The repository offers views of a clinical abstract and results of the most accurate up-to-date information available for a patient, regardless of the treatment location. The INPC Clinical Repository is organized by the patient and segregated by the clinical source institution. It aggregates demographics, insurance information, encounter data, diagnoses, procedures, observations, laboratory, results and clinical observations, social needs, claims, and text reports for pathology, provider notes, and other data in real-time to ensure current patient information is readily available. These individual patient-level data are supplemented by social determinants of health data and other population-level measures.

22.3.7.2 PopCare

IHIE's PopCare products and services provide a complete, coordinated effort to respond to the market's needs and provide insight into population health, allowing providers to track patients, measure progress, and analyze data to meet the demands of an evolving reimbursement structure [16]. Population health managers, including accountable care organizations (ACO), can use the IHIE ADT Alerts service to track where care has been delivered, to support the management of care transitions and follow-up to ensure care has been provided as needed. In one case study, these alerts and subsequent ACO interventions reduced the number of non-urgent ED visits by 53% with a corresponding increase in primary care physician office visits by 68%. The study calculated that this shift in the venue saved the health plan between $2.1 and $4.1 million during the 6-month trial period [17]. The Clinical Value Report service and PopDash population dashboard round out the PopCare bundle of service offerings (Fig. 22.3). The Clinical Value Report service enhances the population health management process by providing aggregated, longitudinal patient data in standard data formats to support quality improvement efforts, care management, risk adjustment, prior authorization, and utilization management. The PopDash services use these same data to provide analytics and visualizations of population-level data, including social determinants, quality measures, and other population-level statistics with relevant stratifications and drill-down capabilities.

Another population service, QHF, was offered from 2008 until 2013; however, the long-term sustainability of QHF proved elusive due primarily to challenges in gaining participation at the needed scale. QHF provided patient-level data for two purposes. First, it gave feedback on individual patients' healthcare needs, such as whether they are due for a screening test. Second, it provided monthly reports on physician performance quality by utilizing aggregated clinical and claims data. QHF was developed by physicians, hospital networks, health insurers, Regenstrief Institute, Employers' Forum of Indiana, Indiana State Medical Association, IDOH, and Indianapolis Medical Society.

The QHF program provided physicians with disease management, preventive care, and reporting services that delivered patient-specific and population-based reports, alerts, and reminders based on participating providers' or payers' needs or incentives. This program combined clinical data, medical and drug claims, and point-of-care data to monitor patients' health and wellness (e.g., cholesterol, diabetes, and asthma), including Physician Quality Reporting Initiative reporting. Physicians were able to compare their results to the rest of the physician community. There was no charge to physicians and no technology or software required for participation in QHF. Payers provided participating physicians with financial incentives for performance improvement and funded QHF by paying a fee to IHIE on a patient per month basis.

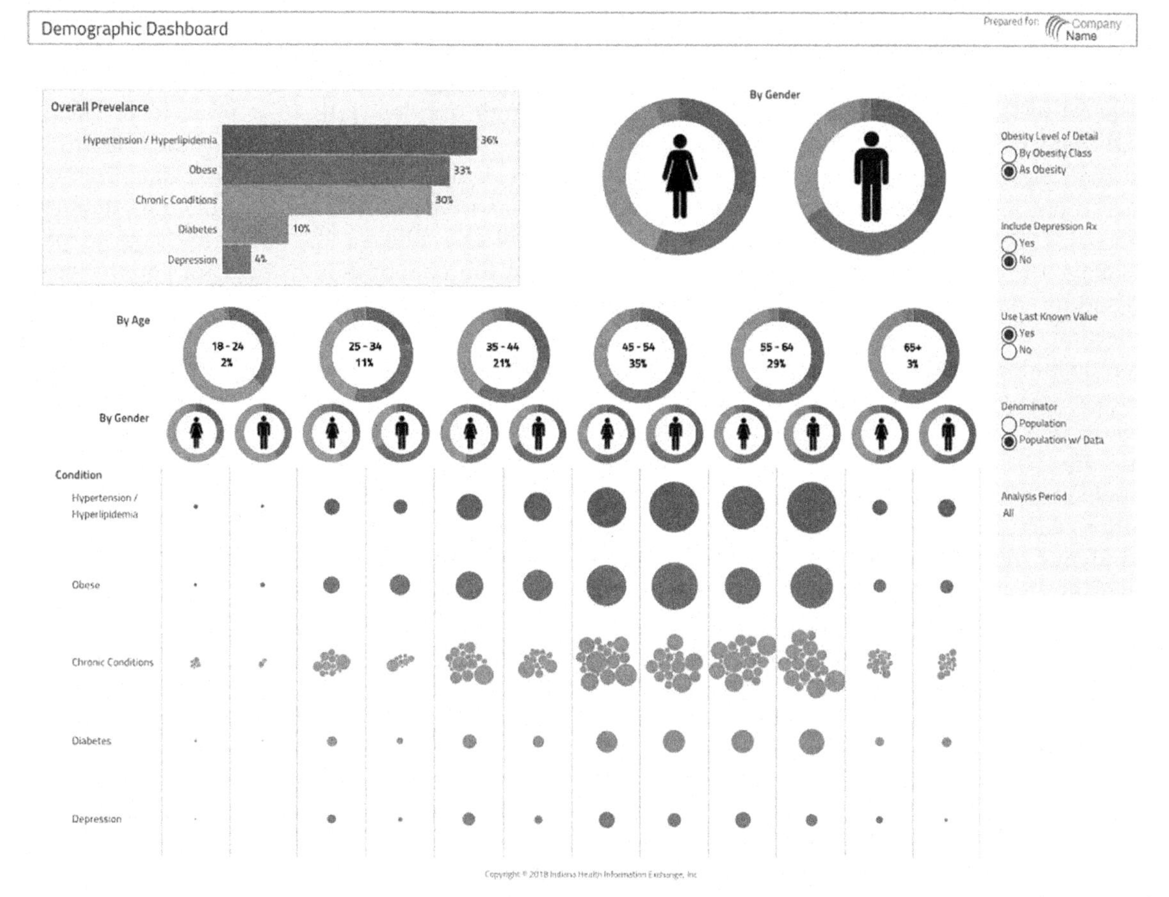

FIGURE 22.3 The PopDash population dashboard provides a number of summary views of specific populations as well as drill-down capabilities.

This report provided physicians and payors with information about the quality of the physicians' care across all patients regardless of payor, which improved the accuracy and value of the information.

22.3.7.3 *GovCare*

GovCare is IHIE's most recent bundle of service offerings that support bi-directional data exchange with State agencies, including IDOH and Family and Social Services Administration (FSSA). This service operates much like government-facilitated HIE models in other states, as the HIE network links government information systems and healthcare organizations. However, unlike other government-facilitated HIE networks, GovCare provides value-added services like data normalization and the INPC repository instead of simply sending and delivering messages between governmental and nongovernmental entities.

Connectivity with public health agencies supports syndromic surveillance, electronic laboratory reporting, laboratory results reporting from public health laboratories, and immunization data exchange. Because the INPC provides data flow from so many sources, including laboratories and ED encounters that are of particular interest to public health, investigators from the Regenstrief Institute, with the support of local and state public health agencies, have created systems [18] that support both electronic laboratory reporting [19–21] and syndromic surveillance [22,23]. In addition, the INPC has been leveraged to support infection control efforts by including data across institutions to support infection control [24]; Regenstrief investigators demonstrated significant improvements in the management of methcillin-resistant staphylococcus aureus and vancomycin-resistant enterooccus [25–27]. Most recently, the INPC served as a single statewide source of testing and hospitalization data to support the IDOH's COVID-19 pandemic response and modeling and dashboarding done by the State and the Regenstrief Institute (https://www.regenstrief.org/covid-dashboard/) [28]. In addition, IHIE utilized the INPC infrastructure to make patients' COVID-19 vaccination information available to clinicians and payors across Indiana. Subsequently, vaccination data were integrated with ED and hospitalization data to enable sharing of information with Centers for Disease Control and Prevention to measure COVID-19 vaccine effectiveness [29–32].

GovCare services also support Medicaid policy and planning and analytics and visualization of combined data from the INPC and the state's Management and Performance Hub (https://www.in.gov/mph/), which aggregates and manages all state government data. The state's Medicaid program, based at FSSA, can leverage clinical and social determinant data from IHIE to enhance its efforts at understanding Medicaid populations' access to care and outcomes.

22.3.7.4 Other services

Through collaboration with other HIE networks, IHIE participates in interstate HIE, including the Patient-Centered Data Home (PCDH) (an initiative of Civitas Networks for Health). PCDH is an inter-HIE notification and data sharing system that allows a patient's data to be shared from their "data home" HIE, through another HIE to a practice or facility where the patient is receiving care (https://strategichie.com/patient-centered-data-home/). Similar to the INPC's original ED data delivery, the PCDH utilizes the ADT message created when the patient is registered for care to locate their "data home" HIE, after which the HIE that serves the treating institution can generate a query to the "data home" HIE and deliver the data to the treating practice or facility. The service also alerts and provides data access for providers at facilities or practices served by the "data home" HIE to data available from the new encounter.

The INPC also serves biomedical research. Researchers at IU, especially the IU School of Medicine, have long used the INPC repositories to estimate patients with particular diseases' number and demographic characteristics for research planning and grant writing. Under institutional review board–approved rules, they use the data to verify that candidates qualify for a study before inviting them and collect patient outcomes for active investigations. The data are also used for epidemiologic studies. One example is a study that discovered the associations between erythromycin and pyloric stenosis among newborns [33]. Research administrators at the IU School of Medicine estimate that more than 2000 of their human subject–based research studies use data from the INPC repository at any given time. Nearly 200 published studies in the biomedical literature as of 2015 explicitly referenced the use of the INPC for retrospective analyses that inform clinical or population health [34]. The heavy utilization of the system for research is unique among HIE networks, mainly due to the INPC's legacy as a research effort. Research use is also facilitated by the Regenstrief Institute, which is a nationally recognized neutral, honest data broker for researchers seeking to use INPC data.

IHIE believes that a variety of services built on standard technology and operations base is the best vehicle for HIE sustainability. The model IHIE created was predicated on the principle that sustained funding would require funders to achieve sustained value. The initial service provided was result delivery through the DOCS4DOCS service.

Organizations paid to have the data they produced delivered to providers. In addition to supporting the costs of interfacing, developing, and maintaining relationships with physician practices and some administrative overhead, the service raised the importance to the participating organizations of preserving the integrity of the interfaces. The ensuing 18 years have involved building several value-added services to fulfill IHIE's mission while maintaining a financially sustainable not-for-profit business.

22.3.8 Lessons learned

While we can abstract some powerful lessons (Table 22.1) from the IHIE experience, we firmly believe that the most challenging (and valuable) work required to develop an HIE network is engaging health systems and other healthcare data holding organizations and operationalizing the data sources. No matter what interoperability technology or approach is adopted, the data created, stored, and managed in various healthcare IT systems need to be freed and normalized, and this work is largely the result of persistent engagement and everyday "blocking and tackling." In addition to freeing the data, there must be trust, collaboration, and connectivity between providers.

22.4 Summary

The Indiana Health Information Exchange has pioneered many fundamentals of technology, policy, and business models for health information exchange. More significantly, IHIE has improved the care of the citizens of Indiana. Looking forward, the organization will continue to identify additional services to

TABLE 22.1 Five powerful lessons to guide organizations implementing health information exchange (HIE).

Lessons	Brief description
Do not make it overly complicated	There are technical complexities and many issues to be addressed in HIE but understanding and articulating clear and straightforward value propositions is essential to obtain the engagement of stakeholders.
"Free" the data—get it out of the silos and establish trust in your community	A major impediment to creating value through the exchange of data is a lack of trust between members of the healthcare ecosystem. Building that trust enables a free flow of data and the creation of the analyses and services that improve care.
Aggregate the data and do something with it	Aggregating data is not enough. Utilizing the data to improve care and produce value for stakeholders is a critical step.
Do not boil the ocean	There are many opportunities but realizing the value of each option requires time and effort, so focusing on a few high-value opportunities is critical to success.
Data reuse is the key	Data are a nonrivalrous good; its supply is not diminished by consumption. HIE organizations can create substantial value by taking advantage of that unusual characteristic and creating value for different stakeholders in different ways from the same data asset.

leverage the data and connections to providers and other key health data sources that they have developed to improve the efficiency, safety, and effectiveness of healthcare delivery and by engaging additional participants in the healthcare ecosystem. IHIE will also continue to navigate the evolution of policy, and continuously adapt and extend its reach in ways that are consistent with its mission.

Questions for discussion

1. Interoperability can only be achieved when provider organizations do the work necessary to participate. Do provider organizations have the incentives required to do that work?
2. Vendor-based HIE networks seem to be growing faster than community-based HIE networks. Community-based HIE networks should arguably offer more value to patients and lower costs to provider organizations. Why the discrepancy?
3. The INPC originated as a research project, was initially funded by grants, and one of the ongoing value propositions is the research use of the data. Is research necessarily critical to the success of a health information exchange?
4. Establishing and operating a HIE network requires various investments, including computing and network infrastructure, software systems of multiple types, and legal and operational costs. Would you agree that data capture and normalization is the most significant investment required?
5. Computing infrastructure, networking technology, software, and clinical information standards will continue to evolve rapidly, and investments in the technology will depreciate relatively rapidly. What are the core assets of an HIE, if not these things?

References

[1] Overhage JM, Tierney WM, McDonald CJ. Design and implementation of the Indianapolis network for patient care and research. Bull Med Libr Assoc 1995;83(1):48.
[2] Biondich PG, Grannis SJ. The Indiana network for patient care: an integrated clinical information system informed by over thirty years of experience. J Public Health Manag Pract 2004;10:S81–6.
[3] McGowan JJ, Overhage JM, Barnes M, McDonald CJ. Indianapolis I3: the third generation integrated advanced information management systems. J Med Libr Assoc 2004;92(2):179.
[4] McDonald CJ, Overhage JM, Barnes M, Schadow G, Blevins L, Dexter PR, et al. The Indiana network for patient care: a working local health information infrastructure. Health Aff 2005;24(5):1214–20.
[5] Overhage JM. Health information exchange: 'lex parsimoniae'. Health Aff 2007;26(5):w595–7.
[6] Zafar A, Dixon BE. Pulling back the covers: technical lessons of a real-world health information exchange. Stud Health Technol Inform 2007;129(Pt 1):488–92.
[7] Overhage JM, Dexter PR, Perkins SM, Cordell WH, McGoff J, McGrath R, et al. A randomized, controlled trial of clinical information shared from another institution. Ann Emerg Med 2002;39(1):14–23.
[8] Finnell JT, Overhage JM, Dexter PR, Perkins SM, Lane KA, McDonald CJ. Community clinical data exchange for emergency medicine patients. AMIA Annu Symp Proc, 2003. 2003. p. 235–8.
[9] Grannis SJ, Overhage JM, McDonald C. Real world performance of approximate string comparators for use in patient matching. Stud Health Technol Inform 2004;107(Pt 1):43–7.
[10] Zhu VJ, Overhage MJ, Egg J, Downs SM, Grannis SJ. An empiric modification to the probabilistic record linkage algorithm using frequency-based weight scaling. J Am Med Inform Assoc 2009;16(5):738–45.
[11] West DM, Friedman A. Health information exchange and megachange, Governance Studies at Brookings [Internet]. [cited July 21, 2015]. Available from: <http://www.brookings.edu/research/papers/2012/02/08health-info-exchange-friedman-west>.
[12] Deloitte Center for Health Solutions. Health information exchange (HIE) business models: the path to sustainable financial success [Internet]. [cited July 21, 2015]. Available from: <http://www.providersedge.com/ehdocs/ehr_articles/Health_Info_Exchange_Business_Models.pdf>.
[13] Rahurkar S, Vest JR, Finnell JT, Dixon BE. Trends in user-initiated health information exchange in the inpatient, outpatient, and emergency settings. J Am Med Inform Assoc 2021;28(3):622–7.

[14] Economides N, Himmelberg C. Critical mass and network evolution in telecommunications. In: Brock GW, editor. Toward a competitive telecommunications industry, selected papers from the 1994 telecommunications policy research conference. Mahwah, NJ: Lawrence Erlbaum; 1995.

[15] Byrne CM, Mercincavage LM, Bouhaddou O, Bennett JR, Pan EC, Botts NE, et al. The Department of Veterans Affairs (VA) implementation of the Virtual Lifetime Electronic Record (VLER): findings and lessons learned from health information exchange at 12 sites. Int J Med Inform 2014;83(8):537–47.

[16] Anand V, Sheley ME, Xu S, Downs SM. Real time alert system: a disease management system leveraging health information exchange. Online J Public Health Inform 2012;4(3).

[17] Indiana Health Information Exchange. ADT alerts for reducing ED admissions: a case study. Indiana Health Information Exchange. [cited July 12, 2015]. Available from: <http://mpcms.blob.core.windows.net/bd985247-f489-435f-a7b4-49df92ec868e//4f798bc84c8f-4dce-b145-cab48f3d8787/ihie-adtalerts-casestudy.pdf>.

[18] Dixon BE, Grannis SJ. Information infrastructure to support public health. In: Magnuson JA, Dixon BE, editors. Public health informatics and information systems. Cham: Springer International Publishing; 2020. p. 83–104.

[19] Overhage JM, Grannis S, McDonald CJ. A comparison of the completeness and timeliness of automated electronic laboratory reporting and spontaneous reporting of notifiable conditions. Am J Public Health 2008;98(2):344.

[20] Dixon BE, McGowan JJ, Grannis SJ. Electronic laboratory data quality and the value of a health information exchange to support public health reporting processes. AMIA Annu Symp Proc, 2011. 2011. p. 322.

[21] Fidahussein M, Friedlin J, Grannis S. Practical challenges in the secondary use of real-world data: the notifiable condition detector. AMIA Annu Symp Proc, 2011. 2011. p. 402.

[22] Mandl KD, Overhage JM, Wagner MM, Lober WB, Sebastiani P, Mostashari F, et al. Implementing syndromic surveillance: a practical guide informed by the early experience. J Am Med Inform Assoc 2004;11(2):141–50.

[23] Grannis S, Wade M, Gibson J, Overhage JM. The Indiana public health emergency surveillance system: ongoing progress, early findings, and future directions. AMIA Annu Symp Proc, 2006. 2006. p. 304.

[24] Dixon BE, Jones JF, Grannis SJ. Infection preventionists' awareness of and engagement in health information exchange to improve public health surveillance. Am J Infect Control 2013;41(9):787–92.

[25] Kho AN, Doebbeling BN, Cashy JP, Rosenman MB, Dexter PR, Shepherd DC, et al. A regional informatics platform for coordinated antibiotic-resistant infection tracking, alerting, and prevention. Clin Infect Dis 2013;57(2):254–62.

[26] Kho AN, Lemmon L, Commiskey M, Wilson SJ, McDonald CJ. Use of a regional health information exchange to detect crossover of patients with MRSA between urban hospitals. J Am Med Inform Assoc 2008;15(2):212–16.

[27] Rosenman MB, Szucs KA, Finnell SME, Khokhar S, Egg J, Lemmon L, et al. Nascent regional system for alerting infection preventionists about patients with multidrug-resistant gram-negative bacteria: implementation and initial results. Infect Control Hosp Epidemiol 2014;35(S3):S40–7.

[28] Dixon BE, Grannis SJ, McAndrews C, Broyles AA, Mikels-Carrasco W, Wiensch, et al. Leveraging data visualization and a statewide health information exchange to support COVID-19 surveillance and response: application of public health informatics. J Am Med Inform Assoc 2021;28(7):1363–73.

[29] Thompson MG, Stenehjem E, Grannis S, Ball SW, Naleway AL, Ong TC, et al. Effectiveness of Covid-19 vaccines in ambulatory and inpatient care settings. N Engl J Med 2021;385(15):1355–71.

[30] Bozio CH, Grannis SJ, Naleway AL, Ong TC, Butterfield KA, DeSilva MB, et al. Laboratory-confirmed COVID-19 among adults hospitalized with COVID-19-like illness with infection-induced or mRNA vaccine-induced SARS-CoV-2 immunity – nine states, January-September 2021. MMWR Morb Mortal Wkly Rep 2021;70(44):1539–44.

[31] Embi PJ, Levy ME, Naleway AL, Patel P, Gaglani M, Natarajan K, et al. Effectiveness of 2-dose vaccination with mRNA COVID-19 vaccines against COVID-19-associated hospitalizations among immunocompromised adults – nine states, January-September 2021. MMWR Morb Mortal Wkly Rep 2021;70(44):1553–9.

[32] Ferdinands JM, Rao S, Dixon BE, Mitchell PK, DeSilva MB, Irving SA, et al. Waning 2-dose and 3-dose effectiveness of mRNA vaccines against COVID-19-associated emergency department and urgent care encounters and hospitalizations among adults during periods of delta and omicron variant predominance – VISION network, 10 states, August 2021–January 2022. MMWR Morb Mortal Wkly Rep 2022;71(7):255–63.

[33] Mahon BE, Rosenman MB, Kleiman MB. Maternal and infant use of erythromycin and other macrolide antibiotics as risk factors for infantile hypertrophic pyloric stenosis. J Pediatr 2001;139(3):380–4.

[34] Dixon BE, Whipple EC, Lajiness JM, Murray MD. Utilizing an integrated infrastructure for outcomes research: a systematic review. Health Info Libr J 2016;33(1):7–32.

CHAPTER

23

Using health information exchange to support public health activities in Western New York: a case study

Saira N. Haque[1] *and Robert F. Bailey*[2]

[1]North America Medical Affairs, Pfizer Inc., New York, NY, USA [2]RTI International Translational Health Sciences Division, Research Triangle Park, NC, USA

LEARNING OBJECTIVES

- Outline uses of health information exchange to support public health functions
- Describe challenges faced by health information exchange to support public health activities
- Explain success factors for health information exchange to support public health

23.1 Introduction

This case study outlines an expanded use of HEALTHeLINK, the western New York health information exchange (HIE), for population health. Chapter 1 outlines different types of HIEs: community based, government facilitated, private, and vendor based. HEALTHeLINK was initially developed by payers and providers for administrative data exchange that expanded to become a community-based HIE to also include clinical data. HEALTHeLINK is governed by health care providers, insurers, and other western New York community health organizations. Using a publicly funded grant program, HEALTHeLINK expanded its role to support public health in several ways: reporting to public health agencies, providing public health alerts, and supporting clinical care and public health services. Specific activities in these areas include identification, investigation, treatment, and tracking of sexually transmitted infections (STIs), tuberculosis (TB), possible rabies exposures, HIV-positive patients, and hepatitis patients. In addition, HEALTHeLINK facilitated provision of public health services including quality control and investigations. Thus less effort is needed for administrative duties, freeing resources for service provision to vulnerable populations. These innovations in routine public health work have allowed public health professionals to save

Health Information Exchange
DOI: https://doi.org/10.1016/B978-0-323-90802-3.00015-0

money through time savings, avoided medical treatment and associated indirect costs, and improved health outcomes.

23.2 Background and context

HEALTHeLINK is an established HIE network that connects data sources and enables querying and data sharing. HEALTHeLINK is the Regional Health Information Organization (RHIO) for the western region of New York State. The major metropolitan area in the region is Buffalo-Niagara [1]. The HIE serves western New York's eight rural and urban counties [2]: Allegany, Cattaraugus, Chautauqua, Erie, Genesee, Niagara, Orleans, and Wyoming.

HEALTHeLINK connects clinical data from all 26 hospitals in an 8-county western New York region as well as 8 radiology providers, 3 independent laboratories, 4 home health care agencies, 4 long-term care facilities, 3 medication history sources, and the Veterans Health Administration [3].

The total population in the region is approximately 1.5 million people. Out of those, approximately 42% have consented to participate in the HIE [4]. The median income is slightly below that of the rest of the state, and the median age is higher. The region is characterized by high socioeconomic and health disparities, particularly among minority and elderly populations [4]. In addition, approximately 30% of the adult population is obese, as well as almost 20% of children. Health concerns in the area include cardiovascular disease, diabetes mellitus, behavioral health, asthma, HIV/AIDS, perinatal care, palliative care, and renal care.

The HIE was established by a consortium of partners representing hospitals and payers. It has since expanded to include other clinical providers, long-term and postacute care, laboratory services, public health, and pharmacy. To expand the HIE and focus on public health, HEALTHeLINK and its community partners applied for, and subsequently received, Beacon Community Cooperative Agreement Program funding. This 3-year grant from the Office of the National Coordinator for Health Information Technology (ONC) supported expansion of HIE infrastructure to include community-based health initiatives [5]. The Beacon Community funding was used to strengthen HEALTHeLINK by connecting additional partners and data sources and to develop new functionality to increase HEALTHeLINK's value to users, including the New York State Department of Health (NYSDOH) and the Erie County Department of Health (ECDOH). Since then, HEALTHeLINK has also received funding from the Strengthening the Technical Advancement and Readiness of Public Health via Health Information Exchange Program entitled "Improving COVID-19 Vaccination Data: Connecting Immunization Information Systems (IIS)" to HIEs from ONC, funded through the CARES Act [6].

HEALTHeLINK has strong community support. Partners include the P2 Collaborative of Western New York (the New York eHealth Collaborative regional extension agent, a nonprofit dedicated to improving health in western New York) and 40 community partners. Over 1200 participant sites and 1.4 million patients are connected through HEALTHeLINK [7]. HEALTHeLINK is governed by health care providers, insurers, and representatives from the western New York community, including the local Catholic Health System, the Erie County Medical Center, HealthNow New York, the Independent Health Association, Kaleida Health, the Roswell Park Comprehensive Cancer Center, Univera Healthcare, and the Health Care Efficiency and Affordability Law for New Yorkers Capital Grant Program from New York State (known as HEAL NY).

Expansion of HEALTHeLINK had several public health impacts for managing patient and population health. Public health officials leveraged the local HIE infrastructure to streamline and improve the effectiveness of communicable disease epidemiologic investigations. These processes allowed public health staff to overcome traditional challenges such as delayed reporting, incomplete information, and resource limitations to acquire more of the demographic and clinical information they need more quickly and with less effort. They use this information to identify significant clinical or behavioral risk factors, complete surveillance reports, and intervene with patients and contacts more effectively when needed.

HEALTHeLINK does not generate or "push" reports or alerts about public health events. Instead, these come from the Electronic Clinical Laboratory Reporting System (ECLRS), via fax or telephone from clinical laboratories and providers. Once NYSDOH identifies an issue in ECLRS, or another one of its databases, it accesses HEALTHeLINK to acquire additional clinical and demographic data. Investigators from ECDOH receive these reports and access HEALTHeLINK to fill in missing clinical data and retrieve demographic and contact information that can aid their investigations [8].

23.3 Health information exchange and public health

Public health activities rely heavily on information sharing and analysis. Improving access to information can support public health services such as surveillance and monitoring immunization coverage [9]. HEALTHeLINK coordinates with other HIEs to share best practices around the exchange of health information and specifically for public health. It is a founding member of the Strategic Health Information Exchange Collaborative, the national association of HIEs. In addition, there is HEALTHeLINK participation in the Statewide Health Information Network of New York (SHIN-NY). policy committee, charged with updating and drafting proposed SHIN-NY policy measures to protect personal health information while expanding the State's ability to share electronic health records between health care providers, consumers, and other community resources.

Public health–specific information exchange activities include the public health–oriented Meaningful Use objectives [10], the National Syndromic Surveillance Program (NSSP) [11], and the Public Health Information Network [12]. In addition to efforts specifically focused on health information technology, some community-based funding initiatives include information exchange such as the Centers for Medicare & Medicaid Services–funded Health Care Innovation Awards [13].

New York State developed a program to help support RHIOs [14], which are described in **Creating a 21st Century Health Information Technology Infrastructure: New York's Health Care Efficiency and Affordability Law for New Yorkers Capital Grant Program**. This program has helped provide infrastructure to overcome barriers to HIE including structures, formats, and vocabularies [15].

These efforts focus on various aspects of public health and information exchange. The following sections discuss ways in which information exchange can support public health.

23.3.1 Uses of health information exchange in public health

Public and population health activities rely on information sharing among health care providers [16]. Facilitating information availability supports HIE to improve public health activities [16,17]. A discussion of several ways in which information exchange can be used to support public health follows (adapted from Shapiro and colleagues in Box 23.1) [17].

BOX 23.1

Uses of health information exchange in public health.

Catastrophic events

- Mass-casualty events
- Disaster medical response
- Pandemics

Reporting to public health agencies

- Reporting of laboratory diagnoses
- Nonmandatory reporting of laboratory data
- Nonmandatory reporting of clinical data
- Reporting of physician-based diagnoses
- Immunization
- Surveillance

Public health alerting

- Public health alerting—patient level
- Public health alerting—population level

Clinical care

- Clinical care in public health clinics

Public health services

- Public health investigation
- Quality measurement

23.3.2 Public health emergencies

Public health emergencies take on many forms, such as pandemics, natural disasters, or other mass-casualty events. In these cases, communication among providers, public health officials, and the public is vital. HIEs provide the infrastructure needed to share information throughout the community to protect the public interest.

The Southeast Regional HIT-HIE Collaboration (SERCH) project on Health Information Exchange in Disaster Preparedness and Response was developed to facilitate sharing health information among participating states in response to a declared national disaster [18]. This is particularly relevant for highly contagious diseases such as TB or COVID-19.

During the coronavirus disease 2019 (COVID-19) pandemic, there was some confusion about when personal health information related to COVID-19 could be disclosed and to whom. In response, the Office of Civil Rights within the US Department of Health and Human Services released guidance related to the Health Insurance Portability and Accountability Act of 1996 (HIPAA) [19]. This announcement allowed covered entities to release information without their HIPAA authorization to provide treatment, protect those on the front lines so that they can take precautions, and support activities to reduce threats. This allowed for real-time information to be shared to protect the public interest [20] and support public health activities.

All of these uses of HIEs can help better coordinate public health activities. By having more information available electronically and a mechanism to share it, public health agencies can have more accurate, timely information.

23.3.3 Reporting to public health agencies

Because public health agencies depend on accurate and timely reporting, activities that facilitate information sharing are extremely important. HIEs can help improve the reporting rate and timeliness of these activities. Types of reporting certified electronic health records support include immunization, syndromic surveillance, reportable laboratory results, cancer reporting, and specialized registries [21].

HIEs can support public health reporting. It is a mandatory requirement to report some positive laboratory test results [15,22]. As the COVID-19 pandemic continued, many organizations and government agencies added COVID-19 to the laboratory results that were reported [23]. Other results are not mandatory but can be helpful for public health activities. HIEs can help improve the reporting rate and timeliness of these activities. With electronic reporting, data are more likely to be complete [24,25]. For nonmandatory reporting, having information available can help identify patterns [17].

Electronic laboratory reporting does not include reporting of physician diagnoses. Such reporting is a separate process with physician-based diagnoses that are mandatory to report and others that are not. Some pieces of clinical information can supplement a diagnosis that is identified through laboratory testing [15,17]. HIEs can facilitate this reporting on the basis of diagnoses, medications, or other identifying factors, which can provide valuable situating information to guide public health activities.

Implementation of HIEs can avoid significant administrative costs of this mandatory reporting to public health departments. Walker and colleagues [26] estimate that national implementation of interoperable HIEs could reduce reporting costs by $195 million (2003 dollars) annually.

Syndromic surveillance depends on exchange of health information. Programs such as the NSSP [11] provide a platform to collect and share information. The Kansas Health Information Network connected to the NSSP at the Centers for Disease Control and Prevention in November 2012 [27]. Previously, the Kansas Department of Health and Environment had been manually collecting and reporting information, such as influenza data, using a system built for another purpose. Through this connection, Kansas can now use the NSSP Platform to track this type of information, rather than collecting it manually.

HIEs can also support immunization registries, which can result in improved supply chain management of vaccines and well as tracking and reporting vaccination rates and preventable disease. With the proposed move to barcoding of vaccine data, exchanging those data will become more important for tracking and reporting [28]. In addition, the COVID-19 pandemic saw an increase in vaccines and in mass vaccination campaigns, where individuals were vaccinated outside of their usual health care provider's office [29]. Linking vaccination information to the IIS and to the provider is an important piece of the HIE's function. Including planning for information sharing is an important piece of mass vaccination readiness [30] to support activities related to vaccine rates, safety, and supply.

23.3.4 Public health alerting

Because of the importance of timeliness and accuracy in public health reporting, HIEs can be extremely useful. At the patient level, sharing information can help identify other affected individuals in the case of a reportable diagnosis. At the population level, HIEs can help ensure that public health alerts are accurate and sent in a timely fashion [31].

Paper-based methods of alerting are time consuming, rely on information that might be out of date, and are not immediate [31,32]. Thus clinicians may not receive alerts at all or receive them too late to affect their clinical practices. In Indiana, HIE was used to facilitate a clinical messaging service to deliver public health alerts with improved efficiency and effectiveness of messaging [32].

23.3.5 Clinical care

Clinical care is managed through public health agencies for some diseases, but it varies by jurisdiction. These diseases are typically communicable, such as TB, COVID-19, and STIs, or characterized by settings with many people such as schools, jails, or shelters [17]. HIEs can ensure that referrals are made accurately and promptly. In addition, HIEs can support information sharing so that full identifiers and history are available. This exchange of information can facilitate coordination and improve outcomes [33]. HEALTHeLINK added alert notifications via Direct messaging between laboratories and providers of record for COVID-19 testing during the pandemic [34], which helped facilitate clinical care through transmission of results. In addition, this helped promote coordination across providers and with the local health department since both would receive results at the same time.

23.3.6 Public health services

HIEs also support public health services such as investigations and quality measurement. Investigations rely heavily on information gathering and synthesizing. By having information about the patient and any other individuals available, public health agencies can conduct better epidemiological investigations. HIE can support public health investigations through improved information availability [15]. This can support activities such as contact tracing and identifying disease clusters [35].

Similarly, quality improvement activities such as chart audits are facilitated through HIEs. Electronic chart audits have been shown to provide reliable data [36]. However, these chart audits could not be completed off site without a system login or access through an HIE. Paper chart audits are manual and time intensive. With electronic information, chart reviews do not require travel to a site for review of copied paper charts, thus improving efficiency and effectiveness of review. HIEs support public health activities in many ways, including catastrophic event response, reporting, alerts, and clinical care and public health services.

23.4 Intervention, planning, and assessment

Although representatives from state and local public health departments were on the board of HEALTHeLINK, the HIE was not developed with public health in mind. Rather, public health officials used existing infrastructure to support public health activities. The improvements in communicable disease epidemiologic investigations were not the result of a planned intervention but were used by public health officials to leverage the capabilities of a well-conceived, robust HIE.

In 1999 a core group of stakeholders defined the vision for HEALTHeNET as a for-profit network for the exchange of administrative data, which went live in 2002. HEALTHeNET is a collaboration that includes as stakeholders the three major payers (BlueCross BlueShield of Western New York, the Independent Health Association, and Univera Healthcare) and four major hospital systems (the local Catholic Health System, the Erie County Medical Center, Kaleida Health, and the Roswell Park Comprehensive Cancer Center) [37].

HEALTHeNET allows all providers (hospitals, clinics, and provider practices) in western New York to access administrative information such as eligibility and claim status. Providers could find the insurance information they needed quickly, easily, and in one place, which allowed them to improve efficiency. Insurance companies benefited from the decrease in telephone calls from providers requesting information. The effort demonstrated to key stakeholders in the region that collaboration could work. The number of participants, data sources, and functionalities continued to grow, when, in 2004 and 2005, these same key stakeholders defined the vision for HEALTHeLINK.

In 2004 a collaborative group conducted the Upstate New York Professional Healthcare Information & Education Demonstration Project and developed a white paper outlining a plan for regional interoperability. Participants included members of the physician community, the State University of New York at Buffalo, the county and state public health departments, and HEALTHeNET. With additional support from the Agency for Healthcare Research and Quality and the Health Foundation for Western & Central New York, the group conducted a 1-year effort to establish and implement a 5-year plan. They hired IBM to conduct an independent feasibility study and develop the business case to improve quality through a financially sustainable model. The support of these organizations individually and collectively culminated in western New York receiving funding from HEAL NY to create HEALTHeLINK.

HEALTHeLINK's success in sharing administrative data led to buy-in for sharing clinical data. Today, its mission is to create and maintain a secure and reliable infrastructure for the timely and accurate electronic exchange of clinical information among health care providers, insurers, and other medical professionals. HEALTHeLINK's vision is for western New York to have an electronic system for real-time sharing of clinical information among health care professionals to promote collaboration, limit duplication, control health care costs, and improve the delivery of services, clinical outcomes, and patient safety [38]. Community partner support and engagement have allowed HEALTHeLINK to continue to build trust among the community and increase the number of participating data sources connected to the HIE.

New York is an opt-in state regarding patient consent to share protected health information. HEALTHeLINK leveraged partnerships so that patients could opt in at the community level. This means that if patients consent at a physician's office, they are also consenting for other participating locations in western New York and do not have to sign a consent form at every clinical location at which they receive care. Patients can also designate practices that do not have access to their information. This degree of specificity in opting in has enabled the HIE to gain traction and acceptance among providers and patients. As an indication of public acceptance, the number of patients consenting to share data via HEALTHeLINK rose from just less than 300,000 to more than 500,000 between 2010 and 2013, while the number of patient record queries rose from 100,000 to 600,000 during that time.

Health departments have access to all HEALTHeLINK data without consent, which is consistent with the HIPAA Privacy Rule. Therefore the high rate of patient consent ensures the robustness and utility of the data but is not required for public health access and use. High rates of provider participation ensure the completeness and utility of the data for public health investigations [3].

23.4.1 Uses of HEALTHeLINK to provide public health services

HEALTHeLINK has been used in a variety of ways to improve public and population health, including communicable disease epidemiologic investigations conducted by the county and state departments of health, which routinely work closely together.

Laboratory results of reportable communicable diseases are reviewed by NYSDOH via ECLRS. NYSDOH staff receive automated reports, then manually sort them and send them to the appropriate counties for follow-up investigation. In Erie

County, these reports go to the Epidemiology/ Disease Control Program.

Erie County public health staff evaluate reports from NYSDOH for completeness of demographic information, such as address. If information is missing, they use HEALTHeLINK to identify or confirm the patient's city of residence, so the appropriate county can be notified and follow-up can be routed accordingly. This process decreases the amount of time needed to identify the correct county, eliminating the time that would otherwise be needed to contact the ordering laboratory or associated physician to obtain basic demographic information. Staff indicated that time to obtain and correct information decreased from hours to minutes.

Although HEALTHeLINK does not generate reports of laboratory diagnoses, physician-based diagnoses, or immunization or surveillance data, it is used to follow up on reports and facilitate investigation. Public health staff receive automated reports of diagnoses through other surveillance systems and use HEALTHeLINK to follow up. Staff use HEALTHeLINK to access treatment information, patient contact information, and clinical encounter and laboratory test results that are relevant but not reportable. Examples of these uses follow.

23.4.1.1 COVID-19

HEALTHeLINK was already in place with high uptake prior to the COVID-19 pandemic. This helped in making sure that the HIE was able to collect and disseminate data across all relevant sectors. In New York, telehealth expansion, which included verbal consent,

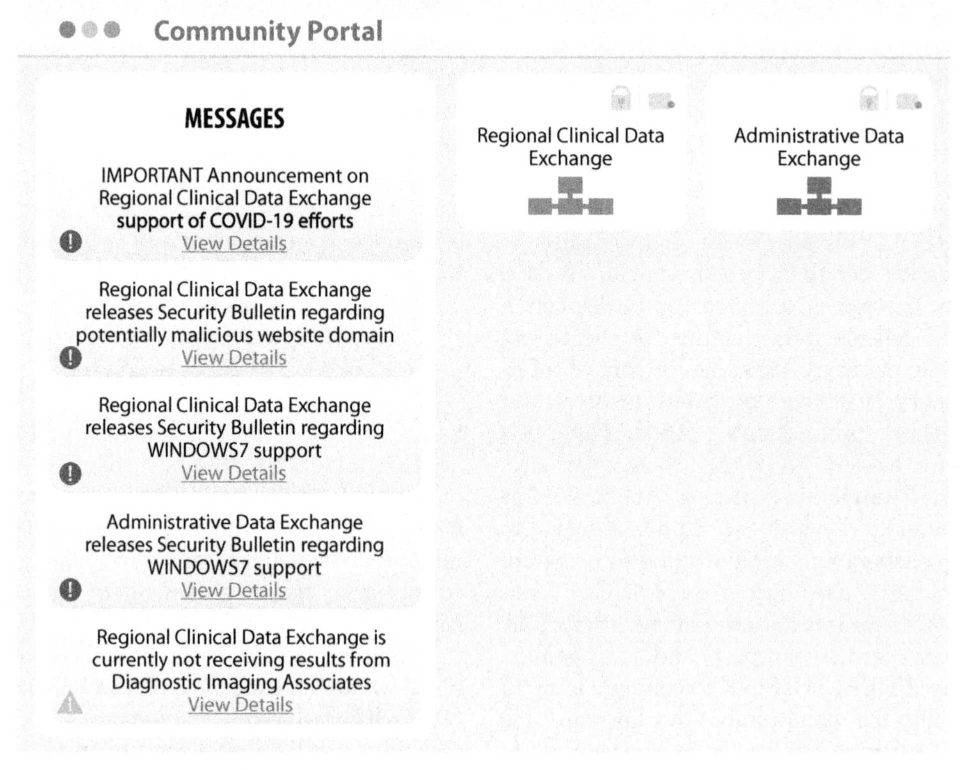

FIGURE 23.1 HEALTHeLINK screen.

occurred during the COVID-19 pandemic. HEALTHeLINK implemented verbal consent during this time to increase participation and improve access to care.

HEALTHeLINK was also used to share COVID-19 laboratory test results performed in western New York. Participating providers were able to receive all COVID-19 tests performed in western New York [39] and could turn on alerts for their patients. In addition, HEALTHeLINK added alert notifications via direct messaging for COVID-19 testing if providers opted for those [40]. During this time, patient consent for sharing was not required due to the public health emergency *unless* patients had previously chosen not to have their information shared. Once a person was identified with a positive test, ECDOH was able to use HEALTHeLINK for contact tracing to identify others at risk such as household members and to provide information and services [40]. At log in, users see each application and practice with messages that show where users see important information. A representation is shown in Fig. 23.1 [41].

High HEALTHeLINK participation coupled with high opt-in rates for providers receiving COVID-19 testing alerts allowed for aggregation and dissemination of key demographic information that was used to better inform public health responses. In addition, HEALTHeLINK coordinated with Hixny, an HIE organization in New York. Hixny facilitated aggregated reporting of COVID-19 populations and hospital beds in different regions of New York outside of the catchment area of HEALTHeLINK. Hixny's analysis also helped better identify populations with underlying conditions to help predict provider capacity.

23.4.1.2 Chlamydia

HEALTHeLINK allows ECDOH to identify and follow up on priority chlamydia cases. Cases are manually identified using criteria including all untreated cases, pregnant females, repeaters (more than once in 90 days), and youth 16 years of age or younger. In 2012 Erie County had 5088 cases of chlamydia, of which 634 were assigned to epidemiologists for further investigation. Erie County uses HEALTHeLINK to look at pharmacy records to identify filled prescriptions. Thus ECDOH can rapidly access information on treatment, treatment compliance (filled prescriptions), and the appropriateness of prescribed therapy. ECDOH can review the prescribed and filled prescription data to determine whether the clinician has prescribed a correct medication effective against chlamydia. Additionally, if the patient is of childbearing age, the HIE can be queried for information on pregnancy status.

23.4.1.3 Gonorrhea

HEALTHeLINK allows ECDOH to identify and follow up on gonorrhea cases. In 2012 Erie County had 1781 cases of gonorrhea, of which 1313 were assigned to disease investigators for investigation. ECDOH staff use HEALTHeLINK to retrieve pharmacy data on filled prescriptions, confirm appropriateness of treatment regimen, verify the name of the ordering physician if it is not on the laboratory report, and verify patient demographic information. This enables ECDOH to resolve cases quickly. ECDOH staff can also intervene quickly to treat close contacts in a timely way.

23.4.1.4 Syphilis

ECDOH staff use HEALTHeLINK to retrieve pharmacy data on filled prescriptions, confirm treatment compliance and appropriateness of the treatment regimen, verify the name of the ordering physician if it is not on the laboratory report, and verify patient demographic information. Negative test results available through HEALTHeLINK are valuable to health department staff. The date of the last negative test can often allow investigators to stage the disease, which determines treatment. In the case of syphilis, if they can determine that the disease is in stage 1, only one treatment injection is required. If the disease stage is unknown, three injections will be required, tripling the cost of treatment. ECDOH staff can further intervene quickly to treat close contacts in a timely way.

23.4.1.5 *Hepatitis surveillance*

HEALTHeLINK allows health department staff to review all viral hepatitis laboratory tests, including negative results, which are not reportable but do encompass case definitions of reportable hepatitis. Staff can also review liver function tests to identify acute cases and prioritize cases. These data are also not reportable but are needed for case classification and follow-up. Staff use HEALTHeLINK to view the date of diagnosis and determine whether the case is new, which again enables them to prioritize their work. Being able to prioritize cases is critical: health department staff can intervene quickly and treat family members and close contacts in a timely way. In addition, they use HEALTHeLINK to view pregnancy test results and to determine hepatitis B status in pregnant and postpartum women, which is required for the perinatal hepatitis B surveillance program. These cases require high-intensity follow-up. Health department staff need to ensure that the child is vaccinated for hepatitis B and subsequently tested to confirm antibody response to vaccination. Using HEALTHeLINK allows health department staff to manage these cases more effectively.

23.4.1.6 *Rabies investigations*

ECDOH staff use HEALTHeLINK to access the most up-to-date information regarding addresses and phone numbers of the exposed victim, potential other victims, and the animal's owner (when applicable). HEALTHeLINK is a rich source of contact information because of the number of connected data sources. This information allows health department staff to begin public health work sooner by telephone and significantly reduces the number of field visits requested by epidemiologists.

23.4.1.7 *Foodborne illness outbreaks*

ECDOH staff access the HIE to retrieve contact information for persons to investigate outbreaks and conduct food history interviews in the case of outbreaks related to foodborne illness. Staff also use it to retrieve laboratory testing on people involved. Improving the timeliness and completeness of these investigations allows ECDOH staff to complete mandatory reporting, follow up with providers, and prevent infected people from handling food and infecting others.

23.4.1.8 *Tuberculosis*

ECDOH epidemiologists send TB reports to a separate group of nurses at a TB clinic dedicated to these investigations. Nurses access HEALTHeLINK to view information on chest X-rays, see other laboratory tests and results, track admission and discharge dates, see medications prescribed, and review discharge notes. They follow these techniques to rule out cases, follow the clinical path, and ensure proper treatment. Before HEALTHeLINK, ECDOH would either send a nurse to the hospital to look through charts for this information or call the hospital to request visit information by fax. Both approaches were labor-intensive and inefficient, requiring nurses to search through entire medical records.

23.4.1.9 *Quality audits to track infection control in hospitals*

One state public health function is quality auditing and reporting, which includes auditing and validating reports from hospitals, reviewing infection prevention practices, and ensuring consistent data across reporting hospitals. HEALTHeLINK allows NYSDOH to conduct audits remotely, significantly reducing time and expense. Before HEALTHeLINK, auditing required ECDOH staff to travel to 40 hospitals and review 60–70 charts per hospital. On-site auditing required travel, lodging for 1–4 days, and per diem expenses. Chart review occasionally identified the need for hospital staff to pull additional charts, requiring additional time. In addition to reducing costs associated with travel, HEALTHeLINK allows staff to monitor the details of admissions and readmissions, ensuring accurate reporting. Remote auditing has enabled staff to spend more time in the office and less time traveling, allowing them to keep pace with an increase in the types of surgical procedures that require reporting despite staffing reductions.

23.4.1.10 Tracking nursing home and long-term care infections

NYSDOH staff use HEALTHeLINK to support tracking and follow-up on health care–associated infections in nursing homes and long-term care facilities. Staff use HEALTHeLINK to check address information to determine whether a patient is a resident of such a facility (which can be challenging because this population may not have a consistent address). Staff use HEALTHeLINK to conduct investigations in response to trends such as an increase in multidrug-resistant organisms. One such investigation of vancomycin-intermediate *Staphylococcus aureus* involved reviewing health information for 25 patients, including admission and discharge, underlying medical condition, demographics, laboratory results, and primary care physicians. HEALTHeLINK was particularly useful in these cases because these patients often travel from rural areas to cities for health care.

23.4.1.11 HIV investigation and contact tracing

Upon notification of HIV-positive status, NYSDOH staff use HEALTHeLINK to look up information needed to investigate cases. This includes identifying those with potential exposure to HIV. HEALTHeLINK can be used to provide demographic information such as spousal or household documentation to identify close contacts who might be exposed. Once an HIV-positive individual has identified relevant contacts, health department staff can use HEALTHeLINK to look up information and contact those individuals and ensure that they get the testing and treatment they need.

In addition, ECDOH staff follow up with HIV-positive individuals who have not received treatment for the disease in the last 13 months. HEALTHeLINK provides an additional source of contact information for these individuals, allowing public health professionals to reach patients more quickly and avoid time-consuming field visits. In addition to time savings, further information in HEALTHeLINK such as toxicology screens and provider comments on other medical conditions provides greater situational awareness to public health staff and allows them to target their approach to patient follow-up.

23.4.2 Challenges

Several challenges were associated with using HEALTHeLINK to support public health services, including access to information by public health workers, integration with other state regulatory requirements, and education for both providers and patients.

One reason for the high uptake is that users (e.g., providers, provider staff, payer staff) have role-based access control. This means that there is a mechanism to restrict HIE access to authorized users and to further restrict it so that people can see only the information they need for their jobs. Because the HIE was designed primarily for payers and providers, access for public health workers was not initially considered, and they did not have a profile for role-based access. This means that there was no set protocol for giving public health workers access. This issue, coupled with an initial misunderstanding of the HIPAA Privacy Rule, made access to data challenging for public health workers.

To combat concerns, NYSDOH established a workgroup consisting of its legal, public health, and IT staff, and included county public health representatives to help develop policies that would allow public health access to all RHIOs in New York State. The legal staff additionally developed one uniform public health contract statement based on input from the workgroup, which was designed to be incorporated by every RHIO when granting public health access to their systems. The policies were then submitted for review to the commissioner's advisory council on HIE, and after their input, the commissioner.

In the interim, the western region's associate commissioner used a workaround to grant access and spent a great deal of time on education and awareness. Public health staff were then given specific, role-based access to do public health work. This workaround was eventually addressed, and the staff were given access. This issue is not unique to western New York, and other communities may need to consider similar issues for public health access.

Although the users of public health data made accessible via the HIE were pleased with the benefits realized to date, they identified opportunities to improve the usefulness of the data: more complete data, real-time availability, and improved access. Several changes could be made to improve effectiveness, some of which will be addressed through the most recent round of funding related to the COVID-19 pandemic:

- Include vaccine information for children and adults.
- Connect additional area practices and hospitals to the network.
- Automate nightly updates of reportable disease diagnoses to ensure timely reporting.
- Automate alerts to public health staff based on prescribing certain drugs such as TB drugs so that public health staff can follow up.

Improvements in these areas would increase the timeliness and effectiveness of public health investigations and would simultaneously decrease the number of telephone calls to providers, which are often disruptive. Negative test results would allow regional public health agencies to calculate denominators needed for aggregate reporting. Otherwise, they are not easily able to determine, for example, if a doubling in positive test results represents an increase in disease or an increase in testing. In addition, access to total numbers tested for recommended preventive health screenings, such as mammograms, Pap tests, and colorectal cancer screenings, can provide community measures for compliance with recommended preventive health screenings among those who are eligible.

As mentioned previously, there is a continuing need to educate providers and consumers to explain public health workers' right to access the data and the privacy and security regulations they follow. Such clarification would help address vague uneasiness based on inaccurate perceptions of unlimited access to data.

23.4.3 Contributors to success

Building on the vision of the core group of payers and hospitals that founded HEALTHeNET and demonstrated value from the outset, HEALTHeLINK now enjoys the participation of pharmacies, radiologists, laboratories, and physicians, and HEALTHeLINK itself participates in SHIN-NY.

Developing and following a 5-year plan allowed the participants to apply successfully for funding and use it strategically to establish governance and policies as a foundation for trust. Representation of stakeholders in governance and oversight has enabled HEALTHeLINK to establish community-wide trust that data will be protected and used appropriately. Trust among providers has led to high rates of participation, which has yielded a critical mass of clinical information. Trust among patients has ensured low rates of opting out. Successful planning also allowed strategic engagement of data holders and addition of new data sources.

The result is an easy-to-use network that provides secure access to timely and accurate data. HIE users can define workflows that improve operational efficiency. Relationships between public health officials and physicians have been strengthened because physicians are not burdened with retrieving information, and calls placed by health departments can focus on more urgent issues.

23.5 Summary

HEALTHeLINK is a case study of an existing, robust HIE network for clinical care that was able to build on a solid foundation to support public health activity. This allowed public health officials and providers to respond to the COVID-19 pandemic. Supporting population health was possible because of several factors beyond funding, including technical infrastructure, interdisciplinary stakeholder involvement, and patient- and provider-facing education. To support the provision of core public health services, HIEs must have high levels of participation from a wide variety of providers. Previous efforts to increase participation in HEALTHeLINK facilitated its use for public health activities before and during the COVID-19 pandemic.

Although HEALTHeLINK streamlined many public health functions, additional potential to improve public health remains untapped for the future. This includes automated reporting, improved connections with IIS, and support for mass vaccination. Going forward, automated, electronic public health case reporting and HEALTHeLINK could be integrated more seamlessly. Using HEALTHeLINK for automated mandatory and nonmandatory public health reporting could streamline follow-up and research efforts. In addition, HEALTHeLINK could be used more broadly to facilitate chronic disease management throughout the region, not just for diseases for which the public health department provides care. The role of HEALTHeLINK can be identified and specified for disaster recovery planning. Integration of systems and automated reporting would add more value. Other public health departments should consider how HEALTHeLINK can help to provide public health services.

Lessons learned

HEALTHeLINK was in place before the COVID-19 pandemic, and the pandemic highlighted the need for HIE. Federal funding also supported expansion of functionality to add to public health use cases. One reason HEALTHeLINK was successfully used for public health activities related to the COVID-19 pandemic is due to its structure. To maximize an HIE's public health benefit, there needs to be high participant uptake. Consequently, HEALTHeLINK's initial efforts to focus on participation provided the foundation needed to support use of public health. However, public health uses were not initially a large part of the HIE's activities; thus changes were needed. Therefore including public health stakeholders in design and implementation from the start could have helped in designing the HIE to support public health challenges. This would include developing a role profile for public health access, developing automated alerts, and sharing information. The board of directors had some representatives from the public health sector to facilitate public health access once the HIE had matured.

Other considerations include educating providers and patients about HEALTHeLINK. When HEALTHeLINK was first implemented, stakeholders were concerned about creating and controlling access to a huge repository of data. Although HEALTHeLINK is not a repository, a great deal of education was needed to explain how it works, who is authorized to access it, and how access is controlled. Stakeholders such as patients and clinicians had some concerns about public health staff having access to data, which further supports the importance of public health involvement. HEALTHeLINK had a champion in the NYSDOH associate commissioner, who conducted educational sessions and other activities to secure access for public health staff.

Questions for discussion

1. What are some other ways in which HEALTHeLINK could be used to support public health activities?
2. What would be necessary in other communities to use their health information exchange or Regional Health Information Organizations to support public health?
3. What are ways in which the use of HEALTHeLINK could be improved to maximize public health benefit?
4. Describe the efficiencies achieved by using HEALTHeLINK.
5. Is the use of HEALTHeLINK synchronous or asynchronous? Why?
6. How would involving public health stakeholders from the outset have changed uses of HEALTHeLINK for public health?
7. What are other ways in which health information exchange can be used for public health beyond what HEALTHeLINK is doing?
8. If you were a public health official involved in HEALTHeLINK, what would your next steps be?
9. How could health information exchanges such as HEALTHeLINK be used to support public health–related activities to manage a pandemic?

Acknowledgments

A portion of this work was funded under Contract 200-2011-F-40207 from the Centers for Disease Control and Prevention to RTI International. The authors gratefully acknowledge the participants who shared their time and expertise with the study team.

References

[1] New York State's Empire State Development. Western New York Regional Office: inside Western New York, <http://esd.ny.gov/RegionalOverviews/WesternNY/InsideRegion.html>; n.d. [cited 31.08.21].

[2] HEALTHeLINK. FAQs, <http://www.wnyhealthelink.com/WhoWeAre/FAQs>; n.d. [cited 31.08.21].

[3] HEALTHeLINK. HEALTHeLINK participants, <https://wnyhealthelink.com/physicians-staff/current-participants/participating-healthelink-providers/>; n.d. [cited 27.07.21].

[4] New York State Department of Health. Western New York Community Health Needs Assessment: Delivery System Reform Incentive Payment (DSRIP) program: volume one: CNA summary, <http://www.health.ny.gov/health_care/medicaid/redesign/dsrip/pps_applications/docs/erie_county/3.8_millenium_-collaborative_care_pps_cna.pdf>; 2014 [cited 2015].

[5] HealthIT.gov. Beacon Community Program, <http://www.healthit.gov/policy-researchers-implementers/beacon-community-program>; 2015.

[6] HEALTHeLINK. HEALTHeLINK awarded federal funding from Office of the National Coordinator for Health Information Technology (ONC) to expand immunization information sharing, <https://wnyhealthelink.com/news/news-releases/healthelink-awarded-federal-funding-from-office-of-the-national-coordinator-for-health-information-technology-onc-to-expand-immunization-information-sharing/>; 2021 [cited 31.08.21].

[7] HEALTHeLINK. Current participants, <https://wnyhealthelink.com/physicians-staff/current-participants/>; 2021 [cited 31.08.21].

[8] Western New York Beacon. The Western New York Beacon Community report, <http://www.wnybeacon.com/>; 2014 [cited 27.01.14].

[9] Calderwood MS, Platt R, Hou X, Malenfant J, Haney G, Kruskal B, et al. Real-time surveillance for tuberculosis using electronic health record data from an ambulatory practice in eastern Massachusetts. Public Health Rep 2010;125(6):843–50. Available from: http://www.ncbi.nlm.nih.gov/pubmed/21121229.

[10] Overhage JM, Grannis S, McDonald CJ. A comparison of the completeness and timeliness of automated electronic laboratory reporting and spontaneous reporting

of notifiable conditions. Am J Public Health 2008;98 (2):344–50.

[11] Centers for Disease Control and Prevention. National Syndromic Surveillance Program, <https://www.cdc.gov/nssp>; 2010 [cited 26.11.13].

[12] Centers for Disease Control and Prevention. Public health information network: guides, <http://www.cdc.gov/phin/resources/PHINguides.html>; 2013 [cited 27.01.14].

[13] Centers for Medicare & Medicaid Services. Health Care Innovation Awards round two, <http://innovation.cms.gov/initiatives/Health-Care-Innovation-Awards/Round-2.html>; 2014 [cited 27.01.14].

[14] Kern LM, Kaushal R. Health information technology and health information exchange in New York State: new initiatives in implementation and evaluation. J Biomed Inform 2007;40(6 Suppl):S17–20 PMID: 17945542. Epub 2007 Sept 7.

[15] Shapiro JS. Evaluating public health uses of health information exchange. J Biomed Inform 2007;40(6 Suppl):S46–9. Available from: http://www.ncbi.nlm.nih.gov/pmc/articles/PMC2137930/.

[16] Kass-Hout TA, Gray SK, Massoudi BL, Immanuel GY, Dollacker M, Cothren R. NHIN, RHIOs, and public health. J Public Health Manag Pract 2007;13 (1):31–4.

[17] Shapiro JS, Mostashari F, Hripcsak G, Soulakis N, Kuperman G. Using health information exchange to improve public health. Am J Public Health 2011;101 (4):616–23.

[18] RTI International. ONC State Health Policy Consortium Project: health information exchange in disaster preparedness and response. Washington (DC): Office of the National Coordinator for Health Information Technology, U.S. Department of Health and Human Services. Available from: <http://www.healthit.gov/sites/default/files/pdf/SERCH-White-Paper.pdf>; 2012 [cited 27.01.14].

[19] U.S. Department of Health and Human Services. OCR issues guidance to help ensure first responders and others receive protected health information about individuals exposed to COVID-19, <https://public3.pagefreezer.com/content/HHS.gov/31-12-2020T08:51/https://www.hhs.gov/about/news/2020/03/24/ocr-issues-guidance-to-help-ensure-first-responders-and-others-receive-protected-health-information-about-individuals-exposed-to-covid-19.html>; 2020 [cited 31.08.21].

[20] U.S. Department of Health and Human Services, Office of Civil Rights. COVID-19 and HIPAA: disclosures to law enforcement, paramedics, and other first responders and public health authorities, <https://www.hhs.gov/sites/default/files/covid-19-hipaa-and-first-responders-508.pdf>; n.d. [cited 31.08.21].

[21] Tandon S, Adhi S. Summary of public health objectives in stage 2 meaningful use ONC and CMS final rules. n.d. [cited 2019 Jan 27]. https://www.cdc.gov/datainteroperability/doc/historical/summary-of-ph-objectives-in-stage-2-mu-onc-and-cms-final-rules_04_01_2014.pdf.

[22] Centers for Disease Control and Prevention. 2013 National notifiable infectious conditions, <http://wwwn.cdc.gov/nndss/script/conditionlist.aspx?type=0&yr=2013>; 2014 [updated 17.01.14].

[23] Centers for Disease Control and Prevention. COVID-19 testing overview, <https://www.cdc.gov/coronavirus/2019-ncov/symptoms-testing/testing.html>; 2021 [cited 31.08.21].

[24] Overhage JM, Suico J, McDonald CJ. Electronic laboratory reporting: barriers, solutions and findings. J Public Health Manag Pract 2001;7(6):60–6.

[25] Silk BJ, Berkelman RL. A review of strategies for enhancing the completeness of notifiable disease reporting. J Public Health Manag Pract 2005;11 (3):191–200.

[26] Walker J, Pan E, Johnston D, Adler-Milstein J, Bates DW, Middleton B. The value of health care information exchange and interoperability. Health Aff (Millwood) 2005;2005(Suppl Web Exclusives):W5-10–18.

[27] Kansas Health Institute. Kansas HIE first to connect to CDC surveillance system, <http://www.khi.org/news/2012/nov/21/kansas-hie-first-nation-connect-cdc-outbreak-surve/>; 2012 [cited 21.11.12].

[28] O'Connor AC, Haque SN, Layton CM, Loomis RJ, Braun FM, Amoozegar JB, et al. Impact of a two-dimensional barcode for vaccine production, clinical documentation, and public health reporting and tracking. Atlanta, GA: Centers for Disease Control and Prevention; 2012. Available from: http://www.cdc.gov/vaccines/programs/iis/activities/downloads/2d-barcode-trkg-rpt.pdf.

[29] World Health Organization. Framework for decision-making: implementation of mass vaccination campaigns in the context of COVID-19, <https://www.who.int/docs/default-source/coronaviruse/framework-for-decision-making-implementation-of-mass-vaccination-campaigns-in-the-context-of-covid19-slide-deck.pdf?sfvrsn=438dccc8_2>; n.d. [cited 31.08.21].

[30] American Society of Health-System Pharmacists. Essential elements of a successful mass immunization program, <https://www.ashp.org/-/media/assets/pharmacy-practice/resource-centers/Coronavirus/docs/COVID-19_Successful-Mass-Immunization-Program_FINAL.ashx>; 2021 [cited 31.08.21].

[31] Dixon BE, Gamache RE, Grannis SJ. Towards public health decision support: a systematic review of

bidirectional communication approaches. J Am Med Inform Assoc 2013;20(3):577–83.
[32] Gamache R, Stevens KC, Merriwether R, Dixon BE, Grannis S. Development and assessment of a public health alert delivered through a community health information exchange. Online J Public Health Inform 2010;2(2) Epub 2010 Oct 29.
[33] Mäenpää T, Asikainen P, Gissler M, Siponen K, Maass M, Saranto K, et al. Outcomes assessment of the regional health information exchange: a five-year follow-up study. Methods Inf Med 2011;50 (4):308–18.
[34] HEALTHeLINK. COVID-19 information, <https://wnyhealthelink.com/physicians-staff/covid-19-information/>; n.d. [cited 31.08.21].
[35] Centers for Disease Control and Prevention. COVID-19: frequently asked questions, <https://www.cdc.gov/coronavirus/2019-ncov/faq.html>; 2021 [cited 31.08.21].
[36] Muehlenbein CE, Hoverman JR, Gruschkus SK, Forsyth M, Chen C, Lopez W, et al. Evaluation of the reliability of electronic medical record data in identifying comorbid conditions among patients with advanced non-small cell lung cancer. J Cancer Epidemiol 2011;2011:983271 PMCID: 3134088.
[37] Western New York HEALTHeNET. Welcome to WNY HEALTHeNET, <http://www.wnyhealthenet.org/>; 2001 [cited 27.01.19].
[38] HEALTHeLINK. Mission and history, <https://wnyhealthelink.com/who-we-are/mission-and-history/>; n.d. [cited 31.08.21].
[39] HEALTHeLINK. Statement from HEALTHeLINK Executive Director Daniel Porreca regarding updated COVID-19 capabilities, <https://wnyhealthelink.com/news/news-releases/statement-from-healthelink-executive-director-daniel-porreca-regarding-updated-covid-19-capabilities/>; 2020 [cited 31.08.21].
[40] Erie County Department of Health. ECDOH COVID-19 isolation and quarantine documents, <https://www2.erie.gov/health/index.php?q = ecdoh-covid-19-isolation-and-quarantine-documents>; n.d. [cited 31.08.21].
[41] HEALTHeLINK. HEALTHeLINK training guide, <https://wnyhealthelink.com/wp-content/uploads/HEALTHeLINK-Training-Guide.pdf>; 2020 [cited 17.09.21].

CHAPTER

24

Creating a 21st century health information technology infrastructure: New York's Health Care Efficiency and Affordability Law for New Yorkers Capital Grant Program

Joshua R. Vest[1,2] *and Erika G. Martin*[3]

[1]Department of Health Policy and Management, Richard M. Fairbanks School of Public Health, Indiana University, Indianapolis, IN, USA [2]Center for Biomedical Informatics, Regenstrief Institute, Inc., Indianapolis, IN, USA [3]Rockefeller College of Public Affairs and Policy, University at Albany, Albany, NY, USA

LEARNING OBJECTIVES

- Contrast the strengths and weaknesses of a geographically defined approach to exchange.
- Discuss the advanages and disadvantages of grant funding to support health information organizations.
- Discuss the motivations for and against mergers between health information organizations.

Major themes

- Organization design of health information exchange
- Public funding
- Program evaluation
- Policy development and implementation
- Governance of health information exchange

Health Information Exchange
DOI: https://doi.org/10.1016/B978-0-323-90802-3.00003-4

24.1 Introduction

Health information exchange (HIE), the electronic sharing of patient information among providers, began in the United States as local activity. Starting in the 1990s, numerous collaborations of health care organizations, community organizations, and government agencies started the technical infrastructure and organizational relationships necessary to share patient information within their communities. These initiatives differed in their technology architectures, types of leading organizations, and community sizes, but all focused on supporting HIE for a local community or geographically defined population [1]. These efforts had high failure rates, but throughout the decade, organizing HIE activity at the community level was the consistent approach [2]. HIE organizations serving local communities even demonstrated some ability to impact the cost of care [3,4].

In the early to mid-2000s, a small but growing number of operational local HIE organizations were serving as effective success stories [5] and the United States began formulating a national HIE strategy. The Office for the National Coordinator (ONC) for Health Information Technology's Framework for Strategic Action envisioned a "consumer centric and information-rich" health care industry, where health data follow patients and are used for medical decision making. Strategic goals included: improving the adoption and use of electronic health records in clinical practice, developing an interoperable health information technology infrastructure to connect clinicians, promoting the use of information to personalize health care, and improving public health surveillance and monitoring. The second goal, to interconnect clinicians, focused on fostering regional collaborations as the organizational mechanism for this activity [6]. The label applied to these local HIE organizations was "Regional Health Information Organizations" (RHIOs).

Organizing exchange activities around RHIOs offered several operational and political advantages over the approaches that had failed in the previous decade [1,7]. First, RHIOs were collaborative organizations with multistakeholder governance, allowing them to act as neutral third parties between competing health care organizations [8]. RHIOs were focused on quality and "improving health and care in that community" [9]. Finally, RHIOs served defined geographic areas, usually a collection of adjacent counties, a metropolitan area, or a state [1], consistent with the idea that HIE should be a locally organized and controlled activity.

The national strategy envisioned at this time was a "network of networks" [10,11]. Numerous autonomous local organizations, primarily RHIOs, would be responsible for HIE activity within their communities and subsequently connected together at a national level [12]. RHIOs were identified as the "building blocks" [13] of this network, with the federal government providing standards and guidance on technology, interoperability, and policy to facilitate HIE across RHIOs [11]. By focusing on organizations providing service locally, the United States adopted a "bottom up" approach to HIE [14].

At the same time, researchers, practitioners, and policy makers were increasingly aware of the barriers inhibiting widespread HIE. Adopting health information technology is costly (including financial costs, retraining staff, and changing clinical workflow), the quality of vendor products can be difficult to assess, and adopters face negative externalities (i.e., although providers purchase technologies, the benefits mostly accrue to patients and payers) [15]. The potential benefits to patient and public health, combined with limited financial incentives, made public funding to establish and maintain a data sharing infrastructure a logical option [1,16,17]. Consequently, funding and national coordination could further support a vision of broader information

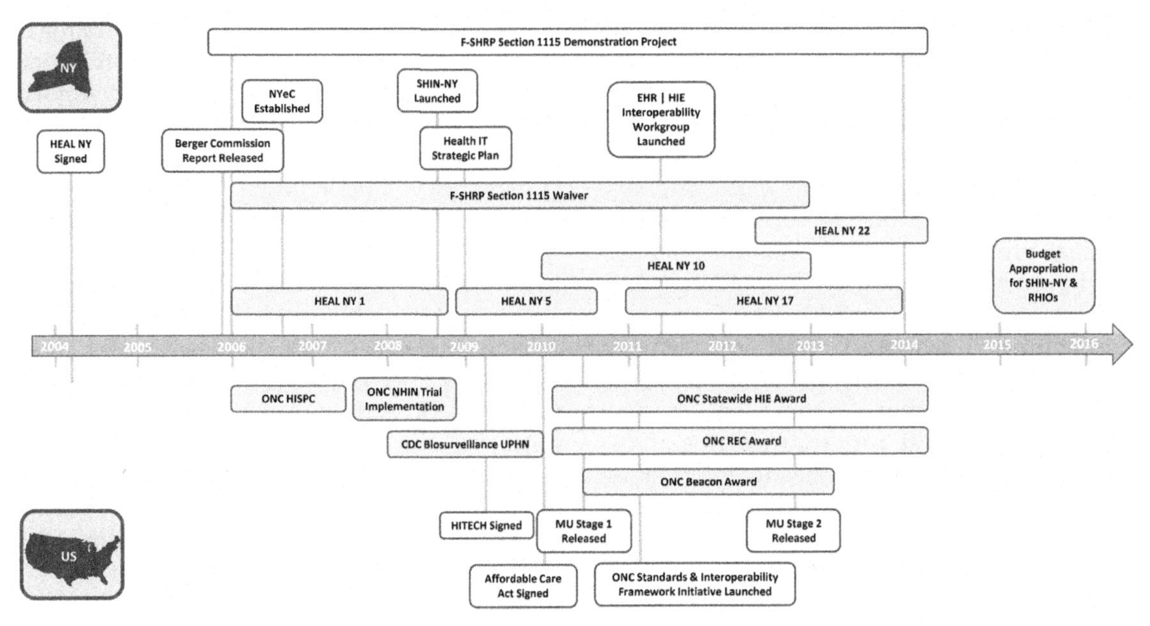

FIGURE 24.1 Chronology of HEAL NY Health Information Technology Grants. *Notes*: Green boxes represent funding sources, and white boxes represent policies and activities. *EHR*, Electronic health records; *F-SHRP*, Federal-State Health Reform Partnership; *HEAL NY*, Health Care Efficiency and Affordability Law for New Yorkers; *HIE*, health information exchange; *HISPC*, Health Information Security and Privacy Collaboration; *MU*, meaningful use; *NHIN*, Nationwide Health Information Network Exchange; *NYeC*, New York eHealth Collaborative; *ONC*, Office of the National Coordinator for Health Information Technology; *REC*, Regional Extension Center, *SHIN-NY*, State Health Information Network of New York; *UPHN*, Universal Public Health Node. (For interpretation of the references to color in this figure legend, the reader is referred to the web version of this book) [25]. Source: *Adapted with permission from the New York State Department of Health.*

exchange [6]. It is within this context that New York State launched the nation's largest (at the time) single public investment in developing a health information technology infrastructure to support HIE.

24.2 Background: the Health Care Efficiency and Affordability Law for New Yorkers Capital Grant Program

In 2004, New York State passed the Health Care Efficiency and Affordability Law for New Yorkers Capital Grant Program (HEAL NY) [18]. HEAL NY was designed to "encourage improvements in the operation and efficiency of the health care delivery system within the state" [19] and part of a broader interest by the governor's office and legislature in improving New York State's health care system [20]. Although most capital grants funded activities such as hospital conversions and debt retirement [21], 5 of the 22 phases aimed to expand the adoption and implementation of interoperable health information technology and HIE [22]. HEAL NY was jointly administered by the New York State Department of Health and the Dormitory Authority of the State of New York.

HEAL NY funds were disbursed through a series of competitive grant opportunities released in so-called "Phases"[1] (Fig. 24.1). In addition to funding health information technology, phases

[1] Only those phases of HEAL NY related to health information technology are described here.

were responsive to the hospital and nursing home reconfiguration recommendations in the Berger Commission report [21] and goals of the Federal-State Health Reform Partnership (F-SHRP) Medicaid Section 1115 waiver, which aimed to right-size the acute care system, shift long-term care to community-based settings, promote health information technology, improve the provision of ambulatory and primary care, and expand Medicaid managed care [23]. HEAL NY and F-SHRP, representing a mix of state and federal funds, were used to implement the Berger Commission's recommendations on health care restructuring across six regions and to expand health information technology. In 2006, HEAL NY Phase 1 provided $52.9 million to 26 projects. In 2008, 21 projects received $104.9 million under HEAL NY Phase 5. HEAL NY Phase 10's $99.9 million went to 11 projects in 2009. HEAL NY Phase 17 made $116.8 million in funding available to 14 projects in 2010. Finally, HEAL NY Phase 22 made $38.2 million available to two projects (Table 24.1) [24].[2] The focus and intent of each phase differed.

Phases 1 and 5 were most directly related to establishing the state's initial HIE structure and promoting the adoption of electronic health records. These phases funded RHIOs and supported community-wide adoption of electronic health records and other interoperable health information technologies. Phases 10 and 17 focused on health information technology for Patient Centered Medical Homes and care coordination. The last phase (22) supported electronic health records for behavioral health (Table 24.2) [18].

Although certain elements remained constant, HEAL NY was dynamic. For example, a goal of sharable patient information through interoperable health information technology was explicitly articulated in every HEAL NY phase [15,26–28]. In addition, under a requirement of "statewide geographic distribution of funds" [19], each HEAL NY phase funded communities across the state, with each Berger Commission region receiving at least one award (Table 24.1). Importantly, RHIOs were the model of HIE organization. Even later phases that did not provide direct funding to support RHIOs required grantees to be participants in one of the HEAL NY-funded RHIOs [15,28].

However, HEAL NY did evolve over time, with later phases building on prior work (Table 24.2). Although Phase 1 had a large focus on e-prescribing and electronic health records [29], Phase 5 introduced the idea of and funding for the Statewide Health Information Network of New York (SHIN-NY), a statewide "network of networks" to connect RHIOs [30]. As Patient Centered Medical Homes were promoted through the Affordable Care Act, subsequent phases focused on implementing electronic health records and facilitating HIE in these organizations especially among behavioral health and long-term care providers. This shift from building technology infrastructure to encouraging HIE across specific health care organizations was intended to "integrate this infrastructure with reimbursement reforms and innovative delivery reforms" [15].

24.3 Case study: the evolution of health information exchange organizations in New York State

The landscape of HIE organizations in New York State changed dramatically over a relatively short period of time. In the summer of 2006, HEAL NY Phase 1 provided $52.9 million to 26 projects. By 2015, New York State was home to nine HIE organizations, a public–private statewide exchange entity and a total

[2] In Phases 5, 10, and 17, two awards each were made to the New York eHealth Collaborative and Health Information Technology Evaluation Collaborative for evaluation and implementation; these awards are included in these counts.

TABLE 24.1 HEAL NY funding for health information technology by phase and Berger Commission region.

Characteristic	Awards, *N* (%)	Funding, $
Phase		
1	26 (35.1)	52,875,000
5	21 (28.4)	104,944,003
10	11 (14.9)	99,914,713
17	14 (18.9)	116,775,701
22	2 (2.7)	38,200,000
Berger Commission region		
Central	9 (12.2)	35,311,990
Hudson Valley	7 (9.5)	31,985,788
Long Island	9 (12.2)	49,798,625
New York City	25 (33.8)	174,100,093
Northern	8 (10.8)	17,713,669
Western	11 (14.9)	61,494,205
Statewide	5 (6.8)	42,305,047
Types of health information technology		
Adoption or promotion of e-prescribing	12 (16.2)	73,070,183
Adoption or promotion of EHRs	56 (75.7)	312,453,255
Adoption of new EHRs	43 (58.1)	250,824,226
Expanded capacity of existing EHRs	33 (44.6)	184,204,077
Adoption or promotion of health information exchange	65 (87.8)	341,818,279
Adoption or promotion of consumer-mediated health information exchange	25 (33.8)	170,475,694
Evaluation	3 (4.1)	11,820,505
Implementation	3 (4.1)	51,684,542
Total, all awards	74 (100)	412,709,417

Rockefeller Institute of Government's analysis of HEAL NY grant materials [24].

public–private investment nearing $1 billion. New York's current state of HIE is the result of the interaction of HEAL NY with changes in state administration, changes in state and federal policy, new technology developments, sustainability needs, and organizational growth and development.

24.4 HEAL NY Phase 1 (2005–08)

Phase 1 funded three categories of health information technology projects: HIE, e-prescribing technologies, and EHR adoption and implementation. HIE funding provided capital costs and targeted projects committed to interoperability.

TABLE 24.2 Categories of HEAL NY grants for health information technology, by phase.

Phase	Start year	Application categories
1	2006	• Creating e-prescribing capabilities • Furthering the use of EHRs • Developing community-wide clinical data sharing
5	2008	• Reference architecture and pilot implementations of the Statewide Health Information Network for New York (SHIN-NY) • Pilot implementations of Clinical Informatics Services, automated tools that aggregate, analyze, measure, and report clinical data for uses such as quality and population health reporting • Pilot implementations of community-wide interoperable EHRs
10	2010	• Implementing EHRs and facilitating HIE for patient-centered medical homes for patient populations with chronic and complex health conditions
17	2011	• Implementing EHRs and facilitating HIE for patient-centered medical homes for patient populations with chronic mental health conditions
22	2012	• Facilitating EHRs for behavioral health

Rockefeller Institute of Government's analysis of HEAL NY grant materials [24].

In contrast to the later phases (which were more focused on HIE and promoting health information technology adoption more generally), e-prescribing received a heavy emphasis because at the time this activity had more advanced standards and clearer quality and efficiency returns [29].

There were a few additional requirements, also included in subsequent phases. Each project required 50% matching funding (with reductions for financially distressed organizations) and applications described the financial viability and sustainability of their business models. This matching requirement was designed to ensure that applicants would be committed to the continued use of health information technology after HEAL NY grants ended [24]. In addition, projects had to be collaborative. Grantees had to involve multiple stakeholders, at least one independent organization (i.e., all organizations on the project could not be controlled by the same entity), and organizations of different types (e.g., hospitals, physician groups, etc.) [26]. Last, all phases sought a "broad" geographic distribution of funds [31], which was accomplished by allocating funds to all six Berger Commission regions (Table 24.1).

The result was a very diverse set of initiatives by 26 grantees across the state (Fig. 24.2). New York City alone was home to nine projects. The average award was $2 million and ranged from about $175,000 up to $5 million [32]. Nearly all grantees reported supporting some type of HIE and described their activities as "regional connectivity," "community exchange," "regional information network," "clinical data exchange," or "information sharing" [32,33].

HEAL NY Phase 1 projects were led by two types of grantees: existing health care organizations and health information organizations created to facilitate HIE [33]. The health care organizations leading Phase 1 projects were hospitals, academic medical centers, health systems, and large physician practices. However, projects also included many other organizations such as physician offices, imaging centers, long-term care providers, and health plans. Eleven of the grantees had the governance structure and activities to be classified as

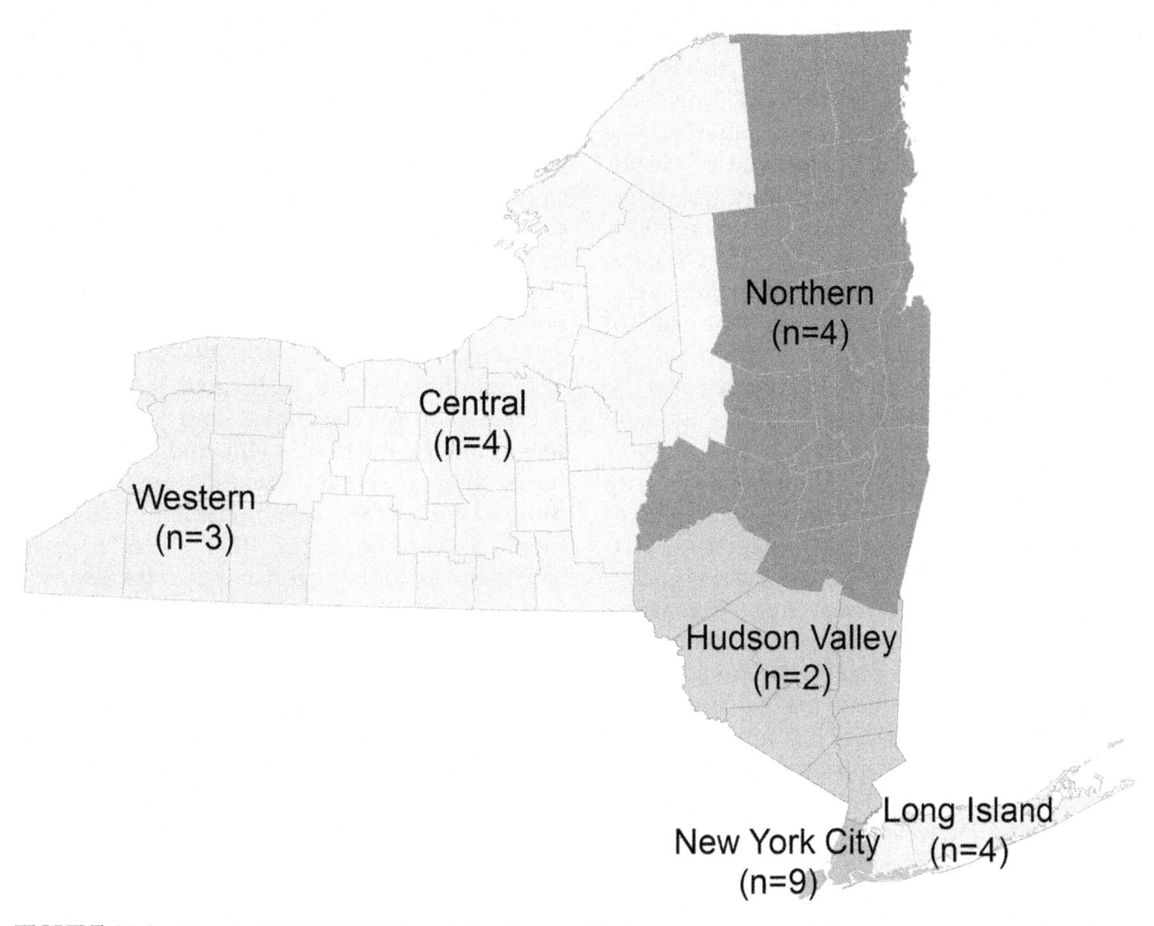

FIGURE 24.2 Number of HEAL NY Phase 1 Grantees per Region.

RHIOs [22]. After 2 years, all 26 grantee organizations were still in existence, but only 11 would subsequently receive funding under HEAL NY Phase 5 [33].

24.5 HEAL NY Phase 5 (2007–10)

With HEAL NY Phase 5, New York State adopted a much more coordinated approach to health information technology policy and funding [22]. The new governor established the Office of Health Information Technology Transformation within the Department of Health to coordinate health information technology policies and programs [27]. In addition, in line with the new administration's policy, New York State would establish a public–private partnership to develop and govern statewide HIE rather than having the health department assume policy guidance [34,35]. Overall, the long-term goal was a health information technical infrastructure to enable statewide information sharing and widespread EHR adoption, and support public and population health [36]. Phase 5 funding reflected this new policy direction.

HEAL NY Phase 5 articulated New York's network-of-networks approach to HIE across the entire state [27]. This phase funded RHIOs as the foundational components for developing cross-sectional interoperability. Grants fell into three categories with corresponding use cases developed by the Department of Health (Table 24.1). The first grant category was reference architecture and pilot implementations of the SHIN-NY. As described by the Office of Health Information Technology Transformation, the SHIN-NY was envisioned as "the sum of interoperable regional HIEs governed by RHIOs" [37]. These grants supported the 10 RHIOs with common software protocols, core services, and standards that could later support HIE through the SHIN-NY. The second category of grants funded pilot implementations of clinical informatics services, tools to aggregate, analyze, measure, and report clinical data for quality and population health reporting. Remaining grants funded pilot implementations of community-wide interoperable electronic health records. Overall, this phase moved away from the initial focus on e-prescribing and toward the creation of RHIOs and improved penetration of electronic health records (Table 24.1).

At the onset New York State envisioned HIE as a local activity. "Design globally, implement locally" was a common refrain among those leading HEAL NY [15,38]. New York's conceptualization of the SHIN-NY as a network of networks reflects this all-health-care-is-local perspective and the political necessity of ensuring a statewide distribution of public funding.

RHIOs were the cornerstone of developing a statewide HIE. To receive state funding, RHIOs had to be nonprofit (and nongovernmental), have multistakeholder governance and participation, serve a defined geographical area, have a sustainability plan, provide matching funds, agree to be interoperable, and participate in a statewide collaboration process to develop common exchange protocols, services, and standards [27]. New York allocated $60.4 million to 8 RHIOs (minimum $4.7 million and maximum $10 million) under Phase 5 as part of the SHIN-NY development [36]. All funded RHIOs had also received Phase 1 funding [22] (Fig. 24.3).

To support the SHIN-NY development, Phase 5 funded the New York eHealth Collaborative (NYeC) to facilitate the statewide collaboration process [27]. NYeC was founded in 2006 as a nonprofit organization with funding and oversight from New York State (e.g., a public–private partnership) focusing on policy and standards development [39]. Under Phase 5, NYeC became the designated independent organization to coordinate and obtain consensus among the RHIOs [40], and continues to serve this function. Funded organizations directed 5% of their reimbursable or matching funds to support NYeC [27]. NYeC's early activities including convening stakeholders (vendors, health care organizations, patients, public health departments, etc.) to formulate statewide HIE policies, including the consent policy that specified an opt-in model with exceptions for emergency access [41].

Phase 5 funded two additional entities that supported the adoption and implementation of health information technology. First, the program introduced a new type of entity called a Community Health Information Technology Adoption Collaboration (CHITA). CHITAs were less formally organized than RHIOs, typically alliances of local providers working to adopt health information technology tools. The HEAL NY Phase 5 request for grant applications describes CHITAs as "primarily responsible for achieving adoption and effective use of health IT tools, especially EHRs, by clinicians at the point of care" [27]. CHITAs purchased software licenses for quality reporting, point-to-point exchange connections, and EHR adoption [35]. With their focus on technology adoption, the eight CHITAs were in some ways a precursor to the ONC's Regional Extension Centers.

Phase 5 also developed new processes to improve effectiveness and accountability. First,

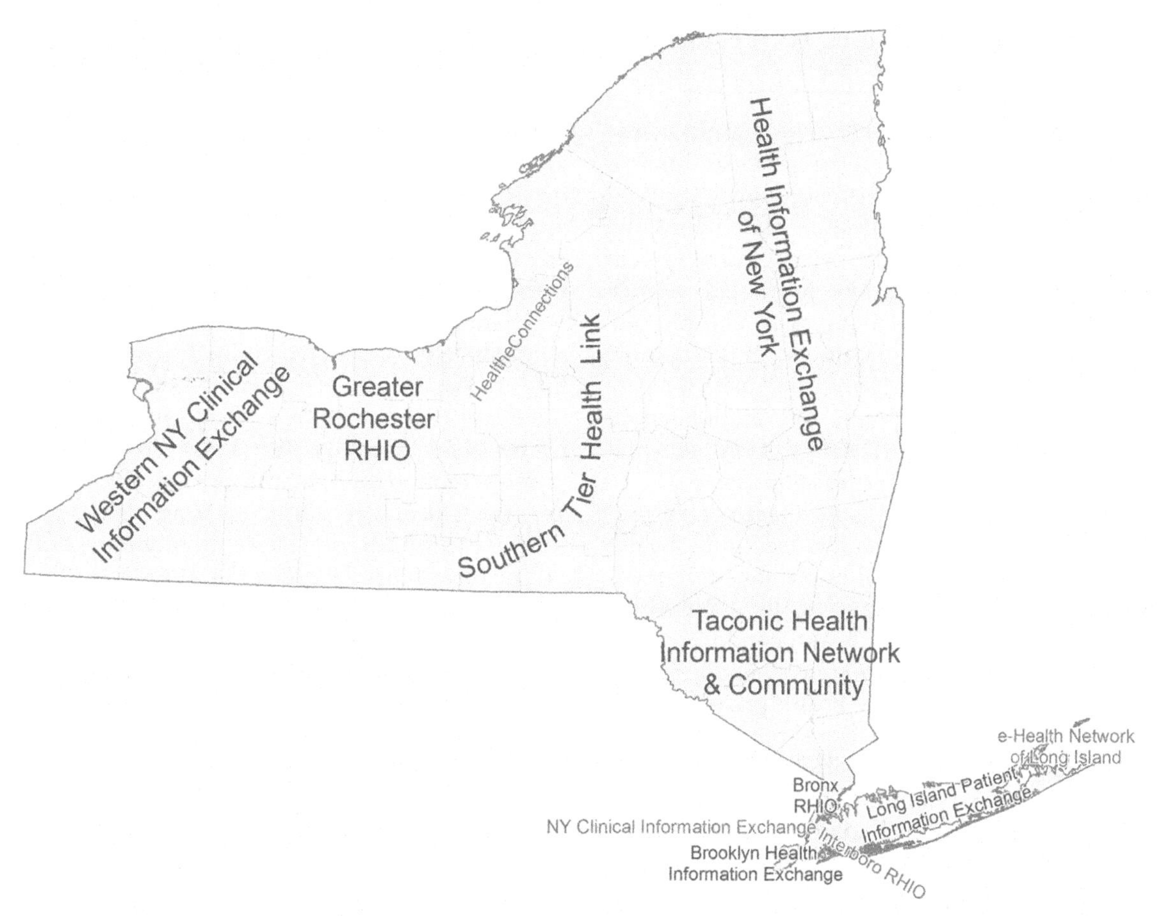

FIGURE 24.3 New York's Regional Health Information Organizations c.2008–09. *Note*: RHIOs funded under HEAL Phase 5 as part of the Statewide Health Information Network for New York are in blue. (For interpretation of the references to color in this figure legend, the reader is referred to the web version of this book).

the Health Information Technology Collaborative (HITEC) was formed to provide consistent statewide evaluation, which differed from the more informal final reports from Phase 1 grantees. HITEC, an academic collaborative of Cornell University, Columbia University, the University of Rochester, the State University of New York at Buffalo, and the State University of New York at Albany, was tasked with establishing common measurement approaches and conducting evaluations of policy, implementation, and impact [42]. HITEC evaluated cross-cutting issues across projects such as adoption, implementation, costs, utilization, safety, and quality. All HEAL NY grantees had to cooperate with these evaluation activities [27]. Second, the HEAL NY program office developed a new pay-for-performance approach to manage grants. Staff created "GAP Tool" spreadsheets that listed all activities that grantees committed to completing in their applications, which were used to track milestones. Grantees submitted documentation or else demonstrated a technical capability in a webinar as evidence of each activity's completion. Ten percent of committed grant funds were withheld until the completion of all deliverables.

24.6 HEAL NY Phases 10, 17, and 22 (2009–14)

Starting in Phase 10, HEAL NY grants were more targeted and followed national interest in medical homes, which received funding through the Patient Protection and Affordable Care Act. This new health care delivery system and reimbursement model promoted coordinated care for people living with chronic diseases or high-cost diagnoses. Interoperable electronic health records were requisite for providers to exchange clinical information about these patients, who often saw multiple clinicians at different health care facilities.

Whereas HEAL NY Phase 10 supported projects to develop interoperable electronic health records and promote HIE in primary care medical homes, Phase 17 specifically focused on populations with mental health conditions [28]. Phase 17 aimed to integrate mental health, long-term care, and home health providers into medical homes. There were two categories: "limited" projects that expanded patient-centered medical homes to include at least one mental health diagnosis and "expanded" projects that included at least one chronic disease associated with mental health disorders in addition to a combination of mental health, long-term care, and home health care providers [28]. Phase 22, the last HEAL NY grant, provided funding to the state's two regional extension centers to facilitate electronic health records for behavioral health, a disease area with limited use of electronic health records [43]. Because behavioral health and long-term care providers were ineligible for Meaningful Use incentives, these phases helped address a gap in HIT adoption in New York State [44].

Overall, grants in Phases 10, 17, and 22 built off the infrastructure developed in earlier phases, "moving [emerging health IT systems] from infancy to childhood" (p. 6) [15]. Applications became more sophisticated, following the incremental adoption of health information technology across the state. As an example, one Phase 17 applicant described how the award would build on Phases 1, 5, and 10, a past federal Beacon Community Program award, and initiatives from the Medical Society for the State of New York (Box 24.1). Other applicants from these later phases proposed advanced capabilities for their existing electronic health records, such as quality metrics and immunization reports that could be automatically generated and transmitted to the Department of Health, incorporating Medicaid administrative data into clinical charts, and clinical decision tools ranging from pop-up reminders to sophisticated algorithms and visualizations about patients' risks for future complications. These capabilities built off the emerging HIE networks (Box 24.2).

24.7 New York State's evolution during the period of federal action: HITECH Act and Meaningful Use Stages 1 & 2 (2008–14)

From the beginning, New York sought consistency with national approaches [26]. For example, HEAL NY Phase 5 envisioned the SHIN-NY as part of the federal Nationwide Health Information Network (NHIN) [27] and both state policy makers and RHIO leaders looked to follow technology standards being adopted by the federal government, when available [45]. Also, Phase 5 use cases aligned with both the ONC's and the Centers for Disease Control and Prevention's HIE use cases. However, midway through Phase 5, federal health information technology policy changed dramatically with the introduction of the Meaningful Use Program under the Health Information Technology for Economic and Clinical Health (HITECH) Act of 2009.

The introduction of this large program had consequences for HIE activities within New York State. Immediately, the state moved to

BOX 24.1

Example of a Phase 17 applicant building off prior HEAL NY Phases.

HEAL 1 provided funding needed to implement HEALHeLINK's Health Information Exchange (HIE) technology platform and to execute ePrescription (eRx) and Diagnostic Data Exchange (lab and radiology results reporting). Through HEAL 5, HEALTHeLINK is accelerating the expansion of the integrated HIE platform in WNY [(Western New York)], standardizing connections and transactions, and leveraging CHIxP [(common HIE protocols)] through the SHIN-NY architecture. This supports the transfer of NYS Immunization Records, Medicaid Medication History Information, and Public Health data. HEAL 10 currently supports EHR adoption to: improve chronic care management as demonstrated by improved clinical outcomes performance measures; proactive patient self-management facilitated by patient portals; and increase care coordination. HEALTHeLINK's MSSNY grant is enabling physician practice EHR interoperability by facilitating the two-way flow of patient referral data via Continuity of Care Document (CCD) exchange. Adding HEAL 17 to these initiatives, which by design build on and enhance each other, will have a significant impact on the provision of mental health care in Erie County that can be replicated throughout WNY.

become more aligned with the Meaningful Use Program. This is most evident in the language and expectations for the HEAL NY phases released during this period. Phases 10 and 17 required that grantees adopt certified EHRs and to ensure that health IT usage complied with the Meaningful Use Program so that the health care providers benefiting from the state grant program would also be eligible for incentive payments [15,28]. Also, RHIOs saw certification, the requirements for interoperability, and a stronger federal role in standard setting necessary and beneficial [45]. The Meaningful Use Program also increased the adoption of EHRs within communities, thereby creating more potential participants for the RHIOs.

Yet not all effects of the Meaningful Use Program were welcome or beneficial. For one, Meaningful Use became the top health information technology priority. For individual physicians and hospitals, resources and time were often allocated toward adopting EHRs or attestations for incentive funding, not for connections with RHIOs [46]. This did not necessarily reflect devaluation of the RHIOs, but with limited resources, achieving Meaningful Use was perceived as more important. Likewise, health information technology vendors had more financial opportunities from the federal Meaningful Use Program, making them less responsive to HEAL NY [45]. This had predictable effects on operations as RHIOs reported challenges with vendor responsiveness. More importantly, the shift in attention limited the RHIOs' ability to grow and innovate. As single entities with less funding, RHIOs reported difficulty in finding vendors willing, or able, to develop new interfaces or tools [46].

The challenges from Meaningful Use were even more pronounced with respect to the federal Direct Project and the Stage 2 criteria.[3] The Direct Project's point-to-point, single-patient approach to HIE was different than the

[3] For more on the Direct Project, see chapter "Standardizing and Exchanging Messages."

BOX 24.2

Examples of Phase 10 applicants coordinating health care services through interoperable electronic health records and health information exchange.

HeR EMR: a PCMH Model for High Risk Obstetrics Using Electronic Medical Records will improve the coordination and management of (high-risk pregnancy) patients through the use of interoperable health information. Participating providers in the (care coordination zone) will implement practice-based EMRs in their offices that will connect to specialists to whom they refer their high-risk patients (e.g., cardiologists for hypertensive pregnant women, endocrinologists for patients with pre- and post-gestational diabetes), pediatricians, laboratories, and home care. In addition, individual practices will be able to connect electronically to the labor and delivery units and the well-baby nurseries and neonatal intensive care units of North Shore University Hospital, Long Island Jewish Medical Center, and Schneider Children's Hospital where an EMR is currently being deployed.

Under the [Southwest Brooklyn Patient Centered Medical and Mental Health Home Project], select outpatient primary and mental health clinics...will utilize electronic health records (EHRs) and portal access to connect to the Brooklyn Health Information Exchange (BHIX) and the State Health Information Network of New York (SHIN-NY) to access information about their patients from disparate sources and to communicate/coordinate with necessary caregivers along the care continuum, thereby enabling them to provide patient centered medical and mental health home services to their schizophrenic patients...Inpatient, specialty, home health, case managers, and other providers and caregivers involved in the care of the target population will also be connected to BHIX and the SHIN-NY and will be provided a secure care coordination plan template (CCPT), brokered through BHIX, that offers a presentation layer that aggregates relevant patient diagnostic information and recommended next steps in care, and that enables providers to add relevant documentation and orders to the plan throughout the patient's course of care...Finally, the project proposes to enable certain stakeholders to provide their patients with access to a Personal Health Record ("PHR") and to supplement the connectivity above with videoconferencing abilities to further enable the provision of truly coordinated care.

centralized data approach taken by most New York RHIOs and the states' focus on the application of information for public health purposes [47]. In New York, RHIOs had adopted query-based exchange [35]. Direct was a challenge because, while all RHIOs eventually offered Direct services, this additional approach did not necessarily further their use of query-based exchange nor address their existing operational challenges. Importantly, the Direct Program meant that providers could meet Meaningful Use Program's expectations for interoperable patient information and HIE without participating in a RHIO [47].

In part because of Meaningful Use, this period also saw significant changes in the national thinking on the organization of HIE activities. For most of the decade, and throughout Phases 1 and 5, the US Department of Health and Human Services promoted a "network of networks" approach for HIE [48]. In 2009, that approach was abandoned [11]. RHIOs were no longer identified as the primary building blocks for national exchange activities and fewer federal resources were dedicated to RHIOs [12].

The HITECH Act also promoted increased centralization of HIE activities within New York State by funding states or their "state-designated entities" (SDEs) to "facilitate and expand the electronic movement and use of health information among organizations" [49]. To be eligible to receive federal funding, an SDE had to be named by the state, a nonprofit with collaborative governance, and focused on health information technology and exchange to improve care [49]. In 2009, NYeC was named as the SDE, due to its nonprofit status and existing work in facilitating collaboration among RHIOs [38].

In part to comply with the federal requirements, NYeC revised the state's Policy and Governance Structure to establish a certification process for organizations that could participate in the SHIN-NY. Organizations that met these criteria were known as "Qualified Health IT Entities" or QEs. Qualified Health IT Entities requirements were very similar to the organizational and governance structure of the state's existing RHIOs, although Qualified Health IT Entities membership was not restricted to RHIOs [50].

The New York HIE experience became marked by consolidation and moved toward centralization. Mergers between RHIOs were not new; two HEAL NY Phase 1 grantees merged to become a Phase 5 RHIO [9]. However, consolidation was more pronounced and focused in the downstate region. In 2011, the Manhattan-based New York Clinical Information Exchange (NYCLIX) and the Long Island Patient Information eXchange (LIPIX) merged to form Healthix. Within 2 years, the Brooklyn Health Information Exchange (BHIX) became part of Healthix, resulting in an RHIO with more than 9 million patients [51]. In 2014, Southern Tier Healthlink (STHL) and the Taconic Health Information Network and Community (THINC), Phase 5 RHIOs, formed HealthlinkNY to serve southern New York [52].

In another move toward centralization that coincided with many of the mergers, NYeC assumed responsibility for consolidating and operating core technology services for the QE/RHIOs. To participate in the SHIN-NY network, QE/RHIOs could either maintain their own existing technology infrastructure or else contract to use the infrastructure supplied by NYeC [50]. A total of six QE/RHIOs signed service agreements to use NYeC's shared service platform; all of these "service Qualified Health IT Entities" were downstate. However, 2 years later in 2014, NYeC, in conjunction with the New York State Department of Health and the leaders of the "service Qualified Health IT Entities," decided to discontinue offering technology services for Qualified Health IT Entities. After this change, each Qualified Health IT Entitieswas again responsible for contracting its own technology services, which was a slight shift from centralization.

24.8 The current state of health information exchange in New York State

By 2015, New York State was home to nine Qualified Health IT Entities (QEs), a public–private statewide exchange entity and a total public–private investment nearing $1 billion. In addition solidifying the HIE infrastructure, the 2015–16 state budget included $45 million for NYeC and the nine RHIOs [53], and the New York State Department of Health proposed regulations requiring all providers using ONC-certified EHRs to connect to the SHIN-NY. Continuing support for the RHIO's role in state health objectives was further evidenced by the Delivery System Reform Incentive Payment Program Medicaid Section 1115 waiver requirements that recipient health care organizations connect to an RHIO [54]. The Qualified Health IT Entities currently offer HIE

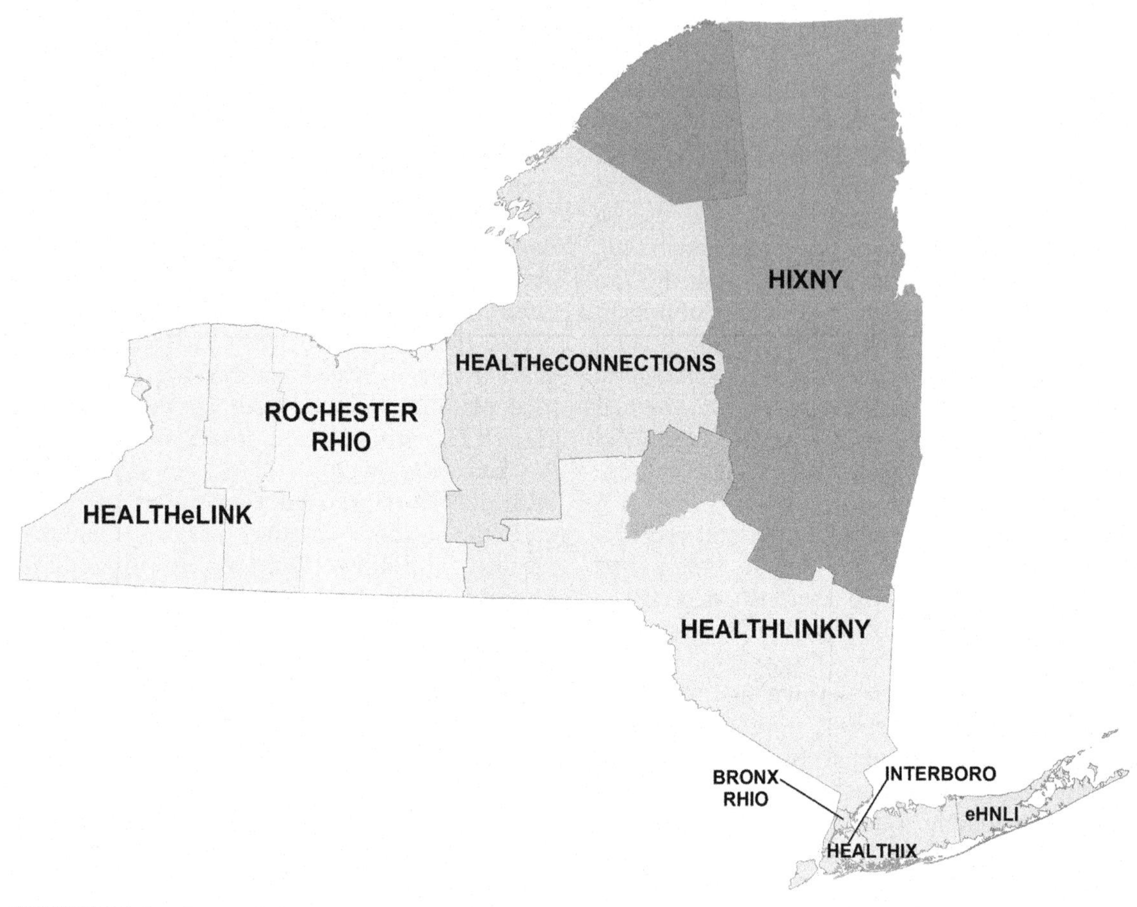

FIGURE 24.4 New York State's Regional Health Information Organizations (Qualified Entities), 2015.

services to health care organizations and are largely supported by membership dues. To create sustainable business plans, Qualified Health IT Entities have also been developing "value-added" services for participating health care organizations, such as electronic master-patient index (eMPI) technologies. Together, these activities have allowed New York to have continuing HIE activity even after HEAL NY funding ended (Fig. 24.4). There is no RHIO-to-RHIO data exchange to date, but the SHIN-NY standards, policies, and relationships are in place to support a genuine statewide network.

24.9 Summary

While HEAL NY's full impact will probably not be evident for several years, the program has been a successful policy intervention on numerous fronts. At a minimum, it expanded the adoption and implementation of interoperable health information technology and HIE across the state. More than 10 years later, the state is home to not only operational HIE organizations, but also some of the leading HIE activities in the nation and is a Centers for Medicare & Medicaid Services innovation grantee. When the ONC began measuring national HIE activity in 2012, New York State led the adoption of query-based HIE and was also a leader in directed exchange [55]. Providers who benefited from HEAL NY funding were more likely to become Meaningful Users of EHRs, compared to other New York State providers [56]. Along the way, the evaluations of grantees' adoption and implementation efforts provided important insights into the usage of health information technology [35,57,58], the integration of technology into workflows [59,60], patient perspectives on privacy and technology [61], success factors in health IT implementation [62], policy and implementation barriers to new HIE initiatives [63], the functioning of organizations in response to health information technology policy [33,46,48], and the practice of community-based research [42,64].

Substantial evidence exists to conclude that the program made significant progress toward the goal of encouraging "improvements in the operation and efficiency of the health care delivery system within the state" [19]. For example, studies of the Rochester RHIO found that HIE usage was associated with reduced hospital admissions via the emergency department, readmissions, and repeat imaging [65–67]. The public health benefits of the state's investment in health information technology included improved reporting efficiency and use of an immunization registry from EHRs [68] and that Southern Tier HealthLink provided emergency access to medical records for individuals displaced during the 2001 flood [69]. In addition, NYeC participated in the NHIN Trial Implementations project [70].

No health policy, nor technology project, is implemented in a vacuum, and over time HEAL NY was influenced by and changed in response to internal and external developments. During the course of the HEAL NY program, New York State experienced multiple changes in executive leadership and program staff. The role of the public–private partnership increased and became formalized at the SDE. Most importantly, the federal government changed the entire industry landscape with HITECH and the Meaningful Use Program.

While the many of the experiences of New York State are similar to those had by other states and organizations working to facilitate HIE, in total New York's experience with health information technology and exchange adoption is unique. It stands alone in its cumulative scope, scale, total financial investments, public sector leadership, evolution, and interaction with federal policy.

Questions for discussion

1. Is the assertion "all health care is local" valid?
2. What are the strengths and weakness of a centralized versus a decentralized approach to health information exchange organization within a state?
3. What are the challenges or advantages for states on the cutting-edge of new policies?
4. Given the history of the HEAL NY program, what would you have changed, when, and why?
5. What factors contributed to the success of the HEAL NY program?
6. What should other states take away from the HEAL NY program? What lessons are applicable to the ongoing effort to develop nationwide HIE?

Acknowledgments

Thanks to Jessica Ancker, Thomas Campion Jr., and Alex Low for their comments and insights. Parts of this chapter have been adapted from *Evaluation of New York's Federal-State Health Reform Partnership (F-SHRP) Medicaid Section 1115 Demonstration* (Albany, NY: Rockefeller Institute of Government, 2015, Unpublished). Co-author E. G.M. was a coprincipal investigator on the Medicaid evaluation report.

References

[1] Vest J, Gamm LD. Health information exchange: persistant challenges & new strategies. J Am Med Inf Assoc 2010;17(3):288–94.

[2] Rubin RD, O'Carroll PW, Yasnoff WA, Ward ME, Ripp LH, Martin EL. The community health information movement: where it's been, where it's going. In: O'Carroll PW, Yasnoff WA, Ward ME, Ripp LH, Martin EL, editors. Public health informatics & information systems. New York: Springer; 2003.

[3] Overhage J, Deter P, Perkins S, Cordell W, McGoff J, McGrath R. A randomized, controlled trial of clinical information shared from another institution. Ann Emerg Med 2002;39(1):14–23.

[4] Lassila KS, Pemble KR, DuPont LA, Cheng RH. Assessing the impact of community health information networks: a multisite field study of the Wisconsin Health Information Network. Top Health Inf Manage 1997;18(2):64–76.

[5] eHealth Initiative. Emerging trends and issues in Health Information Exchange: select findings from eHealth Initative Foundation's second annual survey of state, regional and community-based Health Information Exchange initatives and organizations. Washington, DC: Foundation for eHealth Initative; 2005.

[6] Brailer DJ. The decade of health information technology: delivering consumer-centric and information-rich health care. Washington, DC: US Department of Health and Human Services; 2004.

[7] Adler-Milstein J, McAfee AP, Bates DW, Jha AK. The state of regional health information organizations: current activities and financing. Health Aff 2008;27(1): w60–9.

[8] Vest JR, Menachemi N. A population ecology perspective on the functioning and future of health information organizations. Health Care Manage Rev 2019;44 (4):344–55.

[9] The National Alliance for Health Information Technology. Report to the Office of the National Coordinator for Health Information Technology on Defining Key Health Information Technology Terms. Department of Health & Human Services. Available from: <https://www.nachc.org/wp-content/uploads/2016/03/Key-HIT-Terms-Definitions-Final_April_2008.pdf>; 2008 [updated April 28, 2008; cited November 19, 2021].

[10] National Committee on Vital Health & Health Statistics. Functional requirements needed for the initial definition of a Nationwide Health Information Network (NHIN). Hyattsville, MD; 2006.

[11] Office of the National Coordinator for Health Information Technology (ONC), Department of Health and Human Services. Nationwide health information network: conditions for trusted exchange. Federal Register 2012;77(94):25843 8560.

[12] Lenert L, Sundwall D, Lenert ME. Shifts in the architecture of the Nationwide Health Information Network. J Am Med Inf Assoc 2012;19(4):498–502.

[13] Conn J, Robeznieks A. IT at center stage: HIMSS conference draws record attendees, vendors. Modern Healthcare. Available from: <http://www.modernhealthcare.com/article/20060220/MAGAZINE/602200301>; 2006 [cited November 17, 2021].

[14] Coiera E. Building a national health IT system from the middle out. J Am Med Inf Assoc 2009;16(3):271–3.

[15] New York State Department of Health and The Dormitory Authority of the State of New York. HEAL NY Phase 10—Improving Care Coordination and Management Through a Patient Centered Medical Home Model Supported by an Interoperable Health Information Infrastructure; 2009.

[16] New York eHealth Collaborative. SHIN-NY the Network of Networks: 'Better Healthcare through Technology'. Available from: <https://www.health.ny.gov/health_care/medicaid/program/medicaid_health_homes/webinars/docs/2014/2014-10-01_hh_shiny_webinar.pdf>; 2014 [cited November 17, 2021].

[17] Adler-Milstein J, Bates DW, Jha AK. U.S. regional health information organizations: progress and challenges. Health Aff 2009;28(2):483–92.

[18] New York State Department of Health. Health Care Efficiency and Affordability Law for New Yorkers Capital Grant Program. Available from: <https://www.nysenate.gov/legislation/laws/PBH/2818>; 2014 [cited November 17, 2021].

[19] Health Care Efficiency and Affordability Law of New Yorkers (HEAL NY). Capital grant program, Stat. 28 (2004).

[20] Governor George Pataki's Remarks. 2005 Budget Address. Gotham Gazette. Available from: <http://www.gothamgazette.com/index.php/economy/2678-governor-george-patakis-remarks-2005-budget-address>; 2005 [cited November 17, 2021].

[21] Commission on Health Care Facilities in the 21st Century. A plan to stabilize and strengthen New York's Health Care System: final report of the Commission on Health Care Facilities in the 21st Century. Available from: <https://nyhealthcarecommission.health.ny.gov/docs/final/commissionfinalreport.pdf>; December 2006 [November 17, 2021].

[22] Kern LM, Barron Y, Abramson EL, Patel V, Kaushal R. HEAL NY: promoting interoperable health information technology in New York State. Health Aff 2009;28 (2):493–504.

[23] New York State Department of Health. Federal-State Health Reform Partnership (F-SHRP). Available from:

<https://www.health.ny.gov/health_care/managed_care/appextension/docs/2015-09-16_f-shrp_demonstration_rpt.pdf>; September 16, 2015 [cited November 19, 2021].

[24] Rockefeller Institute of Government, Evaluation of New York's Federal-State Health Reform Partnership (F-SHRP) Medicaid Section 1115 Demonstration. Rockefeller Institute of Government, Albany, NY. 2015.

[25] What is the SHIN-NY?. Available from: <https://www.nyehealth.org/shin-ny/what-is-the-shin-ny/>; 2020 [cited November 19, 2021].

[26] New York State Department of Health and The Dormitory Authority of the State of New York. HEAL NY Phase 1: Health Information Technology (HIT) Grants; 2005.

[27] New York State Department of Health and The Dormitory Authority of the State of New York. HEAL NY-Phase 5 Health Information Technology Grants: Advancing Interoperability and Community-wide EHR Adoption; 2007.

[28] New York State Department of Health and The Dormitory Authority of the State of New York. HEAL NY Phase 17: Expanding Care Coordination Through the Use of Interoperable Health IT; 2010.

[29] New York State Department of Health. Request for grant applications. HEAL NY Phase 1: Health Information Technology (HIT) Grants. Available from: <https://www.health.ny.gov/funding/rfa/inactive/0508190240/>; 2005 [November 17, 2021].

[30] New York State Department of Health. HEAL NY—Phase 5: Health Information Technology Grants. Applicant conference. Available from: <https://www.health.ny.gov/funding/rfa/inactive/0708160258/applicant_conference/docs/transcript.pdf>; 2007 [cited November 17, 2021].

[31] New York State Department of Health. HEAL NY hit RGA questions and answers—Set 1. Available from: <https://www.health.ny.gov/funding/rfa/inactive/0508190240/questions_and_answers.pdf>; 2005 [November 17, 2021].

[32] New York State Department of Health and The Dormitory Authority of the State of New York. Health Information Technology (Health IT) Grants—HEAL NY Phase 1. Available from: <https://www.health.ny.gov/funding/rfa/inactive/0508190240//>; 2006 [November 12, 2021].

[33] Kern LM, Wilcox AB, Shapiro J, Yoon-Flannery K, Abramson E, Barron Y. Community-based health information technology alliances: potential predictors of early sustainability. Am J Manag Care 2011;17 (4):290–5.

[34] Conn J. EHR systems key to Spitzer's healthcare agenda. Modern Healthcare. Available from: <http://www.modernhealthcare.com/article/20080111/NEWS/717373599>; 2008 [cited November 17, 2021].

[35] Campion TR, Vest JR, Kern LM, Kaushal R. Adoption of clinical data exchange in community settings: a comparison of two approaches. AMIA Annu Symp Proc 2014;2014:359–65.

[36] New York State Department of Health. HEAL NY—Phase V Health IT Grant Program: Advancing Interoperability and Community-wide EHR Adoption. Available from: <https://www.health.ny.gov/funding/rfa/inactive/0708160258/>; 2008 [November 17, 2021].

[37] New York State Office of Health Information Technology Transformation. Technical discussion document: architectural framework for New York's health information infrastructure; 2007.

[38] New York State Department of Health. State HIE cooperative agreement program: strategic plan; 2009. Available from: https://www.health.ny.gov/funding/rfa/inactive/0903160302/health_it_strategic_plan.pdf [cited June 8 2022].

[39] New York eHealth Collaborative. About NYeC. New York eHealth Collaborative. Available from: <https://www.nyehealth.org/about/>; 2015 [cited November 17, 2021].

[40] Beaton BJ. Walking the Federalist Tightrope: a national policy of state experimentation for health information technology. Columbia Law Rev 2008;108(7):1670–717.

[41] Anonymous, Privacy and security policies and procedures for RHIOs and their participants in New York State, v 2.2. New York eHealth Collaborative and the New York State Department of Health, Albany, NY 2010.

[42] Kern LM, Ancker JS, Abramson E, Patel V, Dhopeshwarkar RV, Kaushal R. Evaluating health information technology in community-based settings: lessons learned. J Am Med Inform Assoc 2011;18 (6):749–53.

[43] New York State Department of Health and The Dormitory Authority of the State of New York. HEAL 22 questions and answers; 2012.

[44] Abramson EL, Edwards A, Silver M, Kaushai R. Trending health information technology adoption among New York nursing homes. Am J Manag Care 2014;20(11 Spec No. 17):eSP53–9.

[45] Vest JR, Campion TR, Kern LM, Kaushal R. Public and private sector roles in health information technology policy: insights from the implementation and operation of exchange efforts in the United States. Health Policy Technol 2014;3(2):149–56.

[46] Vest J, Kash B. Differing strategies to meet information sharing needs: the publicly supported community health information exchange vs health systems' enterprise health information exchanges. Milbank Q 2016;94(1):77–108.

[47] Vest J, Campion TR, Kaushal R. Challenges, alternatives, and paths to sustainability for health information exchange efforts. J Med Syst 2013;37(6):9987.
[48] US Department of Health & Human Services. Office of the National Coordinator. Summary of Nationwide Health Information Network (NHIN) Request for Information (RFI) Responses. Washington, DC; 2005.
[49] American Recovery and Reinvestment Act of 2009: law, explanation and analysis : P.L. 111-5, as signed by the President on February, 17. Chicago: Ill. :CCH; 2009. p. 2009.
[50] New York eHealth Collaborative. Policy and governance structure; 2012. Avaialble from https://www.colleaga.org/sites/default/files/attachments/NYeC_Policy_and_Governance_Paper_v5final.pdf [cited June 8 2022].
[51] Healthix. Healthix, Inc. and the Brooklyn Health Information Exchange (BHIX) announce their merger, effective December 1. Available from: <http://healthix.org/wp-content/uploads/Healthix_Merger-Press-Release_20131201.pdf>; 2013 [cited November 17, 2021].
[52] healtheconnections. About us. Available from: <https://healtheconnections.org/about-us/>; 2019 [cited November 19, 2021].
[53] New York eHealth Collaborative. Final State Budget Funds Statewide Health Information Network of New York. Available from: <https://www.nyehealth.org/final-state-budget-funds-statewide-health-information-network-of-new-york/>; 2015 [cited November 17, 2021].
[54] New York State Department of Health. New York State Delivery System Reform Incentive Payment Program Project Toolkit. Available from: <http://www.health.ny.gov/health_care/medicaid/redesign/docs/dsrip_project_toolkit.pdf>; [November 17, 2021].
[55] Vest JR, Unruh MA, Shapiro JS, Casalino LP. The associations between query-based and directed health information exchange with potentially avoidable use of health care services. Health Serv Res 2019;54(5):981–93.
[56] Jung H-Y, Unruh MA, Kaushal R, Vest JR. Growth of New York physician participation in meaningful use of electronic health records was variable, 2011–12. Health Aff 2015;34(6):1035–43.
[57] Campion TR, Vest JR, Ancker JS, Kaushal R. Patient encounters and care transitions in one community supported by automated query-based health information exchange. AMIA Annu Symp Proc 2013;2013:175–84.
[58] Vest J, Grinspan ZM, Kern LM, Campion TR, Kaushal R. Using a health information exchange system for imaging information: patterns and predictors. AMIA Annu Symp Proc 2013;2013:1402–11.
[59] Kierkegaard P, Kaushal R, Vest J. Patient information retrieval in multiple care settings: examining methods of exchange in emergency departments, primary care practices, and public health clinics? Am J Manag Care 2014;20(11 Spec No. 17):SP494–501.
[60] Kierkegaard P, Kaushal R, Vest JR. How could health information exchange better meet the needs of care practitioners? Appl Clin Inf 2014;5(4):861–77.
[61] Ancker JS, Edwards AM, Miller MC, Kaushal R. Consumer perceptions of electronic health information exchange. Am J Prev Med 2012;43(1):76–80.
[62] Ancker JS, Singh MP, Thomas R, Edwards A, Snyder A, Kashyap A. Predictors of success for electronic health record implementation in small physician practices. Appl Clin Inf 2013;4(1):12–24.
[63] Ancker JS, Miller M, Patel V, Kaushal R. Sociotechnical challenges to developing technologies for patient access to health information exchange data. J Am Med Inf Assoc 2013;21(4):664–70.
[64] Ancker JS, Kern LM, Abramson E, Kaushal R. The Triangle Model for evaluating the effect of health information technology on healthcare quality and safety. J Am Med Inf Assoc 2012;19(1):61–5.
[65] Vest J, Kaushal R, Silver M, Hentel K, Kern L. Health information exchange and the frequency of repeat medical imaging. Am J Manag Care 2014;20(11 Spec. 17):eSP16–24.
[66] Vest J, Kern L, Campion TR, Silver M, Kaushal R. Association between use of a health information exchange system and hospital admissions. Appl Clin Inf 2014;5(1):219–31.
[67] Vest JR, Kern LM, Silver MD, Kaushal R. The potential for community-based health information exchange systems to reduce hospital readmissions. J Am Med Inform Assoc 2014;22(22):435–42.
[68] Merrill J, Phillips A, Keeling J, Kaushal R, Senathirajah Y. Effects of automated immunization registry reporting via an electronic health record deployed in community practice settings. Appl Clin Inf 2013;4(2):267–75.
[69] Southern Tier HealthLink. Southern Tier HealthLink Appreciation Day. Available from: <https://www.healthitoutcomes.com/doc/southern-healthlink-health-new-york-service-platform-0001>; 2012 [cited November 17, 2021].
[70] Kuperman GJ, Blair JS, Franck RA, Devaraj S, Low AF. Developing data content specifications for the nationwide health information network trial implementations. J Am Med Inf Assoc 2010;17(1):6–12.

CHAPTER

25

Use of Health Information Exchanges for value-based care delivery and population health management: a case study of Maryland's Health Information Exchange

Hadi Kharrazi[1,2], *David Horrocks*[3] *and Jonathan Weiner*[1]

[1]Center for Population Health IT (CPHIT), Department of Health Policy and Management, Johns Hopkins School of Public Health, Baltimore, MD, USA [2]Biomedical Informatics and Data Science Section, Johns Hopkins School of Medicine, Baltimore, MD, USA [3]Chesapeake Regional Information System for Our Patients (CRISP), Baltimore, MD, USA

LEARNING OBJECTIVES

- Define the aims and organizational structure of value-based care and accountable care organizations.
- Understand the role of population health in accountable care organizations.
- Explore care examples of utilizing HIE to enhance accountable care.
- Describe various services provided by Maryland's HIE to improve population health efforts.

25.1 Introduction

Continued growth in healthcare costs is unsustainable [1]. Poor levels of efficiency and mixed attainment of quality indicators and patient outcomes have accelerated the adoption of value-based care among US healthcare delivery systems [2]. The Affordable Healthcare Act (ACA) propelled the adoption of value-based care by promoting and incentivizing new care delivery models such as so-called Accountable Care Organizations (ACOs) and Patient-Centered Medical Homes (PCMHs) [3]. These value-based

Health Information Exchange
DOI: https://doi.org/10.1016/B978-0-323-90802-3.00011-3

healthcare delivery models focus on the achievement of the "Triple Aim" of patient satisfaction, improved population health, and increased cost efficiency [4,5]. The US Centers for Medicare and Medicaid Services (CMS) sponsored ACOs attempt to achieve this in large part through a "shared saving" model, where clinicians receive increased incentive payments when their services to a target population are lower in cost and higher in quality [6,7].

ACOs, PCMHs, and other similar "integrated" delivery systems have experienced challenges in collecting and analyzing the information needed to better manage the populations they serve. This has been partly due to a lack of alignment of the Meaningful Use (MU) program with most ACO/PCMH goals [8]. The MU program—funded by the HITECH Act and managed by CMS—has been the main driver to increase the adoption of electronic health record (EHR) systems among professionals and hospitals [9], but it was never intended to provide a turnkey solution for value-based healthcare systems. Consequently, ACOs have often found themselves working closely with a diverse set of healthcare providers who do not necessarily have interoperable information with which to draw a comprehensive picture of their attributed patient populations.

Health Information Exchange (HIE) networks have the potential to fill in the population-wide informational gap for ACOs and play a pivotal role to enhance value-based care [10,11]. An HIE can collect, analyze, and provide critical information from a range of information systems about patients associated with an ACO network. HIEs can also provide information about the events that ACO patients experience out of the ACO's network. Furthermore, HIEs can provide ACOs with broader population-wide health information that goes beyond the ACO providers' medical data (e.g., information derived from the surrounding community) [11]. This will enable ACOs to strategically plan for potential patient populations that might be attributed to them in the future.

Maryland underwent major healthcare payment reform in 2014 [12]. The all-payer waiver program, where all public and private payers pay the same rate for inpatient and outpatient hospital services, is now extended to all Maryland hospitals, which now face a fixed cap for any annual increase in expenditures [12,13]. This cap is set relative to the state's gross domestic product (GDP) and, consequently, most Maryland hospitals now operate under a value-based global budget [12]. This global budget is adjusted based on various metrics including population health measures within the hospital's target communities, as well as inpatient quality indicators [12,13]. One of the key tools being used to achieve such an ambitious value-based program in Maryland is a statewide HIE. The Maryland HIE offers a set of informational and health information technology (HIT) resources to assist hospitals and other organizations to better manage their patient populations [14,15].

Maryland's designated HIE network is known as the Chesapeake Regional Information System for our Patients, or CRISP for short [16]. CRISP covers a diverse set of stakeholders such as hospitals, ambulatory settings, and ancillary providers. CRISP is one of the few HIE networks with 100% real-time participation of all hospitals [16]. CRISP provides several services that are deemed essential to the operations of the inpatient all-payer waiver program and are also quite valuable to ACOs/PCMHs and other organizations moving toward value-based models. Some of these initiatives include real-time encounter notification of significant events, a centralized care coordination infrastructure, automated reporting of quality metrics, and population-based health risk stratification and predictive analytics [17–20].

The remainder of this chapter will discuss the role of information exchange, and population health analytics support, for value-based initiatives including ACOs. The role of Maryland's HIE—CRISP—will be featured within the context of Maryland's unique population-based value-based reform initiative.

25.2 Value-based care and Accountable Care Organizations

25.2.1 Background

US healthcare has historically been delivered based on a fee-for-service (FFS) basis [6]. In this model, healthcare providers are incentivized to focus on each distinct encounter, diagnosis, or procedure regardless of the broader population health implications. Most policy experts agree that the major ramification of this model has been an increasing number of clinical interventions with minimal improvement in population health. Indeed, by adopting a volume-driven FFS model, overall US healthcare expenditures have risen from $2 trillion to more than $3 trillion in less than a decade [1]. The FFS model also spurred fragmentation in care as parties involved in the care process have few effective means to coordinate care [21]. The net effect of FFS has led the US healthcare system to become the costliest system in the world, accounting for close to 20% of the nation's GDP in 2020 [1].

The "Triple Aim" is a unifying framework that describes an approach to optimizing health system performance [4,5]. The three dimensions of the Triple Aim include: (1) improving the patient experience of care (including quality and satisfaction), (2) improving the health of populations (and not just patients under care), and (3) reducing the per capita cost of care [5]. Unfortunately, until recently, most US healthcare delivery systems and providers (other than a few Health Maintenance Organizations where payment and delivery of care are integrated) were not accountable for all three dimensions of the Triple Aim. For example, hospitals were not responsible for the overall health of their target population which would entail a focus on community determinants of health, empowering patients and their families, and an emphasis on community-based primary care [22]. Recent initiatives, in part promoted by the ACA, have propelled the establishment of healthcare delivery systems that are "accountable" for all dimensions of the Triple Aim. ACOs and PCMHs, as well as several dozen CMS-sponsored "innovations" such as the Maryland Waiver, are the most widely adopted emerging models of value-based delivery systems [23].

25.2.2 Accountable Care Organization concept

ACOs are networks of providers with unified governance that assume risk for the quality and total cost of the care they deliver. ACOs may include a variety of healthcare providers from inpatient or outpatient settings. Participation in an ACO is voluntary, and the main goal is to achieve the Triple Aim. Some of the priorities of ACOs include operational tasks such as: effective care coordination of patients with chronic conditions, avoiding duplications of services, and preventing medical errors [24].

Though several non-Medicare ACOs exist, CMS has been the main gateway to support ACOs. CMS reimburses most ACOs through a type of pay for performance (P4P) program termed the "Medicare Shared Savings Program" (MSSP), although there are also similar ACOs termed as Advanced Payment ACO Models, and the Pioneer ACO. The MSSP model basically shares the "savings" with physicians for a target "attributed" Medicare patient population when actual cost FFS are lower than risk-adjusted predicted costs for the cohort, and when quality targets are also met [3,7].

There are predefined conditions that CMS uses to approve providers as an MSSP ACO [7]. These include:

1. ACO providers must coordinate care for their attributed Medicare FFS beneficiaries and be accountable for quality and cost of these patients.

2. ACOs must meet or exceed a minimum cost saving rate established by CMS to receive shared savings payments.
3. ACO participants should include at least one provider/supplier from a specific type of delivery network.
4. ACOs must be a legal entity with an identifiable governing body, and at least 75% of the ACO's governing board must be held by ACO participants.
5. The ACO must include primary care professionals that are sufficient for the attributed Medicare population.
6. ACOs should promote evidence-based medicine, focus on patient-centeredness, have an established quality assurance program, evaluate their process regularly, coordinate care across participating providers, and promote patient engagement.
7. An ACO must have at least 5000 Medicare beneficiaries who receive most of their care from them.
8. ACO providers may not participate in other ACOs.

The total number of registered ACOs under the CMS programs has grown since 2011, reaching 483 Medicare ACOs as of 2022 [25]. The population covered under ACOs (Medicare, Medicaid, and commercial) has also grown considerably, with CMS ACOs serving over 11 million beneficiaries as of 2022 [25]. Since 2016, ACOs have operated in all 50 US states, Washington DC, and Puerto Rico [25]. The number of ACOs correlates strongly with the underlying population of each state; hence California, Texas, and Florida have the highest number of ACOs. However, it is important to note that on a smaller geographical scale, some regions still have negligible ACO activity. Besides CMS, commercial payers also contract with ACOs and their numbers have also risen over time covering 28 million lives in 2016 [25].

25.2.3 Value-based metrics

Tracking the quality of care provided by ACOs is critical to ensure that quality is not compromised while achieving reduced cost. CMS, National Committee for Quality Assurance (NCQA), National Quality Forum, and other organizations that promote quality measurement have published their set of metrics to track the performance and outcomes of ACOs in achieving value-based care. CMS measures for ACOs include several quality metrics that cover various domains such as: patient and caregiver experience, care coordination, patient safety, preventative health, and at-risk populations of certain chronic conditions [26]. CMS envisions that the ACO metrics, which currently focus on performance and outcome attributes, will be further refined by comprehensive population health measures since they are the most appropriate approach to evaluate the population health dimension of the Triple Aim [27].

25.2.4 Role of population health

Population health is a major but yet ambiguous target of value-based care [28]. As discussed earlier, value-based care intends to address each of the three Triple Aim dimensions, including the one that emphasizes the improvement of population health. This aim, however, has not been well defined in the past mainly due to the ambiguity of what exactly population health is, what outcomes should be measured, and what interventions are available to improve it [29,30]. Despite efforts to identify various aspects of population health and to standardize related concepts and terminologies, the theoretical and operational complexities of population health have led to lack of clarity associated with its application within the value-based care context. Some challenges have included: unclear definition of the theoretical population "denominator"; complex population attribution algorithms; lack of standardization of population-focused metrics, outcomes and timelines; and the overlapping population health goals of value-based medical providers, public health, and social services government agencies [31,32]. Perhaps the main distinction between traditional public health and population health relies on two factors: (1) population health is less directly tied to governmental public health agencies, and (2) population health requires the involvement of the healthcare delivery system, thus making it relevant to value-based operations of ACOs [27,33].

Population-focused "care management" is a subset of broader population health activities, and it is essential to the long-term operations of value-based delivery systems. Population healthcare management is an organized, data-supported approach that emphasizes the achievement of health outcomes of individuals in a group, while assessing the distribution of outcomes across the target cohort. Population health management is also critical for ACOs to effectively manage the care of a defined patient population across the continuum of care [34]. Currently the main users of population health management programs are large integrated delivery systems or advanced health maintenance organizations, such as Kaiser Permanente and the Veterans Health Administration, which have robust, centralized HIT infrastructures. Most emerging ACOs, however, often do not have an advanced HIT infrastructure to support the case finding and monitoring essential for such an intervention. This lack of HIT infrastructure will likely be a major challenge that new ACOs will face. Specifically, without adequate HIT support, there will be several challenges for ACOs to achieve such as: adequate risk stratification and case identification, effective cross provider care coordination, efficient care management across the population cohort (and not just focusing on presenting patients), impactful patient and caregiver empowerment (e.g., by sharing information), and meaningful community engagement (e.g., to identify community needs) [33–35].

25.2.5 Accountable Care Organization's information technology needs

As discussed earlier, the ACA has incentivized healthcare providers to achieve value-based care. However, existing HIT policies, such as the "Meaningful Use" incentive program, have not been fully aligned with value-based care. For example, MU criteria, the metrics that establish whether or not an eligible hospital or provider receives an incentive payment for using certified EHR systems, have not for the most part emphasized population health—a cornerstone of an ACO concept [33]. So even though MU has resulted in the wide adoption of EHR systems among eligible hospitals and professionals, more work is needed in support of ACOs who need to address essential HIT challenges.

To operationalize population health, value-based providers need to perform a wide range of information management activities including: capturing population-wide health and medical information; linking, analyzing, and sharing patient-level information among participating providers; integrating nonclinical and clinical information; aggregating population-level data; measuring population health performance from multiple data sources and analyzing the outcomes from different perspectives; delivering actionable information to the population health management team as well as to the clinicians at the point of care; interacting effectively with the population (patients, caregivers and the larger community); and using the generated knowledge to effectively change practice patterns when needed. These data-related activities are all essential for ACOs to become a population-oriented healthcare system [34,35].

To address these and other related information support challenges for ACOs, HIT action items can include: (1) interoperability of the diverse set of HIT systems across all key ACO units, (2) consensus on the definition of population denominators and its extraction from local datasets, (3) reliability and validity of population health metrics that go beyond medical performance and outcome quality measures, (4) certified analytical tools that can provide in-depth risk stratification and "predictive modeling" of the covered population, (5) adoption of HIT solutions within the operational workflows of other non-ACO providers, and ultimately, (6) the integration of population health findings as part of the broader learning health system seeking to gain evidence on what care is linked to increase effectiveness and efficiency.

Current US HIT standards and incentives at-large do not always align with ACO mandates to use information to improve population health. For example, measuring and improving the quality of care provided to the covered population of an ACO require the interoperability of HIT systems across all ACO units, not just a single hospital or physician practice. The interoperability challenges include both the effective integration of data generated or needed by ACO services across the continuum of care (e.g., care coordination across various ACO units) and the effective exchange of data between ACO and other healthcare stakeholders (e.g., sharing ACO data with out-of-ACO entities). As depicted in Fig. 25.1, a variety of HIT systems are used to manage patients within an ACO, including information from organizations external to the ACO that can affect the health of those patients (e.g., payers, public health departments). These challenges have prevented many ACOs from managing their patients effectively due to their incomplete population health data and unreliable analytics [36,37].

Multiple drivers associated with value-based models of care are now offering incentives and facilitators in support of population HIT solutions, thereby focusing attention and resources on the types of population health enhancing systems outlines above. Some of these drivers include: the consolidation of data exchange standards and their increased adoption by the vendor community (e.g., health level 7, HL7 fast healthcare interoperability resources, FHIR) [38], supporting new interoperability initiatives for HIE networks to connect disparate health data sources [39], and advancements in the utilization and integration of disparate data sources for population health analytics [40–42].

25.2.6 Potential role of Health Information Exchanges for Accountable Care Organizations

HIE organizations can play a central role in supporting the population health IT operations of ACOs and other related value-based care systems. HIEs can support the operations of ACOs by connecting entities that use disparate clinical IT systems by providing some level of interoperability to help enable patient-centered and population-based care. More specifically, HIEs can support key population health domains such as: streamlining patient-centered care coordination efforts among noninteroperable providers, providing population-level clinical decision support, identifying and reporting at-risk populations, spotting patient safety issues and tracking quality measures in real-time, and informing and empowering patients/caregivers to be more involved with their own care [43]. Collectively, these HIE-derived IT capabilities can positively impact the measures that CMS and NCQA have adopted to evaluate ACO performance and outcomes.

HIE organizations have the potential to interconnect different entities that comprise an ACO. These entities will vary depending on the breadth and depth of the HIE and the ACO's existing stakeholders/members (see Fig. 25.1). Hypothetically, different groups of HIE stakeholders may include: (1) Common Core Members: include stakeholders from inpatient and outpatient settings such as

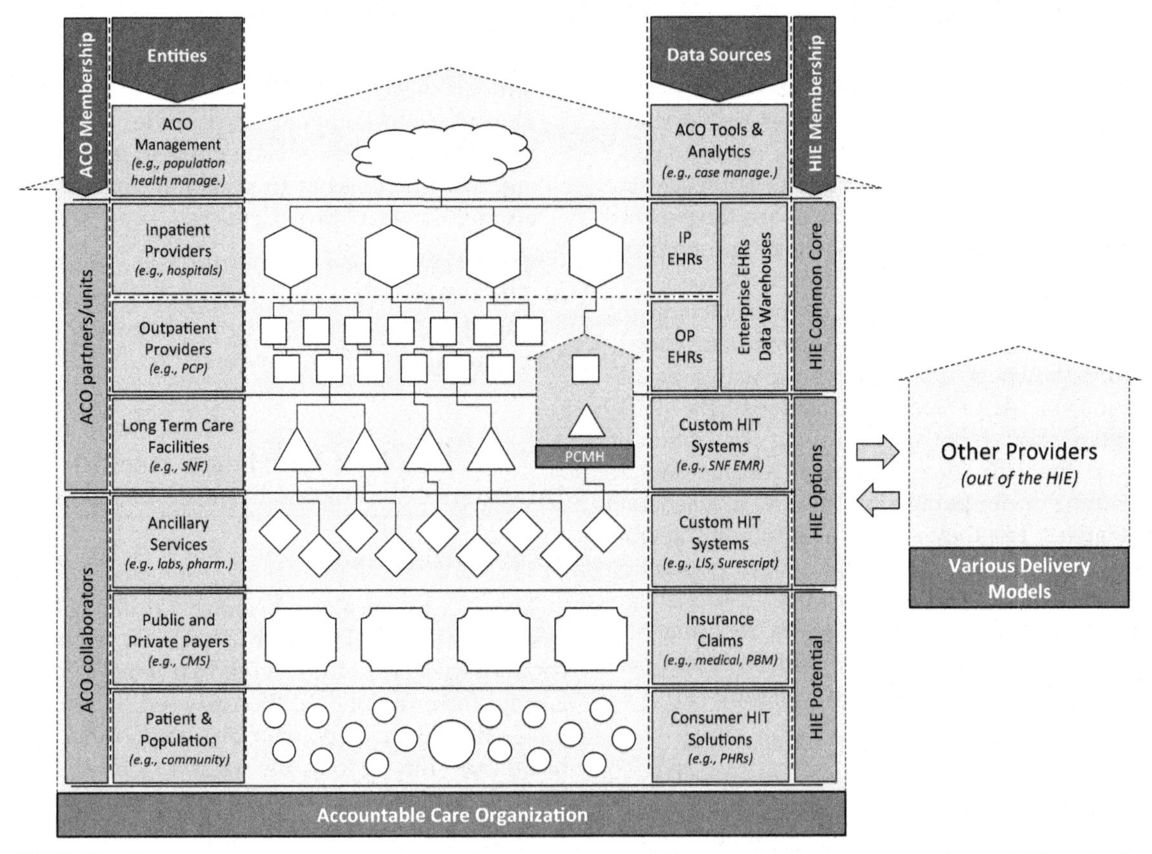

FIGURE 25.1 Diversity of health IT solutions among various healthcare providers operating under an ACO umbrella. Note that the HIE can be a viable solution for integrating the common core members; however, other stakeholders often lack the operational incentives and technical interoperability capabilities to integrate with the broader ACO. *ACO*, Accountable Care Organization; *CMS*, Centers for Medicare and Medicaid Services; *EHR*, electronic health record; *EMR*, electronic medical record; *HIE*, health information exchange; *HIT*, health information technology; *IP*, inpatient; *LIS*, laboratory information system; *OP*, outpatient; *PBM*, prescription benefit management (system); *PCMH*, Patient-Centered Medical Home; *PCP*, primary care physician; *PHR*, personal health record; *SNF*, skilled nursing facility.

hospitals, clinics, and primary care practices; (2) Optional Members: include long-term care facilities (e.g., nursing homes and skilled nursing facilities) and ancillary providers (e.g., diagnostic labs); and (3) Potential Members: include infrequent stakeholders such as payers, community-wide systems, public health departments, and patients/caregivers [44].

If an HIE includes a wide scope of member types and numbers, it will increase the likelihood that the HIE would be able to offer cross-provider services for an ACO entity if most of the component providers fall within the HIE's boundaries. For example, if an HIE integrates optional or potential member groups in addition to its core members, it can provide an ACO with a more comprehensive picture of its attributed population even if those patients have sought care out of the ACO network.

The core ACO entities/units (see Fig. 25.1) often do not possess enterprise-level HIT systems unless they are part of an existing and mature integrated delivery network. Furthermore, most ACOs have very limited capability to integrate their IT systems with non-ACO stakeholders such as payers and individual consumer-level systems. For example, if a patient seeks care out of an ACO network, perhaps the only efficient approach that a provider within the ACO can access the patient's significant medical events—which has occurred elsewhere—is through the HIE services.

The HIE is central to ACOs in achieving the necessary degree of patient-centered care coordination; however, this requires the active participation of ACO members. Indeed, the ACO entities should not only provide the option of using the HIE infrastructure to obtain data to advance their population health management initiatives, but they should also tightly integrate the HIE within their day-to-day population health management workflow (e.g., case management, disease management, quality reporting).

Some of the key services that HIEs can provide to an ACO in this regard include [43]:

1. **Care Coordination**: share clinical data during transitions of care, identify social and community support, support the referral process, and improve clinical information reconciliation.
2. **Cohort Management**: identify cohorts within the ACO patient population, monitor subpopulations for certain significant health events or quality metrics, and provide population-wide decision support.
3. **Patient and Caregiver Empowerment**: provide basic informational services, simplify administrative processes for patients, and improve patient experience of care transition
4. **Financial Management**: enable ACOs to overcome patient attribution hurdles and support value-based case-mixed adjustment of reimbursements.
5. **Reporting**: measure and track ACO quality metrics including the broader population health metrics such as hospital readmissions, streamline public health reporting, and automate the reporting of patient safety issues.
6. **Knowledge Management**: provide population-based decision support and support learning health system initiatives among the ACO providers.

These and other collaborative opportunities of HIEs and ACOs are discussed in further technical detail within the context of Maryland's CRISP HIE network.

25.3 Role of Maryland's Health Information Exchange in value-based care

25.3.1 Background

The "Chesapeake Regional Information System for Our Patients," or CRISP, is a regional, community-based HIE serving Maryland. CRISP is a not-for-profit organization advised by a wide range of stakeholders who are responsible for healthcare throughout the region. CRISP has been formally designated as Maryland's statewide HIE by the Maryland Health Care Commission (MHCC). CRISP has also been named Maryland's Regional Extension Center for Health IT by the Office of the National Coordinator for HIT, with an objective of assisting 1000 primary care providers to deploy EHR systems and achieve MU. CRISP formed an affiliation of other nonprofit HIEs which share technology and certain operational capabilities, called CRISP Shared Services [16].

25.3.1.1 Mission and history

CRISP was chartered to improve health and wellness through HIT initiatives which are best pursued cooperatively. The mission of the organization is to enable and support the healthcare community of Maryland, and the region, to share data appropriately and securely in order to facilitate care, reduce costs, and improve health outcomes. CRISP has achieved a great deal of its original mission since its inception. In 2009, shortly after being designated as the statewide HIE, CRISP implemented its cooperative governance model [16]. In 2010 CRISP started the interconnectivity of hospitals, creating a statewide master patient index (MPI) and implementing a query portal for providers to retrieve past clinical events [17]. By late 2011 CRISP was connected to every hospital in Maryland and focused on increasing its utilization among providers. In 2012 CRISP turned on the encounter notification system (ENS) which notifies providers about significant patient events for enrolled patient populations [18]. By 2013 CRISP achieved financial sustainability of HIE operations, no longer relying on the initial grant/seed funding, and turned its attention to connecting providers in the District of Columbia. In 2014 CRISP started offering population health IT services in addition to providing real-time reports (e.g., hospital readmission reports) and hosting Maryland's statewide prescription drug monitoring program (PDMP) [45]. Between 2015 and 2018, CRISP added new sources of data (e.g., Medicare and Medicaid data), expanded its coverage to include Washington DC's HIE, and offered its care management platform to all participating hospitals. In 2019 CRISP started distributing its products as open source. And, in 2020, CRISP provided the infrastructure for COVID-19 reporting for the state of Maryland (e.g., testing reports). In the same year, CRISP began offering hospitals with real-time hospitalization utilization reports, which was critical for the hospital to manage resources in the face of the COVID-19 pandemic. Over the years, CRISP has established active partnerships with neighboring states to exchange data, including West Virginia, Delaware, and Virginia.

25.3.1.2 Types and number of stakeholders

As of 2021, CRISP serves all 47 Maryland acute care hospitals, all 8 DC hospitals via affiliation, more than 200 long-term care facilities, 15 radiology centers, the national nonhospital labs, and 2 emergency medical facilities [46]. CRISP shares encounter information among all its entities; however, inpatient lab, radiology, continuity of care document, and ENS (admission and disposition) data varies among hospitals. In 2021 CRISP reached 110,000 registered users, 190k + queries per month by clinicians at the point of care, and over 5 million monthly notifications sent through the ENS system to more than 1300 subscribed entities [18].

25.3.1.3 Governance

CRISP strives to build only services which are best pursued through cooperation and collaboration. This has led to operational sustainability of CRISP. In coordination with the MHCC, CRISP has developed a governance model that includes a Board of Advisors to provide guidance and input to the CRISP Board of Directors on certain key decisions during the development of services and operation of the HIE. The Board of Advisors is intended to be broad-based to ensure that a breadth of interested organizations have the opportunity to participate and represent their constituencies. There are currently over 30 organizations represented by 85 individual members in CRISP's several Advisory Board committees [47].

Patient Privacy policies are foundational to HIE networks. CRISP operates under a combination of Federal laws (e.g., Health Insurance Portability and Accountability Act (HIPAA) and 42 CFR Part-2 [48]), State laws and regulations (e.g., MHCC regulations), and Stakeholder agreements (e.g., Participation Agreement). All participating organizations in CRISP HIE are required to (1) update their HIPAA Notice of Privacy Practices to include a paragraph on their participation with CRISP, and (2) make CRISP informational brochures and opt-out forms available at intake areas. CRISP operates an opt-out model, meaning that patients have the right to block electronic access to their information through CRISP. If a

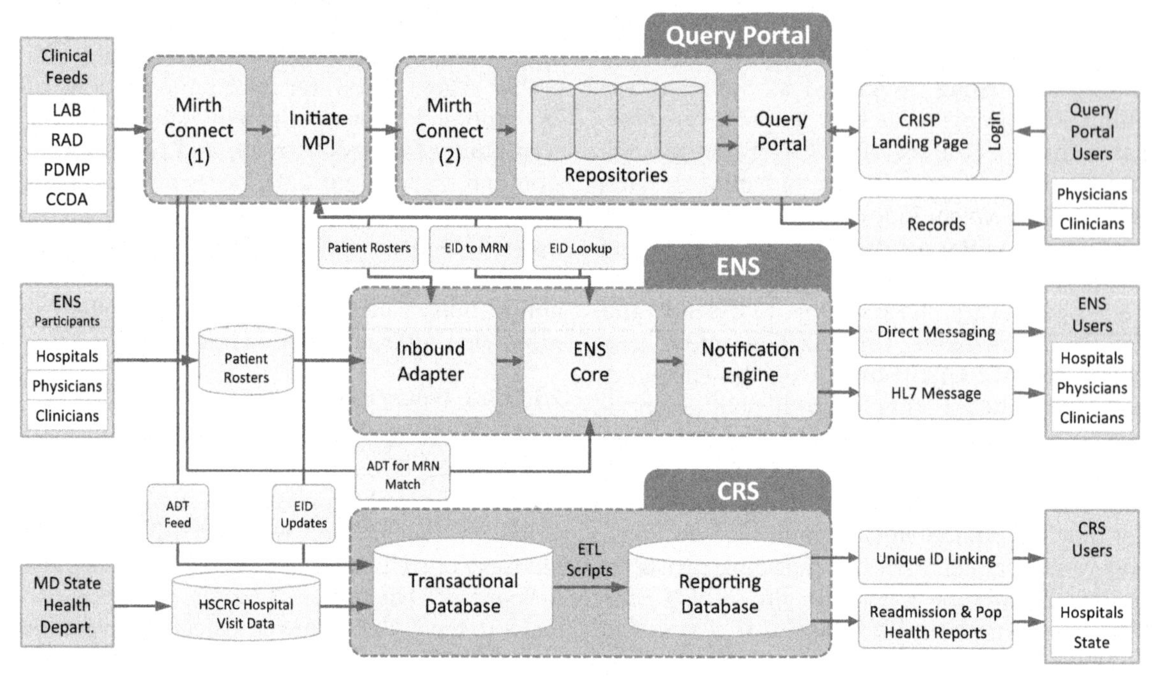

FIGURE 25.2 CRISP's technical and information architecture for its three major services. *ADT*, Admission, discharge, and transfer; *CCDA*, consolidated clinical document architecture; *CRS*, CRISP Reporting System; *EID*, enterprise identifier; *ENS*, encounter notification system; *ETL*, extract, transform, and load; *HL7*, Health Level 7; *HSCRC*, [Maryland] Health Services Cost Review Commission; *MPI*, master patient index; *MRN*, medical record number; *PDMP*, prescription drug monitoring program; *Pop*, population; *RAD*, radiology.

patient opts out, no information will be available through the portal (other than PDMP records, which by statute continue to be available to prescribers and dispensers). Notifications about hospitalizations for opt-out patients will also be blocked, even if a provider has requested them. To drop out, patients must contact CRISP by phone, online, or by mail [47].

25.3.1.4 Information flow and architecture

CRISP uses a federated and harmonized information-architecture. Mirth's open-source interface engine is used as the underlying data connector [49]. CRISP's MPI engine is built on top of IBM Initiate and uses a variety of patient data for matching purposes [50]. As depicted in Fig. 25.2, CRISP delivers three major services to its stakeholders:

1. **Query Portal**: The query portal allows credentialed users to search the HIE for clinical data. Users can search for patients using the patient's last name and date of birth or the medical record number from their practice or a hospital. The initial query returns information from the past 6 months, but the user can query data as far back as 2012 or earlier. While a valuable tool, there are workflow challenges, primarily with the time required to manually check the portal. For ease-of-use, CRISP integrated the portal within selected EHRs, such that clinicians can view information within a tab of their EHR. Over 190k queries are made per month, but this represents only a fraction of the total medical encounters in which a query might be helpful. The following types

of data are available through the portal: patient demographics, lab results, radiology reports, prescription data, discharge summaries, history and physicals, operative notes, and consults.

2. **Encounter Notification System (ENS)**: CRISP receives information pertaining to emergency room (ER) visits and inpatient admissions or discharges in real-time from all Maryland and DC hospitals. Through ENS, CRISP can communicate this information in the form of real-time hospitalization alerts to primary care physicians, care coordinators, and others responsible for patient care. As of 2021, CRISP routes roughly 200,000 notifications per day. Continuity of care documents are also routed through ENS to support transitions of care (including support of hospitals in meeting stage 2 MU measures). Hospitals can also "auto-subscribe" to receive various reports based on certain patient events. Once the sign up is complete, any time CRISP receives admission, discharge, and transfer (ADT) messages for patients on a patient panel, physicians and care coordinators automatically receive an electronic notification. Recipients can receive notifications as read-only PDF attachments in electronic inboxes (like secure email) or merged directly into their EHR systems as HL7 messages. CRISP uses the Direct Project protocol to securely transport the notifications [18].
3. **CRISP Reporting System (CRS)**: The CRS enables linking of healthcare datasets in support of population health reporting and performs statewide health information analytics and reporting. A key element of the infrastructure is the region-wide MPI, used to combine information at a patient level. Furthermore, CRS has evolved in the last few years to support a variety of users ranging from hospitals to state policy makers who need more in-depth analysis of health data for the state of Maryland. The reporting system includes a reporting database that updates routinely. This database is used for analysis and generating reports such as 30-day hospital readmission reports, inpatient and ER utilization reports, and other population health reports. In light of Maryland's new Medicare waiver, which targets controlling costs while improving quality, reducing readmissions, and decreasing the number of unnecessary hospitalizations that can be better and more cost-effectively treated in an outpatient setting, regular reporting from CRS on hospital performance has become especially important. In 2014 CRS began providing monthly reports via a secure web portal. In 2015 an enhanced portal that provides more interactive and sophisticated analysis was launched by CRISP. The scope of CRS has expanded substantially over time by incorporating data from more sources, such as detailed visit information submitted by hospitals for rate setting purposes. Public health data have been an increasing part of the reporting service, and since the start of the COVID-19 pandemic CRISP has served as a COVID-related reporting hub for the healthcare community. CRS is uniquely innovative given the depth and breadth of data available. Moreover, CRS combines data from different sources to allow the analysis of clinical and financial data by demographic groups and geographic regions and to provide more insight into overall healthcare utilization and population health management in Maryland [19].

25.3.2 Maryland all-payer waiver program and CRISP

The state of Maryland recently extended a long-standing CMS Medicare waiver for all its hospitals, authorizing its Health Services Cost

Review Commission (HSCRC) to manage hospital rates for all-payers, while maintaining an annual rate growth cap [12]. Through the efforts of HSCRC, currently all of Maryland's hospitals are operating under a global budget—fixed annual revenue based on the population served, rather than the volume of services. Therefore population health is considered a key, if not the only, approach for Maryland's hospitals to improve financial performance. However, Maryland's hospitals will be challenged to achieve the mandated quality goals without the underlying HIT and analytical tools to provide them with a complete picture of their attributed populations [13]. This challenge is mainly due to the fact that these hospitals cannot track their patient population across multiple providers and payers. To overcome these challenges, the HSCRC recognized the important role of HIT and particularly population health IT solutions, and has decided to invest resources to expand the statewide HIT infrastructure by: (1) developing new population health measures based on existing data captured across various HIT systems; (2) increasing the role of CRISP to capture the data necessary to measure the population health metrics; and (3) utilizing various statewide HIT systems, including CRISP, to provide hospitals with a high-level statewide care coordination platform [51].

25.3.3 CRISP's population health IT services

CRISP offers a range of population HIT services, and it is planning to add more services due to the underlying need created by Maryland's unique waiver program. Fig. 25.3 depicts a framework that lists the current and potential data sources (left), the population health analytics platform (middle), and multiple stakeholders that would use these population HIT services (right).

The main sources of data for CRISP's population health framework are:

1. **Real-time data**: This group of data includes the common core of information that CRISP receives from hospitals, labs, radiology centers, long-term care facilities and pharmacies [46]. These data sources already exist in CRISP. Note that message types differ across the data sources (e.g., hospitals send ADT data while labs send transcripts).
2. **Linked datasets**: These datasets include panels of patients that outpatient providers add voluntarily, HSCRC's hospital case-mix data (structured like claims data), MHCC's all-payer claims database, Medicaid and Medicare datasets, and other sources of data. These datasets include delayed (sometimes by a couple of months) information that will be linked to CRISP's population health data wareshouse. Note that CRISP has already indexed some of these datasets (e.g., MHCC and HSCRC datasets) with CRISP's MPI in order to operationalize the linkages.
3. **Reference data**: Determinants of health data (e.g., social and environmental factors) have shown to be useful in facilitating population health management and improving the identification and risk stratification of high utilizing users [52–55], which is a key to ACO operations. In order to expand population health data with determinants of health, CRISP has linked census and zip-level geo-data with the core population-level data collected from MHCC and HSCRC. The linkage of the reference datasets is mainly based on geo-triangulation methods [56] but actual latitude and longitude distance matching is also planned.
4. **Public health data**: Public health authorities receive data on infectious disease, specific reportable events, immunizations, and the use of certain medications such as opioids. Preventing costly public health events [57]

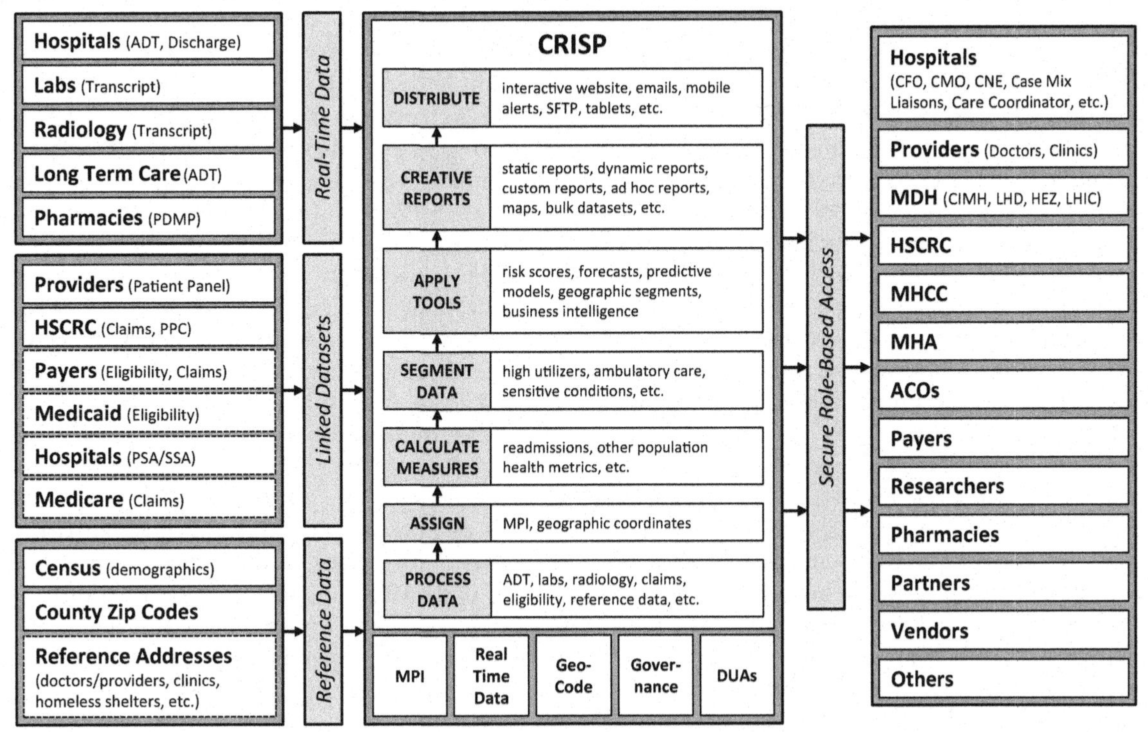

FIGURE 25.3 CRISP's population health IT services framework. ACO, Accountable Care Organization; *ADT*, admission, discharge, and transfer; *CFO*, chief financial officer; *CIMH*, [MDH] Community Integrated Medical Home; *CMO*, chief medical officer; *CNE*, chief nursing executive; *MDH*, Maryland Department of Health; *DUA*, data use agreement; *HEZ*, [MDH] health enterprise zones; *HSCRC*, [Maryland] Health Services Cost Review Commission; *LHD*, [MDH] Local Health Department; *LHIC*, [MDH] Local Health Improvement Coalition; *MHA*, Maryland Hospital Association; *MHCC*, Maryland Health Care Commission; *MPI*, master patient index; *PDMP*, prescription drug monitoring program; *PPC*, potentially preventable complications; *PSA*, professional services agreements; *SFTP*, secure file transfer protocol; *SSA*, Social Security Act (Medicare and Medicaid).

can lower the potential utilization load on ACOs hence improve their outcomes. Within prescribed boundaries, CRISP links and uses such information is support of clinicians and population health purposes.

CRISP's population HIT platform includes the following core processes: ingesting the data, assigning MPIs, calculate value-based measures, segmenting data into relevant categories, applying analytical tools, creating targeted reports, and distributing the reports to stakeholders within an ACO. Depending on the population health goals, CRISP's platform will generate relevant reports/alerts. For example, if the goal of the services fed by the platform is to risk-stratify a subpopulation, all steps from processing the data to distributing the results should be targeted accordingly. In this case, relevant data for risk stratification (e.g., ADT, claims, hospitals discharges) will be segmented into relevant fields for risk stratification (e.g., diagnosis, medications, procedures, utilization, and cost). Then a risk adjustment tool (e.g., Johns Hopkins ACG [58]) will be used to group the population into risk categories and assign them with risk scores. Finally, these scores can be used to generate reports, including geo-adjusted maps, which can be shared with relevant parties such as providers operating under an ACO umbrella. The reports may vary in their timeliness from real-time hospital readmission reports/alerts to monthly inpatient utilization maps. As another example, CRISP combines the patient panel from a specific primary care practice with the state's immunization registry and chronic conditions flags derived from Medicaid and Medicare data. Practices receive reports on the immunization status of their patients, sortable by age and risk factors. Such information supports proactive outreach helpful to improve immunization rates within the community.

CRISP communicates population health results with several healthcare stakeholders in Maryland. Hospitals, mainly due to Maryland's all-payer waiver program, are deeply engaged with CRISP and HSCRC to improve their population health outcomes. Other providers, especially if part of a larger ACO or PCMH system, also receive vital population health information from CRISP. Naturally, state agencies such as the Maryland Department of Health (MDH), HSCRC, and MHCC are also heavily invested to learn from the statewide population health results to adjust various statewide programs including the reimbursement of case-mixed plans under the waiver program. The following are a select number of population health services that CRISP is offering or is planning to offer in the near term to its stakeholders:

25.3.3.1 Hospital readmission reporting and prediction

Maryland's HSCRC measures and tracks 30-day hospitals readmissions annually. The all-payer program has established a readmission reduction target that requires Maryland Medicare rates to be equal or below national Medicare rates. Given resources allocated to reduce readmissions, along with CRISP's support in providing various services to coordinate care, Maryland's readmission rates have gradually decreased over the years. Based on the latest HSCRC report, most Maryland hospitals are ranked below the national average for Medicare's Hospital Readmission indicators. Indeed, Maryland's unadjusted Medicare readmission rate has decreased from ~17.5% in 2012, which was 2% above the national rate, to ~15% in 2019, which is slightly lower than the national rate [59].

CRISP's real-time readmission reports rely on basic inter-hospital readmission logic using ADT data. This allows hospitals an early view of inter-hospital readmissions. CRISP also aligned the readmission logic based on HSCRC's definitions and limitations set by Maryland's all-payer waiver program. Under this methodology, CRISP offers several reports of intra-hospital and interhospital readmissions to help track performance on monthly trends with Medicare FFS, statewide comparisons by clinical service line, and monthly patient-level drill down [60]. This is made possible as each month the CRISP MPI is linked to the inpatient and outpatient case mix data enabling HSCRC to run the CMS readmission logic and to perform other interhospital analysis. CRISP's readmission analysis reports include: (1) monthly reports with patient drill downs; (2) year-to-year and monthly differentials; (3) comparison by hospital, zip, region, county, census block, and health enterprise zones; and (4) grouping by diagnosis or disposition. CRISP is also planning to provide a near real-time county readmission map for HSCRC and MHCC administration.

25.3.3.2 Population health management services

CRISP provides a series of case management and care coordination services. The general strategy of CRISP has been to: (1) identify high utilizer and high risk Medicare patients (~40k beneficiaries) through a combination of case-mix and Medicare data; (2) use a methodology to associate these patients to hospitals (e.g., hospital case-mix data) and to primary care practices (e.g., Medicare data and CRISP's ENS panels); (3) engage hospitals to provide care management for their associated patients, either at a local level, through regional cooperatives, or through a statewide care management program; (4) engage ambulatory clinicians in the care management process; (5) ask clinicians who care for one of the 40k beneficiaries to create a sharable care profile or care plan; and (6) plan for future interventions to benefit a broader group of Medicare patients ~200k beneficiaries [61].

To achieve care management services, CRISP covers the following service categories: (1) statewide reporting services, (2) point-of-care decision support, (3) case management interfaces, and (4) patient engagement initiatives. Currently CRISP offers a cadre of services for statewide reporting and point-of-care decision support and is actively developing case management interfaces [61]; however, CRISP's role in patient engagement, such as patient portals, has been somewhat limited to date.

Several high-level population health reports are also utilized by HSCRC, MHCC, and MDH for statewide health planning. For example, CRISP generates monthly high utilization analysis reports that are categorized by the following: (1) number of visits, length of stay, and date; (2) census tract or neighborhood; and (3) diagnosis, disposition, or charges. See Fig. 25.4 for an

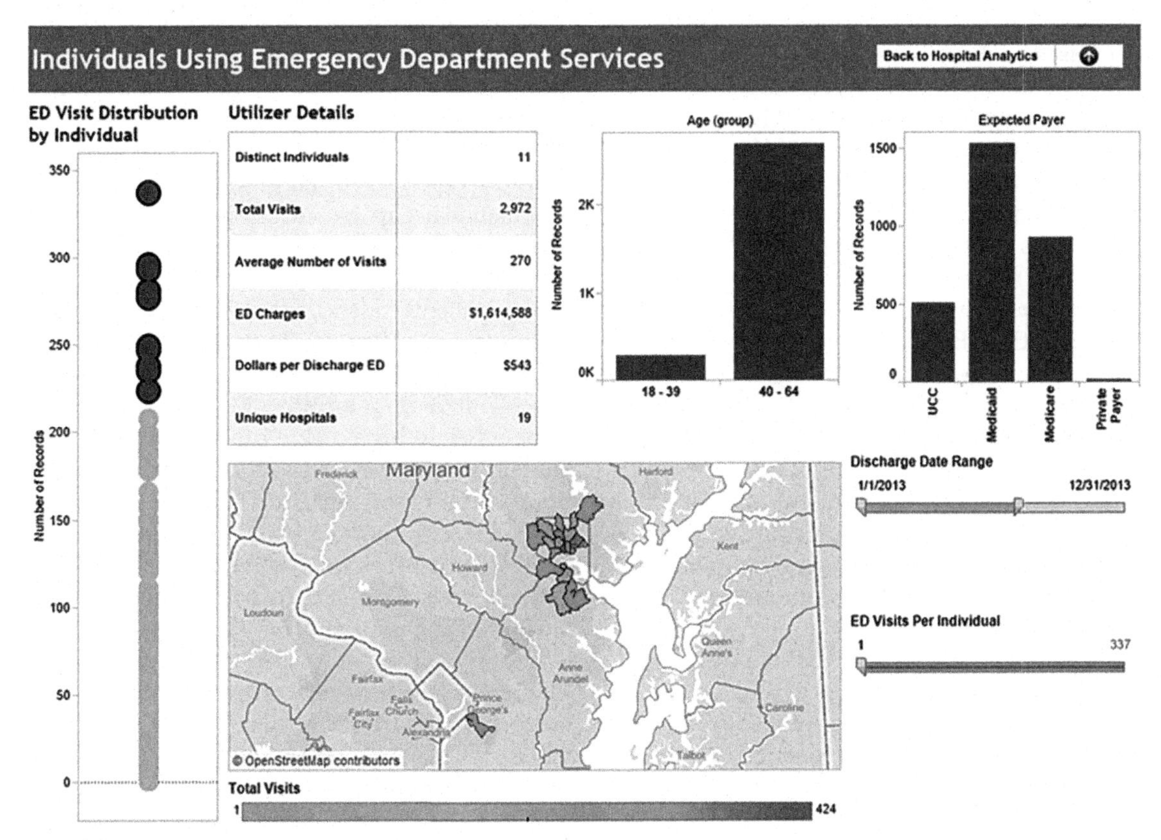

FIGURE 25.4 CRISP's utilization analysis dashboard.

interactive dashboard that is used by state administration to plan accordingly depending on various utilization plans such as ER services.

25.3.3.3 *Other ongoing or planned population health services*

CRISP has developed the capability to generate reports through a combination of CRISP, MDH, and HSCRC data. A number of existing and planned reporting mechanisms include:

- Public health feeds: CRISP interfaces with providers to route certain types of information to MDH, including syndromic surveillance data, immunizations, and reportable conditions [19].
- PDMP: CRISP operates the technical infrastructure of Maryland's PDMP and supports connectivity to every pharmacy licensed to dispense schedule II–IV drugs in Maryland. CRISP also serves as the access point for clinical providers, including prescribers, pharmacists, and other licensed healthcare practitioners [45].
- Overdose analytics: Based on certain overdose related questions, CRISP can produce reports relying on hospital data.
- Newborn early hearing detection and intervention (EHDI) connectivity: CRISP supports hospital integration with the system used by MDH to submit newborn EHDI-related information.
- Patient attribution analysis: CRISP is providing reports with patient attribution levels categorized based on prior visits, percentage of visit allocation by patients, census tract or neighborhood, and by diagnosis or charges.
- Market share analysis: CRISP is providing HSCRC and hospitals with market share reports which include grouping by clinical service line utilization by hospital professional services agreements, by majority of inpatient visits, total visits, and by diagnosis and charges.
- Analysis of potentially avoidable volume: these services include reports on visits with ambulatory sensitive conditions, readmissions, and market share shifts.
- Episode of care analysis: these reports include analyses based on all subsequent hospital visits after discharge, by diagnosis or disposition, and by census tract or neighborhood [61].

25.4 Conclusion/summary

The increasing cost of healthcare has accelerated the adoption of value-based care among US healthcare delivery systems, including adoption of ACOs. These value-based healthcare delivery models attempt to achieve Triple Aim but have experienced challenges in collecting and analyzing the information needed to improve the health of their patient populations.

There are no turnkey HIT solutions available for value-based healthcare systems. HIE networks have the capability to fill in the population-wide informational gap for ACOs and play a pivotal role to enhance value-based care. An HIE can collect, analyze, and provide critical information about patients associated with all providers within and out of an ACO network.

The all-payer waiver program in Maryland has resulted in reforming Maryland hospitals to operate under a value-based global budget. One of the key factors to achieve such an ambitious value-based program in Maryland is its statewide HIE that offers a set of informational and HIT resources to assist value-based organizations such as ACOs to better manage their attributed population.

CRISP is the designated statewide HIE in Maryland which covers a diverse set of stakeholders ranging from hospitals to ancillary providers. CRISP provides several services that are deemed essential to the operations of ACOs in Maryland and, more importantly, to the broader inpatient all-payer waiver program. Some of these population health-IT services include real-time encounter notification of significant events, centralized care coordination infrastructure, automated reporting of quality metrics, and population-based health risk stratification and predictive analytics. CRISP can serve as a health data utility for Maryland's healthcare initiatives.

Questions for discussion

1. List the essential health IT needs of value-based care delivery systems, and discuss which of these requirements can be fulfilled with your statewide HIE services. If you do not have a statewide HIE, pick a state with an HIE and find which of its services can realize these needs. Identify what the technical and operational gaps are and how the HIE can solve them in short term.
2. Discuss the potential services that HIEs can provide to ACO entities if interoperability was not a concern. Explain how such an assumption—full interoperability—can change the role of underlying health IT systems within each of the stakeholders (e.g., EHRs used by hospitals).
3. Identify the recent CMS quality measures for ACOs. Explore the potential data sources and services that HIEs can collect/offer to help the ACOs to calculate/improve these metrics. Determine which type of these ACO measures have a significant application in the HIE context, and propose new ACO metrics that can be easily measured/operationalized by HIEs.
4. Study the main financial reimbursement streams of CMS' Medicare Shared Savings Program (MSSP) for ACOs (e.g., hospital readmissions). Then prioritize the most viable solutions that an HIE can provide to MSSP ACOs. Consider that a certain percentage of the shared savings of the ACO can be shared with the HIE. Identify which of the HIE services are more sustainable in the long run.

References

[1] Centers for Medicare and Medicaid Services (CMS). National Health Expenditure (NHE) fact sheet. Available from: <https://www.cms.gov/Research-Statistics-Data-and-Systems/Statistics-Trends-and-Reports/NationalHealthExpendData/NHE-Fact-Sheet.html>; 2021 [cited 2022 Jan 8].

[2] NEJM Catalyst. What is value-based care? Catalyst 2017;3(1).

[3] Centers for Medicare and Medicaid Services (CMS). Accountable care organizations (ACO). Available from: <https://www.cms.gov/Medicare/Medicare-Fee-for-Service-Payment/ACO/>; 2021 [cited 2022 Jan 8].

[4] Institute for Healthcare Improvement. The IHI Triple Aim. Available from: <http://www.ihi.org/Engage/Initiatives/TripleAim/Pages/default.aspx>; 2015 [cited 2022 Jan 10].

[5] Berwick DM, Nolan TW, Whittington J. The Triple Aim: care, health, and cost. Health Aff 2008;27(3):759–69.

[6] Centers for Medicare and Medicaid Services (CMS). Hospital inpatient value-based purchasing program (Medicare program; final rule). 42 CFR Section Parts 422 and 480. Federal Register 2011;76(88):26490–547.

[7] Centers for Medicare and Medicaid Services (CMS). Shared Savings Programs. Available from: <https://www.cms.gov/Medicare/Medicare-Fee-for-Service-Payment/sharedsavingsprogram>; 2021 [cited 2022 Jan 5].

[8] Walker DM, Mora AM, Scheck McAlearney A. Accountable care organization hospitals differ in health IT capabilities. Am J Manag Care 2016;22(12):802–7 PMID: 27982667.

[9] HITECH Act of 2009, 42 USC sec 139w-4(0)(2) (February 2009), sec 13301, subtitle B: Incentives for the Use of Health Information Technology. Available from: <https://www.hhs.gov/sites/default/files/ocr/privacy/hipaa/understanding/coveredentities/hitechact.pdf>; 2009 [cited 2022 Jan 10].

[10] Balio CP, Apathy NC, Danek RL. Health information technology and accountable care organizations: a systematic review and future directions. EGEMS (Wash DC) 2019;7(1):24. Available from: https://doi.org/10.5334/egems.261 PMID: 31328131; PMCID: PMC6625537.

[11] Nwafor O, Johnson NA. The effect of participation in accountable care organization on electronic health information exchange practices in U.S. hospitals Health Care Manage Rev 2021;. Available from: https://doi.org/10.1097/HMR.0000000000000319 Epub ahead of print. PMID: 34319277.

[12] Rajkumar R, Patel A, Murphy K, Colmers JM, Blum JD, Conway PH, et al. Maryland's all-payer approach to delivery-system reform. N Engl J Med 2014;370(6):493–5.

[13] Sharfstein JM, Kinzer D, Colmers JM. An update on Maryland's all-payer approach to reforming the delivery of health care. JAMA Intern Med 2015;175 (7):1083–4.

[14] Hatef E, Kharrazi H, VanBaak E, Falcone M, Ferris L, Mertz K, et al. A state-wide health IT infrastructure for population health: building a community-wide electronic platform for Maryland's all-payer global budget. Online J Public Health Inform 2017;9(3):e195. Available from: https://doi.org/10.5210/ojphi.v9i3.8129 PMID: 29403574; PMCID: PMC5790428.

[15] Hatef E, Lasser EC, Kharrazi H, Perman C, Montgomery R, Weiner JP. A population health measurement framework: evidence-based metrics for assessing community-level population health in the global budget context. Popul Health Manag 2018;21 (4):261–70. Available from: https://doi.org/10.1089/pop.2017.0112 Epub 2017 Oct 16. PMID: 29035630.

[16] Chesapeake Regional Information System for our Patients (CRISP). Welcome to CRISP. Available from: <https://www.crisphealth.org/about-crisp/>; 2021 [cited 2022 Jan 10].

[17] Chesapeake Regional Information System for our Patients (CRISP). Clinical data. Available from: <https://www.crisphealth.org/applications/clinical-data/>; 2021 [cited 2022 Jan 10].

[18] Chesapeake Regional Information System for our Patients (CRISP). Encounter Notification Services (ENS). Available from: https://www.crisphealth.org/applications/encounter-notification-services-ens/>; 2021 [cited 2022 Jan 10].

[19] Chesapeake Regional Information System for our Patients (CRISP). CRISP Reporting Services. Available from: <https://www.crisphealth.org/applications/crisp-reporting-services-crs/>; 2021 [cited 2022 Jan 10].

[20] Chesapeake Regional Information System for our Patients (CRISP). HIE InContext. Available from: <https://www.crisphealth.org/applications/hie-incontext/>; 2021 [cited 2022 Jan 10].

[21] de Brantes F, Rosenthal MB, Painter M. Building a bridge from fragmentation to accountability – the prometheus payment model. N Engl J Med 2009;36 (11):1033–6.

[22] Kharrazi H, Weiner JP. IT-enabled community health interventions: challenges, opportunities, and future directions. EGEMS (Wash DC) 2014;2(3):1117. Available from: https://doi.org/10.13063/2327-9214.1117 PMID: 25848627; PMCID: PMC4371402.

[23] Rittenhouse DR, Shortell SM, Fisher ES. Primary care and accountable care – two essential elements of delivery-system reform. N Engl J Med 2009;361 (24):2301–3. Available from: https://doi.org/10.1056/NEJMp0909327 PMID: 19864649.

[24] McClellan M, McKethan AN, Lewis JL, Roski J, Fisher ES. A national strategy to put accountable care into practice. Health Aff (Millwood) 2010;29(5):982–90. Available from: https://doi.org/10.1377/hlthaff.2010.0194 PMID: 20439895.

[25] Muhlestein D, McClellan MB. Accountable care organizations in 2016: private and public-sector growth and dispersion. Available from: <https://www.healthaffairs.org/do/10.1377/forefront.20160421.054564/full/>; 2016 [cited 2022 Jan 10].

[26] Centers for Medicare and Medicaid Services (CMS). ACO quality measures. Available from: <https://www.cms.gov/Medicare/Medicare-Fee-for-Service-Payment/sharedsavingsprogram/Downloads/ACO-Shared-Savings-Program-Quality-Measures.pdf>; 2021 [cited 2022 Jan 10].

[27] Stoto MA. Population health measurement: applying performance measurement concepts in population health settings. EGEMS (Wash DC) 2015;2(4):1132. Available from: https://doi.org/10.13063/2327-9214.1132 PMID: 25995988; PMCID: PMC4438103.

[28] Sharfstein JM. The strange journey of population health. Milbank Q 2014;92(4):640–3. Available from: https://doi.org/10.1111/1468-0009.12082 PMID: 25492595; PMCID: PMC4266165.

[29] Kindig D, Stoddart G. What is population health? Am J Public Health. 2003;93(3):380–3. Available from: https://doi.org/10.2105/ajph.93.3.380 PMID: 12604476; PMCID: PMC1447747.

[30] Kharrazi H, Gamache R, Weiner JP. Role of informatics in bridging public and population health. In: Magnuson JA, Dixon BE, editors. Public health informatics and information systems. London: Springer; 2020. ISBN: 978-3-030-41215-9.

[31] Kindig DA. Understanding population health terminology. Milbank Q 2007;85(1):139–61. Available from: https://doi.org/10.1111/j.1468-0009.2007.00479.x PMID: 17319809; PMCID: PMC2690307.

[32] Gamache R, Kharrazi H, Weiner JP. Public and population health informatics: the bridging of big data to benefit communities. Yearb Med Inform 2018;27 (1):199–206. Available from: https://doi.org/10.1055/s-0038-1667081 Epub 2018 Aug 29. PMID: 30157524; PMCID: PMC6115205.

[33] Kharrazi H, Lasser EC, Yasnoff WA, Loonsk J, Advani A, Lehmann HP, et al. A proposed national research and development agenda for population health informatics: summary recommendations from a national expert workshop. J Am Med Inform Assoc 2017;24 (1):2–12. Available from: https://doi.org/10.1093/jamia/ocv210 PMID: 27018264; PMCID: PMC5201177.

[34] Lawrence DM. Analysis & commentary. How to forge a high-tech marriage between primary care and

population health. Health Aff (Millwood) 2010;29 (5):1004–9. Available from: https://doi.org/10.1377/hlthaff.2010.0167 PMID: 20439898.

[35] Handmaker K, Hart J. 9 steps to effective population health management. Healthc Financ Manag 2015;69 (4):70–6 PMID: 26665527.

[36] Wu FM, Rundall TG, Shortell SM, Bloom JR. Using health information technology to manage a patient population in accountable care organizations. J Health Organ Manag 2016;30(4):581–96. Available from: https://doi.org/10.1108/JHOM-01-2015-0003 PMID: 27296880.

[37] Pandya CJ, Chang HY, Kharrazi H. Electronic health record-based risk stratification: a potential key ingredient to achieving value-based care. Popul Health Manag 2021;24(6):654–6. Available from: https://doi.org/10.1089/pop.2021.0131 Epub 2021 Jun 14 PMID: 34129398.

[38] Health Level 7. Welcome to FHIR. Available from: <http://www.hl7.org/fhir/>; 2021 [cited 2022 Jan 10].

[39] U.S. Department of Health and Human Services (DHHS). American Recovery and Reinvestment Act of 2009: advance interoperable health information technology services to support health information exchange. Available from: <http://healthit.gov/sites/default/files/advancedinteroperablehie-foa.pdf>; 2015 [cited 2022 Jan 10].

[40] Kharrazi H, Chi W, Chang HY, Richards TM, Gallagher JM, Knudson SM, et al. Comparing population-based risk-stratification model performance using demographic, diagnosis and medication data extracted from outpatient electronic health records vs administrative claims. Med Care 2017;55 (8):789–96. Available from: https://doi.org/10.1097/MLR.0000000000000754 PMID: 28598890.

[41] Kharrazi H, Ma X, Chang HY, Richards TM, Jung C. Comparing the predictive effects of patient medication adherence indices in electronic health record and claims-based risk stratification models. Popul Health Manag 2021;24(5):601-609. Available from: https://doi.org/10.1089/pop.2020.0306 Epub 2021 Feb 5 PMID: 33544044.

[42] Kharrazi H, Weiner JP. A practical comparison between the predictive power of population-based risk stratification models using data from electronic health records vs administrative claims: setting a baseline for future EHR-derived risk stratification models. Med Care 2018;56 (2):202–3. Available from: https://doi.org/10.1097/MLR.0000000000000849 PMID: 29200132.

[43] Certification Commission for Healthcare Information Technology (CCHIT). A health IT framework for accountable care. Available from: <http://www.healthit.gov/FACAS/sites/faca/files/a_health_it_framework_for_accountable_care_0.pdf>; 2013 [cited 2022 Jan 10].

[44] Dullabh P, Ubri P, Hovey L. The state HIE program four years later: key findings on grantees' experiences from a six-state review. Bethesda: NORC at the University of Chicago. Available from: <http://healthit.gov/sites/default/files/CaseStudySynthesis GranteeExperienceFinal_121014.pdf>; 2014 [cited 2022 Jan 10].

[45] Chesapeake Regional Information System for our Patients (CRISP). Prescription Drug Monitoring Program (PDMP). Available from: <https://www.crisphealth.org/applications/prescription-drug-monitoring-program-pdmp/>; 2021 [cited 2022 Jan 10].

[46] Chesapeake Regional Information System for our Patients (CRISP). Our connected providers – the power behind the CRISP HIE. Available from: <https://www.crisphealth.org/about-crisp/connected-providers/>; 2021 [cited 2022 Jan 10].

[47] Chesapeake Regional Information System for our Patients (CRISP). CRISP policies and procedures. Available from: <https://www.crisphealth.org/wp-content/uploads/2021/05/CRISP-Policies-and-Procedures-DRAFT-updates-v572.pdf>; 2021 [cited 2022 Jan 10].

[48] U.S. Government Publishing Office. Electronic Code of Federal Regulations (eCFR) Part 2 – confidentiality of alcohol and drug abuse patient records. Available from: <https://www.ecfr.gov/current/title-42/part-2>; 2017 [cited 2022 Jan 12].

[49] Mirth Corporation. Mirth connect. Available from: <https://www.mirthcorp.com/community/issues/browse/MIRTH/?selectedTab = com.atlassian.jira.jira-projects-plugin:summary-panel>; 2021 [cited 2022 Jan 12].

[50] Audacious Inquiry (Ai). Master data management within HIE infrastructure: a focus on master patient indexing approaches. Available from: <https://www.healthit.gov/sites/default/files/master_data_management_final.pdf>; 2012 [cited 2022 Jan 12].

[51] Maryland Health Services Cost Review Commission (HSCRC). Improving care coordination and care management: Supporting the all-payer model design by reducing avoidable use of health care, lowering spending, and improving health. Available from: <http://www.hscrc.state.md.us/documents/md-maphs/wg-meet/cc/2015-03-31/2-Care-Coordination-Work-Group-draft-report-3-24-15.pdf>; 2015 [cited 2022 Jan 12].

[52] Hatef E, Searle KM, Predmore Z, Lasser EC, Kharrazi H, Nelson K, et al. The impact of social determinants of health on hospitalization in the Veterans Health Administration. Am J Prev Med 2019;56(6):811–18. Available from: https://doi.org/10.1016/j.amepre.2018.12.012 Epub 2019 Apr 17 PMID: 31003812.

[53] Hatef E, Ma X, Rouhizadeh M, Singh G, Weiner JP, Kharrazi H. Assessing the impact of social needs and social determinants of health on health care utilization:

using patient- and community-level data. Popul Health Manag 2021;24(2):222–30. Available from: https://doi.org/10.1089/pop.2020.0043 PMID: 32598228; PMCID: PMC8349715..

[54] Tan M, Hatef E, Taghipour D, Vyas K, Kharrazi H, Gottlieb L, et al. Including social and behavioral determinants in predictive models: trends, challenges, and opportunities. JMIR Med Inform 2020;8(9):e18084. Available from: https://doi.org/10.2196/18084 PMID: 32897240.

[55] Hatef E, Predmore Z, Lasser EC, Kharrazi H, Nelson K, Curtis I, et al. Integrating social and behavioral determinants of health into patient care and population health at Veterans Health Administration: a conceptual framework and an assessment of available individual and population level data sources and evidence-based measurements. AIMS Public Health 2019;6(3):209–24. Available from: https://doi.org/10.3934/publichealth.2019.3.209 PMID: 31637271; PMCID: PMC6779595.

[56] Fielding NG. Triangulation and mixed methods designs: data integration with new research technologies. Mixed Methods Res 2012;6(2):124–36. Available from: https://doi.org/10.1177/1558689812437101.

[57] Chang HY, Kharrazi H, Bodycombe D, Weiner JP, Alexander GC. Healthcare costs and utilization associated with high-risk prescription opioid use: a retrospective cohort study. BMC Med 2018;16(1):69. Available from: https://doi.org/10.1186/s12916-018-1058-y PMID: 29764482; PMCID: PMC5954462.

[58] The Johns Hopkins University Bloomberg School of Public Health. The Johns Hopkins ACG case-mix system documentation & application manual, Version 11. Baltimore, MD: Johns Hopkins University; 2014.

[59] Maryland Health Services Cost Review Commission. Draft recommendation for the readmission reduction incentive program for rate year 2023. Available from: <https://www.mhaonline.org/docs/default-source/advocacy/hscrc/newsbreak-links/draft-recommendation-for-the-readmission-reduction-incentive-program-for-rate-year-2023.pdf>; 2020 [cited 2022 Jan 12].

[60] Swain MJ, Kharrazi H. Feasibility of 30-day hospital readmission prediction modeling based on health information exchange data. Int J Med Inform 2015;84(12):1048–56. Available from: https://doi.org/10.1016/j.ijmedinf.2015.09.003 Epub 2015 Sep 14. PMID: 26412010.

[61] Chesapeake Regional Information System for our Patients (CRISP). CRISP Care Management Support. Available from: <http://www.hscrc.state.md.us/documents/md-maphs/wg-meet/cc/2015-02-27/3-CRISP-Care-Management-Support-v2-4.pdf>; 2015 [cited 2022 Jan 12].

CHAPTER

26

Health information exchange—the value proposition: a case study of the US Social Security Administration

Sue S. Feldman

Department of Health Services Administration, School of Health Professions, University of Alabama at Birmingham, Birmingham, AL, USA

LEARNING OBJECTIVES

By the end of the chapter, the reader should be able to:

- The learner will identify factors to consider when assessing blended value propositions in a public–private information exchange collaboration;
- The learner will identify secondary uses of data beyond diagnosis, treatment, payment, or operations;
- The learner will understand the influence of governance on technical data sharing and organizational collaboration.

26.1 Introduction

Stakeholder value proposition is not unifocal but comprises multiple factors. Few studies on the secondary use of electronic medical information, as well as associated frameworks and taxonomies, mention using medical record data for benefit determination, disability, or otherwise. Furthermore, explorations into organizational value propositions typically locate the value of Health IT for health information exchange (HIE) in the domains of diagnosis, treatment, and operations—even for providers whose clients may need Social Security Disability Insurance (SSDI) benefits within their lifetimes. Current literature lacks any high-impact value proposition regarding secondary uses of health information for disability determination. This case study addresses that gap, using a framework that examines blended value propositions within enacted collaborations for successful HIE between a public and a private organization. The public entity is the US Social Security Administration (SSA), and the private organization is MedVirigina, a community-based HIE network.

Health Information Exchange
DOI: https://doi.org/10.1016/B978-0-323-90802-3.00002-2

26.2 Theoretical models for examining the value of health information exchange

This case study explores the concept of value in the context of HIE using a conceptual framework based on multiple social science theories. As discussed in Chapter 5, HIE is a business which must deliver value to its customers, which are most often the health care organizations that participate in the HIE network. This section describes the underlying social science (which includes economics and informatics) theories as well as the conceptual framework used to examine the value of HIE for disability determination.

26.2.1 Socio-technical systems approach

A **socio-technical systems (STS)** approach examines social/community links to technical processes [1]. STS design includes several levels of interactions including mechanical (hardware), informational (software), psychological (persons), and social (community). This inclusive approach aims to understand interdependent linkages among a hierarchy of social and technological components. These components interact with social motivations and accomplish a set of social goals that otherwise could not be realized.

Therefore, social motivations and benefits should be examined in a different light than is customary in the return-on-investment economic model commonly used for information exchange in business. This blended value proposition has been defined as the combination of social and economic value used to maximize total returns where, according to Emerson, "the core nature of investment and return is not a tradeoff between social and financial interest, but rather the pursuit of an embedded value proposition composed of both" [2]. Emerson continues: "Societies cannot function strictly on the basis of their economic enterprise. It is social commerce that allows individuals and institutions to pursue the traditional financial returns sought by mainstream financial capital market players" [2].

An STS approach focused on systems that are both technologically sound and socially sustainable [3] has been applied to studying HIE, because of the multiple organizations, user types, hardware and software technologies, and sociopolitical motivations and goals involved in HIE composition. Relatively few studies have examined HIE networks in operation, but a socio-technical approach was previously applied and shown appropriate for studying HIE [4,5].

26.2.2 Interorganizational systems

An **interorganizational system (IOS)** is an IT-based system shared by two or more independent organizations for the purpose of information flows and strategic advantage [5,6]. Prior research on IOS focused on cross-organizational features of an STS [6,7]. While the implementation of IOS has been studied for decades across a wide array of industries, few studies have addressed the value proposition related to health care, and fewer still have considered the value proposition related to HIE [5]. However, consistent with HIE, an IOS creates a virtual value chain for instant encounters or transactions of information between nonpredetermined participants [8]. An important consideration of this value equation is that the participating organizations' values may be unequal as well as interdependent [9].

Historically, the basis for collaborative efforts has been primarily economic, with the goal of information exchange being strategic advantage leading to increased earnings—an easily quantifiable metric [10–12]. Technical performance is crucial and quantifiable in information exchange, but the success of information exchange within interorganizational collaborations frequently hinges on less quantifiable factors such as shared leadership or aligned and dynamic value propositions [13–16]. Governance (see Chapter 4) can also influence the facilitation and coordination of data exchange [17]. For example, knowing who has decision-making power was shown to increase accountability, foster a more cooperative environment, and decrease intra- and interorganizational tensions [18]. Yet, the formal governance structures typical of mature interorganizational collaborations may negatively affect newly established or emerging collaborations [19,20].

26.2.3 Value proposition

Many organizational mission statements include both social and economic factors. In their book, *Ben & Jerry's Double-Dip: How to Run a Values-Led Business and Make Money, Too,* Ben Cohen and Jerry Greenfield describe their corporate social mission as being just as important as their economic mission, and perhaps even more exposed—given that economic audits are written in financial speak, whereas social audits are written in plain English [21]. However, Emerson suggests:

> We must move beyond the traditional belief that an organization's Economic Value is separate and at odds with its Social Value. While one might attempt to track the two (such as by examining the financials of the corporation and then reading the social audit completed by an outside observer), they are wrongly viewed as two separate aspects of the corporation's value proposition [2].

Various research studies have concluded that value propositions in collaborative efforts are supported by the ideal of public good, where social drivers can include elements extending beyond the organization and having a variety of influences for social good; however, such value is diffuse and not easily measured [22,23]. Studies note that an organization's economic needs may be driven by elements that comprise organizational fiscal health and are usually easily quantifiable [16]. Yet another perspective suggests that stakeholder value proposition is not a single-focus proposition, but rather an evolving blend of social and economic factors within a particular context [24].

Value propositions, therefore, may be blended and may change over time. Answering stakeholder value questions such as: "What's in it for me?," "Why is this important?," and "What is needed for sustainability?" is essential for collaboration, especially in HIE networks and public-private collaborations [16,25]. To answer these questions and further understand value proposition changes over time, we must examine evolving social and economic value propositions within the larger context of a blended value proposition.

The highest-order intangible social benefits (human life) of health information sharing are succinctly stated by Porter and Teisberg [26]: "The social benefits of results information will be even greater in health care than in the financial markets, because the physical well-being of Americans is at stake." Social value considerations for collaboration extend beyond those that are actor-based or organizational in nature. In his book on infrastructure delivery in public–private collaborations, Mody [27] draws examples from the railway and transportation systems to suggest that social considerations, such as being able to deliver goods and information to the right place at the right time, might exceed those of economic returns and could exert greater significant pressure.

Social motivations may support economic motivations in some situations but be at odds with them in other situations, a fact that contributes to the need for value propositions to evolve over time in order to sustain the collaboration (or HIE network).

As with supply chain information sharing, health information sharing is a costly investment from which organizations expect an economic return [28,29]. However, with health information sharing at various stages of development and constantly iterating, upfront and continued investments are likely to be very high and a sustained commitment to the collaboration is critical for successful outcomes and sustainability. The healthcare industry could learn about sustainability from other industries such as supply chain management. For example, two studies suggest that factors contributing to positive outcomes and sustainability include cocreating value (relationships being an important component), strategy formation, and competitive advantage [30,31]. A parallel can be drawn with a HEAL NY case study (see Chapter 24) of New York's investment to create an interoperable Regional Health Information Organization (RHIO), which cites "the need to convince stakeholders of the project's value" as a factor in financial alignment and sustainability [16].

In the past, the conceptual basis for exploring collaborative efforts was primarily economic, and the goal of information exchange was increased earnings [10–12]. However, literature suggests that the benefits of interorganizational information sharing can be diffuse and not limited to "the bottom line." For example, Aldrich [32] suggests that collaborating organizations now consider reasons other than economics as drivers for sharing information, and Brynjolffson and Saunders [33] note that the intangible benefits of interorganizational information sharing may be the untapped value proposition for interorganizational information collaborations. The idea that the value proposition may be a blend of intangibles such as social value, and tangibles such as economics, is compatible with the use of blended conceptualizations to understand health information collaborations.

Within the social and economic motivations underlying interorganizational collaborations are multiple dimensions of information sharing. The following are some important studies of HIE implementations examining the elements contributing to value propositions and how they change over time. Delone and McLean [34] note that exploring multiple dimensions can help align organizational needs and bring value to each organization individually and to the collaboration collectively. Riskin et al. [35] included clinical outcomes as an additional metric to fiscal health. Malepeti et al. [36] suggest that value can be found in a wide spectrum of benefits, ranging from organizational fiscal health (changes in market share) to technical performance (getting usable data where needed). While technical performance is crucial in information exchange between organizations, the success of interorganizational collaborations and information exchanges frequently hinges on other factors such as interorganizational alignment, shared leadership, and a blend of value propositions [13,14,16,37]. In the case of HEAL NY (the RHIO mentioned above), a study two years postimplementation revealed that concerns over technical issues increased, but so did the potential for misaligned persistent stakeholder value propositions [16]. And a case study of Virginia statewide HIE implementation found that technical, organizational, and governance elements were critical success factors in collaborations and in realizing a shared value proposition [5]. Now that interorganizational collaborations for the purpose of health information sharing have become more mainstream, many studies are broadening the definition of value to include medication safety [38], adherence [39], workflows [40], and patient satisfaction [39]. Likewise, there is an emerging body of literature on electronic health record (EHR) value in the face of clinician burnout. A systematic review focusing on nurse well-being found that there is an imminent need for multifocal interventions to ease EHR-driven documentation burden [41].

Governance can influence how collaborations facilitate and coordinate data sharing [17]. Governance, in terms of intra- and interorganizational authority (knowing who has decision-making power), has been shown to increase accountability, foster a more cooperative environment, and decrease intra- and interorganizational issues [18]. The nature of the relationships between decision makers is also important in navigating complex governance processes, structures, and sharing decisions [42,43]. A seminal 2010 case study examining the demise of CalRHIO (California Regional Health Information Organization) indicated that a lack of formal governance practices led to the need for subsequent overhaul and eventual restructuring [44].

To summarize: Governance may not be "one size fits all," and newly formed collaborations may be negatively influenced by the formal governance structures that characterize more mature interorganizational collaborations. This is especially true of collaborations involving governmental entities [19], which may need evolving governance that is responsive to change. However, governance is an essential element of collaborations and not one to be viewed as a "footnote" or second-order priority.

A framework depicting HIE relative to public agencies as consumers of EHR data (supplied by private providers) is specific to personal (pertaining to the patient) and public (pertaining to community disease prevention and health promotion) health uses but not to benefit determination, disability or otherwise [45]. SSA was innovative in establishing a public–private collaboration for using Medical Evidence Gathering and Analysis through Health IT (MEGAHIT) across a national HIE network to gather clinical data from EHRs for secondary use (i.e., medical information not used for diagnosis, treatment, or payment). MEGAHIT is an SSA-developed heath IT solution to collect medical records, or medical evidence, electronically through HIE. MEGAHIT is under a larger SSA program called Electronic Evidence and Analysis Program.

Achieving successful public–private collaborations for HIE may require a shared understanding of the changing value orientation and expectations by each collaborating organization as well as a recognition that, over time, the value proposition may shift. One could conjecture that, in some cases, value (like beauty) is in the eye of the beholder—in that each collaborator may have a different opinion of what constitutes value. Furthermore, the value proposition may change as organizational goals change. Therefore both context and perspective are necessary to understand value propositions. Identifying the value proposition—in this context meaning the worth, importance, or utility of the information received through HIE—helps answer the question: "What's in it for me?"

A 2010 report from the eHealth Exchange (eHE) underscores the observation that collaborations designed specifically for sharing health information may have misaligned motivations for sharing data, and more research is needed to clarify the value of HIE as related to stakeholders' motivations and perspectives [46]. For example, a public agency may be satisfied with finding value in sharing health information for the public good (e.g., community disease prevention and health promotion), while the private organization wants to understand the value proposition in terms of business value, with some degree of economic impact (e.g., operational savings or cost avoidance) [16,47,48]. In the context of disability determination, SSA as a public agency may find value in faster disability determinations, which could provide economic benefit to the private organization through decreased uncompensated care losses. Understanding the value that SSA and disability benefit determination collaborators find in the overall process may provide information that can facilitate sustainable HIE.

Research findings on public–private information exchange suggest that unsustainable value propositions (e.g., no economic benefit) and poorly defined governance are key reasons for failures [25,47,49]. Thus it is critical to consider that while the initial value in HIE may have been the technical exchange of data, that value evolves over time and organizational and governance factors begin emerging as critical factors.

Aligned and evolving value propositions related to successful HIE networks have yet to be empirically established, but information from other industries suggests that a strong relationship exists between understanding value propositions and sustained success. For example, a study examining a variety of service industries (e.g., automotive) suggests that initial value may have been in the mere exchange of goods, but over time the value moves to use of the goods [50]. As applied to HIE, the initial value may have been in the technical exchange of data, but that value continues to evolve over time, and organizational factors—such as use and usefulness of the data to impact organizational fiscal health—begin to emerge as critical factors.

The Agency for Healthcare Research and Quality released a vision and strategy document discussing a strong relationship between HIE sustainability and value proposition [51]. The report also identifies the potential for federal programs to contribute to HIE sustainability and comprehensive information exchange but does not discuss this contribution in the context of SSA. Thus the opportunity presents itself to better understand stakeholder value propositions in health data exchange within a high-impact area of disability determination.

26.2.4 Conceptual framework

Enactment theory proposes that a rationale is ascribed to outcomes [5,52]. Fountain's Technology Enactment Framework (TEF) applies enactment theory to IT to suggest that more than the technology produces outcomes; rather, organizational factors combined with the technical factors provide a rationale that is embedded *within* each collaborating organization; it is *how* the technology is enacted that influences outcomes [5,17]. Schooley's Time Critical Information Systems framework suggests that the core components of a public–private collaboration involve more than governance and IT, and also include interorganizational relationships [37]. Robey [53] notes that we can no longer examine IOS as if they were a snapshot of a moment in time, but must revise existing theories to reflect technical evolution.

Based on the previous frameworks of Emerson [2], Fountain [17], and Schooley [15], this case study uses a Blended Value Collaboration Enactment Framework shown in Fig. 26.1 [5]. The framework suggests that, while the output may be seen in terms of quantifiable system performance, the HIE value proposition is influenced by a combination of factors—technical, organizational, and governance—within and between organizations. The value proposition may further be motivated by social or economic considerations.

Within each organization (labeled as Organization A, B, etc.), multiple dimensions influence the Output and subsequent Value proposition. These dimensions are shown as technical and organizational (unique to each organization), which are supported by governance structures and motivations for collaboration within each organization. The value propositions for organizations A, B, etc. are considered to be social or economic, or a blend of the two. The balance beam denotes the dynamic nature of the motivation and allows for motivations changing or evolving over time. As the collaboration evolves (lower axis) the Output and resulting Value (HIE value proposition) result from *what* drives the collaboration and *how* the multiple dimensions of collaboration are enacted. This conceptual framework illustrates that as time passes (denoted by T_1, T_2, and so on), changes occur, and that these events recur (as opposed to occurring at only one moment in time). This Blended Value Collaboration Enactment Framework guided the methodology of this

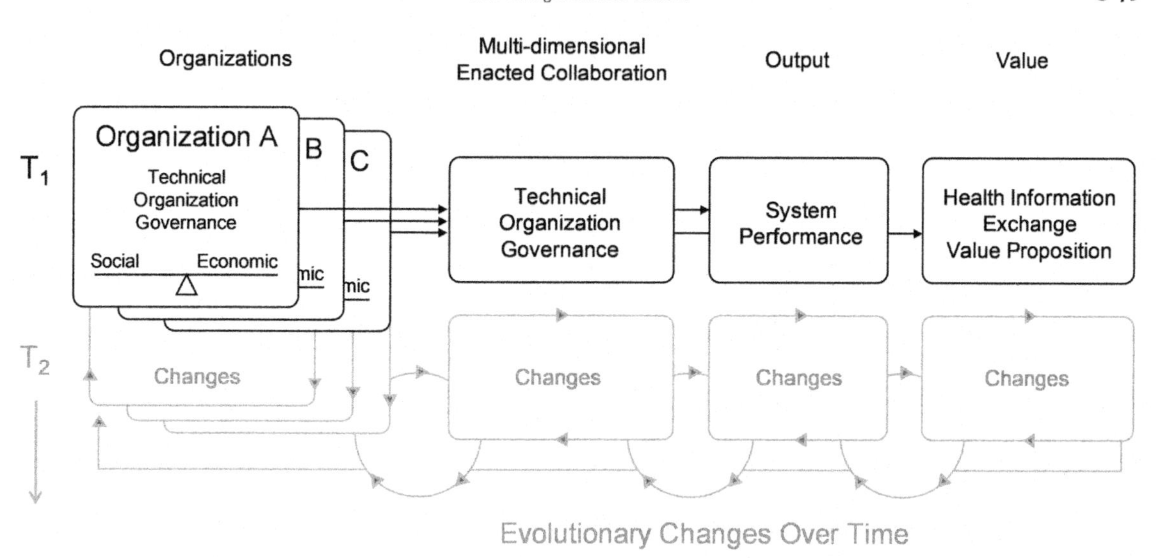

FIGURE 26.1 Blended Value Collaboration Enactment Framework. Source: *From the Journal of Medical Internet Research [5].*

case study. The framework is especially valuable for its consideration of the recursive nature of *how* collaborations are enacted and that changes occur over time—both within each organization and between organizations, influenced by the perceived value proposition.

26.3 Background and context

This case study involves the collaboration between three entities: the Nationwide Health Information Network (NwHIN; the transport mechanism), MedVirginia (the HIE network providing information), and the US SSA (the Federal Agency requesting information).

26.3.1 Nationwide Health Information Network

One of the earliest initiatives of the Office of the National Coordinator for Health IT (ONC) was the NwHIN, designed to be a "network of networks" and the nation's HIE [54–56]. When this case study was originally conducted, NwHIN was managed by ONC. It was later privatized to the Sequoia Project and rebranded as **eHealth Exchange (eHE)**, and then more recently eHE and the Sequoia Project were separated to provide appropriate definition between the two entities. eHE is a national health information network, whereas the Sequoia Project acts as a neutral body, inclusive of diverse participants (not just eHE) operating in the public interest with a governance process to insure transparent oversight.

To keep current, all references to NwHIN are as eHE, except where the context requires NwHIN, such as in a historical context. eHE consists of a set of technical standards, web services, and policies that facilitate secure and interoperable information exchange across multiple entities using the Internet. Participants in eHE must go through a technical certification process as well as a governance review process to ensure their multiorganizational, regional, or national network of facilities can meaningfully exchange data with the other participants while adhering to established policies to protect data as it is exchanged for a range of use cases.

26.3.2 MedVirginia/Bon Secours[1]

MedVirginia, Virginia's RHIO, is an HIE network in Richmond, Virginia, that began in 2001 with a vision of creating communities of care making Richmond the most health data-connected community in the nation. By 2005, using the Internet, MedVirginia launched a HIPAA-compliant portal giving clinicians access to lab, pharmacy, and other patient health information at the point of clinical care; any secondary uses of this information were unrealized potential whose value had not yet been considered.

At the time of this case study, MedVirginia provided services for physicians and hospitals in the Bon Secours Health System, and four Bon Secours hospitals were involved in this study. On February 28, 2009, MedVirginia and SSA began using eHE (then NwHIN) to transmit patient health information for disability determination using MEGAHIT, described earlier. This project was the first instantiation of a much larger initiative that was later expanded with funds from the American Recovery and Reinvestment Act (ARRA). Prior to collaborating with SSA, MedVirginia's data-sharing focused on clinicians, diagnostic laboratories, pharmacies, etc., primarily for purposes of diagnosis, treatment, and payment. The uncompensated care cost recovery in this case study is that of Bon Secours and not of MedVirginia.

In February 2010 MedVirginia received one of SSA's 14 ARRA-funded awards to expand the initial use of MEGAHIT across eHE for collecting medical evidence for disability determination. This meant that more of MedVirginia's current providers could participate in MEGAHIT and provided a unique opportunity, as well as the means, to examine the evolution over time of factors contributing to value propositions.

26.3.3 US Social Security Administration

The US SSA, the nation's primary disability benefit provider, is among the largest US users of medical record information, particularly for determining disability benefits [57]. Disability applications begin when a claim is filed with SSA (Internet, telephone, in person) at a local field office. The field office then sends a signed form (Authorization to Disclose Information to the Social Security Administration or Form 827[2]) to the state Disability Determination Services office, which generates an authorized request to the claimant's healthcare provider(s) for supporting documentation (medical evidence) to be used in deciding the merits of the claim. This begins an arduous process of requests and re-requests for medical evidence. Re-requests are often needed because many responses are incomplete, some are inadequate, and many remain unanswered, resulting in delays and increasing disability determination costs. Fig. 26.2. illustrates the disability application process at the time of this case study.

[1] The content in this case study represents the organizational structure of MedVirgina at the time the case study was completed and their relationship with Bon Secours at that time. It is likely that the structure and the relationship have changed since this original case study was completed. The process and outcomes are still applicable.

[2] SSA Form-827 is an Authorization to Disclose Information to the Social Security Administration (SSA). The purpose of this form is to obtain medical and other information needed to substantiate the merits of a disability claim and render a disability determination.

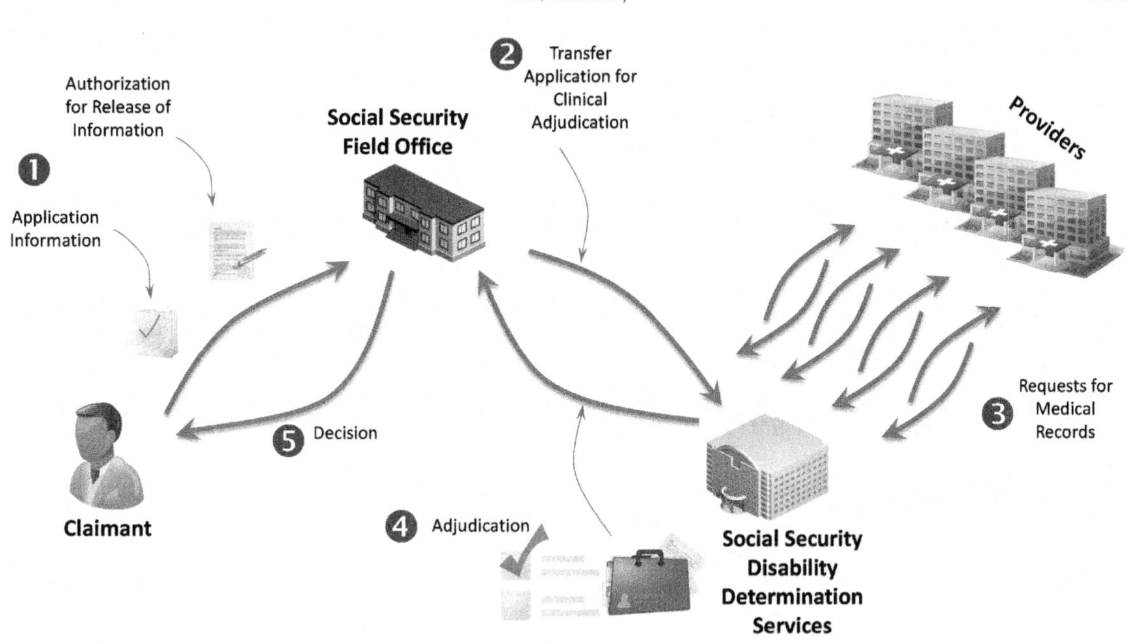

FIGURE 26.2 Disability determination process. Source: *Modified from the Social Security Administration.*

SSA uses health IT solutions to expedite delivery of medical records for disability determination and has dedicated some of its ARRA funds to incentivizing providers to exchange medical information for disability determination. In the context of disability determination, Health IT advances (such as the use of MEGAHIT) provide a secure and interoperable transport mechanism for transporting medical record data to SSA. SSA's goal is to use MEGAHIT (which includes business rules for automated processing) across the eHE, enabled by existing Internet technology, for HIE for disability determination. Doing so changes the lens through which we see HIE and brings into focus the high-impact, high-value motivations for secondary uses of existing EHR data. Using MEGAHIT through the eHE has both social and economic motivations: time savings in disability determination and uncompensated care cost recovery, respectively.

In the context of disability determination, public–private collaborations for HIE offer opportunities to understand the multiple dimensions and evolving organizational motivations of sharing health data information. This opportunity is especially unusual in that the public organization (SSA) is not typically considered a healthcare provider and is therefore frequently left out of the collaboration loop of sharing health information. Therefore examining this collaboration for disability determination changes our image of viable collaborators and consumers of EHR data in HIE and provides a unique opportunity to understand changing and evolving value propositions for sharing health information in a public-private collaboration.

26.4 Case study

26.4.1 The challenge

Relying upon principally manual methods for developing (requesting, receiving, and analyzing) medical evidence for disability determination is an inefficient process [58,59].[3] A Government Accountability Office report suggests that SSA disability claims take too long, the backlog is too large, and the processes are out of step with technological advances [60]. Such factors lead to decreased access to health care,[4] delayed receipt of cash benefits, and increased uncompensated care costs. Note that gains in healthcare coverage provided through the Affordable Care Act have led to a 21%, or $7.4 billion, decrease in uncompensated care costs [61]. However, Medicaid expansion is not mandatory and several states have not participated. States *not* engaging in Medicaid expansion are estimated to decrease uncompensated care costs by only half as much as do those states participating in Medicaid expansion. Thus access to healthcare services made possible through SSA disability benefits remain an important value proposition for healthcare providers.

26.4.2 Opportunity

The inefficient process of medical evidence development for disability determination stands to benefit from the technological advances so well suited to routine and predictable processes: requesting, gathering, and analyzing information [59,60,62]. However, SSA does not collect medical evidence in a vacuum, but depends on healthcare providers to supply the medical evidence. HIEs have emerged as logical candidates with whom SSA could collaborate to collect medical evidence for disability determination.

The collection of the information is only one part of the process. Another critical component is figuring out the degree to which the health information collected can be used to support the case. As health information sharing matures, so too do the technologies supporting the use of the information. Natural language processing (NLP) has been used in linguistics, computer science, and artificial intelligence for some time and is now expanding into different domains. While NLP is not without its potential for biases [63,64], promising work has begun to use NLP in the disability determination domain [65]. Early work by Newman-Griffis [65] suggests that NLP has the potential to hasten the disability determination adjudication process, while increasing its accuracy, by applying NLP relative to triaging cases.

26.4.3 The case: examining social versus economic value propositions

SSA underwent two reorganizations during the course of this study and has further undergone additional reorganization (not reflected in this case study). The first reorganization "institutionalized" Health IT. Instead of Health IT being its own division with a division director, responsibilities were spread across the agency. The second reorganization relocated the accountability for Health IT from the Office of the Deputy Commissioner of Systems to the Office of the Chief Information Officer. Each time, the value of MEGAHIT needed to be resubstantiated, causing delays and miscommunications. Such situations can fracture developing or already accepted value propositions.

Organizational value propositions may be located across several dimensions rather than in a single dimension. Furthermore, organizational value propositions (whether socially or economically motivated) change over time and much of this change can be prompted by the organizational direction. The value in blended value propositions, as described here, is the ability to provide balance within a collaboration. This balance proved beneficial during

[3] When medical records are collected by SSA, they become medical evidence. This process is part of the medical evidence development process (http://www.ssa.gov/disability/professionals/bluebook/).

[4] In most states, a favorable decision for SSDI includes Medicare (after a two-year waiting period).

SSA's reorganization, when key elements of the collaboration were weakened.

The social-economic-dimensional value blend is illustrated in Fig. 26.3. The value proposition is indicated along the social value (x) and economic value (y) axes, with a line equidistant from both axes indicating an equal value blend. The dotted arc provides a reference for changes that occurred for each organization between the first and second instantiations of MEGAHIT. Each organization's location on the diagram is based on the case study findings and represents each organization's value blend associated with the first and second instantiations of MEGAHIT. The nature of each organization's focus (with respect to dimension) is also indicated—tech = technical, org = organization, and gov = governance—reflecting observations in the literature that collaborations should focus on multiple dimensions [34].

As interpreted from the findings of this case study:

- SSA began MEGAHIT for the social value from a technical dimension and migrated toward finding economic value while retreating slightly on the social value scale, but remains below the equal-value line.
- MedVirginia began MEGAHIT from a social value focus from technical and organizational dimensions and has migrated toward an economic value proposition (retaining the focus on technical and organizational dimensions); however, one notes that MedVirginia is now closer to the equal-value line, indicating a more balanced blended value proposition rather than being weighted heavily toward either the social or economic value zones.
- ONC began NwHIN from an almost purely social value proposition and is beginning to think about the business case that might accompany NwHIN sustainability. It is important to note, however, that this paradigm shifted with the privatization to the Sequoia Project and subsequently with the separation between Sequoia Project and eHE.

Note in Fig. 26.3 that all three organizations, regardless of how far to the right they were on the social value scale in the first instantiation, show a leftward shift (i.e., slightly less social value) in the second instantiation. Likewise, all three organizations migrated toward a higher economic value, with MedVirginia crossing the equal-value line so economic value exceeds social value.

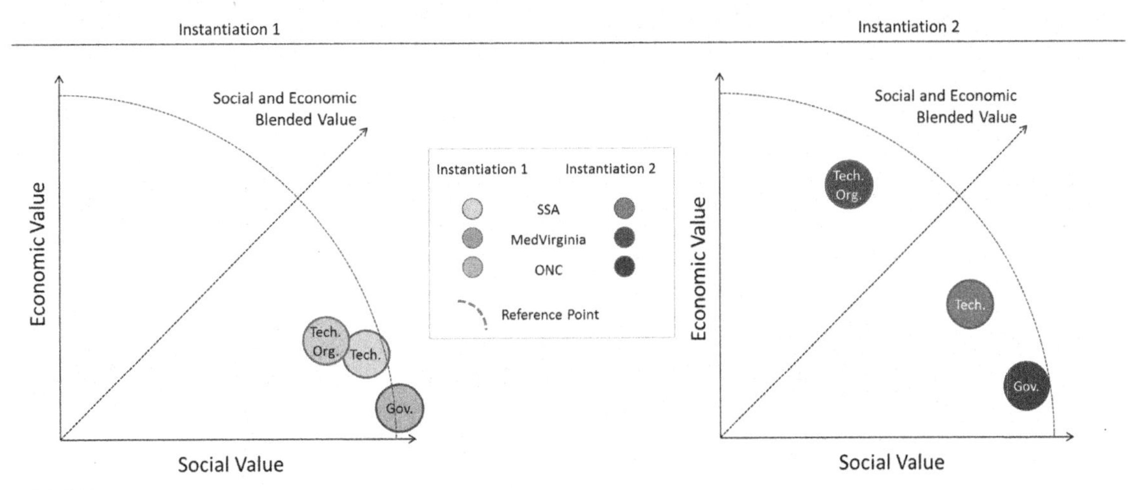

FIGURE 26.3 Social-economic-dimensional value blend by organization.

As time has evolved, MedVirginia and other organizations like them, have found a balanced position on the equal-value dotted line in Fig. 26.3, representing a more balanced social-economic value proposition. Likewise, SSA has appreciated some economic impact as well in terms of faster case adjudication.

26.4.4 The case: examining the blended value collaboration enactment framework

The findings of this case study are a result of analysis from 41 key participant interviews and extensive document analysis and illustrated within the Blended Value Collaboration Enactment Framework (see Fig. 26.3). In Fig. 26.4, advances are indicated by a " + " and setbacks are indicated by a " − ."

26.4.5 Social Security Administration

SSA experienced both advances and setbacks during the project. In terms of advances, (indicated in Fig. 26.4 by +), the findings suggest great progress toward increasing the number of listings or medical conditions for which

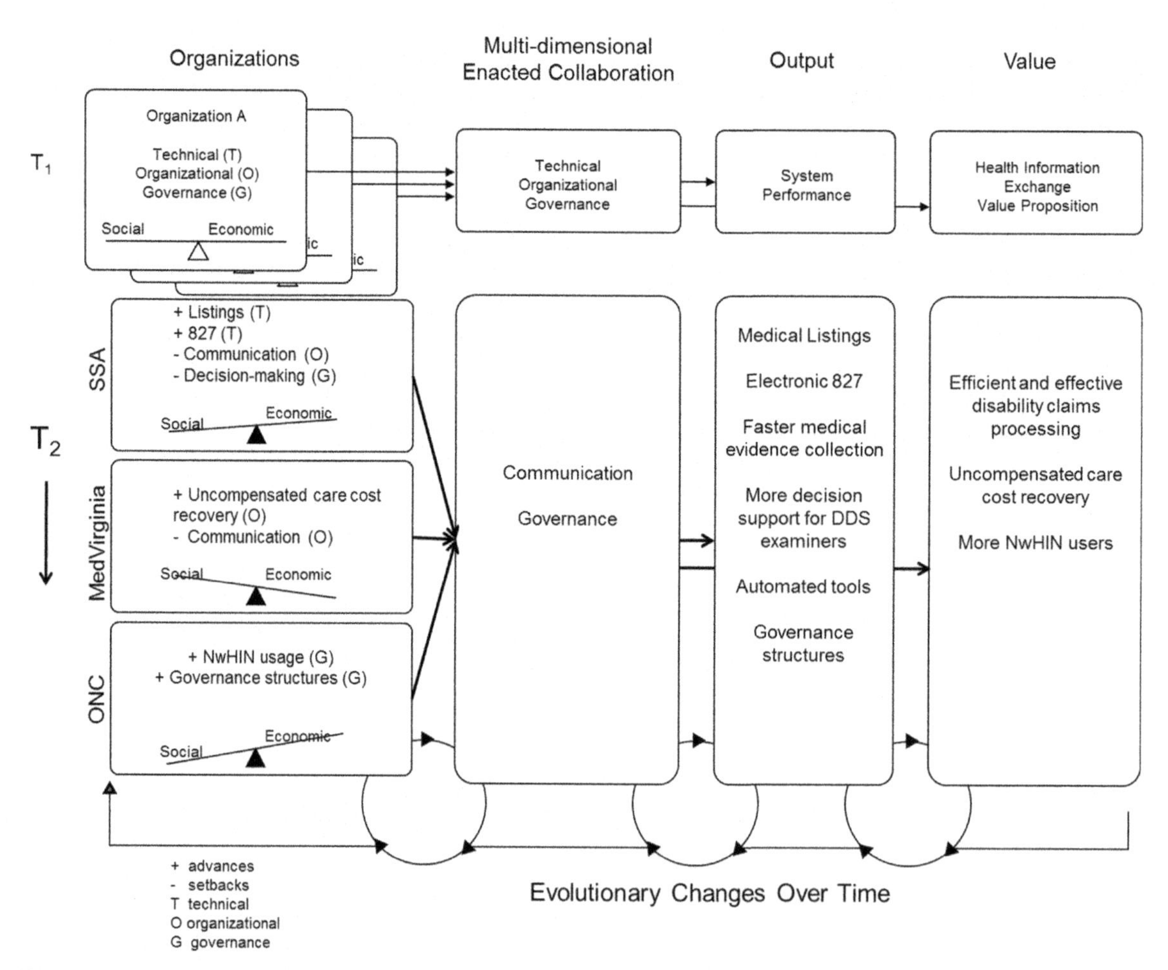

FIGURE 26.4 Blended Value Collaboration Enactment Framework as applied to this case study.

business rules were established within MEGAHIT. Increasing listings provide earlier disability determination on more conditions. This increase enables MEGAHIT to provide preliminary analysis on more conditions and represents SSA's ability to save overall case processing time and make faster disability determinations, thereby getting benefits to claimants sooner.

Findings regarding case processing time suggest that there was a 33% reduction in how long it took to process cases. Faster processing can potentially provide faster benefit payments and increased access to care for the claimant and affect the provider's "bottom line" in terms of uncompensated care cost recovery. This is an example of a social-economic blended value proposition in which SSA gets benefits to claimants faster (social) and the provider gets paid faster (economic). Findings also support the view that Form 827 has been a bit of a conundrum, both as a faxed document in early prototype phases and, later, while trying to find a standard to accommodate "at will" viewing by the provider. The move toward an electronic Form 827 represents great progress.

As discussed by interviewees within and outside of SSA, the main contributor to setbacks (indicated in Fig. 26.4 by −) was communication issues related to multiple changes in Program Directors, staff, and positioning of the program within SSA; these issues stalled decision making. The presentation of a blended value proposition in this area is interesting, as the time delays may have different economic impacts on the public agency and the private agency. While MedVirginia experienced some frustrations, they stayed motivated by continuing similar work with VA and DoD, knowing that time invested with those two agencies held economic value. These results are consistent with the literature, which suggests that a public agency may be satisfied with the social value proposition, but a private organization must find a business value, as measured by economic impact, to support the organization's social mission [16,47,48,66].

26.4.6 MedVirginia

MedVirginia, as an HIE network, provides another lens through which to evaluate HIE. The current situation is that health information organizations (as entities) and HIE (as an activity) are government incentivized (through ARRA funding). Thus HIE networks must struggle to find a sustainable model with the appropriate blend of economic support and governance structure [25,44,67]. Survival is associated with HIE networks that respond to changes brought about by evolving *technical, organizational,* and *governance* dimensions [16]. This collaboration between SSA, MedVirginia, and ONC involved many changes within the three dimensions, requiring that MedVirginia be responsive without being reactive. Most notable, among the changes, were the communication delays reported due to reorganization within SSA. As noted in the literature, communication is critical throughout all phases of a collaboration [68]. Likewise, consistent with the TEF, the output is less about the technology and more about *how* the technology was enacted [17].

While respondents at MedVirginia did not feel that the communication delays due to reorganization within SSA affected the technical processes of the collaboration, they said it did influence their ability to *execute* the technology. The findings show that, early in MedVirginia's collaboration with SSA and ONC, MedVirginia was very heavily motivated by intangible assets such as seeing if the technology to use MEGAHIT *could* work and being the first in the nation to use it. However, as time went on, MedVirginia needed to tip the scales more toward the economic end. Economic considerations for MedVirginia lie in why a provider should subscribe to them as an HIE—their value lies in being able to respond to MEGAHIT queries (for which they are paid $15 each), potentially getting the claimant benefits sooner, and potentially increasing uncompensated care cost recovery to the subscriber, in this case Bon Secours. Across the four Bon Secours facilities participating in this case study, and over the one-year period of time, Bon Secours realized 1.9 million USD in uncompensated care cost recovery. For MedVirginia to keep evolving as an organization directed toward remaining a sustainable HIE, they will have to create and maintain a balanced value proposition. More recent unpublished studies on uncompensated care cost recovery and/or cost avoidance for adult and pediatric participants with SSA suggest annual amounts in excess of 3.0 million USD.

26.4.7 ONC

This study was conducted within a larger and changing national Health IT context in which governance structures related to eHE were evolving. The information in this study provides a better understanding of the evolving governance structures for broader uses of eHE as a transmission vehicle for HIE. The main benefit for ONC resulting from the efforts between SSA and MedVirginia was usage of the eHE. Prior to this collaborative effort, the NwHIN was in a test environment with only theoretical uses. SSA and MedVirginia put the NwHIN into production; SSA continues to drive value in eHE participation for organizations and regional and statewide HIEs. As mentioned earlier, eHE has been privatized and is now operated as a separate entity.

26.4.8 The Sequoia Project/eHE—an update

In 2017 a study was conducted of eHE for the Sequoia Project to understand the sustained value in using MEGAHIT. Twenty-one semistructured interviews were conducted across 10 organizations (hospital systems, statewide HIEs, regional HIEs, vendors, and the federal government). Using a grounded theory approach five main categories and 16 subcategories emerged around value (see Table 26.1).

Interviewees agree the benefits/value and strengths of eHE are:

- a solid proven governance model;
- DURSA, which near eliminates the need for point-to-point legal agreements;
- mature capabilities, processes, operations, testing, and knowledge base,
- connection with federal partners (SSA, VHA, DoD);
- strong vendor partnerships for efficient onboarding; and
- relatively negligible maintenance costs.

Interviewees agree that areas for growth for eHE are the need to address:

- interoperability advancement,
- standards clarity,
- patient matching, and
- provider directory.

Eight core contributors to eHealth Exchange becoming a standard of care are:

- increased usage;
- increased marketing;
- solidifying sustainability;
- ability to get accurate, current, and needed data;
- provider directory;
- increase statewide HIE connectivity;
- organizational leadership commitments; and
- consistent and clear standards.

This study identified three core current perceived value propositions and five potential perceived value propositions—what interviewees expect will happen as eHE evolves and has more participants (see Table 26.2).

Currently, eHE, as a national health information network, has expanded its reach by

TABLE 26.1 Categories and subcategories of value associated with participation in the eHealth Exchange, grouped by category.

Category	Subcategory
eHealth Exchange concerns	Interoperability
	Level of implementation
	Increase statewide health information exchange to eHealth Exchange connectivity
Governance	DURSA
Technical	Technical standards
	Patient matching
	Data usability
	Data integrity
Usage	Increase eHealth Exchange usage
	Who is using eHealth Exchange
	Actual eHealth Exchange usage time
	Number of records exchanged using eHealth Exchange
Value proposition	Value in better care
	Value in avoiding duplication
	Value in lowering costs
	Intangible value

TABLE 26.2 Value propositions of using MEGAHIT for disability determination.

Current perceived value propositions	Potential perceived value propositions
• SSA disability determination (revenue and uncompensated care cost recovery)—this is the only value proposition to have been quantified • Ease with which records are retrieved • Reduction of administrative burden for staff needing to request records	• Statewide HIE connectivity • Avoiding test duplication • Better care • Ability to get accurate, current, and needed data • Decreased costs

HIE, Health information exchange; *MEGAHIT*, Medical Evidence Gathering and Analysis through Health IT; *SSA*, Social Security Administration.

providing connectivity to over 4000 short-term care acute care hospitals nationwide, 4 federal agencies, 61 state and regional HIEs. They currently exchange over 12 billion transactions annually in all 50 states. They supplement their ability to exchange data using Integrating the Healthcare Enterprise technical specifications to also exchange via Fast Healthcare Interoperability Resources. They also require participants to prove the data provided is truly interoperable.

26.5 Summary

The literature is clear about the need to align medical evidence development practices with current technology and the potential benefits thereof [20,59,60,62,65]. Less clear, however, is the value proposition for collaborating organizations to engage in information sharing for secondary purposes, such as disability determination. This study examined three organizations—SSA, MedVirginia, and ONC—to gain insights into the multiple dimensions (technical, organizational, and governance) of the collaboration and the associated evolving value propositions. The SSA MEGAHIT program also provided a context within which to examine the key elements of *how* the collaboration was enacted over a period of time, using the Blended Value Collaboration Enactment Framework.

The findings and the literature suggest that value may be located in different places for different organizations and at different times in their lifecycles. For example, uncompensated care cost recovery is of great interest to care providers, but not for medical records clearinghouses whose only focus is getting the record from point A to point B and being paid for that transmission. Thus, for clearinghouses, value may be located solely in the organizational dimension (human resource and/or capital equipment outlay, etc.). As more diverse organizations exchange clinical information across the eHE, with SSA or other federal agencies, alternative value streams are likely to emerge.

This case study examined uncompensated care cost recovery as a use case for the value proposition of HIE, within the context of SSA disability determination. Fig. 26.5 summarizes key findings related to this context [69]. The Blended Value Collaboration Enactment Framework was used to understand the collaboration between three organizations—SSA, MedVirginia, and ONC – and to gain insight into the factors influencing their collaboration and the associated value propositions.

Questions for discussion

1. Describe the short- and long-term benefits and consequences of Medicaid expansion related to uncompensated care cost recovery.
2. Describe other secondary uses of clinical data.
3. Describe how HIE could facilitate the exchange of clinical data for other secondary

- Reduced case processing times leading to faster benefit determination
  - 32% time savings
  - 50 days saved per disability applicant
- Faster favorable benefit determination
  - 33% time savings
  - 52 days saved per disability applicant
- Changing value propositions over time
  - Original value proposition socially motivated
  - Value proposition eventually stronger toward economic motivations for two organizations (SSA and MedVirginia)
- Uncompensated care cost recovery resulting from faster favorable determination
  - $1.9 million over 12 months

FIGURE 26.5 Summary of case study findings. Source: *Modified from Feldman SS, Horan TA, Drew D. Understanding the value proposition of health information exchange: the case of uncompensated care cost recovery. Health Syst 2012;3:134–46.*

uses (consider other state, federal, or international uses such as a State Department of Health, the Federal Aviation Administration or the World Health Organization). In your description, map out social versus economic drivers for participation and governance structures needed to facilitate streamlined information exchange.

4. In developing and implementing HIE, healthcare entities learned from the banking and transportation industries. Describe potential outcomes from health care that other industries might implement.

Acknowledgments

Fig. 26.1 was first published in the *Journal of Medical Internet Research* [5]. The figure is open-access distributed under the terms of the Creative Commons Attribution License (http://creativecommons.org/licenses/by/2.0/), which permits unrestricted use, distribution, and reproduction in any medium, provided the original work is properly cited with original URL and bibliographic citation information.

References

[1] Whitworth B, Ahmad A. Socio-technical system design. In: The encyclopedia of human-computer interaction, 2nd ed. Interaction Design Foundation; 2013.

[2] Emerson J. The blended value proposition: integrating social and financial returns. Calif Manag Rev 2003;45 (4):35–51.

[3] Whitworth B. The social requirements of technical systems. Handbook of research on socio-technical design and social networking systems. IGI Global; 2009. p. 3.

[4] Unertl K, Johnson K, Gadd C, Lrenzi N. Bridging organizational divides in healthcare: an ecological view of health information exchange. JMIR Med Inform 2013;1(1):e3.

[5] Feldman SS, Schooley BL, Bhavsar GP. Health information exchange implementation: lessons learned and critical success factors from a case study. JMIR Med Inform 2014;2(2):e19.

[6] Cash JI, Konsynski BR. IS redraws competitive boundaries. Harv Bus Rev 1985;63(2):134–42.

[7] Williams CB, Fedorowicz J, editors. A framework for analyzing cross-boundary e-government projects: the CapWin example. In: Proceedings of the 2005 national conference on digital government research. Digital Government Society of North America; 2005.

[8] Benjamin R, Wigand R. Electronic markets and virtual value chains on the information superhighway. Sloan Management Review (Winter, 1995). 1995.

[9] Riggins FJ, Mukhopadhyay T. Interdependent benefits from interorganizational systems: opportunities for business partner reengineering. J Manag Inf Syst 1994;37–57.

[10] Levine S, White PE. Exchange as a conceptual framework for the study of interorganizational relationships. Adm Sci Q 1961;583–601.

[11] Blau PM. Power and exchange in social life. New York: John Wiley & Sons; 1964.

[12] Wright DS. Federalism, intergovernmental relations, and intergovernmental management: Historical reflections and conceptual comparisons. Public Adm Rev 1990;168–78.

[13] Markus ML. Power, politics, and MIS implementation. Commun ACM 1983;26:14.

[14] Geels FW. From sectoral systems of innovation to socio-technical systems Insights about dynamics and change from sociology and institutional theory. Res Policy 2004;33(6–7):897–920.

[15] Schooley B, Horan T. End-to-end enterprise performance management in the public sector through interorganizational information integration. Gov Inf Q 2007;24(4):755–84.

[16] Kern LM, Barron Y, Abramson EL, Patel V, Kaushal R. HEAL NY: promoting interoperable health information technology in New York state. Health Aff 2009;28 (2):493–504 PMID: ISI:000264445100025.

[17] Fountain JE. Building the virtual state: information technology and institutional change. Washington, DC: Brookings Institute Press; 2001.

[18] Phillips N, Lawrence TB, Hardy C. Interorganizational collaboration and the dynamics of institutional fields. J Manag Stud 2000;37(1):23–43.

[19] Mintzberg H, Jorgensen J, Dougherty D, Westley F. Some surprising things about collaboration – knowing how people connect makes it work better. Organ Dyn 1996;25(1):60–71.

[20] Feldman SS, Horan TA. The dynamics of information collaboration: a case study of blended IT value propositions for health information exchange in disability determination. J Assoc Inf Syst 2011;12(2):1 PMCID: PMC4288070.

[21] Cohen B, Greenfield J, Maran M. Ben & Jerry's double-dip: how to run a values-led business and make money, too: Fireside; 1998.

[22] Sen AK. Rational fools: a critique of the behavioral foundations of economic theory. Philos Public Aff 1977;317–44.

[23] Alter C, Hage J. Organizations working together. Newbury Park, CA: Sage Publications;; 1992.
[24] Arthur W. The nature of technology: what it is and how it evolves. New York: Free Press; 2009.
[25] Miller RH, Miller BS. The Santa Barbara County Care Data Exchange: what happened? Health Aff 2007;26 (5):568–80.
[26] Porter M, Teisberg E. Redefining health care: creating value-based competition on results. Boston: Harvard Business School Publishing;; 2006. p. 506.
[27] Mody A. Infrastructure delivery: private initiative and the public good. World Bank Publications; 1996.
[28] Collum TH, Menachemi N, Sen B. Does electronic health record use improve hospital financial performance? Evidence from panel data. Health Care Manag Rev 2016;41(3):267–74.
[29] Jang Y, Lortie MA, Sanche S. Return on investment in electronic health records in primary care practices: a mixed-methods study. JMIR Med Inform 2014;2(2):e25 PMID: 25600508.
[30] Ramaswamy V, Gouillart R. Building the co-creative enterprise. Harv Bus Rev 2010;(October):100–9.
[31] Flint DJ, Golicic SL. Searching for competitive advantage through sustainability: a qualitative study in the New Zealand wine industry. Int J Phys Distrib Logist Manag 2009;39(10):841–60 PMID: 47117776.
[32] Aldrich H. Organizations and environments. Palo Alto, CA: Stanford Business Books;; 2007.
[33] Brynjolfsson E, Saunders A. Wired for innovation. Cambridge: MIT Press; 2010.
[34] Delone WH, McLean ER. The DeLone and McLean model of information systems success: a ten-year update. J Manag Inf Syst 2003;19(4):9–30.
[35] Riskin L, Koppel R, Riskin D. Re-examining health IT policy: what will it take to derive value from our investment? J Am Med Inform Assoc 2015;22 (2):459–64 PMCID: 25326600.
[36] Malepati S, Kushner K, Lee JS. RHIOs and the value proposition: value is in the eye of the beholder. J AHIMA 2007;78(3):24–9.
[37] Schooley BL, Horan TA. Towards end-to-end government performance management: case study of interorganizational information integration in emergency medical services (EMS). Gov Inf Q 2007;24(4):755–84.
[38] Hepp Z, Forrester SH, Roth J, Wirtz HS, Devine EB. Cost-effectiveness of a computerized provider order entry system in improving medication safety: a case study in ambulatory care. Value Health 2013;16(3):A205–6.
[39] Adler-Milstein J, Everson J, Lee SYD. EHR adoption and hospital performance: time-related effects. Health Serv Res 2015;50(6):1751–71.
[40] Peterson LT, Ford EW, Eberhardt J, Huerta TR, Menachemi N. Assessing differences between physicians' realized and anticipated gains from electronic health record adoption. J Med Syst 2011;35 (2):151–61 PMID: 20703574. Epub 2010/08/13.
[41] Nguyen OT, Shah S, Gartland AJ, Parekh A, Turner K, Feldman SS, et al. Factors associated with nurse well-being in relation to electronic health record use: a systematic review. J Am Med Inform Assoc 2021;28(6):1288–97.
[42] Sullivan H, Skelcher C. Working across boundaries: collaboration in public services. Baskingstoke: Palgrave Macmillan; 2002. p. 271.
[43] Greenwald HP. Health for all [electronic resource]: making community collaboration workIn: Beery W, Greenwald H, editors. Chicago: Health Administration Press; 2002.
[44] Ruaber C. CalRHIO closes, but board to help state on IT. 2010 [cited 2010 Jan 15]. Available from: <http://sanfrancisco.bizjournals.com/sanfrancisco/stories/2010/01/11/story7.html>.
[45] Bloomrosen M, Detmer D. Advancing the framework: use of health data—a report of a working conference of the American Medical Informatics Association. J Am Med Inform Assoc 2008;15(6):715.
[46] eHealth Initiative. National progress report on e-Health 2010. 2010. Available from: <http://www.ehealthinitiative.org/sites/default/files/file/National%20Progess%20Report%20on%20eHealth%202010.pdf>.
[47] Adler-Milstein J, McAfee AP, Bates DW, Jha AK. The state of regional health information organizations: current activities and financing. Health Aff 2008;27(1): W60–9 PMID: ISI: 000257188400055.
[48] Kohli R, Grover V. Business value of IT: an essay on expanding research directions to keep up with the times. J Assoc Inf Syst 2008;9(1):23–39 PMID: ISI: 000255118300002.
[49] Walker J, Pan E, Johnston D, Adler-Milstein J, Bates DW, Middleton B. The value of health care information exchange and interoperability. Health Aff 2005;19 W5-10–W5-18.
[50] Vargo S, Maglio P, Akaka M. On value and value co-creation: a service systems and service logic perspective. Eur Manag J 2008;26(3):145–52.
[51] Rosenfeld S, Koss S. Evolution of state health information exchange – a study of vision, strategy, and progress. Rockville, MD: Agency for Healthcare Research & Quality; 2006.
[52] Weick K. Small wins. Redefining the scale of social problems. 1986:29.
[53] Robey D, Im G, Wareham JD. Theoretical foundations of empirical research on interorganizational systems: assessing past contributions and guiding future directions. J Assoc Inf Syst 2008;9(9):497–518 PMID: ISI:000261357800001.
[54] US Department of Health & Human Services. Nationwide Health Information Network (NwHIN).

2013 [cited 2013 Feb 21]. Available from: <http://www.healthit.gov/policy-researchers-implementers/nationwide-health-information-network-nwhin>.

[55] Gravely SD, Whaley ES. The next step in health data exchanges: trust and privacy in exchange networks. J Healthc Inf Manag Spring 2009;23(2):33–7 PMID: 19382738. Epub 2009/04/23.

[56] Rishel W, Riehl V, Blanton C. Summary of the NHIN prototype architecture contracts. Washington, DC: U. S. Department of Health and Human Services; 2007.

[57] Social Security Administration. Nationwide Health Information Network Forum. Washington DC. December 15–16, 2008.

[58] Feldman SS, Horan TA. Innovations and perspectives for streamlining disability determinations. 2009.

[59] Tulu B, Daniels SM, Feldman SS, Horan TA, editors. Role of health information technology (HIT) in disability determinations: when medical records become medical evidence. Washington DC: American Medical Informatics Association; 2008.

[60] United States Government Accountability Office (GAO). Social Security Disability: collection of medical evidence could be improved with evaluations to identify promising collection practices. In: Subcommittee on Social Security, Committee on Ways and Means, editors. Washington DC: GAO; 2008.

[61] Morse S. Uncompensated care costs shrink under Obamacare, especially in Medicaid expansion states. 2015 [cited 2015 Apr 20]. Available from: <http://www.webcitation.org/6ZjOg1iGe>.

[62] Feldman SS, Horan TA. Collaboration in electronic medical evidence development: a case study of the Social Security Administration's MEGAHIT System. Int J Med Inform 2011;80:e127–40.

[63] Shah D, Schwartz HA, Hovy D. Predictive biases in natural language processing models: a conceptual framework and overview. arXiv preprint arXiv:191211078. 2019.

[64] Bender EM, Friedman B. Data statements for natural language processing: toward mitigating system bias and enabling better science. Trans Assoc Comput Linguist 2018;6:587–604.

[65] Newman-Griffis DR. Capturing domain semantics with representation learning: applications to health and function. The Ohio State University; 2020.

[66] Chaudhry B, Wang J, Wu S, Maglione M, Mojica W, Roth E. Systematic review: impact of health information technology on quality, efficiency, and costs of medical care. Ann Intern Med 2006;144(10):E12–22.

[67] >Frohlich J. In Search of ... Health Information Exchange. 2010 [2010 July 30]. Available from: <http://www.ihealthbeat.org/perspectives/2010/in-search-of-health-information-exchange.aspx>.

[68] Fountain JE. Central issues in the political development of the virtual state. In: The network society: from knowledge to policy. 2006. p. 149.

[69] Feldman SS, Horan TA, Drew D. Understanding the value proposition of health information exchange: the case of uncompensated care cost recovery. Health Syst 2013;2:134–46.

CHAPTER

27

Health information exchange—enhanced care coordination: implementation and evaluation of event notification services in the Veterans Health Administration

Brian E. Dixon[1,2,3], *Kenneth S. Boockvar*[4,5] *and Emily Franzosa*[4,5]

[1]Department of Veterans Affairs, Health Services Research & Development Service, Center for Health Information and Communication, Indianapolis, IN, USA [2]Department of Epidemiology, Richard M. Fairbanks School of Public Health, Indiana University, Indianapolis, IN, USA [3]Center for Biomedical Informatics, Regenstrief Institute, Inc., Indianapolis, IN, USA [4]Department of Veterans Affairs, James J. Peters VA Medical Center, Bronx, NY, USA [5]Icahn School of Medicine at Mount Sinai, New York, NY, USA

Major themes

This case study highlights the following themes relevant to health information exchange (HIE):

- Use of HIE by providers to access data across fragmented systems for a specific clinical purpose.
- Event notification services (ENS), an example of a service offered by an HIE network.
- How policy drives the adoption of HIE services like ENS.
- The difference between passive and active HIE services.
- Value of HIE services, specifically the role of ENS in supporting care coordination activities within a health system.
- Barriers to the use of HIE services in clinical workflow and system capacity issues that affect the adoption and use of HIE services.

27.1 Introduction

Coordinating care as patients traverse fragmented health systems remains a significant challenge globally. Many health systems expect primary care providers to synthesize information across the various episodes of care for an

Health Information Exchange
DOI: https://doi.org/10.1016/B978-0-323-90802-3.00021-6

individual patient and coordinate the care delivered to that patient by specialists and other providers. Yet, many patients find it confusing and frustrating that their primary care providers often cannot access the data and information generated by their other doctors, especially when patients end up in the hospital.

In this case study, we explore the use of HIE to support coordination of care as patients received care both within and external to the Veterans Health Administration (VHA), a national system of care delivery funded and managed by the US Department of Veterans Affairs (VA). The case focuses on a specific HIE service that is increasingly used across the United States and other parts of the world to facilitate timely exchange of data and information as patients experience an acute transfer of care, such as an elderly patient discharged from the hospital to their home.

27.2 Background

Health systems around the world are fragmented, requiring patients to navigate a disjointed landscape of providers from which they receive treatment, across multiple insurance networks and health systems. Patients commonly interact with primary care (general practitioners or GPs), specialty care, and hospital-based physicians. In addition, patients interact with multiple nonphysician providers when seeking health and wellness services, including pharmacists, chiropractors, traditional healers (see Chapter 30), occupational therapists, and behavioral therapists. Yet these providers may not share data or information with one another about the patient as each one encounters the patient independently. Moreover, patients must navigate complex health care delivery systems and payers (e.g., insurance plans), especially in the United States and Israel (see Chapter 31), that do not necessarily communicate information with one another.

Fragmentation of care is trending upward. A recent analysis using insurance claims find that older Americans increasingly see more specialists each year, often without coordination from a GP. The cross-sectional study of fee-for-service Medicare beneficiaries (individuals ≥ 65 years) in the United States from 2000 to 2019 found that the number of individuals seeing five or more physicians annually increased from 17.5% to 30.1% [1]. That equates to roughly 1-in-3 older Americans visiting at least five different physicians each year.

Fragmentation is driven by multiple factors. A qualitative study in the United States identified 41 distinct causes of fragmentation [2]. Themes from interviews with patients and providers revealed patient, provider, organizational, and socio-political reasons why patients must see multiple providers, most of which are unrelated to patients' medical needs. For example, patient-level causes included a preference of provider for the convenience of particular locations, availability of appointments, or desire for a second opinion. Provider-level reasons included the amount of time needed to educate a patient versus referring them to a specialist and increasing subspecialization in medicine. Causes at the organizational level included discharge processes that encourage follow-up with various specialists and lack of capacity that results in limited availability when patients call for services. At the socio-political level, participants discussed lack of transparency in costs and benefits that allow for specialist visits without referrals. Some of these reasons are interrelated, but all of them lead to patients receiving care from multiple providers across insurance networks and health systems.

Delivering high quality, coordinated care across fragmented delivery systems requires that clinicians access, manage, and share information efficiently. Retrieving, managing, and sharing health information in the conduct of care coordination, however, remains challenging in most nations.

In a study of internal medical residents, researchers observed providers spending between 5% and 9% of their time looking for information on a patient [3]. During our interviews with primary care providers, one doctor noted that asking patients about care received from other doctors "could take a third of my appointment if somebody is seeing five or six outside docs" [4].

In a care coordination survey of US patients, 27% of respondents reported that their test results were not available or that duplicate tests were ordered during a medical appointment; and 17% reported that information was not shared among their multiple care providers [5]. Similar gaps in care coordination were observed in Canada, Australia, France, the Netherlands, and Norway [5].

Additional evidence from a global systematic review of 33 studies in 14 nations confirms that primary care providers often perceive care delivery to be disjointed, with little flow of information or continuity of care between settings [6]. Coordination is especially important for older adults who experience greater medical comorbidities and disproportionate rates of postoperative morbidity and mortality [7,8].

The VHA is a unique context in which to examine HIE-enabled care coordination, because it is, by design, an integrated delivery network. Integrated networks are designed to address the problems caused by fragmentation of care. Yet, Veterans are increasingly seeking care outside the VHA (due to wait times/need for specialty care/other insurance coverage/), prompting the need for better care coordination as fragmentation increases.

27.3 Event notification

A basic form of HIE, which allows clinicians to query past medical history information for a given patient, can help address the gap in knowledge about what care was provided previously. This form of HIE is important in many contexts, such as an emergency room where a patient may present while unconscious or with limited capacity to recall prior medical care. In other contexts, it is more helpful for the HIE infrastructure to provide some intelligence, recognizing that something has changed about the patient and notifying the patient's primary care provider about their change in health status.

When we asked primary care providers who practice within the VHA about how they learn about their patients' recent acute care events (e.g., emergency room visits, hospitalizations), clinicians (doctors and nurses) generally reported they find out about the occurrence of these events from their patients at their next regularly scheduled appointment. For some patients, this could be weeks or months after their discharge from the hospital or emergency room. As one provider put it, "sometimes I operate a bit in the dark" with respect to previous care received by her patients [4]. Moreover, patient recall is not always precise. One physician relayed that the patient will "say [the visit was] a few weeks ago, but it was, like, two months ago" [4].

Clinicians desire health information technology, especially HIE services, to deliver timely notifications of events relevant to their patients and upon which providers can take appropriate action. Instead of waiting for patients to show up and share details about a hospitalization that occurred six months ago, primary care providers would like to learn about the event shortly after the discharge. The information could then be used to spur action by the provider, such as scheduling a follow-up appointment or coordinating the care of the patient once they are home (e.g., provision of home care services, scheduling rehabilitation services).

ENS, also known as Admission, Discharge, Transfer (ADT) alerting or simply "ADT alerts," is an HIE service that involves the electronic reporting (or pushing) of information pertaining to a clinical event from one provider to another facilitated by a messaging standard. Notification usually pertains to acute care events (e.g., hospitalization, emergency care), and the notifications are typically sent to primary care providers responsible for coordination of care [9].

Recent systematic reviews of HIE do not include any studies on ENS [10,11]. Prior to the work described in this case study, there was just one quantitative study of event notifications sent to ambulatory providers for acute care events over a 3.5 year period using a regional HIE network [12]. That study found a statistically significant 2.9% reduction in 30-day readmissions observed during the intervention period. While the study results are promising, the evidence from this study represents a single before-after cohort study. Therefore our team pursued the implementation and evaluation of ENS within the VHA to generate additional evidence on its effectiveness and usefulness.

27.4 Context

This case study is based on the experiences of implementing ENS as a component of a cluster randomized trial conducted within the VHA system, specifically in two medical centers located in Indianapolis, Indiana, and the Bronx, New York City, New York. The full study protocol is published online [13]. The study was reviewed and approved by the Institutional Review Board of Indiana University as well as the VA Research & Development Committee at both the Indianapolis VA Medical Center and the Bronx VA Medical Center.

The VHA is the largest integrated health care system in the United States, providing care to 9 million enrolled veterans at 1293 health care facilities annually [14]. This includes 171 medical centers and 1112 outpatient sites of varying complexity. VHA primary care operates along a patient-centered medical home model engaging multidisciplinary patient-aligned care teams (PACT) [15]. Still, many VHA-enrolled veterans seek care outside the system [16].

VHA is under increasing pressure to expand access to community providers, and the recently enacted CHOICE and MISSION legislation from the US Congress aim to increase access to out-of-network services for veterans [17–20]. Since the 2015 passage of the CHOICE Act, VHA has authorized 6 million non-VHA visits for nearly 2.4 million unique veterans [19]. Approximately one in six veterans utilize non-VA providers for an acute care event each year, and research suggests this number is higher for veterans over age 65 [21,22].

27.4.1 Overview of the two Veterans Health Administration medical centers

The first medical center is the James J. Peters VA Medical Center (JJP VAMC) located in the Bronx, New York. The JJP VAMC cares for more than 26,000 patients annually via a tertiary care facility providing comprehensive inpatient as well as outpatient care services in addition to four community-based outpatient clinics. The second medical center is the Richard L. Roudebush VA Medical Center (RLR VAMC) located in Indianapolis, Indiana. The RLR VAMC serves more than 62,000 patients annually and consists of a tertiary care facility providing comprehensive inpatient as well as outpatient care services in addition to three community-based outpatient clinics. Both medical centers also serve as teaching hospitals and regional referral sites.

27.4.2 Health information exchange in the Veterans Health Administration

HIE exists in multiple forms within the VHA. Over time, the VHA has developed, implemented, and expanded its HIE capabilities to facilitate clinician access to patient information in coordination with its partners. Effectively VHA HIE operations are like an onion as depicted in Fig. 27.1. Each layer of the onion expands access to medical information for front line clinicians. These layers were developed and implemented over time as technology and policy evolved to enable HIE beyond the VHA.

As depicted in Fig. 27.1, the core information system for the VHA is its EHR system, referred to as Computerized Patient Record System (CPRS). Although all VHA facilities use the common CPRS framework, each facility has a separate instance of the CPRS that allows for local customization and configuration to allow flexibility in the EHR across sites. At the time of writing, the VHA is in the process of migrating its enterprise EHR system to the Cerner Millennium platform [23].

For over 30 years, the VHA has operated an enterprise HIE network (called VistA) in which Veterans' medical records from any VHA facility could be accessed by other VHA facilities [24]. The VHA called its point of care application VistAWeb, which enabled clinicians to look up medical records from other VHA facilities including images [25]. Each night, a common dataset from local CPRS instances is extracted and loaded into central VHA systems. The VistAWeb application retrieves data from the centralized VHA information systems.

Over the past two decades, the VHA has worked with the US Department of Defense (DoD) to exchange medical records for individuals as they are discharged from active duty and transition to care within the VHA system. This facilitates better coordination of care for recently discharged service members as well as their families. Since September 2014, the VHA has used the Joint Legacy Viewer (JLV) as a

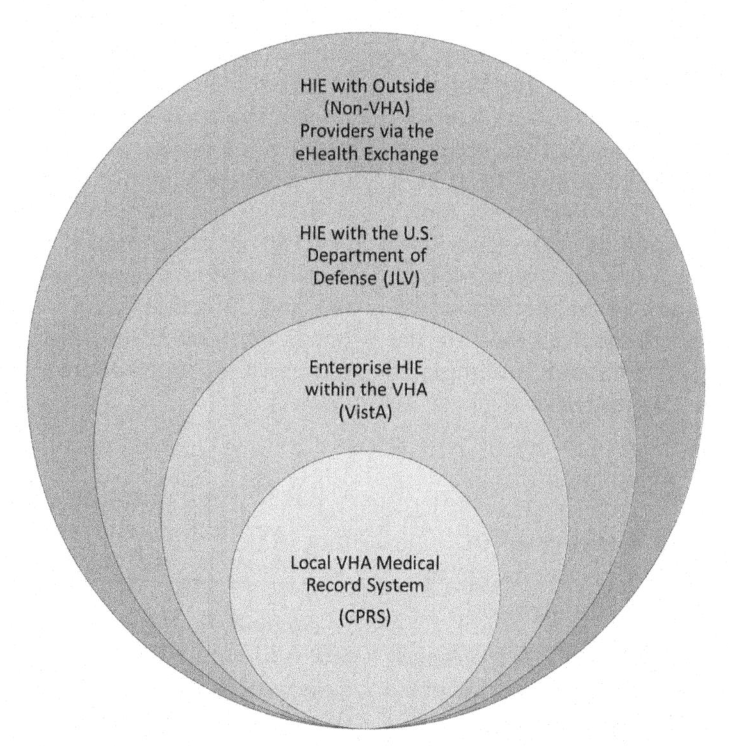

FIGURE 27.1 Venn diagram that peels back the various layers of the Veterans Health Administration's (VHA) health information exchange onion. Providers in the VHA can access external records from a variety of sources.

web-based graphical user interface to view health data from DoD [26]. Data are not transferred from DoD to VHA, but clinicians can access historical records, especially in preparation for the transition to primary care within the VHA system.

The JLV was further expanded beyond DoD to include non-VHA health facilities [26]. Development and implementation of the JLV as well as the backend systems that facilitate HIE within the VHA and across organizational boundaries with other health systems is part of a larger HIE effort referred to as Veterans Health Information Exchange (VHIE) [27]. As a part of VHIE, the JLV connects VHA information systems to the eHealth Exchange, a national network of health information organizations (HIOs; see Chapter 1) in the United States including other federal agencies [28]. By 2019 most VHA facilities could access records from other VHA facilities, the DoD, and eHealth Exchange participants (e.g., outside facilities, community partners) for the Veterans in care within the VHA system.

The VHIE program office further supports VA Direct Messaging, which allows VHA staff to securely send and receive Veterans' health information with community care providers who are a part of the DirectTrust Network [29]. This form of information exchange focuses on sending documents securely over the Internet using established standards, and it eliminates faxing, mailing, or hand-delivering health information.

27.4.3 Strengths and weaknesses of existing health information exchange in the Veterans Health Administration

As of 2022, clinicians in the VHA have multiple ways to access comprehensive information from outside non-VHA providers. They can access JLV to retrieve data from other VHA facilities, the DoD, and participants in the eHealth Exchange. They can also login to their VA Direct inbox to retrieve notes or documents directly sent from providers in the community.

While technically providers in the VHA can access a broad array of information relevant to their patients, the external data are not integrated into either the VHA or clinical workflows. Data exchanged between VHA and non-VHA providers (including the DoD) are not parsed or stored discretely within VHA information systems. Clinicians can retrieve and view the information, but the underlying data cannot be considered by VHA decision support rules, and the data cannot trigger any automated actions. Any action as a result of viewing the data is on the clinician—that is, changing a medication order, ordering a follow-up lab test, scheduling an appointment.

Clinicians typically view the data in the JLV and then go into another information system, such as CPRS, to initiate an action. This extra step requires additional time and mouse clicks for clinicians. It further requires copying and pasting information or transcription from JLV into another system. Moreover, accessing JLV and VA Direct requires clinicians to click out of CPRS or other applications. Active retrieval of information is performed by the providers, not the information system. So while functional, providers must exert extra effort to retrieve the information and then take action upon it.

27.5 Implementing event notification services in the Veterans Health Administration

Against the backdrop of multiple HIE layers and options within the VHA for accessing outside records, we sought to implement and evaluate ENS in support of care coordination for older Veterans (individuals aged ≥65 years). Our aim was to create information and workflows in which events outside the VHA would generate an alert to the patient's primary care team, notifying them of the acute care event. Our hope was that the alert would spur action by the team to initiate follow-up within the VHA. Timely follow-up following discharge can prevent rehospitalization or complications as many patients struggle once home with medication regimens, rehabilitation, etc. [30,31]. This is especially true for older adults.

Our implementation of ENS within the VHA is visualized in Fig. 27.2. Upon utilization of non-VHA acute care, such as an inpatient admission or emergency department (ED) visit, an HL7 ADT message was electronically sent from the non-VHA acute care facility to an HIE network. Each HIE network responded to the ADT message by notifying (or alerting) the VHA that an enrolled patient visited a non-VHA care facility.

For RLR VAMC, the HIE network transmitted the event notification to VA Direct Messaging. Study coordinators at RLR VAMC logged into VA Direct each day to retrieve the notifications. At JJP VAMC, each day study coordinators logged into the HIE network directly to retrieve new ENS notifications using the network's population health tools. These workflows were adapted to meet local VAMC needs as well as the technical infrastructure of each partner HIE network.

Study coordinators at the two VHA sites then created an internal electronic note within CPRS to the Veteran's primary care medical home team (referred to within the VA as a Patient-Aligned Care Team or PACT). This note, which becomes part of the Veteran's medical record, identifies the non-VHA care facility and provides information on the reason for the visit or chief complaint. It further provides details on the external provider and how

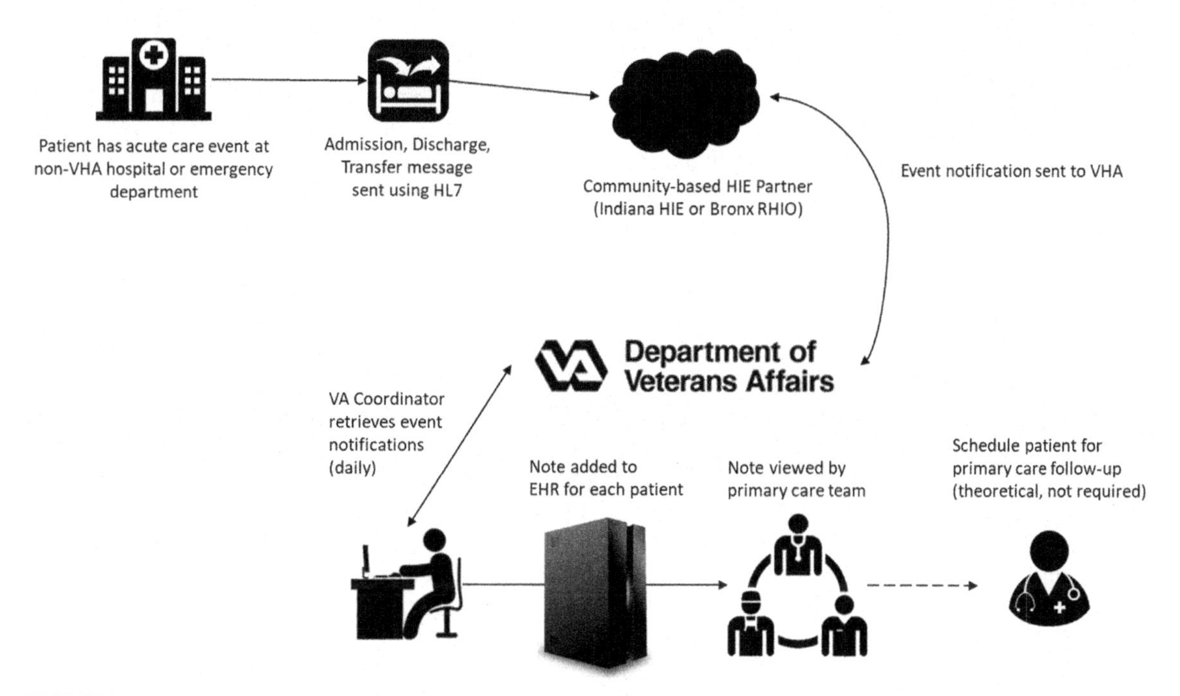

FIGURE 27.2 Architecture as well as information and workflows implemented to enable event notification services in the context of the Veterans Health Administration.

to contact them. Each note required acknowledgment by someone on the PACT team to signal it was read. The individual responsible for reading and acknowledging the note differed by PACT team. No notifications or notes were created for usual care arm patients.

27.5.1 Our community-based health information exchange partners

In New York, the JJP VAMC partnered with the Bronx Regional Health Information Organization (Bronx RHIO). The Bronx RHIO is a HIE that include hospitals, health systems, ambulatory care centers, individual physician offices, long-term care, and home care, as well as community and other organizations. Collectively, these providers deliver the vast majority of the health care received by the borough's 1.4 million residents, including almost all of the borough's annual hospital discharges, over 600,000 annual ED visits and 4.5 million annual ambulatory care visits. Providers at JJP VAMC have accessed the Bronx RHIO since 2008.

In Indianapolis, the RLR VAMC partnered with the Indiana Health Information Exchange (IHIE). IHIE is a community-based HIE network over 117 hospitals. IHIE captures data from >90% of hospitals in the geographic area served by the RLR VAMC. IHIE has exchanged data with the VA since 2011 when it began sending summary of care documents for Veterans enrolled in the Veterans Lifetime Electronic Record program [32], which is now VHIE [27]. Prior to our work, IHIE had joined the DirectTrust network and had experience using ADT alerts with payers in the Indianapolis market who sought to reduce ED utilization. More information on IHIE can be found in Chapter 22.

Implementation required around 9 months to complete. The implementation with JJP VAMC was shorter as the medical center staff already had logins to the population health tools at the Bronx RHIO prior to the study. In Indianapolis, a new contract between RLR VAMC and IHIE as well as data use agreement were required. The documentation and governance to enable HIE therefore required more time to establish.

27.6 Experiences and lessons learned

Alerts were sent from March 2016 until December 2019 for 202 older Veterans (33.4% of the enrolled 605 total study participants who received primary care across 52 distinct primary care teams) who experienced an acute care event (ED visit or hospitalization). In this section, we explore what we learned about the implementation of the ENS alerts in the VHA context.

27.6.1 Characteristics of Veterans with non-Veterans Health Administration care

First, approximately 1-in-3 older adult patients in the VHA received non-VHA care. Given that the VHA currently has over 9 million individuals who receive health care benefits, the VHA should expect to need outside medical records for up to 2–3 million individuals each year. This estimate is on par with previous studies that examined the overlap between VHA and the Medicare program in the United States. Calling, faxing, and waiting on outside records likely consumes significant human and material resources; therefore ENS services would likely significantly reduce administrative burden for VHA clinicians across the nation.

In a focused analysis on the characteristics of those Veterans who had a non-VHA acute care encounter, we found that individuals with higher income, access to private insurance, poorer self-perceived health, and self-reported regular use of a non-VHA provider were associated with a greater likelihood of generating an ENS alert [33]. We also found that older Veterans and those living in a rural area were more likely to generate an alert. Importantly, we found that an increased number of VHA ED visits in the year prior was associated with an increased risk of a non-VHA encounter in the current year. This might be explained by those who have greater real or perceived acute care needs having increased use of both VHA and non-VHA acute care settings.

Although it may seem counterintuitive, we did not find an association with an individual's chronic health status, meaning that individuals with higher numbers of comorbid conditions were not more likely to have acute care events outside the VHA. This finding was consistent with a prior study which found lower ED and hospital use among older adults with multiple chronic conditions seeing the same physicians over time [34].

27.6.2 Impact of event notification services alerts on timely follow-up

A key finding from our research is that when primary care teams are notified of out-of-network acute care episodes, they respond by initiating contact with the patient via phone or by scheduling an in-person visit. Specifically, we observed 2–4 times odds of follow-up by the primary care team for those Veterans with an ENS alert [35]. These findings support the theory that, given the ability of HIE to facilitate access to patient information after a transition of care, HIE can impact care coordination [36], specifically reintegration into primary care following an acute care episode. Our findings also align with quantitative survey research findings from Wiley et al. [37] which found that 53% of non-VHA providers who received ENS alerts reported them as helpful in facilitating "patients' transitions across different settings of care."

In interviews with providers, we found that primary care teams generally perceived alerts as helpful in improving practice operations, including timely follow-up. Several team members said alerts facilitated a "seamless flow" in transitioning from a hospital or ED visit to VHA follow-up care [4]. Physicians also found alerts helpful in guiding patient interviews, since they did not have to use valuable appointment time collecting this information. "They may have all these chronic illnesses, but they were admitted for something more acute," explained one Bronx physician. "So, I can get [the acute issue] out of the way right away, then deal with the others."

27.6.3 Impact of event notification services alerts on hospital usage

While promising, event notifications may not improve patient outcomes. We found that Veterans in the notification group did not have significantly fewer secondary hospitalizations or ED visits within 30 days after an index event. Around 20% of Veterans whose primary care teams received an ENS were hospitalized or had an ED encounter (all cause) within 30 days of discharge compared to 17% of the control group [35]. This difference was not statistically significant when we controlled for factors such as age, race/ethnicity, and Medicaid status at baseline.

Our findings contradict a prior study examining ENS [12], which observed a 2.9% reduction in 30-day readmissions. However, our results were similar to a longitudinal analysis of Medicare fee-for-service claims from a different New York HIE network found that directed HIE services like ENS are neither associated with a reduction in ambulatory care sensitive hospitalizations nor unplanned readmissions [38]. Similarly, a large Danish trial involving older adults (65 +) found that a single follow-up visit postdischarge was not associated with a reduction in all-cause or ambulatory sensitive condition readmissions

[39]. Therefore timely follow-up alone may not be sufficient to prevent readmissions.

These results may also be due to confounders in our trial as well as the prior research, such as how well event notifications were integrated into the clinical workflow, that necessitate further study to better understand when ENS might be useful to reduce secondary acute care utilization. In interviews with providers in our study, we found that many providers were unaware of the alerts or were unable to distinguish them from other messages they receive in the EHR system. For example, one provider said, "it does get a little confusing trying to sort them all out."

We should note that one-half to two-thirds of patients overall did not receive follow-up within 30 days, despite the statistically significant improvement with ENS. Limited overall follow-up by primary care potentially reduced the likelihood of ENS impacting readmissions. This underscores the importance of designing workflows that ensure follow-up after ENS by primary care team members. It further suggests that ENS alerts might need to target acute care encounters with higher likelihood of readmission (e.g., coronary artery disease, stroke, diabetic ketoacidosis). In our study, we included all acute care encounters regardless of their severity. There are other potential confounders, such as provider caseloads, presence (or absence) of caregivers, and patient characteristics not measured in this study that require further examination in future research.

27.6.4 Impact of event notification services alerts combined with a care transitions intervention

In order to test the effect of care coordination above and beyond the electronic ENS alerts on posthospital outcomes, we randomized VHA primary care teams such that in addition to the ENS alerts, some teams' patients also received a care transitions intervention (CTI) [13]. These patients were contacted directly by a trained VA social worker on the study team, who delivered an evidence-based CTI model.

The CTI was adapted from a model developed by Coleman [40,41] and focused on patient activation [42]. This meant the CTI centered on increasing patients' ability to manage their own care, as opposed to having a VHA care team member directly help fulfill patient needs. Thus the social worker did not normally intervene on behalf of patients or communicate with providers, instead providing support for patients and caregivers to intervene on the patients' own behalf—unless there was an urgent clinical need. The CTI was delivered via one home visit 2–3 days after discharge and three additional phone calls within 30 days.

After controlling for multiple factors (e.g., primary care team clustering, race), we observed no differences between those with ENS alerts only and those with ENS alerts plus the CTI with respect to 90-day hospital admission or readmission, ED use, primary care follow-up, patient postdischarge knowledge, or high-risk medication discrepancies [43]. These results suggest that the CTI did not have any added benefit and that the increases in timely follow-up were attributable only to the ENS alerts. The results are disappointing because, although the CTI increased patient activation metrics [42], the intervention did not translate into changes in patient outcomes. These results suggest that other interventions to impact health care utilization and medication discrepancies should be explored when older adults utilize acute care outside of their primary care system.

27.6.5 Barriers to using event notification services

Primary care team members identified several barriers to effectively using ENS, even though many perceived them to make workflow more efficient. The following barriers were identified: content, logging into the HIE network, and capacity.

27.6.5.1 Contents of the event notification services alert message

Several participants requested additional details in the messages they receive in the EHR system, such as a copy of the discharge summary or test results performed by the acute care provider. "It's good to know that [the patient was] on the outside," explained one physician. "But, I probably don't have enough information ... on how to act, or what action to take." Another MD agreed, noting that "I'm not always clear on what to do with that information. To me, it's more like I treat most of them unfortunately like an FYI." Several team members also noted that including a diagnosis code in the ENS alert would be helpful in determining the level of clinical severity and next steps. As one Indianapolis physician explained, "if they have reflux ... the clinical urgency is relatively low vs that they came in with heart failure and ended up in the ICU and really need some close follow up." Although the ADT notifications from the Indiana HIE were supposed to include diagnostic codes, some hospital information systems did not always contain them. Consistency and completeness of data would have enhanced the utility of the messages.

27.6.5.2 Logging into the health information exchange network

Providers also noted that the extra step of logging into JLV to view complete information on the acute care encounter could be a barrier and copying information from JLV into the patient's medical record could interrupt their workflow. As one MD in the Bronx noted, "it takes time to log in and cut and paste information [into the patients' medical chart]." In addition, some team members, particularly medical assistants, did not have access to the community-based HIE network and were dependent on the physician or RN to share information before they could follow up with patients. Some assistants noted this information was not shared with the team. These issues likely stem from governance rules, such as the type of staff that can access the HIE network. Furthermore, there can be issues within the VHA getting approval to access outside web-based information systems. For example, Indianapolis clinicians have not always been able to access the Indiana HIE directly. This change occurred recently, and it required special permission to allow the secure clinician portal used by IHIE to be accessed from the VHA network.

27.6.5.3 Capacity concerns around scaling event notification services

Indianapolis primary care teams had reservations about the capacity implications of ENS alerts if they were to be implemented for all Veterans. Some team members noted that a recent change in scheduling processes for primary care patients meant there might be limited appointments available for patients receiving non-VHA care. Expanding alerts to the larger patient panel was seen as potentially positive, but also an extra scheduling challenge. "My doc has 1,200 [patients] on her panel," explained one team member. "If you've got even 2 percent of that ... it can get overwhelming very easily."

27.6.6 Recommendations for future event notification services development and implementation

Based on feedback from providers in our study, Table 27.1 summarizes several recommendations for improving the design and delivery of ENS alerts to ensure they are noticed, helpful, and used. These suggestions were adapted from a similar table in Franzosa et al. [4].

TABLE 27.1 Perceived barriers to event notification services (ENS) alert adoption and recommendations for improvement.

Perceived barriers to ENS	Recommendations to improve ENS adoption and usage
Next steps not always clear	Add link to discharge summaries; follow-up instructions from doctor
Not always enough information to act on	Include diagnosis, discharge summaries, test results, medications prescribed
Alerts not always on time for follow-up	Include progress notes during hospitalization; send alerts before discharge
Multiple logins can be challenging	Single sign-on
Alerts can be lost in the shuffle; hard to prioritize; information not always shared with team	Use multiple channels (email, text); include multiple team members; grant health information exchange access to multiple team members
Providers unaware of alerts or unclear how to use them	Education and orientation; engage team members in development/ tailoring
Scheduling capacity concerns (Indianapolis)	Prioritize urgency of alerts by severity of diagnosis (e.g., reflux vs cardiac event)

Many participants suggested alerting additional team members beyond doctors and nurses. At the Bronx site, both the team physician and nurse received alerts, while Indianapolis alerts were directed to RNs. Most participants across roles agreed alerts should primarily go to the nurse, who was often responsible for patient follow-up. As an Indianapolis nurse explained, "the medical assistant doesn't really have any kind of medical knowledge ... a nurse needs to be able to [assess the urgency] and then the docs have so much to do that they're going to ... punt it to the nurse anyway." Medical assistants, however, suggested creating redundancies. "I think our whole entire [primary care] team should be involved," noted one Bronx medical assistant. "Just in case the provider and the RN is out that day, we could actually give the patient a follow-up appointment or gather more information."

To facilitate ease of use, many team members suggested streamlining the log-in process with single sign-on. "There are like seven or eight different systems that we're using and signing on ... you're fumbling with your phone, and you're already on like, Outlook and [the EHR system] and secure messaging," explained a Bronx physician. Physicians and RNs also requested ways to prioritize alerts by urgency, and including multiple notification modalities. For instance, one Indianapolis physician suggested alerts could operate similarly to campus safety notifications, where "you get an e-mail, you get a phone call, and you get a text. It's hard to miss that."

27.6.7 Use of event notification services to support COVID-19 response within Veterans Health Administration

During the COVID-19 pandemic, the investigators and study team at JJP VAMC leveraged their experiences with ENS during the trial to support follow-up care for Veterans tested or diagnosed outside the VHA [44]. The JJP VAMC developed a postdiagnosis primary care follow-up protocol for Veterans who were infected with the novel, infectious disease. This protocol worked well for patients tested and treated at JJP VAMC. However, primary care teams also wanted to identify and follow up with Veterans treated outside the VHA for COVID-19.

Using a similar technical architecture and information flow with its partner, the Bronx RHIO, the JJP VAMC implemented a process similar to the ENS trial [44]. Each day, a VHA staff member would login to the Bronx RHIO and query for a list of Veterans recently diagnosed and/or treated for COVID-19 in the ED or hospital. The staff member would then enter a note into CPRS for the patient, which would be cosigned by the primary care team for that Veteran. The primary care team would then initiate the post-COVID protocol for follow-up and document the care provided in the Veteran's electronic health record. Clinicians could query the Bronx RHIO for details about the external care received in the non-VHA ED or hospital.

From April 6, 2020 to June 23, 2020, ENS alerts enabled JJP VAMC primary care teams to identify an additional 88 cases of COVID-19 among Veterans, which represented 11% of all documented cases during that time period [44]. Among the patients tested and treated outside the VHA, 36 (41%) were hospitalized and 12 (14%) died in the outside facilities [44]. While ENS alerts for these patients could not impact the care they received during their acute illness, the alerts enabled VHA clinicians to check in on their patients via telephone and video conference (to a lesser extent). Moreover, it flagged these patients in the system for long COVID monitoring and documented their condition. Such awareness of prior disease and treatment may become important to long-term follow-up with these patients as we learn more about the true impact of COVID-19 on morbidity and mortality.

27.7 Future directions for event notification services

Moving forward, we suggest several steps that developers may consider in implementing event notifications. First, notifications may benefit from standardization. The standard for ENS or ADT notifications is embedded in HL7 Version 2.0. While widely used, this standard has limitations that constrain the amount of information that can be encoded in an event notification message. [45] As event notifications are developed in compliance with the 21st Century Cures Act requirements [46], ADT alerts may benefit from a Fast Healthcare Interoperability Resources profile or Consolidated Clinical Document Architecture template to enable support for expanded content (e.g., discharge summary) as they are implemented across HIE networks. Future work should examine vendor agnostic standards that support event notifications in EHR systems and HIE networks. Second, our study supports previous findings that additional data on patients' diagnosis and discharge instructions would be useful in determining appropriate follow-up care. This is something for commercial EHR vendors to keep in mind when implementing event notifications in compliance with the Interoperability and Patient Access final rule (CMS-9115-F), published in March 2020, which requires hospitals to send electronic ADT notifications "to another healthcare facility or to another community provider or practitioner" [47].

Moving forward, event notification should be further studied as timely follow-up and reintegration into primary care following acute care events are an organizational priority for the VHA and other health systems. In a survey of non-VHA providers in a practice-based research network [48], respondents reported poor communication with VHA colleagues, and their interactions were perceived to be with a "system" rather than a colleague. Moreover, the VHA is under pressure to expand access to non-VHA care for Veterans following legislation from Congress [19]. Likewise other health systems are under pressure to improve coordination as patients move from inpatient to primary care and long-term care settings.

As ENS is implemented across health systems, it will be important to further understand its impact on care coordination and patient outcomes. For example, the quantitative analysis in this paper is not sufficient to explain why ENS reduced readmissions in Unruh et al. [12] but did not impact outcomes in this trial. Moreover, future research should consider additional process as well as proximal outcomes for patients that may be more closely linked to transitions of care. Qualitative methods should examine the implementation of ENS, and future trials or quantitative studies should examine ENS used for coordination of care across a variety of populations beyond older adults. Future research should also help tease out under what conditions ENS best meets care team and patient needs to impact outcomes.

27.8 Summary

We have shown that event notifications sent to primary care teams improve health care delivery processes and are well received by providers and patients. In our study, we observed an improvement in timely follow-up for older patients postdischarge, impacting care coordination. Yet some Veterans still did not receive timely postacute follow-up, and timely follow-up did not directly translate into reductions in secondary hospitalizations or ED visits. This is in contrast to an earlier study in which reductions in rehospitalizations were observed for Medicare patients outside the VHA system. Even if ENS does not definitively reduce rehospitalization, there are strong arguments for its implementation, including more timely follow-up and reduction in complexity as patients navigate fragmented health systems as well as utility in emerging public health emergencies like the COVID-19 pandemic. Yet, there remains additional work to optimize the implementation and use of ENS in support of care coordination and population outcomes. Given recent policies that encourage adoption and use of ENS, over the next 5–10 years this HIE service will likely mature and become an important part of care delivery.

Questions for discussion

1. Compare and contrast ENS notifications with other forms of directed or "push" HIE. Do ENS notifications have any relative advantages over other forms of directed HIE?
2. How did policy or organizational context facilitate adoption and use of ENS within the VHA?
3. What barriers did VHA face internally and externally when implementing ENS? How could these barriers be addressed?
4. How might you improve ENS notifications to better meet health care operational needs?
5. How might ENS notifications be implemented in such a way that they might improve clinical outcomes?

Acknowledgments

The case study described was supported by Merit Review Award Number I01 HX001563 from the US Department of Veterans Affairs (VA) Health Services Research & Development Service of the VA Office of Research and Development. The opinions in this book chapter are solely the responsibility of the authors and do not necessarily represent the official views of the VA.

The authors greatly appreciate the efforts of Ashley L. Schwartzkopf, MSW, Justine May, MSW, Cathy C. Schubert, MD, Jessica Coffing, MPH, and Brian W. Porter, MPH, of the Richard L. Roudebush VA Medical Center in Indianapolis, Indiana, as well as Kimberly M. Judon, MPH, Nicholas Koufacos, MSW, Vivian M. Guerrero, MA, Tanieka Mason, MPH, of the James J. Peters VA Medical Center, who contributed the work described in the case study. We further acknowledge both community-based HIE networks involved in the work: the Indiana Health Information Exchange (IHIE) and the Bronx Regional Health Information Organization (RHIO).

References

[1] Barnett ML, Bitton A, Souza J, Landon BE. Trends in outpatient care for Medicare beneficiaries and implications for primary care, 2000 to 2019. Ann Intern Med 2021;174(12):1658–65.

[2] Kern LM, Safford MM, Slavin MJ, Makovkina E, Fudl A, Carrillo JE, et al. Patients' and providers' views on causes and consequences of healthcare fragmentation in the ambulatory setting: a qualitative study. J Gen Intern Med 2019;34(6):899–907.

[3] Wenger N, Méan M, Castioni J, Marques-Vidal P, Waeber G, Garnier A. Allocation of internal medicine resident time in a Swiss hospital: a time and motion study of day and evening shifts. Ann Intern Med 2017;166(8):579–86.

[4] Franzosa E, Traylor M, Judon KM, Guerrero Aquino V, Schwartzkopf AL, Boockvar KS, et al. Perceptions of event notification following discharge to improve geriatric care: qualitative interviews of care team members from a 2-site cluster randomized trial. J Am Med Inform Assoc 2021;28(8):1728–35.

[5] Schoen C, Osborn R, Squires D, Doty M, Pierson R, Applebaum S. New 2011 survey of patients with complex care needs in eleven countries finds that care is often poorly coordinated. Health Aff (Millwood) 2011;30(12):2437–48.

[6] Damarell RA, Morgan DD, Tieman JJ. General practitioner strategies for managing patients with multimorbidity: a systematic review and thematic synthesis of qualitative research. BMC Family Pract 2020;21(1):131.

[7] Hamel MB, Henderson WG, Khuri SF, Daley J. Surgical outcomes for patients aged 80 and older: morbidity and mortality from major noncardiac surgery. J Am Geriatr Soc 2005;53(3):424–9.

[8] Finlayson EV, Birkmeyer JD. Operative mortality with elective surgery in older adults. Eff Clin Pract 2001;4 (4):172–7.

[9] Moore T, Shapiro JS, Doles L, Calman N, Camhi E, Check T, et al. Event detection: a clinical notification service on a health information exchange platform. AMIA Annu Symp Proc 2012;2012:635–42.

[10] Menachemi N, Rahurkar S, Harle CA, Vest JR. The benefits of health information exchange: an updated systematic review. J Am Med Inform Assoc 2018;25 (9):1259–65.

[11] Rahurkar S, Vest JR, Menachemi N. Despite the spread of health information exchange, there is little evidence of its impact on cost, use, and quality of care. Health Aff (Millwood) 2015;34(3):477–83.

[12] Unruh MA, Jung HY, Kaushal R, Vest JR. Hospitalization event notifications and reductions in readmissions of Medicare fee-for-service beneficiaries in the Bronx, New York. J Am Med Inform Assoc 2017;24(e1):e150–6.

[13] Dixon BE, Schwartzkopf AL, Guerrero VM, May J, Koufacos NS, Bean AM, et al. Regional data exchange to improve care for veterans after non-VA hospitalization: a randomized controlled trial. BMC Med Inform Decis Mak 2019;19(1):125.

[14] US Department of Veterans Affairs. Veterans Health Administration: about VHA, <https://www.va.gov/health/aboutvha.asp>; 2020.

[15] Nelson KM, Helfrich C, Sun H, Hebert PL, Liu C-F, Dolan E, et al. Implementation of the patient-centered medical home in the Veterans Health Administration: associations with patient satisfaction, quality of care, staff burnout, and hospital and emergency department use. JAMA Intern Med 2014;174(8):1350–8.

[16] Liu CF, Batten A, Wong ES, Fihn SD, Hebert PL. Fee-for-service Medicare-enrolled elderly veterans are increasingly voting with their feet to use more VA and less Medicare, 2003–2014. Health Serv Res 2018;53:5140–58.

[17] H.R.3230 - 113th Congress (2013-2014): Veterans Access, Choice, and Accountability Act of 2014. (2014, August 7). http://www.congress.gov/

[18] S.2372 - 115th Congress (2017-2018): VA MISSION Act of 2018. (2018, June 6). http://www.congress.gov/

[19] Dixon BE, Haggstrom DA, Weiner M. Implications for informatics given expanding access to care for veterans and other populations. J Am Med Inform Assoc 2015;22(4):917–20.

[20] VA launches new health care options under MISSION Act [press release], June 6, 2019. 2019. [Accessed 16 Jun 2022]. Available at: https://www.va.gov/opa/pressrel/pressrelease.cfm?id = 5264

[21] Axon RN, Gebregziabher M, Everett CJ, Heidenreich P, Hunt KJ. Dual health care system use is associated with higher rates of hospitalization and hospital readmission among veterans with heart failure. Am Heart J 2016;174:157–63.

[22] West AN, Charlton ME, Vaughan-Sarrazin M. Dual use of VA and non-VA hospitals by Veterans with multiple hospitalizations. BMC Health Serv Res 2015;15(1):1–12.

[23] Ford J, MacTaggart P, Gunnar W. Veterans Health Administration scheduling system: the path to high reliability realization. J Healthc Manag 2021;66(6):421–30.

[24] Brown SH, Lincoln MJ, Groen PJ, Kolodner RM. VistA – U.S. Department of Veterans Affairs national-scale HIS. Int J Med Inform 2003;69(2–3):135–56.

[25] Kuzmak PM, Dayhoff RE. The Department of Veterans Affairs integration of imaging into the healthcare enterprise using the VistA Hospital Information System and Digital Imaging and Communications in Medicine. J Digit Imaging 1998;11(2):53–64.

[26] Legler A, Price M, Parikh M, Nebeker JR, Ward MC, Wedemeyer L, et al. Effect on VA patient satisfaction of provider's use of an integrated viewer of multiple electronic health records. J Gen Intern Med 2019;34 (1):132–6.

[27] Department of Veterans Affairs. VHIE overview. Washington, DC: Department of Veterans Affairs; 2018 [updated 2021 Oct 1]. Available from: <https://www.va.gov/vhie/>.

[28] eHealth Exchange. eHealth Exchange connects healthcare providers. Vienna, VA: eHealth Exchange; 2021. Available from: <https://ehealthexchange.org/what-we-do/>.

[29] Department of Veterans Affairs. For providers. Washington, DC: Department of Veterans Affairs; 2021 [updated 2021 Jun 16]. Available from: <https://www.va.gov/VHIE/For_Providers.asp>.

[30] Tung YC, Chang GM, Chang HY, Yu TH. Relationship between early physician follow-up and 30-day readmission after acute myocardial infarction and heart failure. PLoS One 2017;12(1):e0170061.

[31] Hansen LO, Young RS, Hinami K, Leung A, Williams MV. Interventions to reduce 30-day rehospitalization: a systematic review. Ann Intern Med 2011;155 (8):520–8.

[32] Dixon BE, Luckhurst C, Haggstrom DA. Leadership perspectives on implementing health information exchange: qualitative study in a Tertiary Veterans Affairs Medical Center. JMIR Med Inform 2021;9(2): e19249.

[33] Kartje R, Dixon BE, Schwartzkopf AL, Guerrero V, Judon KM, Yi JC, et al. Characteristics of Veterans with non-VA encounters enrolled in a trial of standards-based, interoperable event notification and care coordination. J Am Board Family Med 2021;34 (2):301–8.

[34] DuGoff EH, Bandeen-Roche K, Anderson GF. Relationship between continuity of care and adverse outcomes varies by number of chronic conditions among older adults with diabetes. J Comorb 2016;6 (2):65–72.

[35] Dixon BE, Judon KM, Schwartzkopf AL, Guerrero VM, Koufacos NS, May J, et al. Impact of event notification services on timely follow-up and rehospitalization among primary care patients at two Veterans Affairs Medical Centers. J Am Med Inform Assoc 2021;28(12):2593–600.

[36] Dixon BE, Embi PJ, Haggstrom DA. Information technologies that facilitate care coordination: provider and patient perspectives. Behav Med Pract Policy Res 2018;8(3):522–5.

[37] Wiley KK, Hilts KE, Ancker JS, Unruh MA, Jung HY, Vest JR. Organizational characteristics and perceptions of clinical event notification services in healthcare settings: a study of health information exchange. JAMIA Open 2020;3(4):611–18.

[38] Vest JR, Unruh MA, Shapiro JS, Casalino LP. The associations between query-based and directed health information exchange with potentially avoidable use of health care services. Health Serv Res 2019;54 (5):981–93.

[39] Lembeck MA, Thygesen LC, Sørensen BD, Rasmussen LL, Holm EA. Effect of single follow-up home visit on readmission in a group of frail elderly patients – a Danish randomized clinical trial. BMC Health Serv Res 2019;19(1):751.

[40] Coleman EA. Falling through the cracks: challenges and opportunities for improving transitional care for persons with continuous complex care needs. J Am Geriatr Soc 2003;51(4):549–55.

[41] Coleman EA, Parry C, Chalmers S, Min S-j. The care transitions intervention: results of a randomized controlled trial. Arch Intern Med 2006;166(17):1822–8.

[42] Koufacos NS, May J, Judon KM, Franzosa E, Dixon BE, Schubert CC, et al. Improving patient activation among older veterans: results from a social worker-led care transitions intervention. J Gerontol Soc Work 2022;65(1):63–77.

[43] Boockvar KS, Judon KM, Schwartzkopf AL, Guerrero Aquino VM, Koufacos NS, May J, et al. Effect of health information exchange plus a care transitions intervention on rehospitalization among primary care patients at two Veterans Affairs medical centers: a randomized clinical trial. J Gen Intern Med 2022;.

[44] Sherman RL, Judon KM, Koufacos NS, Guerrero Aquino VM, Raphael SM, Hollander JT, et al. Utilizing a health information exchange to facilitate COVID-19 VA primary care follow-up for Veterans diagnosed in the community. JAMIA Open 2021;4(1):ooab020.

[45] HL7. Introduction to Hl7 standards, <https://www.hl7.org/implement/standards/>; 2020.

[46] US Food and Drug Administration. 21st Century Cures Act. <https://www.fda.gov/regulatory-information/selected-amendments-fdc-act/21st-century-cures-act>; 2020 [updated January 31].

[47] US Centers for Medicare & Medicaid Services. Interoperability and patient access fact sheet. Baltimore, MD: Department of Health and Human Services; 2020 [updated 2020 Mar 09]. Available from: <https://www.cms.gov/newsroom/fact-sheets/interoperability-and-patient-access-fact-sheet>.

[48] Gaglioti A, Cozad A, Wittrock S, Stewart K, Lampman M, Ono S, et al. Non-VA primary care providers' perspectives on comanagement for rural veterans. Mil Med 2014;179(11):1236–43.

CHAPTER

28

Facilitating HIE in Denmark: the story of MedCom, a Danish health information organization

Brian E. Dixon[1,2], *Thomas Schmidt*[3] *and Christian Nøhr*[4]

[1]Department of Epidemiology, Richard M. Fairbanks School of Public Health, Indiana University, Indianapolis, IN, USA [2]Center for Biomedical Informatics, Regenstrief Institute Inc., Indianapolis, IN, USA [3]Center for Health Informatics and Technology, University of Southern Denmark, Odense, Denmark [4]Department of Planning, Aalborg University, Aalborg, Denmark

Major themes

This case study highlights the following major themes from the book:

- The critical role that a health information organization (HIO) plays in achieving consensus on health IT standards as well as common approaches to data exchange.
- Provides an example of a centralized, government-facilitated health information exchange (HIE) network.
- Demonstrates a path to sustainability where the HIO receives financial support from multiple public and private entities that fund general operations in addition to specific HIE services.
- Demonstrates the role of standards in supporting interoperable exchange across local, regional, and national health IT systems.
- Illustrates how HIE can connect core infrastructure to patient-facing applications like portals.
- Discusses the challenges of moving from legacy interfaces and exchange methods to modern, advanced approaches like FHIR (Fast Healthcare Interoperable Resources).

28.1 Introduction

When most individuals think about Denmark, their minds often focus on images of Vikings, the Little Mermaid statue, bicycles, and delectable pastries sitting in a box on the counter in the office break room. In fact, most people perceive Denmark as an unassuming, small nation that might not have as much to offer as Sweden or Germany, two of Denmark's neighbors. This notion is far from the truth.

Health Information Exchange
DOI: https://doi.org/10.1016/B978-0-323-90802-3.00031-9

Denmark has a richer and more complex history than that taught to most grade school children when they first learn about Europe. Although small, the nation possesses several of the world's most amazing castles and palaces, leads the world in digital governance, and is one of the most environmentally sustainable countries with large numbers of bicycles and wind turbines. There are many other less well known yet impressive facts about Denmark that await those who travel there for business or pleasure.

Another well-kept secret about Denmark is its robust health information exchange (HIE) infrastructure. The nation's health system is highly connected, and it facilitates standards-based exchange among all actors in its health care ecosystem. At the center of this infrastructure is another unassuming entity that is the nucleus of HIE—MedCom. Founded in 1994, MedCom is the health information organization (HIO, defined in Chapter 1) responsible for facilitating HIE in Denmark. Although there are several important players in Denmark's overall digital health landscape, including a now globally renowned patient portal and a National Service Platform that facilitated rapid access to patients' SARS-CoV-2 virus testing results and COVID-19 vaccination records, MedCom is uniquely the Danish Chief Architect and Negotiator when it comes to HIE.

In this case study, we describe the Danish digital health landscape and its HIE infrastructure. We further discuss the critical role MedCom plays in facilitating HIE, including its role in governance and standards development. We further describe aspects of Danish society and health system that support HIE adoption and use. Finally, we look at multiple, exciting HIE efforts that Denmark hopes to work on in the coming years.

28.2 Background

28.2.1 Denmark

As of 2021, Denmark reported a population of 5.86 million with 800,000 individuals residing in its capital, Copenhagen. Denmark is a Scandinavian and Nordic country located in Northern Europe (Schengen Area), bordered by Sweden and Norway to the North as well as Germany to its South. Denmark's total land area is 42,943 km^2 (16,580 sq mi), which makes it roughly equivalent to the State of Maryland in the United States (more land area but slightly smaller population). A unique characteristic of Denmark is its land that is composed of a peninsula (Jutland) plus 443 named islands, including Zealand and Funen (the two largest).

Denmark is a highly developed country whose economy ranks 16th in the world with respect to gross national income per capita, and it is often ranked as one of the most free and competitive markets in Europe. Danish citizens enjoy a high standard of living as the nation also ranks highly on multiple indices for education, health care, and civil liberties. Known as a bicycle nation, Denmark is also progressive in its approach to environmental stewardship with the world's first Ministry of Environment (1971), and 41% of the nation's energy is generated using wind power.

More than 95% of Danes have access to the Internet, and broadband penetration is one of the highest in Europe [1]. Denmark was the first nation to appoint a Tech Ambassador, and it ranks first in digital governance by the United Nations.

Historically, the Danish economy focused on agriculture and shipping given its ports on the North Sea and Baltic Sea. Today, Denmark's economy is service driven, and it is a net exporter of food and energy. The country's main export goods include wind turbines; pharmaceuticals; machinery and instruments (including robotics); furniture and design; and meat, dairy products, and fish.

28.2.2 The Danish health system

Like other Scandinavian countries known for their comprehensive welfare system, Denmark's health system is predominantly public- and government-controlled through regulations and budgetary allocations [2,3]. Danish citizens have universal, free, and equal access to all public hospitals as well as general and specialized practitioner services, all of which is financed through taxes. Dentists, out of hospital medicines, as well as some services are provided under co-payment or through supplemental private insurance.

The organization of the Danish health system is summarized in Fig. 28.1. Although the Ministry of Health provides coordination and supervision, operational responsibilities are distributed across a decentralized administrative structure that consists of 5 regions and 98 municipalities [4]. Regions provide hospital (inpatient, emergency) and primary care (via Public Health Insurance). Municipalities, on the other hand, provide most remaining health services including public health (e.g., epidemiology, prevention programs), postacute care (e.g., rehabilitation, long-term), school-based health services, and social services. The regions and municipalities interface with the national government, European Union, labor unions, and other entities through two nongovernmental associations, Danish Regions and Local Government Denmark, respectively [2,5]. These entities represent the interests of their members, provide consulting services to their members, and negotiate the annual financial arrangements with the government.

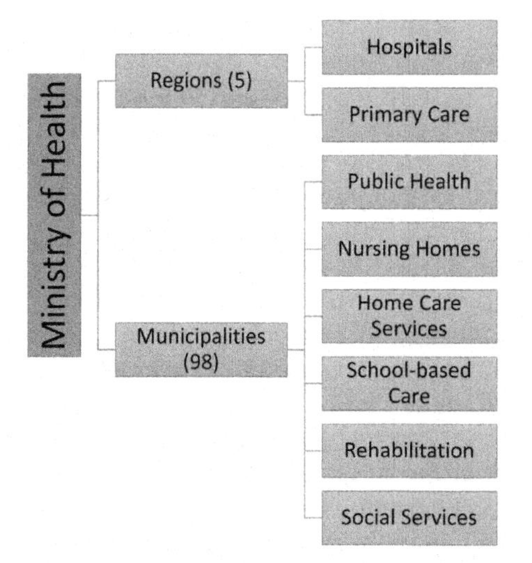

FIGURE 28.1 Structure of Denmark's health system.

Prior to the 21st century, Denmark's health system was plagued by issues of inefficiency and poor quality. Over the past 25 years, the nation systematically transformed its health system through a series of regulatory and operational reforms. Regulations c.2002 that allow citizens to receive care at private hospitals when wait times are too long at public hospitals encouraged reforms that expanded capacity and quality in public hospitals. The current organizational structure was put into place in 2007 as a result of major structural reforms [6] that consolidated counties ($N = 15$) into regions ($N = 5$) and reduced the number of municipalities (from 271 to 98). Currently, life expectancy in Denmark is slightly higher (80.8 vs 80.6 years), the nation spends slightly more per capita on health care (10.4% vs 9.0% GDP), and length of stay in hospitals is lower (5.5 vs 7.8 days) when compared to other OECD nations [7].

28.2.3 Digital health in Denmark

In parallel with its health system reforms, Denmark invested heavily in information technology to support the transformation of health care delivery and public health services. On ICT surveys of OECD countries, Denmark ranks high. For example, Denmark was one of five OECD nations observed to possess mature benchmark ICT capabilities [8], including the percent of general practitioner (GP) practices with electronic systems to store and manage patient information, the percent of hospitals that exchange imaging/radiology results with outside organizations, and the percent of hospitals that have synchronous telehealth capabilities.

Digitization of health data began in the 1970s with patient administration systems as well as laboratory information systems [9]. Electronic health record (EHR) systems started to appear around 1992 [10]. By 2008, EHR systems had wide adoption in Denmark, with "virtually all Danish" providers using EHR systems [3,11]. In 2011, there were 16 different EHR vendors offering systems to more than 3500 GPs and 18 different EHR systems in use by 53 Danish hospitals [12]. Around this time, a report from the Danish National Audit Office [13] detailed technological and organizational challenges to the implementation and adoption of EHRs [6]. As a result, the regional authorities agreed to assume full responsibility for hospital EHR systems, and a plan was made to consolidate the number of EHR systems used in hospitals [6,12]. At this time, the regions formed Regionernes Sundheds it, an eHealth organization focused on collaboration across the five regions with respect to EHR implementation [6].

As of 2022, there were just two EHR vendors supporting systems in Danish hospitals. Epic Systems Corporation (Verona, WI) implemented EHR systems in Eastern Denmark, comprised of the Capital Region (Copenhagen) as well as the Administrative Region of Zealand. Systematic (Aarhus, Denmark) is implemented in Western Denmark, comprised of the North Denmark Region, Central Denmark Region, and Region of Southern Denmark. At the time of writing, GPs and specialists continue to use seven different EHR systems in their practices and all 98 municipalities use three different EHR systems in elderly care.

In parallel with EHR implementation and consolidation, work began in 2003 on *sundhed.dk*, the centralized, governmental eHealth portal for providers and citizens, which remains at the forefront of such efforts in the world [2]. The portal seeks to consolidate relevant information from all parts of the health ecosystem in Denmark and serve as an electronic gateway that facilitates access to the National Health Record (Sundhedsjournalen), a comprehensive view of data across all five regions. The system is hosted by the Danish Health Data Authority, yet the platform is supported by a cross-sector collaboration of many stakeholders across the Ministry of Health, Danish Regions, municipalities, GPs, hospitals, and Public Health Institute [2].

As of 2014, the National Health Record was available for access by clinicians (doctors and nurses) in hospitals as well as patients directly through the Internet [6]. Development required a decade during which the platform expanded from only the data available at the national level to incorporation of data from hospitals, GPs, and municipalities [2]. In many respects, the maturity of eHealth in Denmark occurred in parallel with the maturation of the National Health Record, given that many of the national data systems and interfaces to them were developed to support the portal (*sundhed.dk*).

As of 2022, the eHealth portal provides access to medical records for patients and providers via a mobile application in addition to its Internet site (*sundhed.dk*). Furthermore, the Shared Medication Record (Fælles Medicinkort or FMK) gives health professionals access to a complete, up-to-date prescription information for patients across the entire health system. The COVID-19 Passport, introduced in 2021, enables government agencies, businesses, providers, and patients to verify vaccination records and confirm SARS-CoV-2 testing results of individuals. Upon this robust technological foundation, the Ministry of Health, in its Digital Health Strategy (2018–22), seeks to expand collaboration across providers and engage more patients in becoming active participants in their health [7]. All of these systems (sundhed.dk, FMK, National Health Record) are undergirded by a robust information infrastructure that developed in parallel since the early days of EHRs.

Fig. 28.2 represents a timeline of significant events in the development of the Danish digital health ecosystem, including its HIE infrastructure. While each organization and system represented on the timeline has its own rich history,

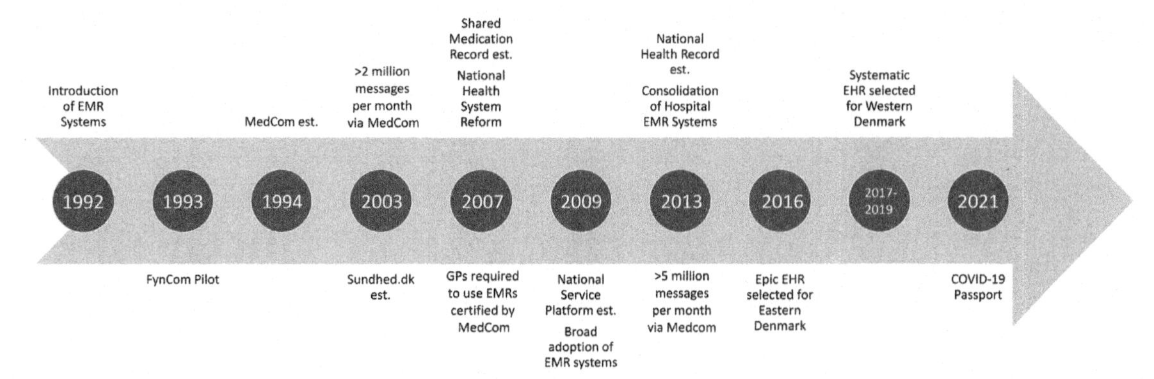

FIGURE 28.2 Timeline of milestones in the development of Denmark's digital health ecosystem.

for example, the story of *sundhed.dk* is featured in Jensen and Thorseng [2], the figure provides an ecosystem view to illustrate the two decades of progress and hard work necessary to achieve development of a robust, national health information infrastructure. The broad availability of health data for clinical and population health purposes would not be possible without the significant contributions of each entity and system represented as well as the underlying infrastructure provided by MedCom that facilitates HIE efforts across the ecosystem.

28.3 Health information exchange in Denmark

HIE started almost immediately after EHRs began to appear in primary care practices. A pathologist and professor at Southern Denmark University in Odense convinced the municipal IT department that electronic clinical messages would benefit primary care physicians [10]. A pilot project, dubbed FynCom, connected two primary practices with a hospital information system and laboratory information system [10]. Lab results and hospital discharge letters (e.g., summaries as they are known in the United States) were delivered to the primary care offices.

The FynCom pilot became a nongovernmental organization, MedCom, by 1994 and continued to work on electronic communications between hospitals, pharmacies, municipalities, and physician offices. In 2000, the Danish national eHealth strategy (now called its Digital Health Strategy) emphasized the need for such communications across all of Denmark [10]. Furthermore, the Ministry of Health elevated MedCom to a central position in connecting health care providers across the nation.

Over the past 30 years, MedCom contributed significantly to the development, implementation, maintenance, and advancement of the national HIE infrastructure in Denmark. MedCom created and maintains the HIE middleware, referred to as the Danish National Health Data Network (SDN), as well as supports the Danish Health Data Authority develop and certify compliance with the health IT standards in use by hospital and GP EHR systems as well as other health information system (e.g., for elderly care in the municipalities). This organization, therefore, undergirds the nation's HIE infrastructure. While other systems and organizations contribute to HIE, the story of HIE in Denmark is centered around MedCom and the SDN network.

28.3.1 Digital health infrastructure

The infrastructure for HIE and digital health in Demark, depicted in Fig. 28.3, is complex and consists of four interconnected layers. In

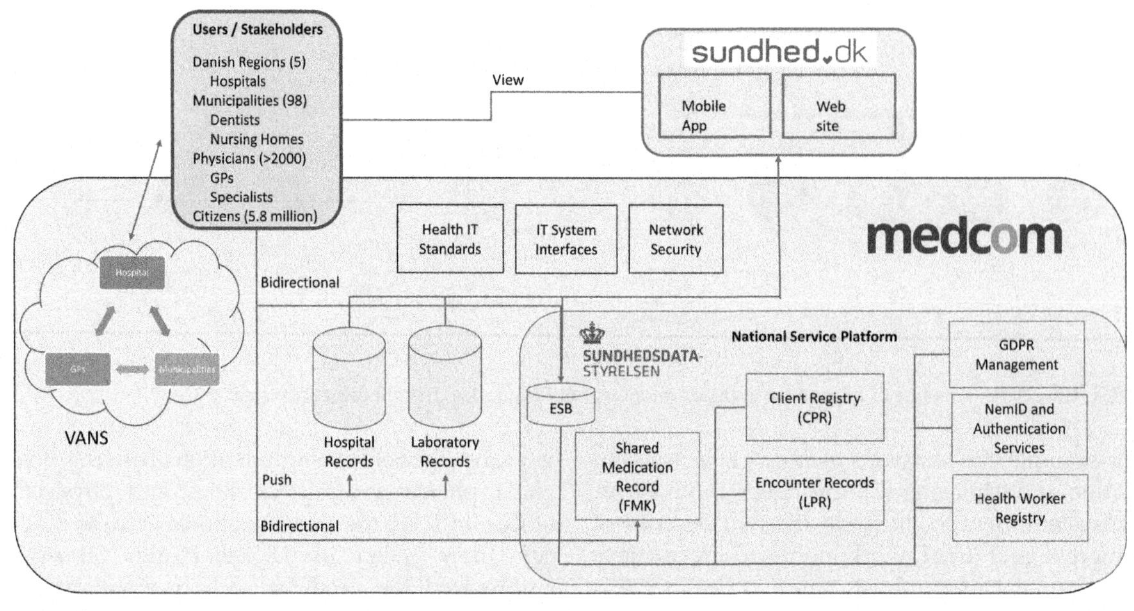

FIGURE 28.3 Denmark's enterprise architecture for major health IT systems and HIE networks. *ESB*, Enterprise service bus; *GDPR*, general data protection regulation; *GP*, general practitioner; *VANS*, Value-Added Network Service.

this section, we break down each layer and describe how it contributes to the national infrastructure. Each layer plays a key role in supporting HIE for use in care delivery as well as payment, operations, patient access to their medical records, and public health.

Briefly, the four layers include:

- Value-Added Network Service (VANS)—these networks operate as wide area networks within a given Danish health region. Each VANS is responsible for operating and maintaining the health IT systems used by hospitals, GPs, and municipalities, including their commercial EHRs.
- MedCom—a publicly funded, nongovernmental (nonprofit) organization that seeks to facilitate cooperation between health authorities, health care organizations, and private firms connected to the Danish health sector. MedCom supports the use of national health IT standards and operates the messaging infrastructure that connects the health care ecosystem of Denmark. Note that this layer spans most of Fig. 28.3, denoting that MedCom is central to nearly all data and information exchange except for limited transactions within the VANS.
- National Service Platform (NSP)—the national health data and authentication platform hosted by the Danish Ministry of Health (specifically the Danish Health Data Authority). The NSP is home to the FMK (Shared Medication Record) as well as the national Client Registry (CPR), Health Worker Registry, National Patient Register (Landspatientregistret in Danish; LPR, which is a claims database of encounter records), and common security services.
- Sundhed.dk—the national eHealth portal [14]. This mobile and web-based platform offers patients as well as clinicians access to medical records gathered from multiple sources, including the NSP, MedCom, and VANS.

The old adage of "all health care is local" applies to the Danish health system. Hospitals, GPs, and municipalities (e.g., nursing homes, public health authorities) all operate within the five Danish regions, closest to their constituents. These entities have strong autonomy and therefore flexibility in the health IT systems they choose to implement in order to meet their workflow and operational needs. The EHR systems are selected and implemented within VANS, which necessitates each VANS hosting its own integration platform to enable exchange within the VANS and between the VANS and the national HIE infrastructure. Applications like Epic's MyChart (patient portal) and EpicCare Link (allows GPs to view hospital EHR data) can be used to facilitate HIE within a region.

Although vendor selection and customization are up to each region, each health IT system contract with a local Danish health authority is required to (1) adopt the national health IT standards established by MedCom and (2) establish a contract with MedCom for HIE services. For example, delivery of a discharge summary from a hospital to a GP requires the use of messaging standards established by MedCom, even though the exchange occurs within a given VANS. Through the VANS' integration platforms, local health IT systems are connected to and exchange data with the national HIE infrastructure using standards established by MedCom. Some of this exchange is bidirectional, like prescription data written to the FMK and also retrieved from the FMK. Other exchange is unidirectional, such as hospitals pushing discharge letters to the national repository hosted by the regions via MedCom, making it available for retrieval by the sundhed.dk portal. Therefore all data exchange within a VANS is guided by MedCom (and those systems certified to be compliant with standards), and all data exchange between the VANSs and the national infrastructure is guided and serviced by MedCom.

National platforms must also subscribe to MedCom HIE services, creating conformity in messaging and data across the national health IT ecosystem. Furthermore, national health IT system contracts are required to adopt the national health IT standards established by MedCom. Moreover, health IT systems at the national level must contract with the VANS to enable bidirectional communication with regional and municipality health IT systems. In Denmark, these common requirements are viewed as part of contributing to the common good—in this case the national digital health infrastructure. And that national infrastructure, it is facilitated by MedCom and the national standards established by MedCom.

Despite the portal (sundhed.dk) being a highly visible health IT application that patients and clinicians access, the portal is primarily a visualization layer that aggregates data from across the Danish health system. Clinicians access the portal using single sign on (SSO) via their EHR system. A button in the Epic or Systematic EHR takes clinicians to the portal, which logs them in and presents the outside data to them using interfaces developed by sundhed.dk. The Danish refer to this approach as "light" (or lightweight) integration between the EHR and the national HIE infrastructure. Patients access the portal primarily through a mobile application, although a browser-based application remains available (initially this was the only method for patients). The transactions between the portal and national infrastructure are facilitated by MedCom messages and standards.

Data available in the portal are primarily sourced from the NSP via an enterprise service bus (ESB). Authentication is also performed through the NSP, using the national identifier, a number unique to each Danish citizen used across governmental services including health care. Some data from the VANSs are stored in national databases, including laboratory results and hospital discharge data. The queries of those databases and pushing of data into national systems, mediated by MedCom using standards established by MedCom. Other databases are stored at the regional level and must also be queried through MedCom using established messaging standards.

The NSP developed around the FMK (Shared Medication Record). Prior to the FMK, in the early 2000s, MedCom facilitated exchange of e-prescribing (eRx) messages between the EHR and a national database of prescriptions (Receptserveren). Although the eRx database was popular with GPs, pharmacies, and patients (who could view their data via the portal), it was challenging to discern when patient medications were changed or updated. In other words, the system did not reconcile patient prescriptions. This frustrated clinical decision-making processes during emergency care and after-hours (urgent) care scenarios [12]. Furthermore, other stakeholders like the municipalities (e.g., public health, nursing homes) did not have access to the electronic medication record. Therefore the stakeholders (regional health authorities, Danish Health Authority, and municipalities), in consultation with MedCom, reached a decision to create the FMK.

The FMK is a database at the national level that provides automated reconciliation whenever any prescriber updates the outpatient medication list for a patient. Upon discharge from the hospital, the FMK is updated by hospital clinicians providing immediate access by GPs. When pharmacists make a substitution, the FMK is updated. When a GP or dentist prescribes a new medication or changes a medication order, the FMK is updated. When long-term care facilities update the medication regimen, the FMK is updated. As one informant stated, "if a patient chooses to refill a prescription using the app [sundhed.dk], within one minute pharmacies can fill the prescription." This statement denotes the rapid availability of data. When patients use the portal to request a refill, it must be approved by the GP before the pharmacy can fill the order. This process typically happens quickly. Furthermore, we note that the inpatient medications are not synced to the FMK. The FMK is designed to house the ongoing medications taken by a patient in home and community settings.

Achieving the FMK required what MedCom describes as "deep" integration, as opposed to the "light" integration of the SSO button in EHR systems. Not only are messages exchanged across the various health IT applications used within municipalities, GP offices, and hospitals, but the NSP must parse the messages and reconcile the information in real time. The system must handle multiple, simultaneous requests for updates and queries. This change necessitated the use of robust syntactic and semantic standards, and all stakeholders had to agree upon these standards as they needed to be implemented consistently across the country. Much of the overhead needed for deep integration for the FMK, including the ESB as well as authentication methods, suggested the development of the larger NSP rather than mechanisms for just one health IT system.

Because of the success of the FMK, the NSP expanded to host a health worker registry (see Chapter 14), client registry (see Chapter 12), and encounter records (claims) database (see Chapter 15). The encounter records (known as LPR) database highlights the uniformity and efficiency of the Danish HIE infrastructure. In order for a provider to be paid for a clinical encounter, the visit must be logged in the LPR. This requires all health IT registration systems to provide a standardized message to the NSP. The standards were established by MedCom through consensus involving the three key stakeholder groups. Because of the standardization and centralized approach, the Danish Health Data Authority has an accurate reflection of all visits to a health care provider, and clinicians can access an accurate, longitudinal medical record of patients' past encounters (Box 28.1).

28.3.2 Security and user authentication

Similar to other HIE networks, including Indiana (**Chapter 22**) and Taiwan (**Chapter 30**),

BOX 28.1

Rapid expansion of infrastructure during COVID-19 pandemic.

During the COVID-19 pandemic, most nations rapidly expanded their digital health infrastructure to utilize telehealth for ambulatory encounters [15,16]. In Denmark, the Ministry of Health asked MedCom and the GP Organization to enable a videoconference service that would allow consumers to have a GP visit remotely from their smartphone, tablet, or other device as depicted in Fig. 28.4. The service needed to be ready in 2–3 weeks.

The videoconference service was established in an already existing application "MinLæge" (MyDoctor), owned by the GP Organization and the Ministry of Health. A virtual waiting room was developed in the application and, luckily, standards and infrastructure to support video conferencing was developed by MedCom decades ago. However, the video conferencing infrastructure was "sleepy," meaning that it supported a few hundred video calls each day requiring a low level of maintenance for the MedCom network. The new service, at its height during the pandemic, would facilitate over 5000 calls each day. MedCom quickly pivoted to expand bandwidth and support for thousands of video conference calls.

More challenging, MedCom needed to enable consumers to connect to the videoconferencing infrastructure using multiple points of connection, including integration with Epic in the Capital Region. Consumers could use MyChart to initiate the telehealth visit. However, the service was facilitated by the MedCom platform, without knowledge to the consumer.

This example highlights the critical role that MedCom plays in the digital health infrastructure for Denmark. The organization serves as the backbone of the video conferencing platform, yet most providers and patients likely don't know about MedCom. They perceived the calls to be hosted in the EHR or tablet application they used to start the session. Meanwhile, MedCom maintains the technical infrastructure that enables the video calls, and it creates the standards used by Epic, Systematic, and other health IT applications to connect to the backbone and leverage it for their customers.

Denmark employs a multipronged approach to security. MedCom establishes security standards and protocols that are used throughout the country when exchanging data. Secure communications channels are established on the backbone operated by MedCom.

Beyond transport security, Denmark employs role-based authentication to enable access to medical information. Performed by MedCom in the early years, the NSP now hosts access databases that enable the portal and other systems to ask the question, "is this person authorized to view this patient's record?" The HIE network ensures that GPs access records for their patients, requiring the network to employ provider attribution algorithms such that the system knows that Dr. Hansen is the GP for Mrs. Petersen. Using admission, discharge, and transfer messages, the NSP is able to determine whether a given patient is currently in a given hospital. Users from that hospital can access data on admitted patients, but they are not allowed access to patients discharged who are no longer in the facility.

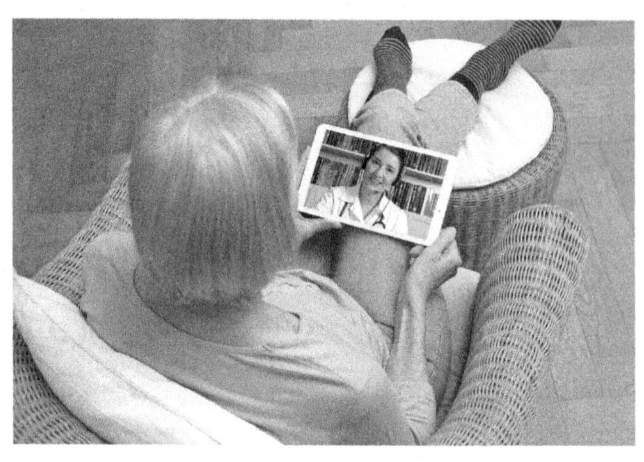

FIGURE 28.4 A senior citizen conducts a telemedicine visit with her GP via a tablet device from the comfort and safety of her home.

28.3.3 A pragmatic approach to engineering HIE solutions

According to the CEO of MedCom, there are three general approaches to HIE: (1) view only, (2) messaging, or (3) integration. These are the options he ponders when challenges are presented by physicians, nurses, ministry officials, or regional authorities. They encapsulate the sage wisdom of someone with more than 25 years' experience in HIE and describe a pragmatic methodology for tackling information challenges faced by evolving health systems.

28.3.3.1 View only

This approach would implement a mechanism by which a clinician would be able to view information from another health system actor (e.g., pharmacy, nursing home). Typically, a View Only approach is the most cost-effective approach as it may not require data transformations or new interfaces. In many scenarios, however, this approach would likely not be a "smart solution" as it would both (1) introduce additional workflow for the clinician who would need to query and retrieve the information and (2) prohibit the use of decision support algorithms or system features that could analyze the information and suggest an action. For example, in the Capital Region, the hospitals chose to implement EpicCare Link, which allows GPs to view data from the inpatient visit of their recently hospitalized patient. The GPs can view hospital data via the national health portal, but EpicCare Link provides them with some additional details of the inpatient stay. However, it requires the GP to login separately to Epic, which is not the EHR they use. They must go outside their usual system to access it, in order to gain some additional information that might or might not be relevant to follow-up care.

In other scenarios, the View Only approach might be optimal because the other approaches might be cost prohibitive for the value gained by the additional information. For example, GPs in Denmark sometimes look at the rehabilitation plan the municipalities develop postdischarge since the municipalities are responsible for care following hospitalization. Would this scenario require the use of electronic messages where the plan is "pushed" into the GP's inbox? Perhaps it should be integrated into the GP's EHR using an interface. Given GPs only sometimes want to look at this information, a View Only approach, which requires retrieving it for viewing, is likely best. The other approaches are feasible, but they increase in cost and complexity.

28.3.3.2 Messaging

This approach relies primarily on standards-based messaging to deliver information to another information system into which it can be stored or retained. For example, think about referral consults where a GP might request a specialist examine his or her patient. After the patient visits the specialist, the GP would like the consultant's exam records and recommendations. This information can be put into an HL7 message and transmitted to the EHR system at the GP office, where it can be stored as part of the legal medical record and available on demand in the EHR system. This form of exchange is bedrock of HIE in Denmark and most nations. In fact, this is likely the default option for most HIE scenarios globally given the plethora of HL7 messages and clinical document types available for use as discussed in other chapters of this book.

Of note, a significant number of messages in Denmark utilize the United Nations rules for Electronic Data Interchange for Administration, Commerce and Transport (EDIFACT) standard. When MedCom was first developing the national HIE infrastructure, Europe was focused on developing EDI-based standards for interoperability within nations and across the continent. Denmark, however, did not want to wait for the European informatics federation to finish its development process. Therefore the Danes developed and implemented their own messaging standards based on EDIFACT. Today messages and documents rely on a combination of EDIFACT, HL7 V2, and HL7 V3 standards.

28.3.3.3 Deep integration

This approach requires that the data in both the sending and receiving systems be integrated such that if the data are updated in one system, changes are harmonized across the HIE network. The FMK in Denmark uses this approach, such that all systems used by prescribers push changes to the medication list immediately to the FMK. The FMK can then be immediately queried to retrieve the new information. In most scenarios, the data would be synchronized across two information systems, such that a change in one system would be immediately replicated in the other system. Unfortunately, this is not yet the case with the FMK but nonetheless medication data is the class with the deepest integration in Denmark.

This approach is often desired, so that all clinicians treating a patient have the same information. In fact, this approach is perceived by MedCom to be true interoperability. Yet, this approach is the most expensive and complex option. Synching with a canonical record hosted on the NSP may sound like the right approach for most scenarios, but it would require significant network bandwidth to handle constant queries of the individual's medical record. It would further require relationships to be defined such that the central database would know which providers and facilities need to be notified when an update occurs. Most of the time this would be the GP but could be nursing homes or specialists, depending on the patient and his or her health status.

28.3.3.4 Value proposition

When MedCom considers the three potential approaches, an important lens it uses is that of the value proposition to the three stakeholders. The CEO considers which entity benefits the most from a proposed approach. If all stakeholders, or the two entities exchanging the data, benefit with the more complex approach then investing in the more costly solution makes sense. If only one stakeholder or party benefits, then a lighter and less costly approach makes more sense given that health system resources are finite. Examining costs and benefits is important to consider when designing a solution at the regional and national levels.

28.4 HIE adoption and use

The HIE infrastructure in Denmark is heavily utilized. The number of messages exchanged on the MedCom SDN quickly grew from less than 1 million per month in 1998 to over 2 million by 2002 and then doubled again to more than 5 million by 2010 [12]. As summarized in Fig. 28.5, overall messaging across hospital, GPs, and municipalities as of 2022 is well over 15 million per month [17].

Because hospital discharge summaries are automatically sent to GP EHR systems and all prescription data are sent to or queried from the FMK, adoption of HIE is universal. Hospitals are the heaviest users of the HIE. They both send the highest volume of data and retrieve the highest volume of data from the national HIE infrastructure. At the local level, GPs use the HIE platform for telehealth, and they can view patient information via the portal. GPs can also access software like Epic CareLink to view hospital data in the two regions that implemented Epic in hospitals. The various uses and data exchanged are summarized in Table 28.1.

Utilization of HIE is mostly uniform across geographic regions as of 2021 as summarized in Fig. 28.6. These two charts represent normalized message volume for hospitals and GPs by geographic regions [17]. When adjusted for population size, message volume is similar, although hospitals in Northern Denmark and GPs in the Capital Region/Central Denmark are heavier users than their peers.

Although adoption is universal, not all clinicians actively use the HIE. Much of the HIE is used passively. Documents are delivered automatically for retrieval via the EHR. Informants estimate that only 20% of physicians use the portal. Medical students are not instructed on how to use it or integrate it into their

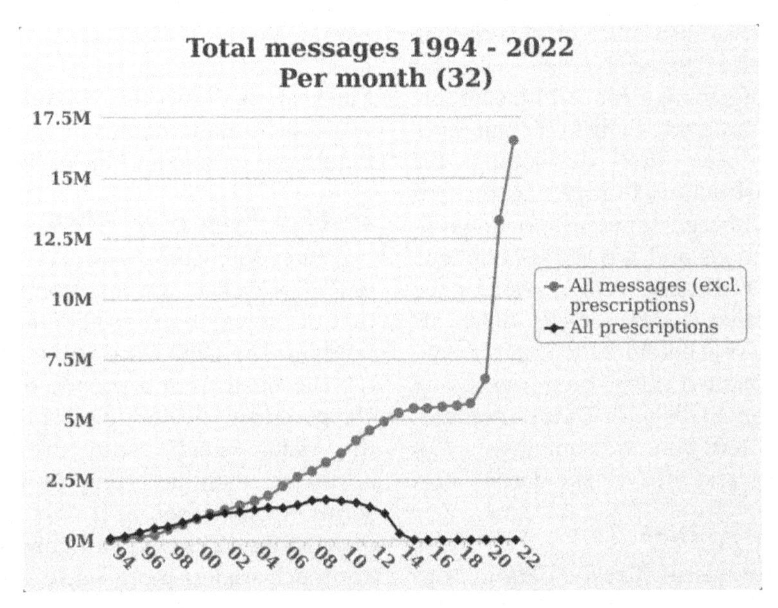

FIGURE 28.5 Average messages per month exchanged by hospitals, GPs, and municipalities across the MedCom network for the years 1992–2022 through February 2022. Source: *Used with permission from MedCom, adapted from MedCom. Overall traffic monitoring 1994 – 2022 Odense, Denmark: MedCom; 2022 [cited 2022 Apr 5]. Available from: https://statistik.medcom.dk/exports/medcom_monitorering_en.pdf [17].*

TABLE 28.1 Uses of the national HIE infrastructure in Denmark as well as the data types available via HIE along with the systems and standards used to facilitate exchange.

Purpose of use	Actors involved	Data exchanged	Standards or system leveraged
Medications: Providers prescribe medications and authorize refills; pharmacists dispense medications; patients request refills	GPs, hospitals, pharmacies, patients	Medication name, dose, route, administration	Portal (sundhed.dk) and FMK
Reimbursement: To be reimbursed, providers must submit encounter data	All providers	Encounter date, diagnostic codes, procedures performed	LPR
Past medical history: Using a variety of systems, providers and patients can view past encounters, lab results, and other medical history information	All providers, patients	Recent encounters, medications, recent laboratory results	Clinicians can view local data in their EHR; patients and providers can access outside data via the portal
Patient reported outcomes	Hospitals, patients	Physiological and psychological parameters [18]	WebPatient [19]
Discharge letters (summaries) to GPs	Hospitals, GPs	Date of admission, free text note from hospitalists	
Administration referrals	GPs, hospitals	Admission, discharge,	EDIFACT, HL7-XML
Rehabilitation	Municipalities, hospitals, GPs	Treatment plans	HL7-XML
Documentation terminology	Municipalities, GPs	Care and treatment procedures	Fælles Sprog 3, SNOMED CT

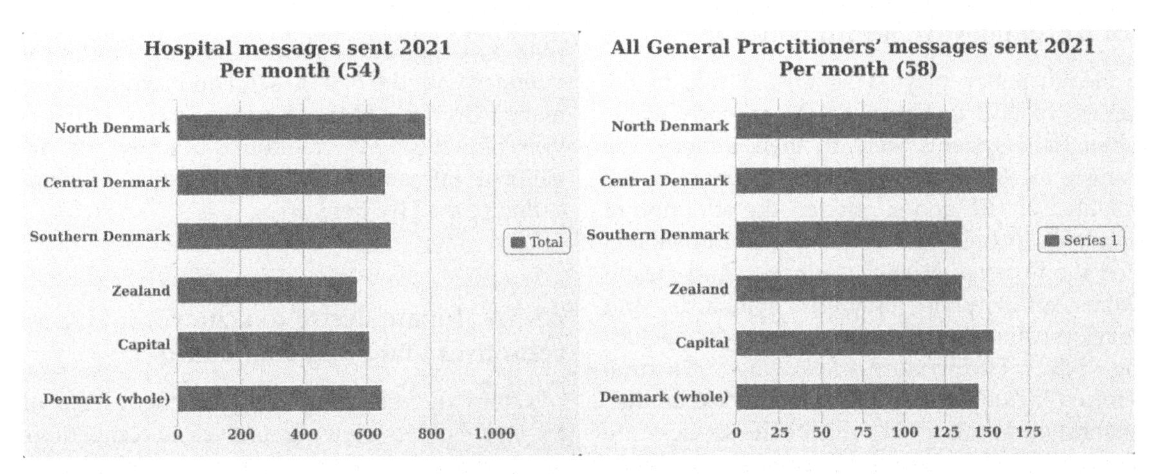

FIGURE 28.6 Average messages per month exchanged by hospitals (left) and GPs (right) across the MedCom network for the year 2021, stratified by Danish geographic region. The figures are normalized based on geographic population and represent the number of messages per 1000 citizens. Source: *Used with permission from MedCom, adapted from MedCom. Overall traffic monitoring 1994 – 2022 Odense, Denmark: MedCom; 2022 [cited 2022 Apr 5]. Available from: https://statistik.medcom.dk/exports/medcom_monitorering_en.pdf [17].*

workflow. Because of the COVID-19 pandemic, informants suspect more physicians are aware of it because the entire nation is more aware of it. There are even commercials for it online, on television, and on buses. Yet, active retrieval of information from the HIE infrastructure is rare. Nursing homes and GPs typically use their local health IT applications, and hospitals almost exclusively use their EHR systems. This might seem bizarre except for the fact that messaging and deep integration are so common that physicians do not need to push buttons or sign into separate applications to view data that come from the national HIE infrastructure.

28.5 Keys to success for Denmark

In this section, we review some of the fundamental keys to success for Denmark. Although the HIE infrastructure is not perfect, it is advanced in comparison to most states and nations. Their keys to success could be useful to other nations seeking to develop or evolve their HIE services or digital health infrastructure.

28.5.1 Supportive health policy

Health policy plays a significant role in the success of HIE in Denmark. At an early stage, when EHR systems were in their infancy, the Danish Health Data Authority recognized the potential of HIE and supported the adoption of standards. Administratively, the government created the National eHealth Authority and Health Data Authority to establish standards and develop national infrastructure resources, including NSP. Furthermore, following structural reforms in 2007, the health system stakeholders established a culture in which HIE services are required for major health IT contracts, establishing a foundational infrastructure upon which HIE can occur when it is needed.

An example of supportive health policy is the National Patient Registry—in Danish LPR, which is the national database of encounter records established by the Danish Health Data Authority. Policy requires hospitals, GPs, and specialists to send encounter records to the LPR in order for providers to be reimbursed for their services to the patient. The LPR functions as an all-payers claims database, since the Danish Health Authority is the single payer for health care. The LPR is further an important research platform, supporting studies [20,21] like in other Scandinavian countries that use population health registries for research.

The encounter records contain service dates, procedures, and diagnostic codes. However, there are no clinical values (e.g., vital signs, lab results) in the database. The requirement of sending records to the LPR using standardized messages via the national infrastructure—MedCom's HIE network—supports the existing infrastructure rather than create a one-off system that requires separate interfaces, messaging, and other technical specifications.

Additional policies also support the common, shared digital health infrastructure. These include the establishment and required use of the FMK as well as the use of the NSP for user authentication. Because pharmacies leverage the FMK to dispense medicines, all providers must interface with the NSP to send and retrieve information from the FMK. Requiring a core HIE service like the FMK reinforces the use of the national infrastructure, which ensures sustainability of the HIE network.

28.5.2 Innate desire to achieve consensus and build community

Danes are very community oriented. None of the stakeholders view themselves as competitors with others in the health system. In fact, perceptions are the stark opposite. Stakeholders see themselves as peers who must work together to lobby the government for what they wish to see happen in the regions, municipalities, etc. The health system uses a global capitation system, which means there is a finite level of resources to spend on digital health. Furthermore, these funds must cover projects at the national, regional, and local levels. Therefore it is the best interest of the stakeholders to achieve consensus around solving challenges rather than each entity working to establish its own solution.

This philosophy carries all the way down to the level of implementation. As one informant explained, if a single GP practice or region is not ready to implement a system or standard, no one in Denmark implements that system or standard. Although frustrating to those who are ready, the culture values a consistent way for each entity to exchange lab data, receive discharge summaries, etc.

This esprit de corps is driven, in part, by MedCom and its CEO, who takes his role as Chief Negotiator seriously. MedCom perceives its role to be that of consensus-builder, so the organization actively works across levels (e.g., national, region) to broker agreement on standards, approaches, and the data to be captured and shared for a given context. When the stakeholders come together to negotiate the financial terms of a new service or IT component, this provides an opportunity for MedCom to advocate for a common, consensus-based approach or standard to be used to achieve the goal. The stakeholders work with MedCom to hammer out a solution that will work for everyone.

Ensuring there is one FMK or one messaging standard for electronic laboratory reporting is a marvel and may seem impossible to individuals in other nations. Yet this approach is efficient, enabling national investment in the most appropriate system using a common approach that is built using standards-based exchange. Think about how much money could be saved in other nations if they used this approach to implement HIE and other population health services.

We note that the spirit of cooperation has carried over to other parts of the Danish eHealth ecosystem. In their profile of *sundhed.dk*, Jensen and Thorseng [2] describe the highly collaborative nature of the governance structure and committees involved in the development and sustainability of the platform. Given that these same stakeholders were engaged by MedCom in earlier eHealth activities including the development of eHealth standards, we believe that the MedCom philosophy spread to other parts of the health system and has become embedded in the Danish eHealth culture. In other words, what started at MedCom is now a guiding principle for digital health in Denmark.

28.5.3 MedCom the white hat organization

MedCom as an organization plays a critical role in the success of HIE in Denmark. Previously, this case study highlighted the important role that the technical infrastructure managed by MedCom plays in the digital health ecosystem. Furthermore, the HIO serves as a standards organization, advocating and establishing requirements for the use of syntactic and semantic standards. Moreover, MedCom serves as the organization that certifies compliance with standards for EHR products, other health IT vendors, and organizations that implement the consensus-based approaches to HIE across Denmark. These three functions are essential to HIE, and they are embodied in one nongovernmental organization.

MedCom contributes even more to the digital health ecosystem in Denmark. MedCom also supports GPs, elder care facilities, and smaller organizations that do not have their own IT department. MedCom connects these entities to the portal and NSP and helps troubleshoot connection issues, even though MedCom does not directly support the national platforms (they have their own IT staff).

For these many reasons, MedCom is perceived to be a "white hat" organization, meaning that it is a trusted, neutral organization that can help all stakeholders achieve their goals. Other HIOs, like the Regenstrief Institute that started the Indiana HIE (see Chapter 22), have been referred to as the Switzerland of HIE for the same reason. Nongovernmental organizations that work to advocate for HIE and standards, and which look for the "most appropriate" solutions to challenges rather than just use a specific technological hammer, are rare and highly valuable. MedCom is highly regarded by individuals across the three key health system stakeholder groups. These entities come to MedCom for advice, and they actively work to support its consensus-building approach to solving challenges.

MedCom performs its many roles with just 40 staff. The organization has an unassuming office in a tech park near the University of Southern Denmark in Odense in the central part of the country. Although it works largely in the background (citizens and physicians alike are unaware of its existence), MedCom's contributions to the Danish health system are enormous.

28.6 Challenges and barriers to HIE and data use

Despite its many successes, there are challenges to HIE in Denmark as well as the use of data from its national HIE infrastructure. Here we discuss some of those challenges reported by informants as well as the published literature.

28.6.1 Failed efforts at interoperability and HIE

During the past three decades, Denmark attempted three times to create a national HIE infrastructure. The first two attempts failed; the third one is in operation and described throughout this case study. The two previous attempts were both major health IT projects initiated by the national ministry of health:

- In 2001, the government attempted to address interoperability among disparate EHR systems in hospitals and GPs by establishing specifications to which all of the EHR vendors and health facilities were expected to adhere. These requirements were too complex for the vendors, and they required significant modifications to organizational workflows. This project was abandoned 5 years later [12].
- In 2011, the national eHealth authority initiated plans to develop a technical platform (National Patient Index) to link all health-related data across Denmark [12]. The approach was top-down and federated, meaning that distributed queries would search across all data sources, which would be required to comply with national specifications. After 2 years, the project was abandoned due to delays and a report questioning the feasibility of success [12].

These two failed attempts share a common theme: top-down approaches from the national government. The robust infrastructure in place today is driven by collaboration with bottom-up approaches in each region and active collaborative approaches across regions. The national government is a partner but does not dictate health IT development at the local and regional levels. This approach has yielded strong national platforms and infrastructure as well as common, standards-based approaches. Perhaps without these high-profile failures, success would not have been possible. Other nations (e.g., United Kingdom, Australia) that have tried heavy-handed national approaches have also learned painful growing lessons.

28.6.2 Using data for research and quality improvement

Like many nations, Denmark seeks to leverage its robust infrastructure to improve clinical and population health. Although like many countries Denmark has leveraged its encounters database (the LPR) for health services research [3], the nation now seeks to use EHR data, particularly at the local level, to create learning health systems and support academic research.

One challenge is in extracting and transforming data from EHR systems into national repositories. Multiple informants suggested that Epic's EHR is nearly impossible to work with, a notion supported by an online article criticizing the rollout of Epic in the Capital Region [22]. Informants complained that naming conventions for data are not standard and that hospitals struggle to extract useful datasets for local analysis. It is unclear whether these same problems exist with the Systematic EHR, although EHR systems in general are known to be challenging when it comes to data extraction.

Another challenge is data quality. There can be multiple dimensions to data quality, including timeliness, completeness, and accuracy. In a study by Geneviève et al. [23] that examined 345 population research studies from Denmark and Switzerland, the authors found that there were more facilitators overall to health data collection, sharing, and linkage reported in Danish studies. Moreover, Danish studies rarely reported political, economic, or ethical barriers to data sharing and linkage for research. However, there were more data quality barriers reported in Danish studies due to the re-use of data whose primary reason for collection was health care delivery versus a prospective cohort study. The review by Geneviève et al. [23] did not specify which dimensions of data quality were more prevalent, but prior work demonstrated that secondary use from EHR systems can often lead to incomplete or missing data challenges [24–27].

28.6.3 Limited awareness of HIE and multiple channels for access can equal confusion

Two phenomena observed about Danish HIE that lack of training and multiple ways to access the same information do not necessarily go well together. First, informants reported that there is limited training on how clinicians should access past medical history and other "outside" information on their patients. Medical students are not trained on the national platforms, only the local EHR in the region in which they are trained during internships. Furthermore, staff clinicians are not provided in service training on how to access the HIE infrastructure. Again, their focus is on the local EHR or information system. In some scenarios (e.g., discharge letter pushed to EHR system in GP office), information is delivered directly to the local EHR, which enables seamless access to the outside information. Yet in most HIE scenarios, clinicians need to use the portal or click a button from the EHR to launch a separate window in which they access data at the regional and/or national levels. At the local level, clinicians may need to log into a separate system, such as Epic CareLink in the Capital Region.

Given that there are multiple ways to access outside information, and the modes of access can vary by clinical scenario, clinicians can be confused leading to situations where available information is not utilized in the care delivery process. This phenomenon was observed in a series of interviews that researchers did with clinicians in multiple nations, including Denmark [28]. The researchers suggested that nations should create single approaches or gateways in which clinicians access external information. In Denmark, this could mean centralizing access via the button in the EHR maintained by MedCom. Instead of offering CareLink and other one-off methods, access to regional and national records outside the local EHR should be streamlined.

If multiple approaches exist, the researchers recommended placement of a "reference card" at each EHR terminal to guide clinicians on available HIE approaches [28]. These cards could detail under which clinical scenario each mode of access would be best to use and how to access outside information via the EHR or external site. Beyond the cards, Denmark should consider integrating training on HIE into medical education as well as in service trainings for staff clinicians.

28.7 Future directions

Although Denmark possesses a truly remarkable and resilient digital health infrastructure, the Danes recognized that their HIE efforts can improve and expand as well as innovate. Interviews with multiple individuals with EHR companies as well as MedCom, regional health authorities, and the NSP revealed a number of future priorities for Denmark. These may not be officially in the nation's eHealth strategy, but they are enhancements that Denmark's HIE and digital health leaders hope to see implemented in the coming years.

28.7.1 Setting Denmark on FHIR

Like many nations, Denmark seeks to evolve its infrastructure in such a way that it supports FHIR (Fast Healthcare Interoperability Resources), the newest set of interoperability standards published by HL7. As discussed in Chapter 10, FHIR uses a RESTful approach to accessing data via application programing interfaces (APIs) as opposed to the existing suite of messaging (Version 2) and clinical document (Version 3) standards. Nations seek to enable FHIR-based approaches to HIE in addition to messaging interfaces and clinical document exchange. The larger goal is to replace and augment existing interoperability methods, eventually maintaining more FHIR-based APIs as opposed to older messaging interfaces.

The CEO at MedCom would like to see several existing EDIFACT messaging methods replaced with FHIR-based approaches. Furthermore, MedCom would like to see FHIR-based approaches for all three important HIE methods: messaging, data sharing (e.g., query), and document sharing. FHIR supports all three common HIE scenarios. The change would improve performance and provide access to data rather than just messages that require parsing and normalization.

The challenge is how best to move the nation toward the use of FHIR. Once MedCom requires that health IT systems, including EHR systems, use FHIR-based APIs, it must certify those systems to ensure they are compliant with the new regulations. However, EHR system vendors have raised concerns, especially financial concerns, about moving to FHIR-based approaches. The vendors informed their customers that it would be very expensive to move to FHIR. The estimated costs are prohibitive for the nation as it comes out of the pandemic and faces limited resources given growing health care spending levels at the national level.

An alternative approach is being discussed wherein the VANSs would provide FHIR-based APIs for accessing information at the regional level. The integration platforms would establish the APIs such that the portal, NSP, and MedCom would use APIs implemented in each region to request data. The regions would extract data from EHR and other health IT systems, putting the data into a data warehouse at the regional level. MedCom could then certify FHIR compliance with the VANSs, and EHR companies would not need to implement APIs.

28.7.2 Quality reporting for specialty providers

Currently, the portal (sundhed.dk) is piloting a new program that calculates quality indicators for specialty physician practices. The goal is to provide these practices with quality reports showing how each provider compares to national benchmarks for specialty care. The service is similar to that of Quality Health First in Indiana (see Chapter 22) and the CRISP Reporting System in Maryland (see Chapter 25).

The program would allow specialty care providers to opt into the program. After consent, the NSP would extract data from the clinic's EHR system for storage in a centralized database. These data would be aggregated with other data sources available, including hospital and laboratory databases as well as the FMK. Aggregate, integrated data would create benchmarks at the municipality, regional, and national levels. The specialty clinics could then see how their patients compare to these benchmarks. At the time of writing, the portal was piloting this program with one–two specialties in the nation to examine adoption and use of the service.

This approach could be expanded in the future to include GP quality indicators. Currently, GP data are not available from the portal. An expanded quality reporting service could enable extraction of GP data into the national infrastructure, and enable better access to GP data by hospitalists, emergency room physicians, and specialists. It would also allow the Danish Health Data Authority to better understand quality of primary care. Expanding the program in the future would need to involve the Danish Organization of General Practitioners to ensure the program meets the needs of GPs in addition to the other stakeholders.

28.7.3 Enabling notifications for data harmonization

Currently, health IT systems query the FMK to retrieve a list of the patient's current medications. While the medication is reconciled and up-to-date, the FMK does not notify subscribers as to medication changes. Therefore, when the patient is discharged from the hospital, new medications are sent to the FMK and reconciled. Although GPs are notified of the event via the Discharge Letter, municipalities are often not informed of such events performed by another health system actor. For example, nursing homes would like to be notified of changes to their patients' medication lists. Recall that municipalities play a critical role of care coordination for patients, especially older and more vulnerable populations.

Another example is demographics updates. If a patient changes his or her mobile number in the GP EHR system, this change is not shared with other systems like the portal. Moreover, other systems cannot query the GP EHR to retrieve the new number. Demographic information is being discussed as a central type of data for which notifications might be beneficial. There is even discussion of a central repository like FMK for demographic information.

Updates to records could be provided using a web standards Publish/Subscribe model, which is used by the eHealth Exchange/Nationwide Health Information Network in the United States [29]. Alternatively, Denmark might consider event notifications, which is described in Chapter 27. Either approach would provide a messaging platform that would notify GPs and municipalities when the patient had a certain type of encounter or when their state (e.g., medication list, mobile number) changed.

28.7.4 Care coordination

Informants emphasized that integration between hospital information systems and the national HIE infrastructure is excellent. However, integration with the other major stakeholders remained limited and could be improved. For example, hospitals cannot view data from GP EHR systems even though GPs can view hospital data using the portal or a local application like Epic's CareLink in the Capital Region. Furthermore, hospital-based providers cannot view records from nursing homes or specialists' EHR systems. Bidirectional integration of these stakeholders is a focus of future efforts.

A specific example involves communication between emergency departments and nursing homes. Providers in the ED do not always understand the motivations for the nursing homes sending patients, especially in the middle of the night. The providers would like to see the nursing homes electronically send a brief note to the ED providers with their concerns. What triggered the nursing home to decide the patient needed to be transferred? What information should the providers know about this patient? This kind of care coordination HIE would improve quality of care in the ED as well as patient outcomes based on evidence from other nations that have implemented HIE in this clinical scenario [30–32].

28.7.5 Saving and parsing discharge summaries

Another key project for the future is updating how discharge summaries (aka letters) are managed. Currently, discharge summaries are sent from the source system (e.g., hospital EHR) to the local GP EHR using standard clinical messaging. However, these data are not stored in a database or repository at the national level. Some details about the inpatient encounter are stored, but not the rich detail available through a discharge letter, which is written by the hospitalist to inform the GP or next care provider about what happened during the inpatient encounter.

MedCom desires to see the discharge summaries captured in a national database by 2030. The goal is to develop a database like the laboratory records database or FMK for discharge letters. Data in each letter would be parsed, normalized, and stored in a persistent way such that the portal and NSP could query the repository for these details. This would enable query capabilities across inpatient visits and over time, enabling trending for an individual patient or a population.

28.7.6 Electronic patient data suitcases

Increasingly patients utilize a variety of medical and health devices in their daily life to support fitness, rehabilitation, or chronic disease management [33]. These devices are quickly becoming part of the Internet of Things, meaning they are connected to home-based Internet networks. This enables the devices to share the data they collect with other devices the patient uses and the patient's providers. Recognizing this trend, regional health authorities in Denmark are anticipating the need to connect these devices to VANSs and develop algorithms to analyze data provided by patient-controlled devices.

Currently, the regions are investigating how best to incorporate patients' device data into the digital health infrastructure. A couple regions are piloting a new solution referred to as "patient suitcases," which represents a bundle of devices that are provided to the patient for their use at home. The devices capture data as they are used by patients. These data are then transmitted to a third-party data center that organizes the data into a common, shared platform accessible to both the regions and municipalities. Clinicians can view data using the platform. The pilot is also developing clinical decision support functions on top of the platform to support decision-making, such as alerts when the patient's disease appears to be exacerbated or vital signs trend downward. Prompts to the patient or their clinicians may better support patient self-management of their chronic illness.

The current pilot is focused on COPD (chronic obstructive pulmonary disease), a chronic inflammation of the lung that results in restricted airflow. Emphysema (often caused by smoking) and chronic bronchitis are two common forms of COPD. Patients often use a rescue inhaler and take oral steroids to prevent further damage to the lung. However, COPD patients often utilize the emergency department or require inpatient services when their disease becomes unmanageable. The goal of the pilot is to reduce health care utilization, enabling patients to manage their disease better at home. The Danish Health Authority plans to expand the pilot to other chronic illnesses in the future based on the success of the pilot and their ability to develop other suitcases.

There are several important challenges to solve moving forward, assuming the pilot is a success. First, how should these data be integrated into the national HIE infrastructure? A third-party data center for every disease is likely not the best option. Decisions will need to be made whether the devices will interact with the NSP or VANSs. Second, patients would most likely want to track their data via the portal rather than a separate application. The portal will need to interact with the data center or ultimate platform in which the data are stored. Finally, not all of the data captured by patient devices will be useful; some are likely to be irrelevant. Providers and regions will need to work together to determine which data are most meaningful and which algorithms are most helpful to support patient self-management while reducing costs and improving health and safety.

28.8 Summary

As evidenced in this case study, Denmark possesses an advanced HIE infrastructure. Local, regional, and national health IT platforms are connected and regularly exchange data vital to care delivery, quality, and safety. A central force in the HIE infrastructure is a small but mighty HIO, MedCom, that facilitates negotiations between the major stakeholders to address critical health system challenges via HIE and interoperability. Certifying systems and establishing standards, this unassuming mediator is slowly advancing and evolving the digital health ecosystem. Respected and valued, MedCom has a strategic view toward the future, aiming to evolve not only the standards leveraged to facilitate exchange but also the HIE services available in Denmark and the more appropriate levels of integration to use to achieve the goals of the nation's digital health strategy.

Questions for discussion

Please provide at least five [5] critical thinking/review questions that require the learner to abstract broader concepts from the contents of the case study. Questions should ask probing questions that require the learner to think critically about the lessons of the case study.

1. What are the advantages and disadvantages of requiring consensus across all stakeholder groups before implementing a new HIE service? How might HIE be different in Denmark if each Region was free to set up its own HIE network?
2. Denmark has a robust HIE infrastructure with several important databases centralized at the national level. Would this approach work in your country or state? Why or why not?
3. Compare and contrast MedCom to another HIO you've read about in the book. Are there roles that MedCom plays in Denmark that the other HIO would benefit from doing? What might be the barriers to the other HIO performing some of the same roles as MedCom?
4. Why is it that Denmark simply has not settled on implementing a single national EHR system? What political, legal, industry, and practical concerns might be at play? Has being dependent on multiple vendors catalyzed Denmark's national HIE service infrastructure?
5. In a context with national HIE standardization institutions—who should bear the cost of compliance? What are

possible solutions if vendors refuse to offer standardized interfaces referencing the cost of doing so?

Acknowledgments

The authors gratefully acknowledge the time and information shared from a number of individuals interviewed for background on this case study. These individuals include:

Name	Title
Hans Erik Henriksen	CEO of Epital Health
Søren Vingtoft, MD	Chief Physician, Region Zealand, Ministry of Health
Steffen Lerche, MS	Principal, Healthcare, Netcompany
Lars Hulbæk	Director of MedCom
Claus Duedal Pedersen, MA	Director of the Sentinel Unit at Sundhed.dk
Mikael Bay Skilbreid, MSc	Engagement Manager at IQVIA
Claus Balslev, MS	Director at NNIT

References

[1] Danish Regions. IT brings the Danish health sector together Odense: MEDCOM; 2010 [cited 2022 Jan 27]. Available from: https://www.medcom.dk/media/1175/it-brings-the-danish-health-sector-together_3.pdf
[2] Jensen TB, Thorseng AA. Building national healthcare infrastructure: the case of the Danish e-health portal. In: Aanestad M, Grisot M, Hanseth O, Vassilakopoulou P, editors. Information infrastructures within European health care: working with the installed base. Cham: Springer International Publishing; 2017. p. 209–24.
[3] Schmidt M, Schmidt SAJ, Adelborg K, Sundbøll J, Laugesen K, Ehrenstein V, et al. The Danish health care system and epidemiological research: from health care contacts to database records. Clin Epidemiol 2019;11:563–91.
[4] Pedersen KM, Andersen JS, Søndergaard J. General practice and primary health care in Denmark. J Am Board Family Medicine 2012;25(Suppl 1):S34–8.
[5] KL. KL - Local Government Denmark [cited 2021 Jan 27]. Available from: https://www.kl.dk/english/kl-local-government-denmark/
[6] Kierkegaard P. Interoperability after deployment: persistent challenges and regional strategies in Denmark. Int J Qual Health Care 2015;27(2):147–53.
[7] Ministry of Health, Danish Ministry of Finance, Danish Regions, Local Government Denmark. A coherent and trustworthy health network for all: digital health strategy 2018–2022. Copenhagen: Sundhedsministeriet; 2018.
[8] Zelmer J, Ronchi E, Hyppönen H, Lupiáñez-Villanueva F, Codagnone C, Nøhr C, et al. International health IT benchmarking: learning from cross-country comparisons. J Am Med Inf Assoc 2017;24(2):371–9.
[9] Nøhr C, Bertelsen P, Vingtoft S, Anderson SK. Digitization of the Danish healthcare system: eyewitness accounts from key players. Odense: University Press of Southern Denmark; 2019. p. 251.
[10] Protti D, Bowden T, Johansen I. Adoption of information technology in primary care physician offices in New Zealand and Denmark, part 2: historical comparisons. Inf Prim Care 2008;16(3):189–93.
[11] Protti D, Bowden T, Johansen I. Adoption of information technology in primary care physician offices in New Zealand and Denmark, Part 3: Medical record environment comparisons. Inf Prim Care 2008;16(4):285–90.
[12] Kierkegaard P. eHealth in Denmark: a case study. J Med Syst 2013;37(6):9991.
[13] Rigsrevisionen. Beretning til Statsrevisorerne om elektronske patientjournalar pa sygehusene. Copenhagen: Rigsrevisionen; 2011.
[14] Nøhr C, Parv L, Kink P, Cummings E, Almond H, Nørgaard JR, et al. Nationwide citizen access to their health data: analysing and comparing experiences in Denmark, Estonia and Australia. BMC Health Serv Res 2017;17(1):534.
[15] Lonergan PE, Washington Iii SL, Branagan L, Gleason N, Pruthi RS, Carroll PR, et al. Rapid utilization of telehealth in a comprehensive cancer center as a response to COVID-19: cross-sectional analysis. J Med Internet Res 2020;22(7):e19322.
[16] Reeves JJ, Pageler NM, Wick EC, Melton GB, Tan YG, Clay BJ, et al. The clinical information systems response to the COVID-19 pandemic. Yearb Med Inf 2021;30(1):105–25.
[17] MedCom. Overall traffic monitoring 1994 – 2022 Odense, Denmark: MedCom; 2022 [cited 2022 Apr 5]. Available from: https://statistik.medcom.dk/exports/medcom_monitorering_en.pdf
[18] MedCom. Patient guides and method sheets 2015 [cited 2022 Apr 22]. Available from: https://www.medcom.dk/projekter/pro-i-almen-laegepraksis/patientvejledninger-og-metodeblade

[19] MedCom. Patient-reported information (PRO) in general practice 2021 [updated Jun 16]. Available from: https://www.medcom.dk/projekter/pro-i-almen-laegepraksis

[20] Matzen J, Bislev LS, Sikjær T, Rolighed L, Hitz MF, Eiken P, et al. The effect of parathyroidectomy compared to non-surgical surveillance on kidney function in primary hyperparathyroidism: a nationwide historic cohort study. BMC Endocr Disord 2022;22(1):14.

[21] Bager P, Wohlfahrt J, Fonager J, Rasmussen M, Albertsen M, Michaelsen TY, et al. Risk of hospitalisation associated with infection with SARS-CoV-2 lineage B.1.1.7 in Denmark: an observational cohort study. Lancet Infect Dis 2021;21(11):1507–17.

[22] Allen A. Lost in translation: epic goes to Denmark Copenhagen: Politico; 2019 [cited 2022 Mar 9]. Available from: https://www.politico.com/story/2019/06/06/epic-denmark-health-1510223

[23] Geneviève LD, Martani A, Mallet MC, Wangmo T, Elger BS. Factors influencing harmonized health data collection, sharing and linkage in Denmark and Switzerland: a systematic review. PLoS One 2019;14(12):e0226015.

[24] Lee SJ, Grobe JE, Tiro JA. Assessing race and ethnicity data quality across cancer registries and EMRs in two hospitals. J Am Med Inf Assoc 2016;23(3):627–34.

[25] Bahous MC, Shadmi E. Health information exchange and information gaps in referrals to a pediatric emergency department. Int J Med Inf 2016;87:68–74.

[26] Dixon BE, Siegel JA, Oemig TV, Grannis SJ. Electronic health information quality challenges and interventions to improve public health surveillance data and practice. Public Health Rep 2013;128(6):546–53.

[27] Liaw ST, Chen HY, Maneze D, Taggart J, Dennis S, Vagholkar S, et al. Health reform: is routinely collected electronic information fit for purpose? Emerg Med Australas 2012;24(1):57–63.

[28] Klapman S, Sher E, Adler-Milstein J. A snapshot of health information exchange across five nations: an investigation of frontline clinician experiences in emergency care. J Am Med Inf Assoc 2018;25(6):686–93.

[29] Office of the National Coordinator for Health Information Technology. Publish and Subscribe Message Exchange Washington: Department of Health and Human Services; 2021 [cited 2022 Mar 6]. Available from: https://www.healthit.gov/isa/publish-and-subscribe-message-exchange.

[30] Cross DA, McCullough JS, Adler-Milstein J. Drivers of health information exchange use during postacute care transitions. Am J Manage Care 2019;25(1):e7–e13.

[31] McCloskey RM. A qualitative study on the transfer of residents between a nursing home and an emergency department. J Am Geriatr Soc 2011;59(4):717–24.

[32] Zive DM, Cook J, Yang C, Sibell D, Tolle SW, Lieberman M. Implementation of a novel electronic health record-embedded physician orders for life-sustaining treatment system. J Med Syst 2016;40(11):245.

[33] Pandita D. Consumer health informatics: engaging and empowering patients and families. In: Finnell JT, Dixon BE, editors. Clinical informatics study guide: text and review. 2nd ed. Springer Nature; 2022.

CHAPTER

29

Addressing data needs for national HIV programs using HIE: case studies from Ethiopia and Nigeria

James M. Kariuki[1], Asaminew Petros[2], Ibrahim Dalhatu[3], Chinedu Aniekwe[4], Minen Sead[5], Gonfa Ayana[5], Adebobola Bashorun[6], Charles Nzelu[6], Bedri Ahmed Mumme[7], Kalechristos Abebe Negussie[8], Dereje Woldehanna[2], Lisa A. Murie[1] and Eric-Jan Manders[4]

[1]US Centers for Disease Control and Prevention, Center for Global Health, Division of Global HIV and TB, Atlanta, GA, USA [2]US Centers for Disease Control and Prevention, Addis Ababa, Ethiopia [3]US Centers for Disease Control and Prevention, Abuja, Nigeria [4]US Centers for Disease Control and Prevention, Center for Global Health, Office of the Director, Atlanta, GA, USA [5]Ethiopian Public Health Institute, Addis Ababa, Ethiopia [6]Federal Ministry of Health, Abuja, Nigeria [7]ICAP at Columbia University, Addis Ababa, Ethiopia [8]Clinton Health Access Initiative, Addis Ababa, Ethiopia

Major themes

- Health information exchange (HIE) implementation approaches in countries are driven by program needs.
- HIE framework enables improvements in the delivery of health service delivery and data use.
- Experience gained when adopting principles of HIE for one health program can inform scale up and application across the health system in a country .

29.1 Introduction

The human immunodeficiency virus (HIV) pandemic, and the international response that it has mobilized, has had an impact on the field of global health that is unprecedented. This response,

Health Information Exchange
DOI: https://doi.org/10.1016/B978-0-323-90802-3.00034-4

now nearing its third decade, represents one of the most significant programs in global public health in low- and middle-income countries (LMICs). It has also resulted in many of innovations in all aspects of the health sciences, and health care. Health services delivery, population health, and all ancillary services have all undergone transformational changes in the availability of health information systems (HIS); this chapter, highlights specific program use cases for the adoption of a health information exchange (HIE) platform in Ethiopia and Nigeria. In the context of this chapter, use case is defined as a unique instance of collecting, sharing, or using specific health information regarding a patient or program for a specific purpose or need, such as care coordination or program monitoring.

As the sophistication and scale of HIV programs have evolved, so have the requirements to measure their performance. The programs can only be improved and refined based on measurements of the programs. Essential metrics still include counting the number of people who are receiving HIV services; others are patient outcomes and measures of how well patients are living with a managed chronic condition. National HIV programs are now extensively monitored with performance indicators that measure progress both in geospatial granularity and at frequent intervals, allowing adjustments to objectives where needed. For example, indicators that track new HIV infections provide data needed for HIV program leaders, managers and staff to make decision on the kind of interventions needed depending on the populations and geographic locations affected. These data are also essential to the US President's Emergency Plan for AIDS Relief (PEPFAR) program to track progress, adjust program objectives, and optimize the design of newer program interventions [1].

Following the science and experience of implementing increasingly sophisticated health intervention programs, HIV programs are shifting toward a patient-centered approach, where a focus on high-quality care and individual patient outcomes, and influencing both at population level, are essential to further drive the progress in an HIV program [2,9]. From the HIS perspective, this means that clinical documentation for HIV services is instrumental to service provision. The need to track an individual for a lifelong episode of care puts a great demand on all aspects of clinical services documentation, and the integration of service delivery. The notion of a structure patient chart has often been introduced for HIV care services where previous documentation was based on unstructured provider narratives.

From the HIS perspective, essential needs in implementing a patient-centered approach include (1) managing the entire continuum of care, from testing through enrollment in an HIV program, and the longitudinal record needed for that; (2) managing the identity of the individual, with an evolving landscape of civil identifiers, health sector-specific identifiers, or even biometric identifiers, to ensure accurate patient identity; and (3) managing linked patient-level data to allow for the generation of information for different uses. These requirements result in the need to link patient-level information systems, manage the identity of patients in a coordinated way, and allow the exchange of clinical data between systems. Establishing an HIE framework provides a systematic solution to evolving the HIS support in a sophisticated national HIV program.

This chapter presents use cases from Ethiopia and Nigeria where HIEs are adopted at the national level and subsequently supported with an implementation that focuses on an essential aspect of HIV data integration. Introduction of HIE in these countries was done in conjunction with the Ministry of Health (MOH) to support HIV epidemic control. This use case, HIV epidemic control, is an important one for LIMCs as it unlocks resources to support HIE while addressing a major population health issue that can be extended to other existing or emerging health issues.

29.2 Background

29.2.1 Working toward adoption of health information exchange in countries

One of the strategic objectives for the global strategy on digital health 2020–2025 by World Health Organization (WHO) is to stimulate and support countries to have a strategy on digital health that suits their vision, context, and health trends. It encourages development of a national digital health strategy through a multistakeholder approach with consideration to the following core components: (1) leadership and governance; (2) investment and operations; (3) services and applications for scaling up; (4) integration and sustainability; (5) standards and interoperability (6) a flexible digital infrastructure; (7) an adaptable health workforce; (8) legislation, ethics policies and compliance; and (9) a people-centered approach.

The global strategy on digital health builds on resolutions adopted by the United Nations General Assembly and the World Health Assembly, related WHO global and regional reports, regional strategies, the two-part report of the ISO Technical Committee on Health Informatics on eHealth architecture, the resolution on ICD-11 and the WHO Family of international classifications and terminologies, the three-part National eHealth strategy toolkit, Member States 'current digital health situation and status, actions, strategies, policies and investments, and recommendations of various United Nations panels on digital and innovation topics [3–5].

Several countries have embarked on a process to develop or update their digital health strategies that have incorporated interoperability and HIE architecture as a core component for exchange and integration of data for patient care and to support monitoring of their health programs. Examples include:

- Ethiopia: The Ethiopia eHealth Architecture and the Information Revolution Strategic Plan 2018–25 identify the development of HIE and interoperability standards as critical components of an HIS enterprise architecture for Ethiopia [6]. In addition, the digital health blueprint identifies data exchange across systems as a priority intervention to build capability for electronic systems to communicate and exchange data through specified data formats and communication protocols based on nationally and internationally accepted standards.
- Cameroon: The 2020–24 National Digital Health Strategic Plan for Cameroon is a catalyst to produce guidelines on standards and interoperability to ensure their implementation and monitoring [7]. The plan includes a strategic objective to develop components that will improve the collection and exchange of consistent and accurate health information across geographical and sectoral boundaries.
- Nigeria: The national Health ICT strategic framework 2015–2020 provides a vision to enable and deliver universal health coverage. It provides a guide for alignment on existing digital health investments with enabling environment components including Leadership and Governance; Strategy and Investment; Architecture, Standards and Interoperability; Legislation, Policy and Compliance; Capacity Building; and Infrastructure and Solutions (Services and Applications) [3]. The framework recommends a national architecture that defines health information services, harmonization of digital information systems, and establishment of functional requirements for standards and interoperability to support consistent and accurate data exchange.

29.2.2 Health information exchange and global human immunodeficiency virus program data needs

People living with HIV receive diverse services to meet their health-care needs over time in different locations. It is important to ensure that they are linked to HIV care and treatment as soon as they are diagnosed and that they are retained in care.

The U.S. President's Emergency Plan for AIDS Relief (PEPFAR) has invested in the global HIV/AIDS response. PEPFAR has been critical in ensuring that that living with HIV are aware of their status so they can begin treatment, which saves lives and prevents HIV transmission to others and accelerating progress toward controlling the global HIV/AIDS epidemic in more than 50 countries. Since its inception, PEPFAR has supported development and implementation of digital health solutions to help manage patient care and programs in these countries. In line with the UNAIDS 95–95–95 goals to fast-track progress toward ending the HIV epidemic, PEPFAR have continued to strengthen HIS and HIE to provide coordinated care for people living with HIV, HIV case-based surveillance (CBS), improvement in program monitoring and systems interoperability to drive effective, efficient, and sustain able health care.

- *Patient care coordination*: HIV patients receive services in different locations over time. It is important to ensure that relevant information is available at the point of service to ensure a patient-centered approach, which integrates and coordinates various elements or aspects of the care they receive. Using information systems with processes, governance, and infrastructure for sharing and integrating data allows health care workers to access relevant information when providing care services for an individual. This helps reduce or eliminate fragmentation and/or duplication services to deliver consistent and appropriate care such as providing correct medication and doses, providing referral services, and informing decisions, such as initiating differentiated service delivery or changing medication based on laboratory results and managing complex cases, such as comorbidities or advanced HIV disease.
- **Case-based surveillance (CBS)**: CBS systematically and continuously collects available demographic and health event data (sentinel events) about persons with HIV infection from diagnosis and, if available, throughout routine clinical care until death, to characterize HIV epidemics and guide program improvement. Surveillance signals, such as high viral load (VL), mortality, or recent HIV infection, can be used for rapid public health action [10].
- **Program monitoring and planning**: Generating aggregate data to develop indicators to monitor and evaluate progress has been key to making decisions in the program. These indicators are used for M&E as well as planning available resources, such as medication, testing commodities, and health workers to be available where they are most needed.
- P**atient identity management**: The ability to accurately identify, track, manage and link individual patients is critical with the increasing quantity of electronic data and need to link healthcare data [11]. Patient matching helps with identification and linking of one patient's data within and across health care data sources in order to obtain a comprehensive view of that patient's healthcare record. At a minimum, this is accomplished by linking multiple demographic data fields, such as name, birth date, phone number, and address. Patient matching is a critical component to interoperability and the nation's health information technology infrastructure.

29.2.3 Key health information exchange technical considerations

Implementation of HIE involves the establishment of key technical infrastructure, human capacity, and procedures/governance that enables efficient and effective exchange of health information between disparate systems. The following are some technical aspects that are suitable and relevant to support implementation of HIE.

- Data standards (terminology and messaging formats): Establishing a standardized set of health data classes and data elements for interoperable HIE is key to implementation of HIE. Through this process, common message formats, and unambiguous, shared meaning for data to be exchanged are defined. This is important in addressing interoperability challenges resulting from variability in health information software products, implementations of those software products, their data models, coding schemes, and tools for extraction and transformation, all of which are burdensome for staff and their organizations and causes delays and data quality issues [8]. Using standards enables integration of data from disparate sources and eliminates the need to collect the same data multiple times. Routine data collected at the health facilities can also be leveraged for secondary purposes, including the establishment of a central repository of longitudinal, patient-level health records. For example, The United States Core Data for Interoperability is a standardized set of health data classes and constituent data elements for nationwide, interoperable HIE. The data class is an aggregation of various data elements by common themes or use cases and data elements are the most granular level at which data are exchanged.
- HIE architectures: Adopting the HIE approach improves efficiency of information exchange workflow by eliminating the need for patient level HIS to have point-to-point communication with other systems. A patient-level HIS only needs to communicate with the interoperability layer, which then mediates communication with other services and systems. This eliminates redundant communication, reduces the overall burden of work, and optimizes use of existing resources.
- HIS readiness to participate in an HIE: Data exchange capability could be integral to software application or platform design or enhanced to include data exchange functionality.
- Health data security, privacy, and confidentiality: Data security is a critical element that should be considered during exchange, storage, and use. Strategies to consider for health data security include defining when access to patient data for different purposes is permitted or limited, creating procedures that specify workforce roles that require access to health data, and developing security requirements and monitoring system use for unauthorized access.

29.3 Case studies

The case studies describe implementation of HIE to support HIV program in Ethiopia and Nigeria (Fig. 29.1). Each PEPFAR-supported country has a well-established national HIV program. Ethiopia and Nigeria have national HIV programs that have achieved or are close to achieving "Epidemic Control" [12]. That measure represents the concept that HIV can be eliminated as a public health threat at the national level. As the countries achieve epidemic control, the focus can shift from improving program performance to ensuring program sustainability. A well-functioning HIS is an essential factor in sustainability. Ethiopia and Nigeria represent two countries that introduced HIE as a concept in their national digital health strategies and followed through with an implementation to address existing challenges in their HIV programs.

29.3.1 Case Study 1 Establishing a HIV viral load data exchange through an HIE in Ethiopia

29.3.1.1 Background

The national viral load (VL) scale-up plan has been operational in Ethiopia since March 2016, with capacity developed at 19 VL testing

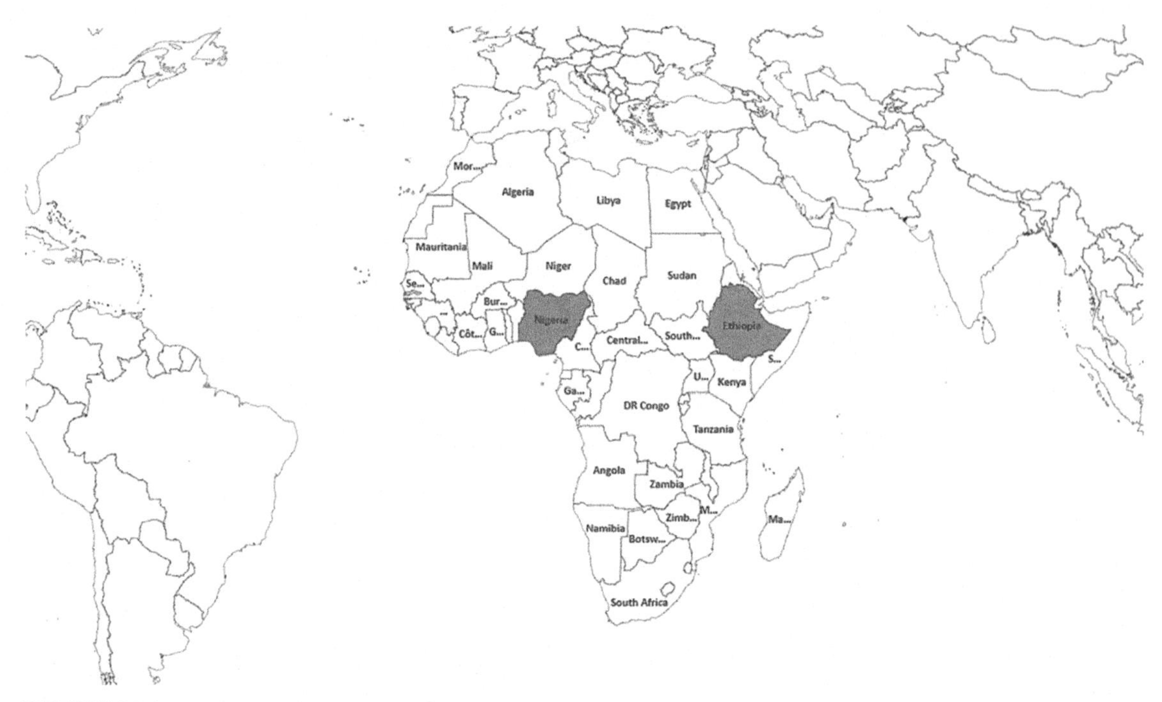

FIGURE 29.1 Map highlighting case study countries.

laboratories and specimen referral system linking the health facilities with testing laboratories. Specimens are collected from referring facilities by courier service and transported to testing laboratories. The results are delivered back to the referring facilities using the same service. Optimizing the system to consider distance between referring and testing facilities has not been straightforward. Preference to link facilities without crossing administrative boundaries may be one of the contributing factors for long turnaround time (TAT) for VL test result delivery. In addition, the paper-based system for VL requests has inconsistent and incomplete clinical and socio-demographic data and is not fully utilized for patient management. Entering data for the VL request and results at facility and testing laboratory using different systems for the same data duplicate the effort and is prone to errors.

Even though several e-health applications have been implemented in the Ethiopian health system, most of them are not capable of exchanging data. Historically, these applications have not exchanged data due to lack of nationally defined health information technology standards to guide development or customization of e-health applications resulting disparate systems. As Ethiopia implements its digital health strategy (since 2018) [6], it seeks to evolve systems toward HIE approaches. Implementing HIE architecture and leveraging available HIE platforms can help the existing HIS to exchange and use data.

The VL database system is locally developed and has been implemented in 19 VL testing sites, including Ethiopia Public Health Institute (EPHI), to capture and manage VL and Early Infant HIV Diagnosis data. At health facilities, SmartCare-ART electronic medical record (EMR) is used to capture and manage antiretroviral therapy (ART) patient data. Electronic VL Test Ordering and Result Reporting System (ETORRS) was introduced by collaborative stakeholders including

EPHI (MOH), CDC Ethiopia, Clinton Health Access Initiative (CHAI), and International Center for AIDS Care and Treatment Program, Columbia University (ICAP), to address the lack of data exchange between these two systems, resulting in longer total VL-TAT, poor data quality, and delayed clinical response for patients with high VL.

29.3.1.2 *Viral load request and return of results before health information exchange*

Clinicians at referring ART clinics order VL tests using a nationally standardized VL test requesting form. The clinician completes a paper form and sends two copies to facility's assigned laboratory. At the laboratory, a technologist collects the sample and fills additional details in the form, such as sample collection date and shipment date, and enters information for each test request and result when received in the VL logbook. At testing site, the receptionist/data clerk preprocesses the samples and submits accepted samples for analysis. The VL test results are filled in the VL requisition form sent with the sample and also entered to the VL database system before a copy is sent back to the facility.

At the referring facility, the test results are recorded in the logbook, the laboratory request form with the results is added to the patient chart, and test date and results transcribed in the follow-up form as well as the EMR by a data clerk at ART clinic.

The manual VL process for requesting and return of results between clinical sites and testing laboratories before HIE is outlined in Fig. 29.2.

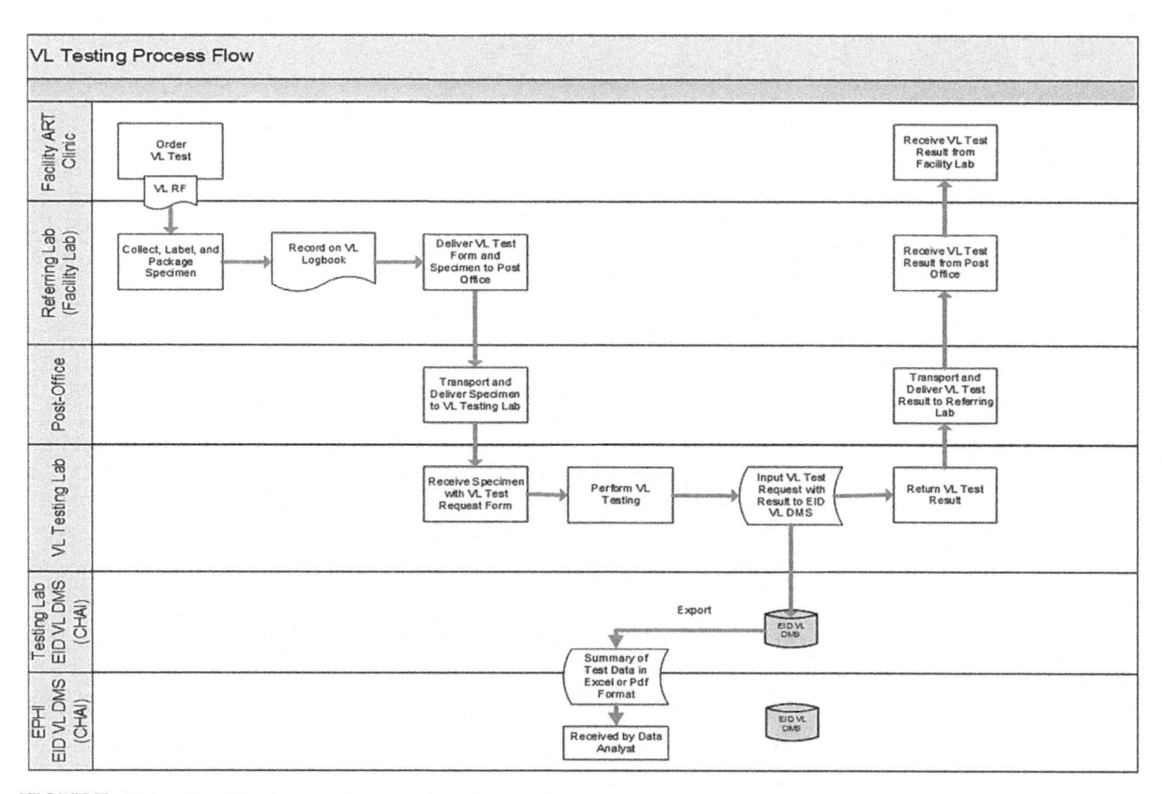

FIGURE 29.2 Viral load testing process flow (manual).

29.3.1.3 *Viral load data exchange using health information exchange*

The goal of ETORRS was to establish an HIE architecture based on OpenHIE, shown in Fig. 29.3, to facilitate the exchange of health records, particularly VL data between health facilities and testing laboratories using existing information systems. This allows health facilities to submit test orders to the VL testing laboratories and receive test results through the same channel to reduce site-specific TAT. In addition, clinical and socio-demographic data of a patient/client are shared with the testing laboratory when VL tests are requested to help improve monitoring of VL testing processes and results to support timely clinical decision-making.

ART provider at ART clinic initiates VL test order using the VL test request paper form, which is sent to the facility laboratory. After collecting the specimen, the laboratory technologist fills the additional information, such as sample collection date and shipment date in the VL request form, then sends it to the ART data clerk through assigned runner. The ART data clerk enters the laboratory request information in the SmartCare-ART EMR and then submits electronic VL test requests from SmartCare-ART EMR to the VL testing laboratory via an interoperability layer (IL). The facility laboratory collects paper copies of the electronically submitted VL test request forms from ART clinic through runner and ships the samples together with the

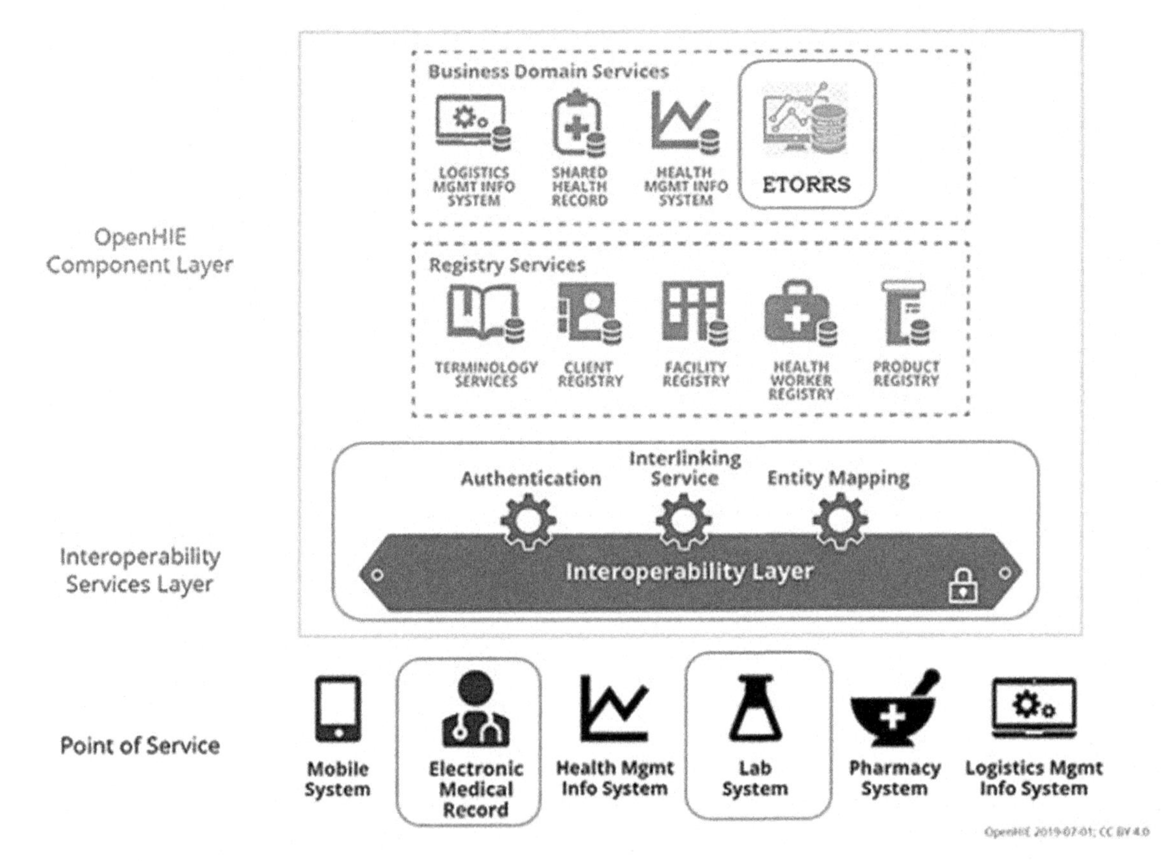

FIGURE 29.3 Electronic viral load Test Ordering and Result Reporting System (ETORRS) as a component in an OpenHIE-based architecture in Ethiopia.

VL test request forms to the mapped testing laboratory using the postal system.

At the testing laboratory, data clerks process the samples received using electronically submitted VL test requests from IL to the VL database. After performing VL test, the laboratory technologist completes the test result in the VL request form and submits it for approval by laboratory quality officer. The approved results are then entered in the VL database system by the laboratory data clerk. Then the laboratory quality officer reviews the results entered in the VL database system and approves release, and submission of the VL test results to health facilities electronically. Once the results are sent to the IL, they are visible in referring facilities' SmartCare-ART system as results ready for uploading. The ART clinic data clerk uploads the results to the facility SmartCare-ART system from the IL and prints copies of the results for ART providers.

ETORRS provides capabilities for electronic VL test and result data exchange between referring facilities and testing sites, Fig. 29.4. The system consists of three main subsystems: EMR-ART, responsible for electronic VL test ordering and result management from referring sites; VL database system, which handles incoming VL test orders and delivers results at testing sites; and OpenHIM, used as IL component and responsible for managing the routing of data exchange between referring and testing sites.

29.3.1.4 Development and implementation process

The development and implementation of VL data exchange between clinical sites and testing laboratories using HIE solution architecture

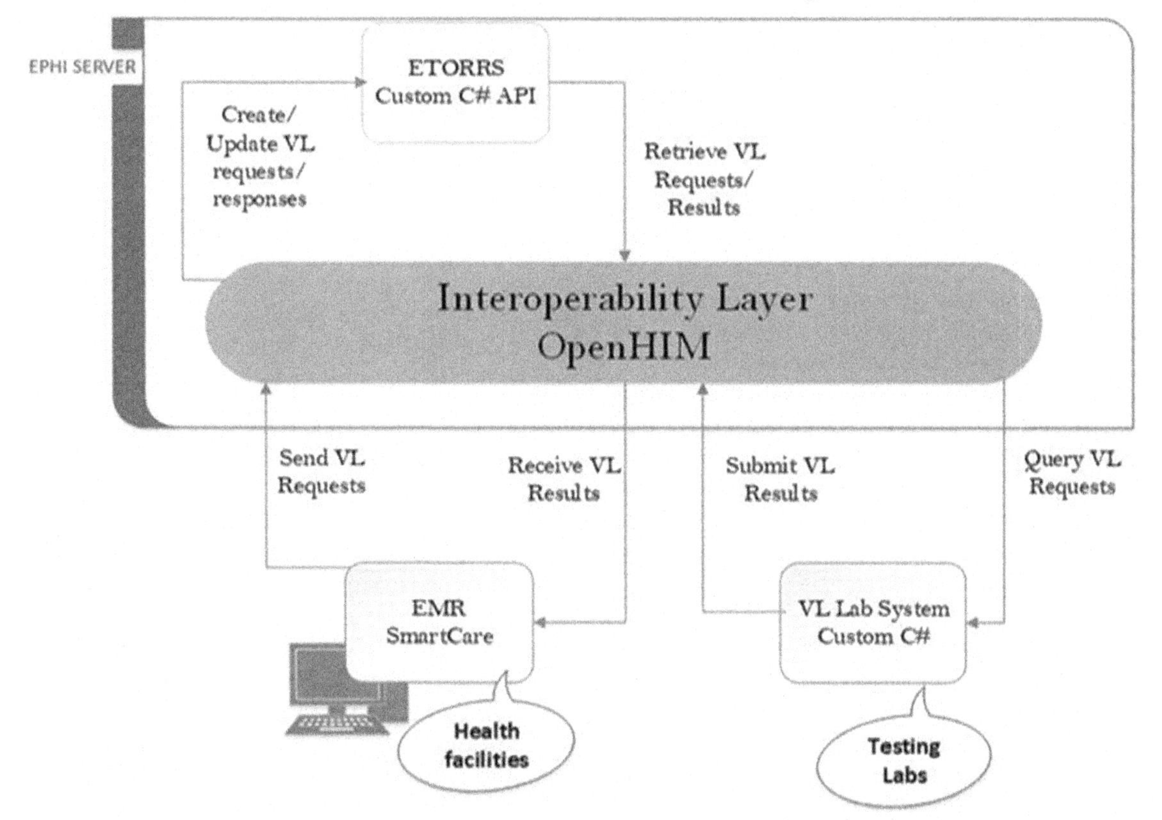

FIGURE 29.4 ETORRS data exchange process. *ETORRS*, Electronic viral load Test Ordering and Result Reporting System.

was led by a Technical Working Group (TWG) formed by all collaborative stakeholders (EPHI, CDC Ethiopia, ICAP, and CHAI). Recognizing that data exchange using a HIE architecture is a complex process and requires a long period of time to design and implement, and the TWG agreed to implement the trimmed version of OpenHIE architecture to focus on laboratory test data exchange between the SmartCare-ART and VL database systems using OpenHIM as the IL component.

After developing and testing ETORRS based on the solution architecture, TWG demonstrated the solution to a larger working group that included EPHI, CDC Ethiopia, ICAP, and CHAI directors for their endorsement. Upon approval, the solution was deployed in a few selected facilities as a pilot and then expanded to more facilities. The pilot was done in 13 health facilities and 3 VL testing laboratories in 2 regions, with close monitoring by the TWG. The pilot was concluded by performing an assessment and producing a preliminary report with pilot deployment findings and recommendations for further deployments.

ETORRS is currently deployed in 60 health facilities and 12 associated VL testing laboratories in 5 regions. Approximately 283 healthcare workers, including clinicians, laboratory technicians, and data clerks, have been trained. There are plans to scale up ETORRS service to 15 additional health facilities and associated VL testing laboratories and to enhance ETORRS service by incorporating additional features including SMS.

The following steps/activities were critical to the implementation of the HIE solution architecture to support VL data exchange between clinical sites and testing laboratories:

1. Establishment of a TWG that comprised of members from all collaborative stakeholders (EPHI, CDC Ethiopia, ICAP, and CHAI).
2. An assessment of ICT infrastructure (hardware, network, and other) readiness at EPHI and facilities (clinical sites and regional/testing laboratories). Issues identified with the LANs at selected facilities were addressed.
3. Analysis, design, and development of the software components, database, web APIs, and other services at the central server (EPHI), SmartCare-ART, and VL database system.
4. Development of system/solution documentations [software requirements specification (SRS), software design document (SDD), user manual, training manual, standard operating procedure (SOP), etc.].
5. Training for software developers on deployment and configuration of OpenHIM, the IL.
6. End-user training.
7. Deployment and configuration of the solution at facilities.
8. Maintenance and support following deployment.
9. Periodic assessment of ETORRS implementation.

29.3.1.5 Challenges

Even though SmartCare-ART and VL database systems can exchange data as part of an HIE architecture with the aim of reducing TAT and improving data quality, several challenges still exist, hindering stakeholders from achieving true interoperability for optimal care delivery and improved patient health outcomes.

The main challenges identified during monitoring and follow-up assessment are as follows.

- Data quality and completeness:
  - Medical Record Number and Unique ART Number discrepancies between paper request form and electronically submitted data, making it difficult to return result from VL Testing Lab electronically,
  - VL paper request forms were not properly completed, for example, incomplete and missing data, such as Date Specimen Collected and Date

Specimen Sent to Reference Laboratory, affecting TAT computation.

- Intermittent internet connection:
  - Most facilities use 3 G dongle as a primary internet source: its slow speed and poor connectivity are discouraging to users.
  - Increased probability of service interruption since 3 G uses mobile network.
- Stakeholders not following SOP:
  - Lack of smooth coordination and collaboration among actors for example the runner not picking shipment-ready VL request forms from facility laboratory or runner assignment is inconsistent.
  - Tight specimen shipment schedule does not allow time for staff to enter all VL requests electronically.
  - Poor communication while making changes to facility referral network (health facility to laboratory mapping) leads to electronic requests being sent to the old testing laboratory.
- Health facilities not using the result delivered in the system:
  - Data clerks not uploading ready results from the ETORR system.
  - Lack of result and report utilization for clinical intervention and decision-making.

29.3.2 Case Study 2 A National Data Repository as the enterprise data store in an HIE in Nigeria

29.3.2.1 Background

Nigeria's vision for digital health is to have healthcare information technology as an enabler toward the delivery of universal health coverage by 2020.[1] Through this vision, health IT will help improve availability of and access to data, patient identity management, human resource for health and coordinated supply chain for health commodities. This is envisioned in an architectural framework (Fig. 29.5) that introduces the concept of interoperability to integrate data from different HIS using HIE layer.

By 2015 Nigeria's HIV program had scaled up EMR systems across more than 90% of health-care facilities providing HIV care and treatment services. This scale up was key to ensure data for program management is available at all levels ranging from the healthcare facilities to state and national government agencies. This wide-spread implementation of EMR systems across the country and the need for data-driven decision making formed the foundation for HIE implementation in Nigeria.

Nigeria's HIE efforts are led by the government through the Federal Ministry of Health. The exchange between the EMR and the NDR is led by the Federal Ministry of Health with support from the United States Centers for Disease Control and funding form PEPFAR. There are several other stakeholders that contribute to this eco-system including the Global Fund, HIV program implementing partners and healthcare facilities. Stakeholders' contributions to HIE activities range from financial to technical as well as governance at different levels of implementation.

Two examples of data exchange use cases are in use

1. Data exchange between the clinical record systems (EMRs) and national repository of clinical records (National Data Repository) which sits within the National Health Management Information system.
2. Data exchange between EMR systems and the laboratory information systems.

These data exchange implementations are at different scales across the different healthcare organizations in the country. This case study

[1] https://www.health.gov.ng/doc/HealthICTStrategicFramework.pdf.

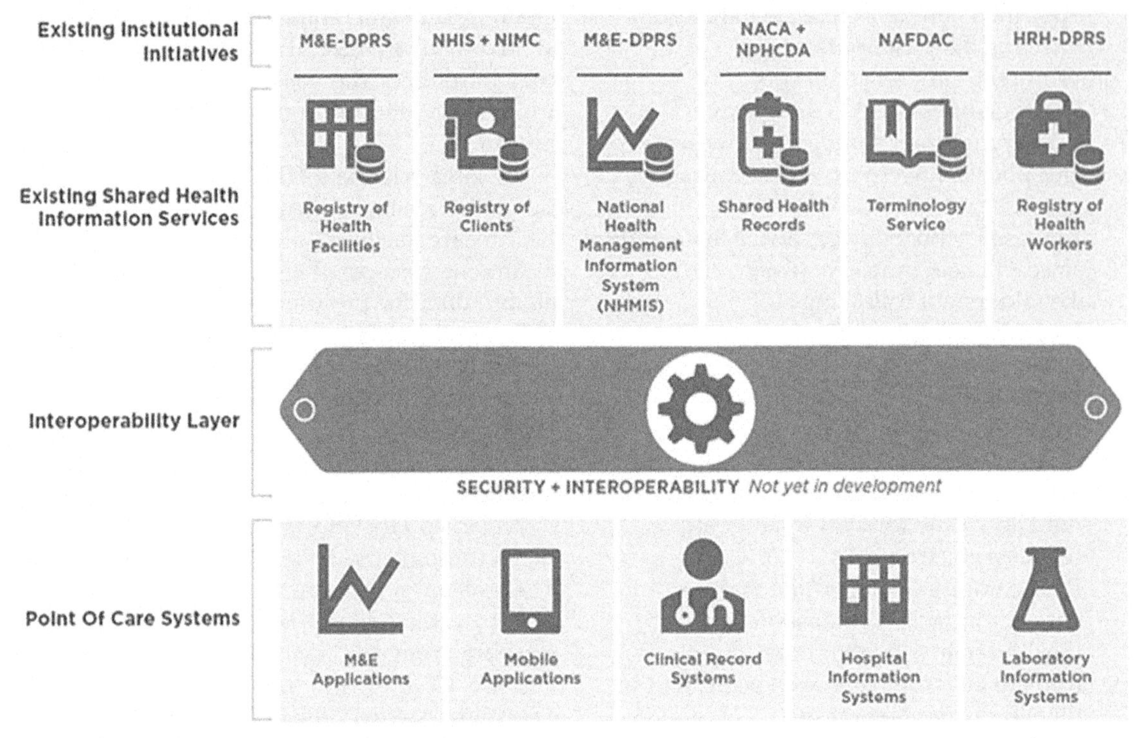

FIGURE 29.5 Interoperability architecture in Nigeria.

focuses on the data exchange between the EMR system and the National Data Repository (NDR).

29.3.2.2 Data exchange

In 2021 the focus for PEPFAR program in Nigeria was on client-centered care. This goal was driven by activities including continuity in HIV treatment, and viral suppression; and are enabled by near-real-time access to program data amongst other clinical strategies. Data exchange between the EMR and the NDR played a significant role in making data accessible to support near real-time tracking of key program indicators for reporting and monitoring program performance across supported health facilities, states, and implementing partners. This data between the EMR systems and the NDR have facilitated bringing together de-identified patient records from across health facilities enabling national de-duplication of records. Duplicates across health facilities are identified and removed or merged which has improved monitoring and evaluation of program goals and support record deduplication use cases. This de-duplication effort has led to discussions on the need to implement other related systems like a national client registry to support a unique identification system for healthcare delivery system across the country.

HIE between the EMR and the NDR also provides support for HIV case surveillance allowing de-identified case-based reporting and cohort monitoring of new and recent HIV infections for public health program monitoring.

Additionally, while not a primary use case, the data exchange has enabled a repository of historical de-identified health data set of persons living with HIV that is used for program evaluation studies.

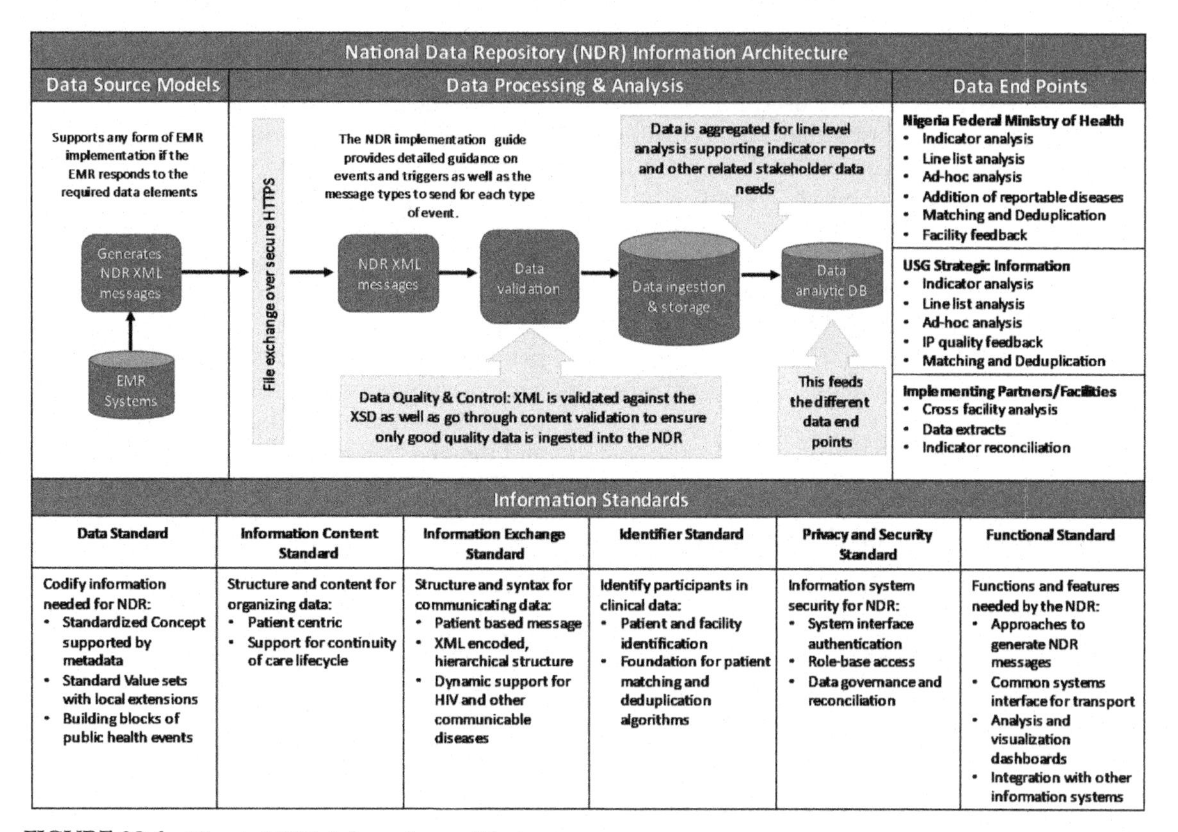

FIGURE 29.6 Nigeria NDR's information architecture.

The NDR's information architecture (Fig. 29.6), describes the data source, transport, data processing, and end points. It also describes information standards guiding data exchange between the EMR systems and the NDR.

29.3.2.3 Development and implementation process

Stakeholders meet routinely to access performance of data exchange between the EMR and the NDR. During these meetings, quality of data exchanged is assessed for fidelity and concurrence, new indicators are proposed, discussed, and included, existing indicators are modified if necessary, and indicators that are no longer needed are deprecated.

The message format for data exchanged between the EMR and the NDR is Extensible Markup Language (XML). The XML is based on an XML schema definition (XSD) document that describes the elements from the data dictionary that are contained in the XML exchanged. The business process for data exchange between the EMR and the NDR is guided by an implementation guide.

For data exchange to occur, data messages generated from the EMR systems are submitted to the NDR via a web interface over secure HTTP. When the data message files are received by the NDR, they are first validated against the XSD and thereafter go through data validation process. Only data message files that pass these validations are accepted and processed on the NDR. The NDR has a feedback mechanism to notify users of any failed files and reasons for failure.

Data messages that are processed successfully in NDR are analyzed using an analytic engine. The analyzed data are used for creating key reports and dashboards that are accessible by stakeholders. Some reports are entered into the national aggregate reporting system.

As of October 2021 more than 5 different EMR systems were used in over 2000 healthcare facilities across all of Nigeria's 36 + 1 states sending data to the NDR. The NDR contains over 1.7 million active HIV client records and receives on the average 650 messages (patient records) daily.

29.3.2.4 Barriers and enablers in the health information exchange implementation

There are several barriers in the implementation of HIE.

- Poor infrastructure is a major concern for most LMICs. Some of these includes lack of reliable and consistent internet access at service delivery sites which affects connectivity between sites and other locations where HIS are hosted. This hinders automated data exchange implementations. Consistent power supply is another infrastructural barrier with HIE implementation in Nigeria. While programs and implementers continue to find solutions to the power problems with alternative power sources, such as generators and solar-driven inverters, its implication is an increased financial cost of HIE implementation.
- Matching and record linkage are a key piece of HIE to help facilitate deduplication and longitudinal tracking of patients. Nigeria's health system does not currently have a unique identification system for health records. Each information system implements different forms of identification process, which makes it difficult to uniquely identify individuals and link records when the data are brought together at a central level. The current HIE implementations established ways to link records using a concatenation of hospital numbers and patient's hospital/treatment number; however, these approaches are not sustainable as individuals who visit a different health facility receive different identification numbers. A more systematic approach to unique patient identification that builds algorithms based on other patient demographic information may present more sustainable solution.
- Lack of defined standards for HIS implementation to facilitate interoperability and data exchange creates significant challenges. Most HIS implementations within the country were not built a priori following any national or international standard. Defining specific HIS and HIE standard is critical for scalability of any data exchange (such as the EMR-NDR exchange) to be implemented within the country's HIE eco-system.

Despite the barriers faced with implementing HIE, there are several factors that are enablers in Nigeria:

- The growing interest in HIE: several stakeholders are investing both technical and financial resources at different levels to implement HIS across different public health use cases, from EMR systems to immunization tracking systems to logistics information management systems, etc. As these systems continue to evolve, the need for data exchange between systems will continue to emerge hence HIE becomes inevitable.
- Local technical capacity: increase in the number of individuals who can design and implement HIS that exchange meaningful information is key to scalability and sustainability.
- Data-driven decision making: A systems thinking approach to health will require high-level program decision making to not

only be based on clinical records but also other related data on supply chain, personal health records, finance, etc. This growing need for wide variety of data from different sources will create a growing need for HIE. Nigeria health ICT strategy intends to support universal health coverage, and this will be made possible through interoperable systems that exchange data.

29.3.2.5 *Monitoring health information exchange and future plans*

Nigeria has two approaches to measure how the HIE is working. The first approach is a part of the routine data exchange monitoring, which runs data fidelity checks on files exchanged between the EMR and the NDR to establish concurrence. The second approach is more detailed and focuses not only on the quality of the data exchanged but also on other key HIE components (data use, funding, governance, privacy, data security, standards, infrastructure, business process, workforce) using a systematic evaluation framework.

Immediate future plan for HIE is implementation of a client registry to support unique identification and Introduction of an IL as a message broker within the current architecture to enable real-time data exchange, scale-up data exchange and ensure secure automated exchange of data between systems.

29.4 Summary

A country's approach to HIE implementation depends on several factors, including programmatic priorities, data exchange use case, stakeholders, existing information systems. The two case studies presented share several aspects that are similar, such as articulation of HIE in the national digital health strategy and implementation work undertaken under a technical working group led by MOH. There are also differences in the data exchange use case they implement; technical exchange implemented, which may be dependent on existing information systems capabilities, program priorities, and ICT infrastructure readiness at national and health facilities (Table 29.1).

A country can start with an HIE component and does not need a full HIE strategy for

TABLE 29.1 Comparison of health information exchange (HIE) implementation approaches in Ethiopia and Nigeria.

HIE implementation aspect	Ethiopia	Nigeria
HIE articulated in the national digital health strategy	Yes—The Ethiopia eHealth Architecture and the Information Revolution Strategic Plan 2018–2025	Yes—The national Health ICT strategic framework 2015–2020
Data exchange(s) use case currently in use	Patients HIV viral load test and result data exchange	Patients HIV clinical data
Information systems participating in data exchange to meet the use case needs	• EMR • Laboratory information system • Interoperability layer	• EMR • National data repository
Organizations leading HIE implementation	Technical Working Group formed by all collaborative stakeholders	Federal Ministry of Health with support from the PEPFAR and other stakeholders—global fund, implementing partners, and health-care facilities
HIE architecture/approach	Submits electronic VL test requests using SmartCare-ART EMR to the VL testing laboratory via and interoperability layer	Data messages generated from the EMR systems are submitted to the NDR via a web interface over secure HTTP

(Continued)

TABLE 29.1 (Continued)

HIE implementation aspect	Ethiopia	Nigeria
Coverage	60 health facilities and 12 associated VL testing laboratories in 5 regions	Over 2000 health-care facilities across all states
Stakeholders' engagement/ involvement process	Development and implementation	Development and implementation
Top priorities for HIV program	Address the lack of data exchange between these two systems resulting in longer total VL-TAT, poor data quality, and delayed clinical response for patients with high VL	Client-centered care to support continuity in HIV treatment, and viral suppression and tracking of key program indicators for reporting and monitoring program performance
How existing applications were accommodated to maximize their value in the HIE	Existing EMR and LIS applications were enhanced to generate information in a format that is exchanged	Existing EMRs were enhanced to produce XML data messages based on an XML schema definition document for exchange with NDR
Future plans for HIE		• Implement interoperability layer as a message broker for the current data exchange use case • Implement a client registry component in the HIE for unique patient identification

implementation to address a health program need or improve existing processes. These two case studies are examples in which priority program use cases enable focus on key components to implement within the HIE architecture. In Ethiopia, two point-of-care systems, EMR and LIS, and the IL participate in HIE to improve TAT of HIV VL data to ensure this information is available for clinicians when providing care. In Nigeria, point-of-care system, EMRs, and a data repository form the HIE to avail data for HIV treatment continuity, VL monitoring, and tracking key program indicators for reporting.

Discussion questions

1. What is the best approach for implementing HIE given that countries are at different points in their implementation?
2. How do you see evolving ICT infrastructure and human resource capacity influencing the future of HIE in your country?
3. How do you see the evolving patient identity management approaches and privacy considerations influencing the future of HIE implementation?
4. How do you see these priority cases evolving because of HIE implementation?
5. What other priority use cases do you see emerging in the future because of HIE implementation?

Acknowledgments

The HIV programs in Ethiopia and Nigeria have been supported in part by the US President's Emergency Plan for AIDS relief. Co-authors and staff from the US Centers for Disease Control and Prevention in Atlanta and at CDC offices in Ethiopia in Nigeria, have supported the HIV program through assistance with the implementation of HIS. The authors acknowledge contributions to this work from individuals the following organizations: ICAP at Columbia University in Ethiopia, Clinton Health Access Initiative in Ethiopia, and Ethiopian Public Health Institute. The authors thank Dana Dolan, TEKsystems/Peraton contractor for CDC, for assistance with technical writing. This publication/chapter has been supported by the PEPFAR through the Centers for Disease Control and Prevention (CDC).

Disclaimer

The findings and conclusions in this publication are those of the author(s) and do not necessarily represent the official position of the funding agencies.

References

[1] The Joint United Nations Programme on HIV/AIDS (UNAIDS), Understanding fast-track: accelerating action to end the AIDS epidemic by 2030. Geneva, 2015.

[2] Porter LE, et al. Beyond indicators: advances in global HIV monitoring and evaluation during the PEPFAR era. J. Acquir. Immune Defic. Syndr. 2012;60(Suppl 3): S120–6.

[3] World Health Organization and International Telecommunication Union, National eHealth Strategy Toolkit. Geneva: International Telecommunication Union World Health Organization; 2012.

[4] Seventy-first World Health Assembly, Resolution WHA71.7Digital Health. Geneva: World Health Organization, 2018.

[5] World Health Organization, eHealth standardization and interoperability, in 66th World Health Assembly. Geneva, Switzerland: World Health Organization, 2013.

[6] Ministry of Health Ethiopia. *Digital Health Blueprint*. Addis Ababa: Ministry of Health-Ethiopia; 2021.

[7] Republic of Cameroon Ministry of Public Health. *The 2020–2024 National Digital Health Strategic Plan*. Yaounde: Ministry of Public Health; 2020.

[8] Holmes JR, et al. Status of HIV Case-Based Surveillance Implementation—39 U.S. PEPFAR-Supported Countries, May–July 2019. Morb Mortal Wkly Rep 2019;68(47):1089–95.

[9] World Health Organization. *Consolidated guidelines on person-centred HIV strategic information: strengthening routine data for impact*. Geneva: World Health Organization.

[10] Kim AA, et al. Tracking with recency assays to control the epidemic: real-time HIV surveillance and public health response. Aids 2019;33(9):1527–9.

[11] Gliklich RE, Dreyer NA, Leavy MB, editors. Registries for Evaluating Patient Outcomes: A User's Guide [Internet]. 3rd edition. Rockville (MD): Agency for Healthcare Research and Quality (US); 2014 Apr. 17, Managing Patient Identity Across Data Sources. Available from: https://www.ncbi.nlm.nih.gov/books/NBK208618/.

[12] The Joint United Nations Programme on HIV/AIDS (UNAIDS). UNAIDS DATA 2021(2021).

CHAPTER

30

Health information exchange in Taiwan: multiple layers to facilitate broad access and use of data for clinical and population health

Hsyien-Chia Wen[1], *Li-Hui Lee*[2], *Nimish Valvi*[3] *and Brian E. Dixon*[3,4]

[1]School of Healthcare Administration, College of Management, Taipei Medical University, Taipei, Taiwan [2]Department of Health Care Management, National Taipei University of Nursing and Health Sciences, Taipei, Taiwan [3]Center for Biomedical Informatics, Regenstrief Institute, Inc., Indianapolis, IN, USA [4]Department of Epidemiology, Richard M. Fairbanks School of Public Health, Indiana University, Indianapolis, IN, USA

Major themes

The following themes from the book are explored in this case study:

- Taiwan provides an example of a government facilitated health information exchange (HIE) network that utilizes a federated architecture.
- The HIE network in Taiwan supports the government's administration of universal health care in which patients can receive health care from a variety of providers, including traditional Chinese medicine doctors.
- Citizens in Taiwan are issued a unique, universal health identification number along with an identification card with an embedded security chip that allows for the provision of healthcare services (e.g., eligibility checking) as well as retrieval of information from the last six visits.
- Policies that require the use of HIE systems for reimbursement compel health facilities and providers to use the technologies, resulting in improvements in quality and safety as well as the reduction in health system costs.
- The national HIE network in Taiwan utilizes syntactic and semantic standards to facilitate the interoperable exchange of clinical documents between electronic medical records (EMR) systems.

Health Information Exchange
DOI: https://doi.org/10.1016/B978-0-323-90802-3.00027-7

- The national HIE network benefits from Taiwan's robust information and communications technology infrastructure, including high-speed internet bandwidth available to medical facilities.

30.1 Introduction

Health information exchange (HIE) in Taiwan emerged in the early 2000s due to three interrelated phenomena: (1) universal health coverage, enabling citizens to receive health care from any provider; (2) broad adoption of electronic health record (EHR) systems, making digital health data available; and (3) Taiwanese culture that embraces technological innovations, including information technologies. The national HIE infrastructure in Taiwan features three related HIE networks managed by the National Health Insurance Administration (NHIA). The governmental-facilitated HIE network is multilayered, patient-centric and distributed, enabling patients and providers to access medical records in support of efficient, safe, and quality health care services. Taiwan saw important health care spending reductions following the introduction of HIE. The HIE infrastructure adapted quickly during the COVID-19 pandemic to facilitate access to information on test results, vaccination, and personal protective equipment.

In this case study, we examine the multipronged HIE infrastructure in Taiwan. First, we examine Taiwan and its universal health system. Next, we explore the three independent but related networks that comprise the complex, multilayered approach to HIE available across Taiwan's health system. We further examine how each network is used and how together, HIE is broadly available to maximize access to patient medical records on demand by providers as well as patients. The case study concludes with planned features as well as challenges Taiwan plans to address in the future.

30.1.1 The Republic of China (Taiwan)

The Republic of China (Taiwan) is located in Southeast Asia and neighbors China, Japan, and the Philippines (Fig. 30.1) [1]. Total population is 23.4 million persons. Land area is 35,808 km^2, resulting in a population density of 648 people per km^2, which ranks 19th in the world [2]. GDP per capita of Taiwan is $32,123 (2021), which ranks 29th in the world, and its national health expenditure to GDP ratio is 6.6% [3] compared to the United States, which spends 18% of its GDP on health care [4,5].

Taiwan's life expectancy is 80.94 years; 77.7 years for males, and 84.2 years for females. The fertility rate is very low at 1.15 births per woman, and adults over 65 years of age account for 16.1% of the total population in 2021, with estimates projected for over 20% in 2026, constituting a demographic shift toward a super-aged society. Cancer, heart disease, pneumonia, cerebrovascular diseases, and diabetes are the top 5 causes of death, making chronic diseases a major health priority [6–8]. Taiwan has a variety of healthcare personnel and medical institutions, including 58,347 physicians (this includes 7,302 traditional Chinese medicine doctors); 172,966 registered nurses; 479 hospitals; and 22,653 clinics [9].

30.1.2 Taiwan's health system

Taiwan implemented its *national health insurance (NHI)* system in 1995. The NHI is classified as a single payer compulsory social insurance plan with a centralization of funds collected by monthly premium from citizens. The NHI is characterized by good accessibility, comprehensive population coverage, short waiting times, low cost, and national data collection systems for planning and research. Although its weaknesses include variable quality of care, a weak gatekeeper role, and increasing financial pressures by overused available medical resources [10], data show that

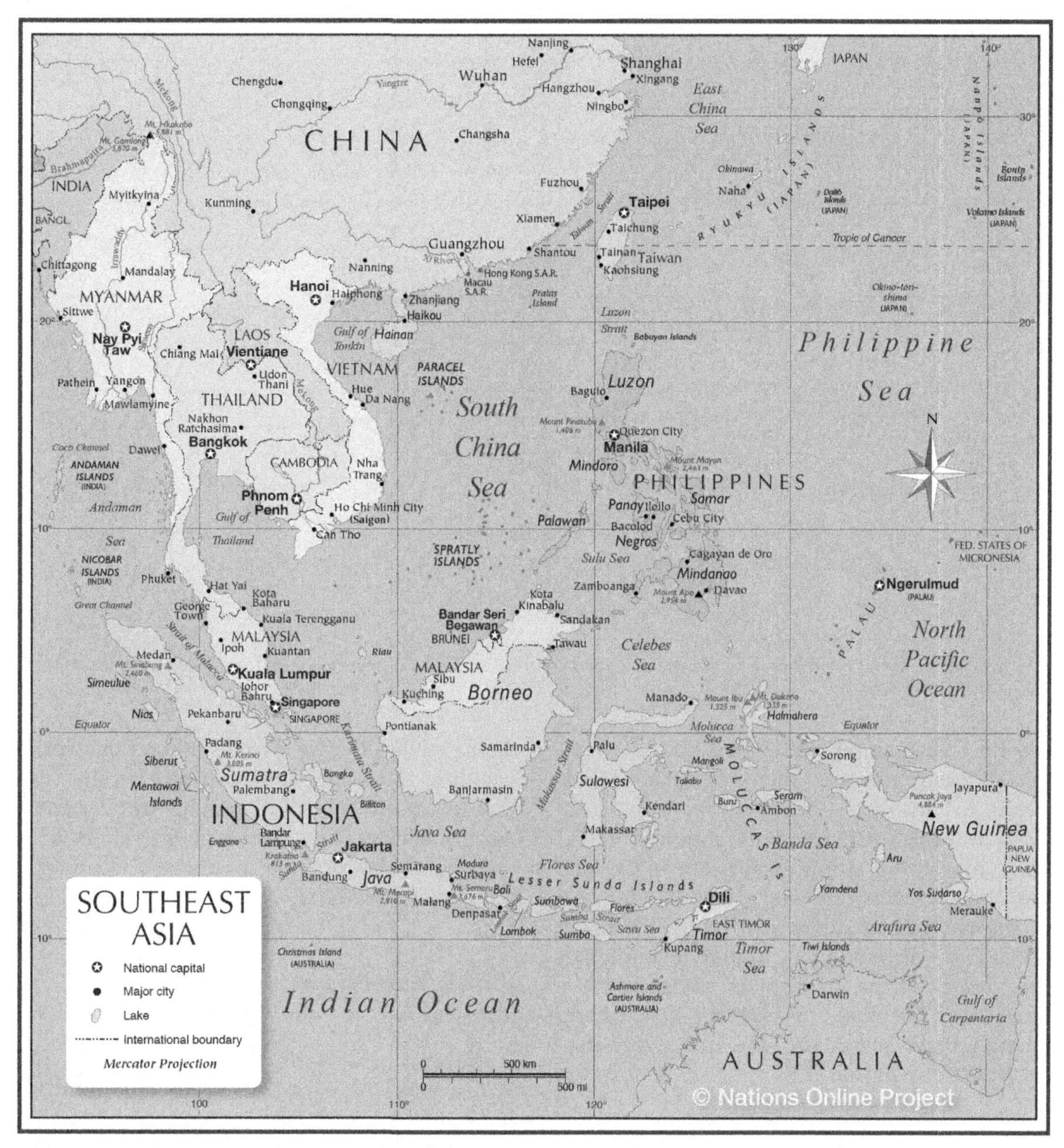

FIGURE 30.1 Map of Southeast Asia that includes the Republic of China (Taiwan). Taiwan is close to Japan, China, and the Philippines. Source: *The Nations Online Project (nationsonline.org).*

Taiwanese people recognize the value of NHI services with satisfaction rates increasing over the years (Fig. 30.2), maintaining an average rating over 80% from 2015 to 2020 [11,12].

To comply with NHI reimbursement policy, hospitals and clinics must claim their medical expenses electronically. Health care providers established *Health Information Systems (HIS)* not

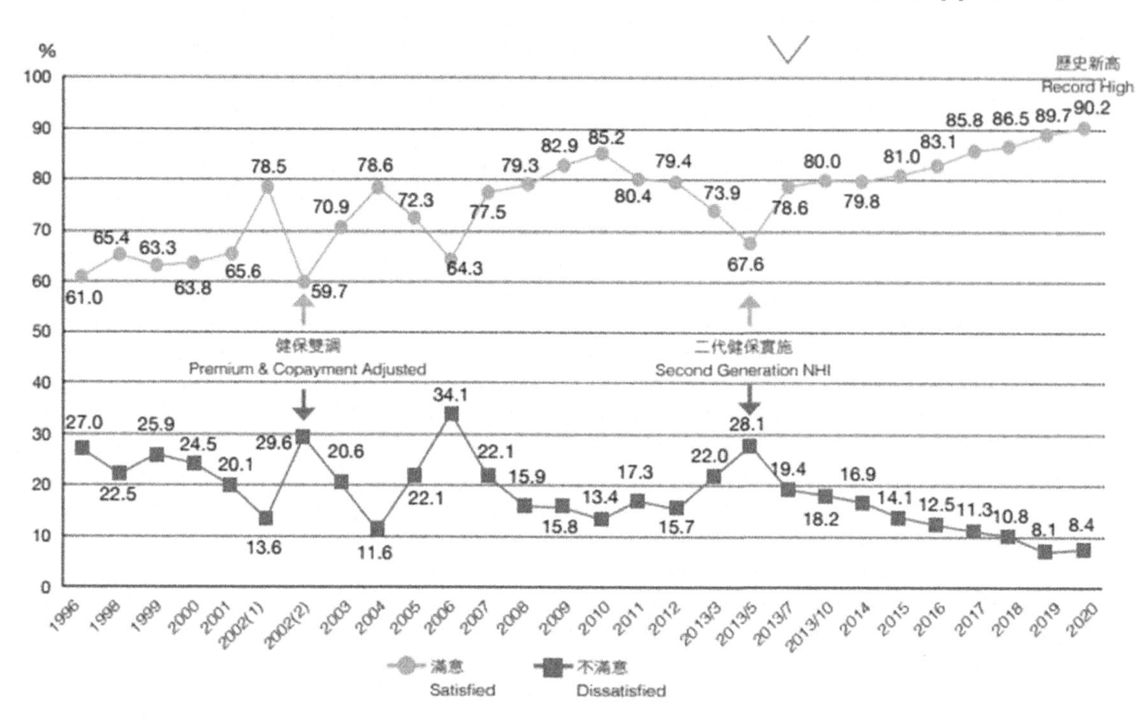

FIGURE 30.2 Trend of NHI Satisfaction rate survey from 1996 to 2020. Source: *2020–2021 National Health Insurance in Taiwan Annual Report.*

only for collecting billing data and daily operations, but they also use HIS for hospital accreditation to improve quality of care [13]. In addition, health information technology (HIT) integrated with a strong healthcare infrastructure and advance planning plays a vital role for the nation's epidemic control [14]. During the COVID-19 pandemic, digital technologies were used for preventing or mitigating the impact of infection disease by identifying potential cases and control the spread of infection in the population [15].

30.2 Background on Taiwan's national health insurance system

Taiwan's HIE network operates within and aligns its goals with the NHI. Taiwan's health policy planners took 7 years to carefully study alternative health care systems around the world, including Germany and Canada. Because the NHI program is critical to the development, implementation, and sustainability of HIE in Taiwan, we describe the context and technology necessary for the NHI.

30.2.1 Enrollment and universal coverage

Taiwan's National Health Insurance Act (Article 8, 9) [16] requires compulsory enrollment of all citizens and foreign nationals living in Taiwan for longer than 6 months. It ensures adequate risk pooling and the broad-based collection of funds to finance the NHI system. Currently, more than 99.6% of Taiwan's population is enrolled and covered, compared to preimplementation when roughly 41% of the population was uninsured [17]. Therefore the NHI system increased healthcare coverage, improving social justice. The NHI system aligns with the World Health Organization's target of universal health coverage (see Chapter 15).

30.2.2 Financing and administration

The NHI system is financed with income-based premiums. A uniform enrollment process and one flat premium rate apply to those insured, regardless of their sex, age, health, or employment status. The insured, employers, and the government contributed 36.92%, 29.30%, and 33.78% of the premiums for the NHI, respectively [18]. The monthly premium pay for insured is affordable. Also, patients need to pay out-of-pocket payments when they encounter health care services, but those who cannot afford co-payments received public assistance.

NHI is run by the *NHIA*, which is a government division of the Ministry of Health and Welfare (MOHW) and the single purchaser of health care services. The single-payer system enables Taiwan to manage health spending more efficiently and effectively. It facilitated the government to negotiate fee schedules under global budgets to contain the growth of NHI expenditures (like Maryland, see Chapter 25). NHIA promptly uses provider and patient profiles to identify and reduce fraudulent claims, overcharges, duplication of treatments and services. Moreover, one uniform reporting procedure and claim filing system greatly reduced transaction costs. For example, the administrative budget for the NHIA was a mere 1.07% of NHI's expenditures in 2014 [18], which is much lower compared to the United States and Canada [19].

30.2.3 Accessibility and comprehensive coverage

Taiwanese citizens can seek treatment from physicians, specialists, or any level of hospitals, directly without a referral. A variety of health care services are provided by 93% of the hospitals and clinics, which have contracts with the NHIA [10,11]. Patients have easy access and complete freedom of choice to these contracted providers, and they enjoy a high degree of timely access to care without worrying about waiting times [18]. All services are reimbursed by NHI from western medicine, traditional Chinese medicine, dental care, medications, telemedicine, and preventive medicine providers.

30.2.4 Information technology

During the creation of the NHI, the government invested in robust information technology (IT) infrastructure, developing centralized and integrated electronic patient databases in Taiwan. All claims from hospitals and clinics are requested to file and process electronically by NHIA, and its claims review process checks for the overall appropriateness of claims. The NHIA recognized early on that it could track utilization and costs by profiling of both patients and providers in near real time.

Taiwan's EHR systems were initially developed by the National Health Informatics Project in 2004. The nation's EHR plan was implemented in three stages: Stage 1 (2008–11) promoted the EHR strategy and adoption of EHR systems; Stage 2 (2010–12) accelerated EHR system adoption in hospitals and clinics; and Stage 3 (2013–15) subsidized the interoperability and application of EHR systems [20]. As of 2019, 411 of 496 hospitals (80.4%) and 5244 of 9782 private clinics (53.6%) were certified as having interoperable EHRs [21].

Moreover, the NHIA implemented two IT initiatives in 2014 aimed at improving quality and empowering patients for better managing their health care [18]. The first is Medi-Cloud program (previously, Pharma-Cloud), developed to enable the prescribing physician to check for prescribed drugs or exams by different doctors that the patient visited within the past 3–6 months. The program sought to avoid potential adverse reactions among multiple drugs, duplication of prescriptions, and unnecessary tests. The second is the "My-Health-Bank," a personal health record (PHR) that contains the patient's complete medical history for the past year, which can be checked from the Internet and mobile phones. The PHR enables insured citizens to check their past treatment history and manage their own health condition. During the COVID-19 pandemic, all citizens were able to use the PHR to check their mask purchase records, laboratory testing results, and vaccinations. This tool enabled the government to identify and track infectious disease outbreaks quickly [15].

30.2.5 Information systems management

The information management division of NHIA is responsible for all NHI information systems, which includes HIE. NHIA has six regional divisions across Taiwan, and each has an information management office to handle insurance enrollments, premium collections, utilization review and reimbursements, and management of contracted medical institutions (Fig. 30.3).

The information management division of NHIA consists of six sections, which are responsible for: insurance information, medical information, administrative information, information services, information engineering, and information planning. The number of full-time employees is about 152 and the details of their tasks in the division of information management are listed below:

1. The overall planning, design, promotion, maintenance, review, and evaluation of information systems and information security, as well as education and training.
2. The planning, installation, and management of computer hardware, software, database, and overall network.
3. The utilization review, monitoring, analysis, and adjustment of computer equipment and network.
4. The operation, management, maintenance, and troubleshooting of the host computer and its peripheral equipment.
5. The establishment, operation, and maintenance of the insurance certificates information management center.
6. Planning and management of internal and external integrated information platforms.
7. Research and development, statistical analysis, and technology promotion of information business.
8. Other issues related to information management.

The information management division of NHIA provides internal and external services to various stakeholders, such as hospitals, clinics, vendors, and departments of civic servant (Fig. 30.4). Clinics and hospitals are requested to follow the NHIA technical guidance and data formats to submit their claims. The annual budget of NHIA offers financial subsidies to providers to expand the network bandwidth of their **virtual private network (VPN)** infrastructures, which facilities pay for, to enhance the efficiency of electronic transactions.

IT forms the backbone for Taiwan's NHI that facilitates the single-payer system to gather comprehensive information on patients and providers, which is used to monitor and improve clinical quality and health outcomes. It is in this context that Taiwan's HIE efforts have developed and evolved over the past 8 years.

30.3 Health information exchange to support the NHI

The NHI system operates three independent, but interrelated, HIE networks that facilitate exchange of administrative as well as clinical data among NHI stakeholders, providers, and patients. Each HIE network plays a unique role within the NHI system in support

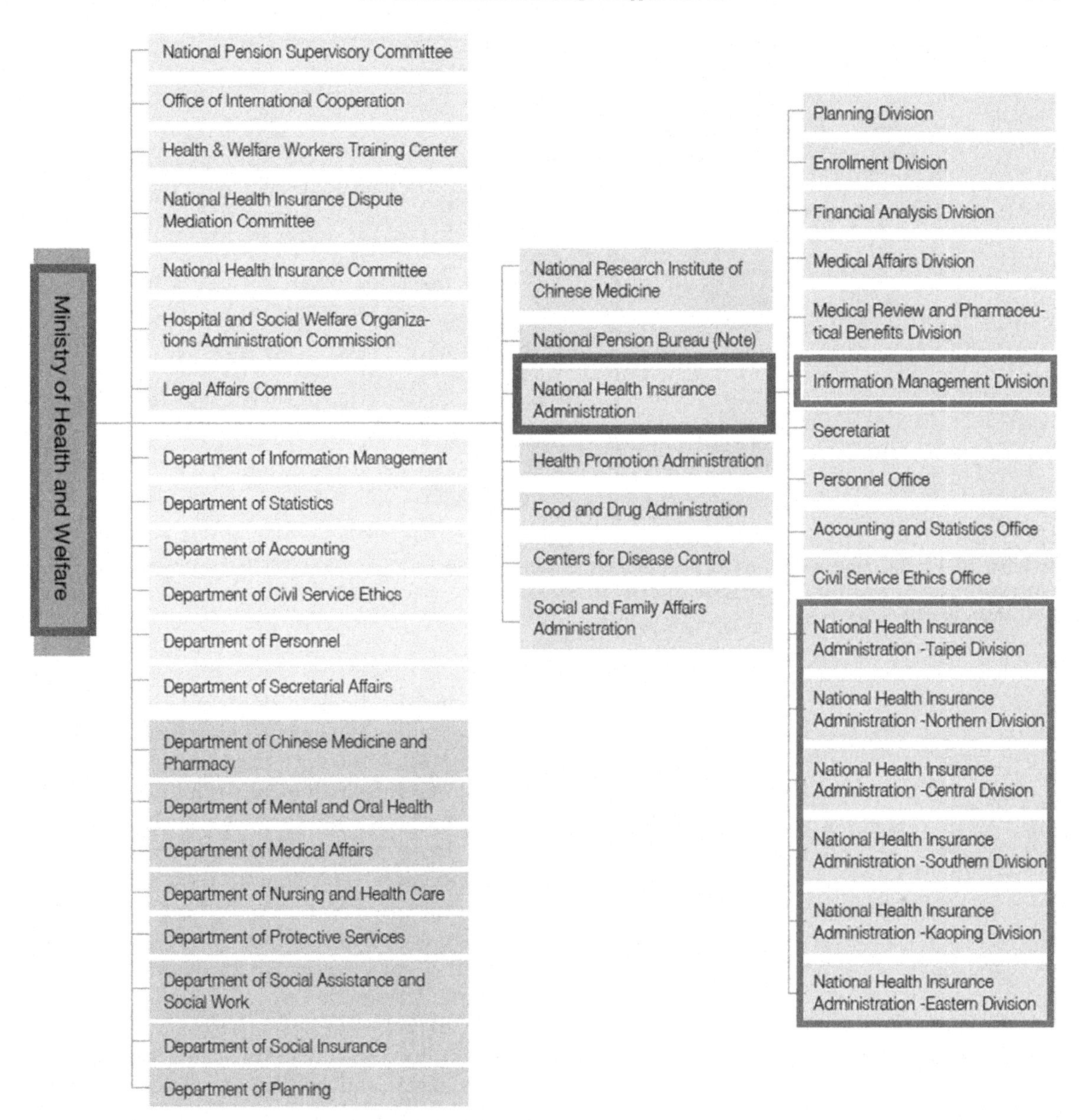

FIGURE 30.3 Organization Chart of the Ministry of Health and Welfare (MOHW) [22].

of claims adjudication, care delivery, and population health. First, we describe each network independently. Then we examine how these networks function together to facilitate universal health access, safety, and quality of care.

30.3.1 The NHI IC card network

All citizens enrolled in the NHI program are issued an identification card (NHI-IC card), which is a smartcard that contains an

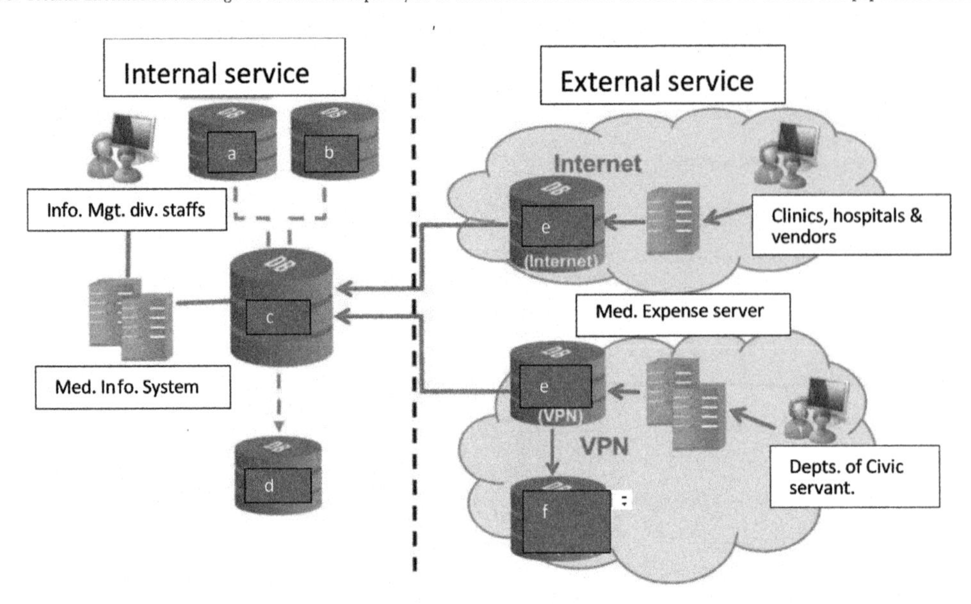

FIGURE 30.4 The framework of National Health Insurance (NHI) information system [23]. **Internal services:** (a) computing server; (b) underwriting server; (c) medical server; (d) warehouse server; **External service:** (e) expense claim server; (f) expense claim backup server.

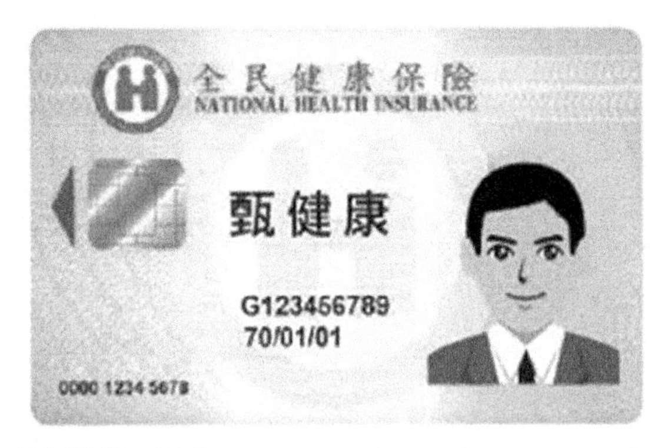

FIGURE 30.5 Example of the National Health Insurance identification card (NHI-IC Card), issued to all citizens of Taiwan who enroll in the national health insurance system [24].

identifiable photo (Fig. 30.5). All individuals must use their NHI-IC card to access healthcare services at every visit.

According to the National Health Insurance Act, NHIA must produce and distribute NHI-IC cards to patients with electronic information processing functions to store and send ambulatory treatment and major laboratory test information [16]. A memory chip embedded in this card stores information regarding the **past six visits** to a health care provider, including **diagnoses, prescriptions, allergies, vaccination, and insurance data**. The NHI-IC card is presented by an individual at a clinic or hospital, and the provider swipes his or her own NHI-IC card through a card reader at the same time, and data are transmitted to the NHIA instantly (Fig. 30.6) [21].

The following functions of the NHI-IC card are beneficial and helpful for patients seeking medical attention:

1. Clinical treatment

The NHI IC card serves as the authoritative record of treatment, recording all physicians' prescription and examination records. It stores records of medication usage and past examinations as a reference for doctors to not duplicate prescriptions,

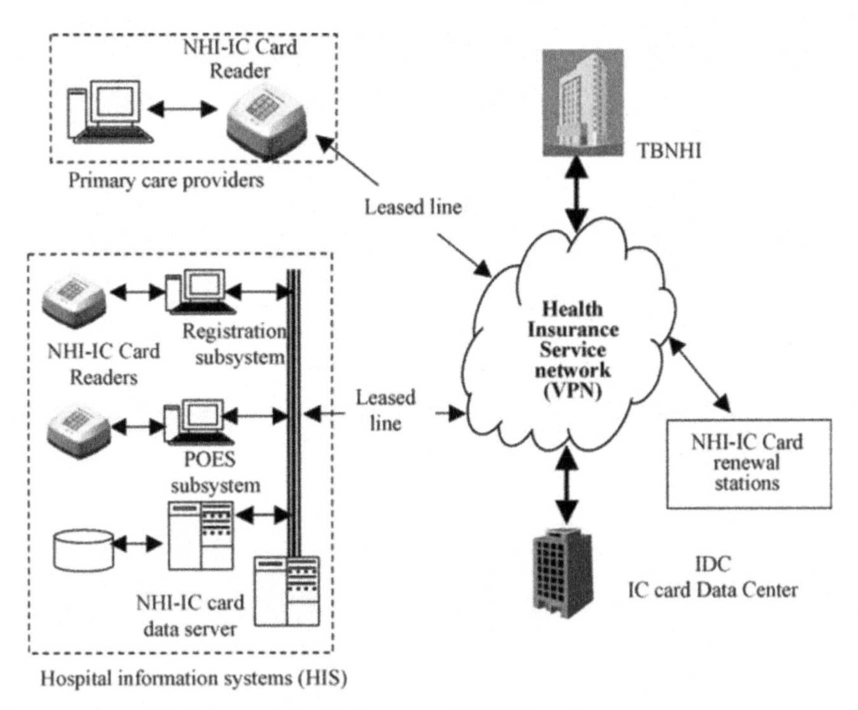

FIGURE 30.6 The framework of National Health Insurance (NHI) IC card system.

exams, or tests. This helps reduce medical errors and enhances the quality of care.

2. **Auditing mechanism**

   NHI IC card ensures patients' completed enrollment procedures for their medical benefits, daily updates to medical visit data for the last six medical visits, and traces or monitors infectious disease. It detects heavy users and provides reminders and alerts of drug prescriptions and allergies, which safeguard patient safety.

3. **Registration for special purposes**

   The card records catastrophic illnesses for patients who are treated without having to pay a co-payment. Organ donation, palliative care, or advance decisions like do-not-resuscitate information are also written onto the card when the NHI database is updated, helping clinicians make timely decisions.

30.3.2 The NHI MediCloud System (NHI-MCS)

To enhance the quality of care and reduce unnecessary treatments using cloud technology, NHIA established the "NHI MediCloud system" to facilitate physicians checking recent patient diagnoses or clinical treatments and assist pharmacists to prepare medications for patients. This system, introduced in 2013, was constructed on the NHI information network service system of a VPN. When patients seek medical attention at 25,885 NHI contracted medical service institutions, physicians can query medical treatment information using the three-card (safety module card, medical personnel card, and patient's NHI-IC card) certification approval.

The MediCloud system (formerly known as the PharmaCloud system) now includes 13 categories of information: western and Chinese medicine records, test/examination records and results,

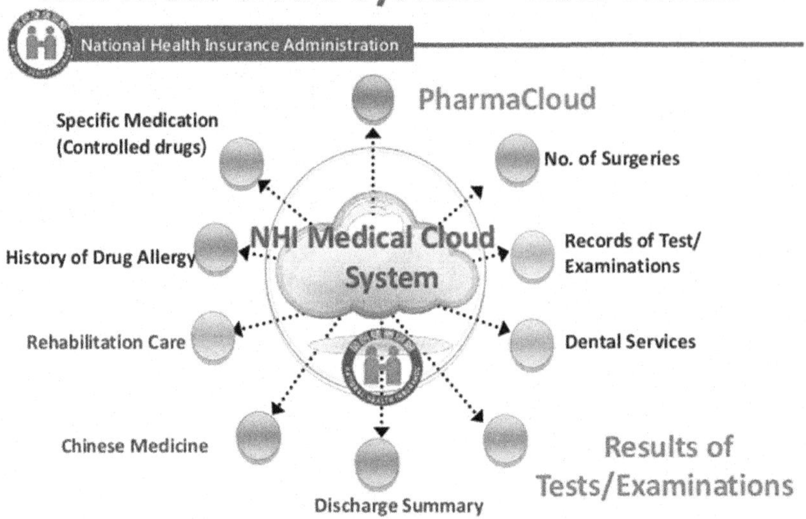

FIGURE 30.7 Services of the NHI MediCloud System (NHI-MCS) [24].

dental treatment and operation notes, specific controlled, coagulation factor or allergy drug usage records, rehabilitation medical records, discharge summary, and vaccination records from the Taiwan Centers for Disease Control. These categories are summarized in Fig. 30.7.

Starting from January 2018, hospitals and clinics were incentivized to provide a timely upload of blood test results, medical examination images and reports, such as computed tomography (CT), magnetic resonance imaging, gastroscopy, colonoscopy, ultrasound, and X-ray, etc. Failing to upload data would result in the loss of payment from NHIA for the service delivered to the patient. Physicians use this system to retrieve medical reports and images to avoid unnecessary medications, exams, and improve the medical service quality [25].

30.3.3 EEC health information exchange

This section describes the EMR Exchange Center (EEC), the third and newest HIE network developed to support the Taiwan health system.

30.3.3.1 Organization

EEC authority is the Department of Information Management (DOIM), Ministry of Health and Welfare (MOHW), Taiwan. The organizational structure for DOIM is shown in Fig. 30.8 [26]. There are three core managers, including a director, a deputy director, and a senior analyst. The director leads four divisions: (1) infrastructure and information security, (2) common information systems and services, (3) public HIS, and (4) social administration information systems.

For the maintenance and execution of EEC, DOIM has authorized and contracted with EBM Technologies Incorporated. To maintain and develop the clinical document architecture (CDA) specifications required by the EEC, DOIM uses a Project Management Office (PMO) through a contractor. HL7 Taiwan ran the PMO from 2001 to 2019. From 2020 onward, the Taiwan Hospital Association has continued to maintain the CDA specifications.

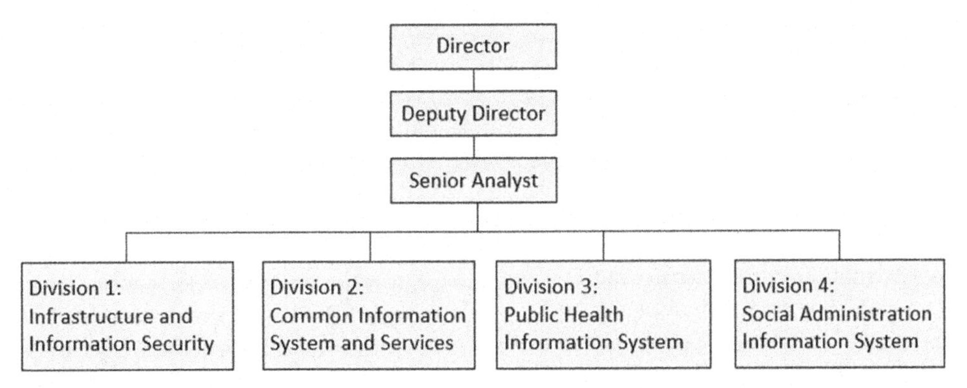

FIGURE 30.8 The organizational structure of the Department of Information Management in the Ministry of Health and Welfare (MOHW) of Taiwan.

30.3.3.2 Regulation

The regulations for EEC exchanging health information are listed below [25].

1. **Medical Care Act Article 70** [27]: Medical care institutions shall provide a copy of the patient's medical records or Chinese summary of medical records when necessary in accordance with the patient's requests and shall not delay or refuse without cause. The fee for the copy of paper medical records shall be paid by the patient.
2. **Medical Care Act Article 72** [27]: Medical care institutions and their staff shall not disclose without causing any information regarding a patient's illnesses or health, which are acquired by virtue of practice.
3. **Medical Care Act Article 74** [27]: When treating a patient, the hospital or clinic may contact any previous hospitals or clinics where the patient was treated for copies of medical records, medical record summary, and other examination reports as necessary, but only after obtaining the consent of the patient or his/her legal agent, spouse, kin, or interested party. The previous hospital or clinic shall not refuse to provide said information, and the patient shall pay the cost.
4. **Physician Act Article 23** [27]: In addition to the regulations in the previous article, a physician may not without reason reveal information about a patient's condition or health information that he or she is aware of or in possession of as a result of his or her practice.
5. **Nursing Personnel Act Article 28**: Unless otherwise provided for above, permitted by law or agreed by the person concerned or his/her legal representative in writing, nursing personnel or nursing institutions and their staff shall not disclose the confidential information of others acquired or held by them during practice.
6. **Regulations for the Production and Management of Electronic Medical Records of Medical Care Institutions** [28]: All signatures in legal EMR have to adopt verified electronic signatures and be signed within 24 hours after completing an EMR.
7. **Personal Data Protection Act** [29]: This Act addresses any personal data protection requirements, including the protection of personal information in EMR.

30.3.3.3 *Stakeholders engagement*

Government, patients, and medical care institutions are principal stakeholders of EEC. Each of these is described below.

1. Government

   Since 2001, the MOHW of Taiwan has implemented several 2–4 year projects to enhance information infrastructure and software capabilities for national health and medical data exchange. These projects include the Internet Health Services Promotion Project (2001–05), the Health Bureau Office Web-based Services Project (2003–06), the National Health Informatics Project (NHIP, 2008–11), the Accelerated Medical Care System Implementation Program (2010–12), Taiwan Health Cloud (2016), and Health Cloud 2.0 (2017–20). Notably, the Regulations for the Production and Management of Electronic Medical Records of Medical Institutions came into effect in 2009. The EMR is officially recognized as a digital document with legal status. Where a digital medical record using electronic signatures conforms to the Regulations, the document is a legal EMR [30].

   Subsequently, DOIM replaced the original Medical Image Exchange Center, initially by NHIP, with the **EEC**. The EEC content expanded from medical images to laboratory tests records, discharge notes, and outpatient notes. Due to occupational obligations, some workers from other authorities are also required to read the EHRs of specific patients. Since 2017, the demand for access to the EEC has broadened from medical care institutions to other authorities, including Taiwan Centers for Disease Control (TWCDC), the Ministry of Labor Taiwan (TWMOL), Air Referral Review Centers (ARRC), and Drug and Alcohol Addiction Systems (DAAS). As Taiwan has added additional governmental stakeholders, the number of document types available in the EEC has gradually increased from 4 to 15. Details of the document types are described below and summarized in Table 30.2.
2. Patient

   Beyond governmental authority users, the primary users of the EEC are physicians who provide diagnoses for patients. However, patients are the direct applicants who request access to view the latest 6-month EEC-based virtual medical record with the custodial medical care institutions. Patients can either apply for querying their EHR before an encounter or apply for their EHR at the point in time of admission, discharge, or transfer from inpatient or emergency settings.
3. Medical care institutions

   The number of institutions that joined the EEC project in different hospital accreditation levels and clinical types in 2016 is listed in Table 30.1 [30]. Almost all medical centers and regional hospitals were involved in the project. As of November 2021, 404 hospitals (479 nationwide,

TABLE 30.1 The number of participating institutions in different hospital accreditation levels and clinical types in 2016.

	In Taiwan	Participating in the EEC Project	
Characteristic	*N*	*n*	(%)
Accreditation levels of hospitals	476	406	(85.29)
Medical centers	26	25	(96.15)
Regional hospitals	84	83	(98.81)
District hospitals	366	298	(81.42)
Service types of clinics	23,053	5541	(24.04)
General practitioners	11,834	4459	(37.68)
Dentists	7119	1076	(15.11)
Chinese medicine	4100	6	(0.15)

December 2019 statistics [31]), 5,872 clinics (22,653 nationwide), and 352 public health centers (374 nationwide) are currently participating in the EEC.

30.3.3.4 Technical approach

Next, we explore the EEC technology in terms of the EEC HIE framework, the method of evaluating and subsidizing hospitals' EHR uploads, and the EHR content and semantic standards used.

30.3.3.4.1 EEC HIE structure

The EEC's quasi Integrating the Healthcare Enterprise (IHE) Cross-Enterprise Document Sharing (XDS) structure is shown in Fig. 30.9 [32]. The main actors include EEC, medical care institutions (hospitals, clinics, and public health centers), and other governmental authorities (TWCDC, TWMOL, ARRC, and DAAS). Four types of gateways exist in medical care institutions and authorities. The Lite Gateway is designed for clinics, Cloud Lite Gateway is for public health centers, Gateway is for hospitals, and Cloud Gateway is for other governmental authorities. The Lite Gateways allow users to query and view the EHR (documents) online, whereas the Gateways for hospitals and governmental authorities (Cloud) enable users to query, view, and download the EHR as well as store the EHR documents locally for sharing. Although hospital users have the option to download, most documents are simply viewed by users online. For the EEC itself, its core features include the generation of indexes for the EHR documents and provision of index query and EHR (document) access [33]. All messages are transmitted over the proprietary NHI VPN to ensure information security.

When a hospital generates any of the 15 types of EHRs due to providing care, it should save the EHR in its Gateway within 7 days. A valid EHR must have a legal electronic signature by Medical Care Institutions IC Card (MCI IC Card) certificate or Server Application Certificates, which were issued by Healthcare Certification Authorities (HCAs). In this way, patients can proactively ask their physicians to

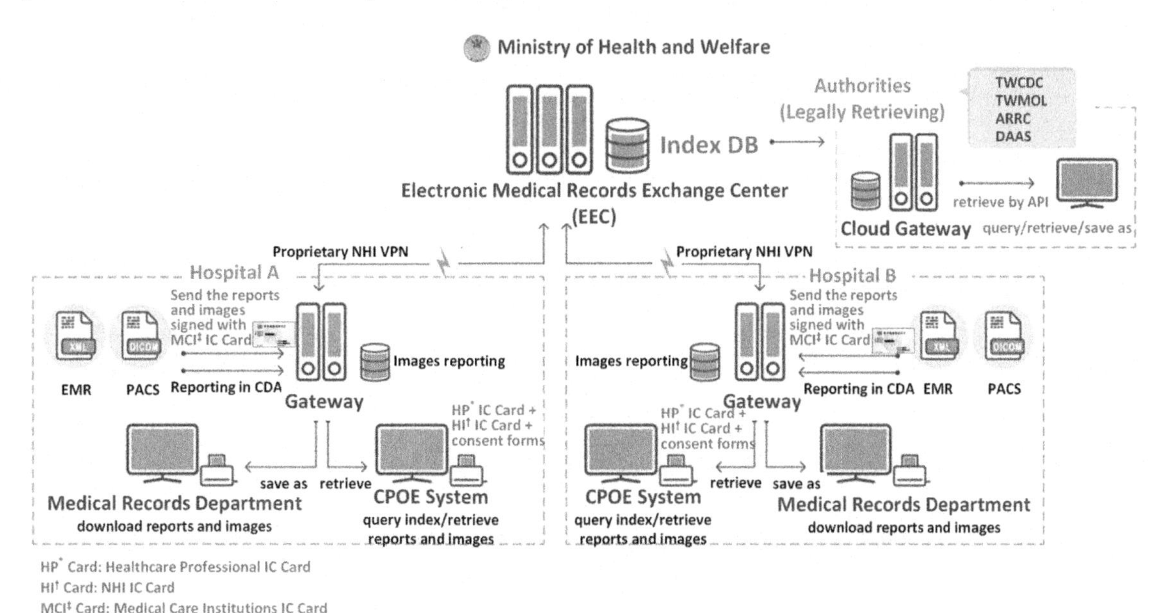

FIGURE 30.9 The health information exchange structure of EEC [6] (translated by Li-Hui Lee).

check the EEC for EHR related to their care at other facilities during encounters. Suppose the physician thinks to refer to the EHR and have the patient's agreement. In that case, a quick read can be made by inserting the patient's NHI IC Card and the physician's Healthcare Professional IC Card (HP IC Card) in a card reader. However, users from authorities must use the certificate issued by Government Certification Authority (GCA) to query and read EHR. Also, they do not need to use the patient's NHI IC Card when reading the EHR.

30.3.3.4.2 Evaluation and subsidization of the EMR uploads

It is crucial to ensure medical care institutions keep uploading EHR. The EEC requests batches of institutions claim statistics from NHI for comparison. For example, Hospital A has claimed 100 outpatient visits to NHI. However, Hospital A has only uploaded 10 Outpatient Notes to the EEC Gateway. Only 10% of the EHR has been shared in EEC. Hospital A, therefore, does not have a high level of involvement. As a result, DOIM has a financial assistance mechanism to encourage active participation by institutions. Once an organization uploads 60% or more than 60% of the interoperable EHR, it will receive additional incentive payments from DOIM.

30.3.3.4.3 Content and semantic standards

Since 2009, at least 108 types of CDA R2-based EHR document types, such as discharge notes, admission notes, and progress notes, have been prepared and produced to develop EEC EHR content and format standards. Up to December 2021, only 15 EHR types presented in Table 30.2 were modified for adoption in the EHR exchange [34]. These documents are

TABLE 30.2 The 15 clinical document types (EMR format standards) adopted by the EEC.

Purposes	Types	Version (date)
For the exchange of EMRs among medical care institutions and authorities	**1.** Medical Images and Reports	V5.0 (August 19, 2019)
	2. Discharge Notes	V3.1 (August 19, 2019)
	3. Laboratory Tests Reports	V2.1 (November 16, 2021)
	4. Outpatient Notes	V3.1 (November 25, 2021)
	5. Surgical Records	V1.0 (August 19, 2019)
	6. Pathology Reports	V1.0 (August 19, 2019)
	7. Chronic Disease Continuous Prescription	V1.0 (January 01, 2021)
	8. Physical Examination Report	V1.3 (December 19, 2016)
	9. Emergency Care Summary	V1.1 (November 16, 2021)
	10. Discharge Care Summary	V1.1 (November 16, 2021)
	11. Out-of-Hospital Cardiac Arrest (OHCA) Summary	V1.4 (December 13, 2021)
	12. Traumatic Injury (TRAUMA) Summary	V1.4 (December 13, 2021)
For medical care institutions in the addiction medicine sector	**1.** Addiction Medical Initial Assessment Record	V1.1 (December 15, 2020)
	2. Addiction Medical Follow-Up Assessment Records	V1.1 (December 15, 2020)
	3. Alcohol use disorders identification test (AUDIT) records	V1.1 (December 15, 2020)

available to users for viewing (all users) and download (hospitals and governmental authorities) via the gateways.

30.3.3.4.4 Gateway installation environment requirements for the EEC

All participating hospitals and clinics must follow the workflow designed for Gateway installation. As illustrated in Fig. 30.10, three major tasks are presented in preparation, and launch [30]. The first task is that the participating organization must apply the EEC contractor, and the EEC and PMO contractors will verify that the applicant organization has passed the regular MOHW audit of the information security environment. Only those who pass the audit will be able to request an organization account on the EEC platform to access Gateway-related information.

In the second preparation task, successful applicants must begin testing the EEC Test Gateway and EEC Web functionality. Their operating hardware and software specifications along with NHI VPN IP will be provided to the

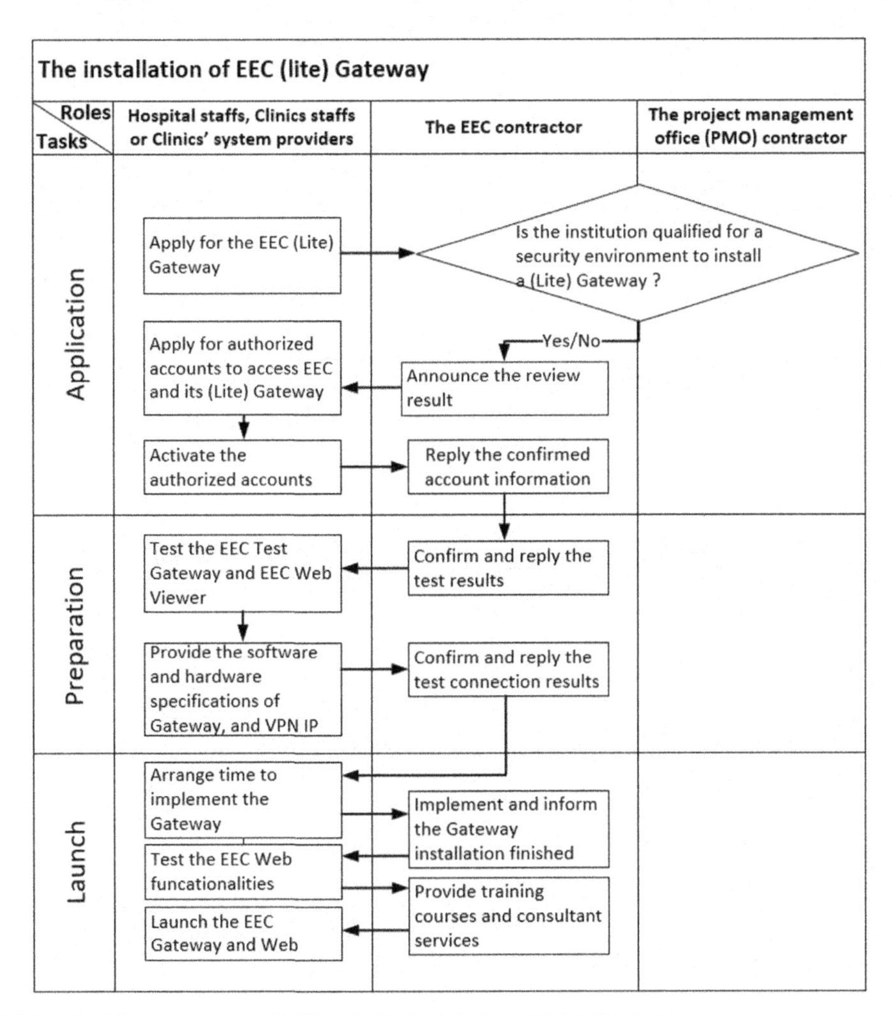

FIGURE 30.10 Workflow and responsibilities for the installation of EEC (Lite) Gateway.

EEC contractor to test the connection. The final task is for the EEC contractor to install the EEC (lite) Gateway and Web at the applicant's workplace. The applicant's personnel must conduct postinstallation functional tests. Furthermore, the EEC contractor will provide education and consultation services so that all users of the applicant organization can learn to use the system as soon as possible. Once local users can independently manage the system, the system will move into production.

30.4 Security and privacy across the NHI system

Privacy and security are the foundation upon which HIE services create trust among organizations, users, and patients. In this section, we describe the strong security and privacy protections in place within the various NHI HIE networks.

30.4.1 Security

To encourage medical care institutions, which document and store medical records by means of electronic records, the Medical Care Act [27] bestows these medical records exempt from producing another written copy. **The Regulations for the Production and Management of Electronic Medical Records of Medical Care Institutions** [28] defined specifically the criteria, production method, content, and other observances for EMR. Furthermore, these electronic records are required to use a **digital signature**, an electronic signature generated by the use of mathematic algorithm to create digital data encrypted by the signatory's private key, and capable of being verified by the public key [35].

30.4.1.1 Electronic signature and access control

HCA, contracted to the Department of Information Management, issues four kinds of certificates, including (1) HP IC Card, (2) MCI IC Card, (3) MCI IC additional Card, and (4) Server Application Certificates. These certificates are frequently used in daily encounters and EHR access (see Figs. 30.6 and 30.9). Since 2011, the certificate hashing algorithm has been adopted in the SHA-256 with RSA and 2048 key length [36]. Another, EEC users from other authorities must verify their GCA certificates, the 4096 RSA with SHA-256, are authorized for access [37]. Otherwise, they would not be able to use EEC services.

For data security, physicians at NHI contracted medical service institutions use a three-card certification approval process (safety module card, HP IC Card, and patient's NHI-IC Card) to query medical treatment information when patients present for medical attention. The HIE network employs various detection and defense features. NHIA adopted a single gateway design, and leverages various defense in-depth mechanisms, such as firewall, intrusion detection, application firewall, antivirus, and antispyware. Any identifiable personal data, which are stored in the database, are encrypted by information security systems to guarantee its safety [11].

Based on the law, NHIA examined the item, quantity, and quality of the medical service provided by the contracted medical care institutions. These medical and administrative reviews mandate providers to upload specific information, such as basic information, medical service, and health administration data, and all information transacted under the NHI information network service system of a VPN to accelerate the process and assure the security.

30.4.2 Privacy

Since NHI contracted medical institutions routinely upload patients' diagnosis and treatments via NHI IC card, and filed claims for reimbursement under VPN in Taiwan, the electronic transactions through HIE became a critical issue for NHIA to protect patients' privacy. Unlike Health

Insurance Portability and Accountability Act (HIPAA), the laws and rules regarding privacy in Taiwan are more decentralized, without a single centralized law [33]. Legal articles related to privacy protection are enacted in many laws, such as the Medical Care Act [27], the Electronic Signature Act [35], Personal Data Protection Act [29], and the Criminal Code.

Medical institutions are mandated to protect patients' rights, so they must comply with all current, relevant laws and regulations. Hospitals assign dedicated personnel to implement security and maintenance measures to prevent personal data from being stolen, altered, damaged, destroyed, or disclosed [29]. Under the law and principle of respect and notification, providers must get patients' informed consent before releasing any information, and providers must collect medical information from patients or their legal representatives directly. Also, providers must follow the law and the minimum necessary principle, all medical and relevant staff should make reasonable efforts to reduce the scope of collecting, using, or disclosing the medical information to the minimum as needed all the time [33].

Encounter-based and administrative claims data, once collected and de-identified, can be used for statistical purposes, including population health, and academic research. In fact, universities and research organizations in Taiwan leverage the National Health Insurance Research Database [34], which contains registration files and original claim data for reimbursement, regularly for academic research. Between 2004 and 2021, over 6,550 articles have been published in academic journals using data from this national database [38].

Physicians can read the EHR only when the patient visits them and when the patient gives permission to use their NHI IC Card to access information. Also, before a physician queries or reads the EHR, patients must sign consent forms in agreement with (1) physicians from which medical care institution can view their EHR, (2) what types of EHR can be viewed, and (3) what the valid time duration of the consent form is. All consent forms are considered part of the EHR and kept in medical care institutions. All-access to the EHR must conform to the consent provided.

30.5 Comparison of the NHI IC Card, Medi-Cloud, and EEC HIE Networks

The NHI IC Card, Medi-Cloud system, and EEC EHRs are all used for HIE in Taiwan. Although the purposes and functions of these tools are different, they complement each other quite well. The comparison among these tools (Table 30.3) shows the features and performance of each network. In brief, here are the similarities and differences between the three networks:

1. NHI IC Card, Medi-Cloud system, and EEC EHRs belong to government agencies but are operated and maintained by different divisions.
2. The IC Card and Medi-Cloud are mandatory under the laws, but EEC EHRs is elective for hospitals and clinics to use. However, only EEC EHRs are treated as legal documents because they use a digital signature through the KPI mechanism.
3. Medi-Cloud contains more information than NHI-IC Card and EEC EHRs, such as western and Chinese medicine, test/examination results, operations, and dental treatment.
4. The available period of data inquiry for NHI IC Card is the patient's recent six visits, but Medi-Cloud and EEC EHRs can provide 3–6 months. Last, the utilization of NHI IC card and Medi-Cloud by clinicians are significantly higher than EEC EHRs due to the laws that hospitals and clinics must follow to get reimbursements.

TABLE 30.3 Comparison of health information exchange among NHI IC Card, Medi-Cloud system, and EEC EHRs.

	NHI IC Card	Medi-Cloud	EEC EHRs
Operation agency	NHIA	NHIA	Ministry of Health and Welfares
Usage condition	Mandatory	Mandatory	Elective
Legal document	No	No (only for clinicians' reference)	Yes (digital signature)
Contents	Diagnoses, prescriptions, allergies, vaccination, and insurance data	Western and Chinese medicine records, test/examination records and results, dental treatment and operation notes, specific controlled, coagulation factor or allergy drug usage records, rehabilitation medical records, discharge summary, and vaccination records from Centers for Disease Control	15 clinical document types as shown in Table 30.2
Available period of data inquiry	Recent six visits	3–6 months	6 months
Utilization by clinicians	High	High	Low

30.6 Results and lessons from two decades of HIE in Taiwan

The three HIE networks in Taiwan collectively exchanged data for 20 years. The NHI-IC cards have been used since 2003, MediCloud since 2013, and the EEC since 2009. Over the past two decades, Taiwan has measured the adoption and use of HIE, and it has learned a lot about the development and implementation of HIE services. In this section, we examine the findings from two decades of HIE research.

30.6.1 MediCloud network impact

The "NHI MediCloud system" is a patient-centered system, integrating the medical treatment records of patients across different hospitals and clinics, and the network can assist physicians in obtaining a thorough understanding of past test/examination results and drug use status of patients. It reduces medical risks of repetitive blood collection, examination, and drug use and reduces exposure to multiple X-ray radiation, and physical discomfort due to endoscopic examinations. It can assist physicians in making relatively more precise diagnosis and prescription while reducing harm and waste of medical resources due to repetitive prescription or repetitive examination/test on patients. It reduces time for seeking medical attention across different hospitals and saves costs on the application of medical record summary photocopies and image optical disk preparation, so repeated prescriptions and waste will be reduced to a minimum and utilize NHI resources more effectively. This helps patients save time and money spent on traveling and retrieving films, too.

Measures used by MediCloud prevent repeat prescriptions for commonly used drugs for indications such as hypertension, hyperglycemia and hyperlipidemia, and hypnotics and sedatives. NHIA estimated that sharing information via MediCloud has saved as much as NT$7.4 billion (US$264 million) in NHI-covered drugs over the past 6 years (2013–18) and around NT$2.6 billion (US$92.9 million) on laboratory testing (examinations) in 2018. The MediCloud system not only lowered NHI medical expenditures, but also reduced the health risks brought by drug interactions and allergies [39].

30.6.2 EEC network utilization and performance

This section discusses the achievements of the EEC network from three perspectives: EHR utilization, access performance, and application status.

First, statistics for January 1, 2015, to June 1, 2017 [21] show that the quarterly average volume of EHR uploads to hospitals was 52,790,721. The quarterly average EHRs view by physicians from hospitals and clinics were 650,323 and 218,230. The upload-to-view EHR ratio was approximately 81:1. Medical centers and clinics primarily read the overall EHRs volume to 54% (318.717) and 45% (269,082). The central branch read was highest, accounting for 21% (305,230), compared with other NHI branches. Laboratory tests reports and outpatient notes account for 50.3% and 40.9% of viewing times, which were much higher than medical images and discharge notes. In addition, to encourage hospitals to upload EHR, the viewing times ranking statistics of EHR uploads is published twice a month on the EEC website [40]. Since 2017, other authorized users have become the primary users of EEC. Their index query volume was extremely higher than those of medical care institutions.

Second, the download time showed the average for medical images from 9.92 to 32.05 seconds in the early phase [21]. However, access performance has been improved over recent years due to the upgrade of the NHI VPN.

Finally, although the download volume is not high, EEC is the first national HIE mechanism to apply an electronic signature to EHR in Taiwan. All EHRs delivered via the Intranet and Internet are verifiable. Digital signatures enhance the "confidentiality" of EHR by ensuring that the signer of the EHR is the person, the "integrity" of the EHR will not be tampered with after signing, and the "nonrepudiation" of the source after signing the EHR. To maximize the use of EHR, DOIM has also continually encouraged government units with EHR access needs to use the EEC platform to read the EHR in recent years.

30.6.3 Facilitators of HIE in Taiwan

There are several factors that led to the successes (e.g., impact, use) of HIE in Taiwan. This section describes those and places them in the context of the book.

30.6.3.1 *Universal health access and identifiers*

A major driver of HIE in Taiwan is the organization of NHI and the use of the NHI IC Card. Broad access to health care by citizens allows individuals the freedom to choose where they seek care. This creates necessity for HIE as data must be shared across providers across the health system. Unique identification of patients facilitates easier linkage of individuals across EHR systems.

30.6.3.2 *Policy and breadth of data that compels use of HIE network*

Requiring providers to use MediCloud in order to receive reimbursement for health services is a major motivator for health systems to adopt HIE, and it explains why providers use this system more than the EEC. However, the MediCloud system also offers a broader array of data types than the EEC. Clinicians need information to care for patients, and their strong utilization of MediCloud indicates they utilize a resource that provides them access to critical, comprehensive information, such as pharmacy records, traditional Chinese medicine records, and laboratory results all available through MediCloud. It is likely that if the EEC had equally expansive data available, clinicians might increase their utilization of that system.

30.6.3.3 Engagement of consumers in HIE access

Another facilitator of HIE is the engagement of Taiwanese citizens in the various HIE networks. Patients must consent to clinician access of their past medical history by providing their NHI IC Card to clinicians or indicate consent in advance of the visit. This step, while cumbersome, makes citizens aware of the HIE activity. It further directly engages patients in the process, likely stimulating conversations about prior medical tests/exams/imaging between the patient and doctor. Engagement likely influences positive patient self-management behavior, as patients are aware of their health care utilization patterns. Doctors, for example, might use the information to help patients with asthma better understand what triggers their exacerbations "attacks" that drive patients to utilize emergency care. Reducing the attacks will reduce emergency care utilization, leading to lower costs and happier patients. Moreover, patients have access to their medical records in the system via the My Health Bank application. This also enables patients to take a more active role in their care plans and self-management [41].

30.6.4 Barriers and lessons learned

Although CDA is the standard for exchange in the EEC network, there are few value-added EHR-based applications in Taiwan that parse or utilize the data within the exchanged documents. The national HIE has not led to the expansion of industry (vendor) applications. The main factors are the long learning curve of the CDA standard and the low flexibility of interfacing and extension of existing EHR products. As a result, the EEC is not supported by the HIT industry.

The following lessons from Taiwan's experience may benefit other countries' HIE efforts:

1. Strong, robust infrastructure of health information and communications technology (ICT) in Taiwan supports adoption and use the national HIE networks. Most health care providers have EMR systems, and they can submit and share their health information with sufficient network bandwidth.
2. NHIA offers financial incentives to health care providers for using the MediCloud system, and subsidizes them to expand the network bandwidth, which helps providers raise VPN speed in submission of claims. Also, for those providers who choose not to cooperate, NHIA delays their reimbursements.
3. The NHIA administered the MediCloud system to facilitate physicians checking recent patient diagnoses or clinical treatments and assist pharmacists to prepare medications for patients. This cloud technology enhanced patient safety, quality of care, and reduced unnecessary treatments.
4. HIE helps integrated care services provided in hospitals for elder care, so physicians can get effective and timely information from different specialties and hospitals to treat old people.
5. The pandemic control system used the NHI IC card and MediCloud links with immigration data immediately, which enabled effective alerts in real-time and precision testing for suspected and infected COVID 19 cases. Taiwan has developed digital solutions to contact-tracing, monitoring, and isolation/quarantine during the pandemic [14,15].

30.7 Future directions

MOHW continues to apply ICT while expanding and deepening applications of medical information. The following are NHIA and EEC working to meet the needs of society and achieving the goal of building a smart and healthy Taiwan.

30.7.1 Using services online by virtual NHI IC card

Taiwan is a highly tech-savvy country with over 98% of population owning smartphones in 2019 [42]. Enabling people to apply for mobile insurance services, NHIA has set up a "Personal NHI Online Services" network website and implemented a trial plan for using virtual NHI IC card in 2021. People can download the "NHI Mobile Access" app at Google Play or Apple Store and enjoy e-services through virtual NHI IC card (Fig. 30.11) by a mobile device.

FIGURE 30.11 Example of a virtual NHI Card to replace physical smart cards.

30.7.2 Using NHI cloud technology to tackle pandemic

Health ICT integrated with a solid healthcare infrastructure and advance planning can be a powerful tool for a nation's epidemic control [14]. NHI MediCloud system played a vital role as COVID-19 pandemic hit Taiwan. It not only proved instrumental in facilitating rationed surgical masks, but medical institutions were also linked through the cloud system to exchange any information necessary by asking patients' travel history, occupation, contact history, and cluster (TOCC) (Fig. 30.12). Although the NHI database and cloud system constructed over the years have proven effective in pandemic prevention, the NHI MediCloud system still has room to improve and develop to meet the ultimate goal for maximizing public health benefits and minimizing intrusion of privacy.

30.7.3 Building up systemwide interoperability

Although all hospitals and clinics applied and shared medical information provided by NHI IC card and MediCloud system, owing to a lack of common international standards, NHI still has no fully systemwide interoperability in Taiwan [43]. Unlike the United States, Centers for Medicare and Medicaid Services declared "meaningful use" EHR Incentive Programs in 2011, required hospitals and eligible professionals to complete a set of core objectives, such as "Maintain an up-to-date problem list of current and active diagnoses based on ICD-10-CM/PCS or SNOMED CT" [44]. Thus the lack of agreement on the definition of a problem list leaves each medical institution to

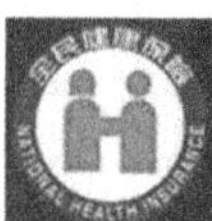

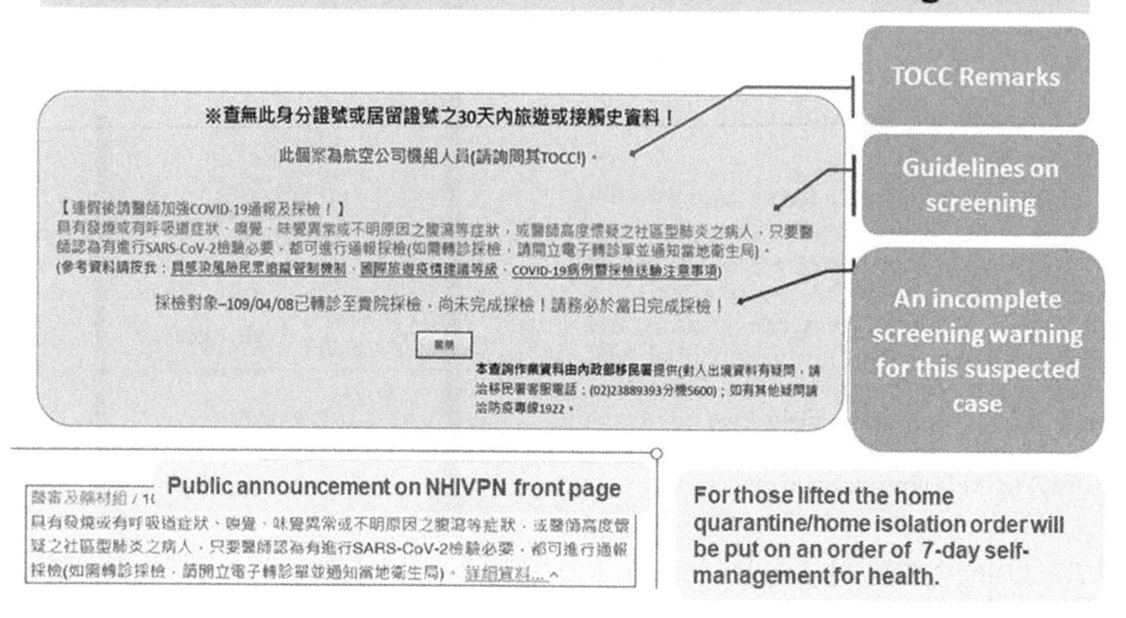

FIGURE 30.12 COVID-19 pandemic inquiry on MediCloud system. *TOCC*, Travel history, occupation, contact history, and cluster.

determine its own problem list policy, which makes the interoperability between institutions more difficult to share and apply in patient treatments [45]. Therefore MOHF needs to overcome the challenge to implement various international interoperability standards, and educate physicians, nurses professionals to adopt them in their medical practices.

The population aging has led to a growing number of people with chronic diseases in Taiwan. In order to avoid the NHI reserve fund being run out due to the increasing expenses incrementally, adjustment of higher premiums might be inevitable. Thus, the premium rate has raised from 4.69% to 5.17% in January 2021 [46]. For the sustainability of the NHI program, considering the nation's economic and political situation, and knowing that increasing NHI funding is difficult, the best solution is to cut unnecessary expenses. Hopefully, effective and timely HIE would help NHIA share information through the cloud, prevent additional expenses caused by unnecessary checkups or exams and build an effective referral system.

30.7.4 Evolving standards to FHIR

On the other hand, there may be an opportunity for the next generation of HIE standards, for example, FHIR, to support mobile applications and scalability. MOWH will adopt HL7 FHIR and convert EHR content and format standards from CDA-based EHR API to FHIR-based EHR API. Also, the FHIR-based API will be applied in related projects to reduce the information security risks arising from numerous interfaces [36,37]. It is recommended that the government follow the recommendation of HL7 International first to develop Taiwan's core profiles and implementation guide. Then gradually convert the CDA-based EHR to FHIR-based EHR. This will facilitate and activate the national HIE and progressively enhance the global competitiveness of medical information vendors and medical institutions in applying information technology.

30.7.5 Incentivizing provider use of EEC

In contrast to the subsidized incentives for EHR uploads, there are no relative incentives for clinicians downloading and reading EHR documents via the EEC [47]. Electronic signatures help secure communication and accessing the information in CDA-based documents can benefit physician diagnostics. With the existing NHI MediCloud system and claims incentives of the NHI, it may not be possible to raise physician willingness to read or download EHRs via EEC. In addition to enhancing the user group of EEC, through the long-term promotion and application of FHIR, the industry should provide solid value-added application capability in EHR systems. This will provide greater opportunity to achieve the ecosystem of the medical information application market. Stakeholders can easily access the complete EHR and maximize the benefits of HIE through various applications or in their existing systems.

30.8 Summary

Over the past three decades, the Republic of China (Taiwan) has systematically replaced paper charts with EMR and developed a robust ICT infrastructure that supports broad HIE accessible to patients, providers, and governmental authorities in support of clinical and population health. The exchange of data is driven by government policy and regulations rooted in universal health coverage. Three distinct and complementary HIE networks facilitate access to a broad range of data, including western and traditional Chinese medical information across outpatient clinics, emergency departments, and inpatient wards. Smart cards provide robust security and rapid access to data from recent medical encounters. Secure VPNs enable exchange of large volumes of data. A newer, standards-based exchange network enables querying and download of clinical documents. Investment in HIE yielded reductions in redundant testing and duplicate medications, which resulted in cost savings as well as improved patient safety and quality of care for the Taiwanese people. Future directions further expand access to information for patients and indicate an evolution toward newer standards like FHIR. The lessons and challenges from Taiwan serve as an example for other nations who may be earlier in their digital health journey but nonetheless can achieve similar outcomes in the coming decades.

Discussion questions

1. A government-facilitated HIE network requires a federated architecture. What aspects of the Taiwan infrastructure facilitate HIE?
2. Compare the NHI IC Card, Medi-Cloud system, and EEC EHRs in Taiwan's HIE. How could they be improved? How could they be expanded?
3. Population aging has led to a growing number of people with chronic diseases in

Taiwan. How could effective and timely HIE reduce unnecessary exams and enhance the quality of care?

4. Due to the lack of interoperability standards, patient information is difficult to share among Taiwan's medical institutions because its HIE is based on a government-facilitated network. How could Taiwan enhance its infrastructure to adopt and leverage available, common international standards?

5. How does the approach to HIE in Taiwan compare to the approaches used in Denmark (Chapter 28) and Israel (Chapter 31)?

References

[1] Taiwan | History, Flag, Map, Capital, Population, & Facts | Britannica. Available from: https://www.britannica.com/place/Taiwan [accessed 18.11. 21].

[2] National Statistics, Republic of China (Taiwan). Available from: https://eng.stat.gov.tw/point.asp?index = 9 [accessed 24.02. 22].

[3] Taiwan GDP per capita 2021 - StatisticsTimes.com. Available from: https://statisticstimes.com/economy/country/taiwan-gdp-per-capita.php [accessed 24.02. 22].

[4] Anderson GF, Hussey P, Petrosyan V. It's still the prices, stupid: why the US spends so much on health care, and a tribute to Uwe Reinhardt. Health Affairs 2019;38(1):87–95. Available from: https://doi.org/10.1377/HLTHAFF.2018.05144.

[5] U.S. health spending as share of GDP 1960–2020. Available from: https://www.statista.com/statistics/184968/us-health-expenditure-as-percent-of-gdp-since-1960/ [accessed 18.11.21].

[6] Life expectancy at birth in Taiwan 1990–2030. Available from: http://www.cdway.com.tw/gov/mhw2/book109/bk109e/index.html; 2021 [accessed 18.11.21].

[7] 2020 Taiwan Health and Welfare Report. Available from: http://www.cdway.com.tw/gov/mhw2/book109/bk109e/index.html [accessed 24.11.22].

[8] Healthcare in Taiwan. Available from: https://en.wikipedia.org/wiki/Healthcare_in_Taiwan; 2021 [accessed 18.11.21].

[9] Ministry of Health and Welfare, Statistical yearbook of the Republic of China 2020, 2021. [Online]. Available from: https://eng.stat.gov.tw/public/data/dgbas03/bs2/yearbook_eng/y021.pdf.

[10] Wu TY, Majeed A, Kuo KN. An overview of the healthcare system in Taiwan. Lond J Prim Care (Abingdon) 2010;3(2):115. Available from: https://doi.org/10.1080/17571472.2010.11493315.

[11] National Health Insurance Administration of Ministry of Health and Welfare. 2020–2021 National Health Insurance in Taiwan Annual Report, Taipei, 2021. [Online]. Available from: https://www.nhi.gov.tw/resource/Webdata/2020-2021全民健康保險年報.pdf.

[12] National Health Insurance Administration. "2020–2021 Handbook of Taiwan's National Health Insurance," 2021. [Online]. Available from: https://ws.nhi.gov.tw/001/Upload/293/RelFile/Ebook/English.pdf

[13] Liao MC, Lin IC. Performance evaluation of an information technology intervention regarding charging for inpatient medical materials at a regional teaching hospital in Taiwan: empirical study. JMIR mHealth uHealth 2020;8(3). Available from: https://doi.org/10.2196/16381.

[14] What we can learn from Taiwan's response to the covid-19 epidemic - The BMJ. Available from: https://blogs.bmj.com/bmj/2020/07/21/what-we-can-learn-from-taiwans-response-to-the-covid-19-epidemic/ [accessed 18.11.21].

[15] Summers DJ, et al. Potential lessons from the Taiwan and New Zealand health responses to the COVID-19 pandemic. Lancet Reg Heal - West Pac 2020;4:100044. Available from: https://doi.org/10.1016/J.LANWPC.2020.100044/ATTACHMENT/A429F7EB-B128-4329-9F2C-757D3123965B/MMC1.DOCX.

[16] National Health Insurance Act - Article Content - Laws & Regulations Database of the Republic of China. Available from: https://law.moj.gov.tw/ENG/LawClass/LawAll.aspx?pcode = L0060001 [accessed 18.11.21].

[17] Cheng TM. Taiwan's new national health insurance program: genesis and experience so far. Health Aff (Millwood) 2003;22(3):61–76. Available from: https://doi.org/10.1377/HLTHAFF.22.3.61.

[18] Cheng TM. Reflections on the 20th anniversary of taiwan's single-payer national health insurance system. Health Aff 2015;34(3):502–10. Available from: https://doi.org/10.1377/HLTHAFF.2014.1332/ASSET/IMAGES/LARGE/2014.1332FIGEX4.JPEG.

[19] Himmelstein DU, Campbell T, Woolhandler S. Health care administrative costs in the United States and Canada, 2017. Ann Intern Med 2020;172(2):134–42. Available from: https://doi.org/10.7326/M19-2818.

[20] 2020 International Profiles: Country Responses COVID-19 Pandemic | Commonwealth Fund. Available from: https://www.commonwealthfund.org/blog/2020/2020-international-profiles-useful-resource-interpreting-responses-covid-19 [accessed 18.11.21].

[21] Wen HC, Chang WP, Hsu MH, Ho CH, Chu CM. An assessment of the interoperability of electronic health record exchanges among hospitals and clinics in

Taiwan. JMIR Med Inform 2019;7(1). Available from: https://doi.org/10.2196/12630.

[22] National Health Insurance Administration Ministry of Health and Welfare-NHIA Organization Chart. Available from: https://www.nhi.gov.tw/english/Content_List.aspx?n = 48001B3696391F5C&topn = ED4A30E51A609E49 [accessed 09.03.22].

[23] Toward the cloud: a win-win for patients and physicians - Health Care Reform Diary 2.0." Available from: https://www.nhi.gov.tw/resource/NHIb2/482/index.html#zoom = z [accessed 09.03.22].

[24] National Health Insurance Administration Ministry of Health and Welfare-NHI MediCloud System. Available from: https://www.nhi.gov.tw/english/Content_List.aspx?n = 02BA04454AED80E0&topn = BCB2B0D2433F6491 [accessed 09.03.22].

[25] National Health Insurance Administration Ministry of Health and Welfare-NHI MediCloud System. Available from: https://www.nhi.gov.tw/english/Content_List.aspx?n = 02BA04454AED80E0&topn = BCB2B0D2433F6491 [accessed 24.02.22].

[26] 2020 International Profiles: Country Responses COVID-19 Pandemic | Commonwealth Fund. Available from: https://www.commonwealthfund.org/blog/2020/2020-international-profiles-useful-resource-interpreting-responses-covid-19 [accessed 24.02.22].

[27] Medical Care Act - Chapter - Laws & Regulations Database of The Republic of China. Available from: https://law.moj.gov.tw/ENG/LawClass/LawParaDeatil.aspx?pcode = L0020021&bp = 7 [accessed 10.11.21].

[28] Regulations for the Production and Management of Electronic Medical Records of Medical Care Institutions. Available from: https://law.moj.gov.tw/LawClass/LawAll.aspx?pcode = L0020121 [accessed 24.02.22].

[29] Personal Data Protection Act - Article Content - Laws & Regulations Database of the Republic of China (Taiwan). Available from: https://law.moj.gov.tw/ENG/LawClass/LawAll.aspx?pcode = I0050021 [accessed 24.02.22].

[30] Ministry of Health and Welfare. EMR exchange center promotion. Available from: http://sc-dr.tw/news/105/04/04250304.pdf; 2016.

[31] Statistics of Medical Care Institution & Hospital Utilization 2020- Ministry of Health and Welfare. Available from: https://www.mohw.gov.tw/cp-5255-63398-2.html [accessed 24.02.22].

[32] Ministry of Health and Welfare, EMR format standards for EMR exchange center. Available from: https://emr.mohw.gov.tw/emr/emrstd.aspx [accessed 06.10.21].

[33] Yang CM, Lin HC, Chang P, Jian WS. Taiwan's perspective on electronic medical records' security and privacy protection: lessons learned from HIPAA. Comput Methods Prog Biomed 2006;82(3):277–82. Available from: https://doi.org/10.1016/J.CMPB.2006.04.002.

[34] National Health Insurance Research Database: Taiwan. Available from: https://nhird.nhri.org.tw/en/index.htm [accessed 09.03.22].

[35] Electronic Signatures Act - Article Content - Laws & Regulations Database of the Republic of China (Taiwan). Available from: https://law.moj.gov.tw/ENG/LawClass/LawAll.aspx?pcode = J0080037 [accessed 24.02.22].

[36] Ministry of Health and Welfare. Healthcare Certification Authority (HCA) 2.0. Available from: https://hca.nat.gov.tw/ [accessed 26.12.21].

[37] National Development Council. Government certificated portal. Available from: https://gcp.nat.gov.tw/views/AnnDownload/download_2-1.html [accessed 26.12. 21].

[38] National Health Insurance Database Journal Papers Taiwan: National Health Service. Available from: https://www.nhi.gov.tw/Query/Query_AcademicResearch.aspx [accessed 09.03.22].

[39] Enhanced Patient Safety and Information Security Both through the NHI MediCloud System. Available from: https://www.nhi.gov.tw/english/News_Content.aspx?n = 996D1B4B5DC48343&sms = F0EAFEB716DE7FFA&s = 148EAC979AAE3F75 [accessed 25.02.22].

[40] Ministry of Health and Welfare, EEC news. Available from: https://eec.mohw.gov.tw/new [accessed 20.12.21].

[41] P.D. Consumer health informatics: engaging and empowering patients and families. In: Finnell J, Dixon B, editors. Clinical informatics study guide: text and review. 2nd ed. Springer Nature; 2022.

[42] Smartphone market in Taiwan - Statistics & Facts | Statista. Available from: https://www.statista.com/topics/6038/smartphone-market-in-taiwan/ [accessed 25.02.22].

[43] How does universal health coverage work? https://www.commonwealthfund.org/international-health-policy-center/countries/taiwan [accessed 25.02.22].

[44] Promoting Interoperability Programs | CMS. Available from: https://www.cms.gov/Regulations-and-Guidance/Legislation/EHRIncentivePrograms [accessed 01.01.22].

[45] Krauss JC, Boonstra PS, Vantsevich AV, Friedman CP. Is the problem list in the eye of the beholder? An exploration of consistency across physicians. J Am Med Inform Assoc 2016;23(5):859–65. Available from: https://doi.org/10.1093/JAMIA/OCV211.

[46] Taipei Times. NHI premium being raised to 5.17 percent: ministry. Available from: https://www.taipeitimes.com/News/front/archives/2021/01/01/2003749736 [accessed 06.28.22].

[47] Department of Information Management- Ministry of Health and Welfare. Available from: https://www.mohw.gov.tw/cp-377939364-2.html [accessed 24.02.22].

CHAPTER

31

Israel's national HIE network Ofek: a robust infrastructure for clinical and population health

Brian E. Dixon[1,2], *Ofir Ben-Assuli*[3] *and Yaron Denekamp*[4,5]

[1]Department of Epidemiology, Richard M. Fairbanks School of Public Health, Indiana University, Indianapolis, IN, USA [2]Center for Biomedical Informatics, Regenstrief Institute, Inc., Indianapolis, IN, USA [3]Faculty of Business Administration, Ono Academic College, Kiryat Ono, Israel [4]Clalit Health Services, Tel Aviv, Israel [5]School of Public Health, Haifa University, Haifa, Israel

Major themes

This case study highlights the following major themes from the book:

- Grassroots development and expansion of HIE across a state/nation
- Working example of a SOA-based, federated architecture
- A clear focus on delivering value to clinicians
- Sustainability of HIE through services that provide value to health systems and pivoting to meet evolving socio-political needs
- The role of a national identifier in facilitating HIE
- The importance and role of evaluation to HIE use and sustainability
- Implementation of a clinical or HIE system
- Usage of HIE by providers for a specific clinical or public health case/reason
- Improving medical and managerial outcomes following HIE adoption

31.1 Introduction

The national health information exchange (HIE) in Israel is one of the most robust HIE networks in the world, yet few are familiar with it. This case study aims to put a spotlight on a small but determined country that seeks to be a global leader in health information technology.

Most Israelis do not know it exists or how it operates, yet Ofek (as it is called in Hebrew) works 24/7 in the background to connect the nation's hospitals and ambulatory facilities in support of patient care and population outcomes.

Health Information Exchange
DOI: https://doi.org/10.1016/B978-0-323-90802-3.00018-6

The HIE network began around the turn of the 21st century as an effort to connect hospitals and community clinics within Clalit Health Services, the largest health maintenance organization (HMO) in Israel. Today, the HIE network is used extensively throughout the Israeli health system, seamlessly facilitating access to comprehensive medical records. During the COVID-19 pandemic, the health system leveraged the HIE network to facilitate clinician awareness of the epidemiology of disease in the nation as well as the status (disease and vaccination) of patients in each health facility.

The case study begins with the background and history on the development of Israel's national HIE network. The case study then describes the organization and technical architecture of the network. Next, the case study highlights the facilitators and barriers to HIE in Israel. The network, despite broad adoption and use, remains a work-in-progress. The case study, therefore, concludes with an overview of the network's future, one in which a new system will replace Ofek.

31.2 Background

31.2.1 Israel

As of 2022, Israel's population is estimated to be 9.45 million, most of whom live in one of the country's four major metropolitan areas: Tel Aviv, Jerusalem, Haifa, and Beersheba. Located in southwest Asia (aka the Middle East), Israel is a Mediterranean country bounded by Lebanon to the north, Syria to the northeast, Jordan and the West Bank to the east, and Egypt and the Gaza Strip to the southwest. Its total land area under Israeli law is 22,072 km^2 (8522 sq mi), which is roughly equivalent to that of New Jersey in the United States.

Israel's economy is ranked high when compared to most nations, and the nation is considered by many to have the most advanced economy in the Middle East. Important industries include software, tourism, and agriculture. Its technology sector is considered very robust, often invoking comparisons to Silicon Valley [1]. The nation has research and development (R&D) facilities owned by Intel, Microsoft, Google, Apple, Meta, and Cisco Systems. It also has one of the highest concentrations of start-up technology companies in the world; a nickname for Israel is "Start-up nation." A major contributing factor: Israel is first in the world with respect to its gross domestic spending on R&D [2].

31.2.2 The Israeli health system

Based on the National Health Insurance Law of 1995, Israel uses a universal health coverage scheme. Israeli citizens are required to be insured through one of four health insurance organizations (HMOs): Clalit Health Services, Maccabi Healthcare Services, Meuhedet Health Fund, and Leumit Health Fund. The HMOs are nonprofit organizations (e.g., they do not seek to make profit for shareholders). Among these institutions, Clalit is the largest covering 51.5% of the population [3].

Citizens pay a compulsory health tax (often deducted from their wages by their employer) to the National Insurance Institute, which redistributes the funds to the HMOs based on several criteria, including a capitation formula. Each HMO also receives some direct funding from the government. There are several exclusions from the health tax, including active-duty military and disabled Veterans whose health insurance is covered by the Ministry of Defense.

The law requires that the four HMO's offer a regulated "health basket" or set of health care services to their members. Insurance coverage covers all costs of medical diagnosis and treatment in the areas of family medicine, hospitalization (general, maternity, psychiatric, and chronic), preventive medicine, surgery (including elective surgery), transplants, drug abuse, and alcoholism; medical equipment and appliances; first aid and transportation to a medical facility; obstetrics and fertility treatment; chronic diseases; and mental health. The basket further includes coverage for most medications, updated annually, and medication copays can apply in certain circumstances.

Supplemental insurance plans can also be purchased through the HMO to some extent of insurance level, and private insurance plans that go beyond the regulated health basket can also be purchased from commercial insurance companies. Citizens choose to which HMO they will subscribe, and they can easily change that election.

Hospitals and health care clinics, including specialty and outpatient facilities, are managed by the four HMOs. The Ministry of Health (MOH) also operates several prenatal, postnatal, and geriatric care services. Private hospitals also exist and offer amenities such as private rooms, fast access to medical services, and beds for visitors who wish to stay overnight.

Israel has one of the most technologically advanced health systems in the world, and the nation seeks to be a leader and innovator in digital health. Adoption of electronic health record (EHR) systems is ubiquitous. Paper does not exist in primary care, and 90% of secondary care is digitized. Given the proliferation of EHR systems, the Government invested $300 million into a big data utilization initiative [4]. The funding spurred innovation in creating digital solutions to de-identify (or anonymize) clinical data for use in large-scale analytics that will enable researchers to develop new treatments and understand underlying etiologies of disease. An example is MDClone [5], an Israeli company whose data platform was selected to serve as the research data enclave for the National COVID Cohort Collaborative (NC3) [6], funded by the US National Institutes of Health [7]. Such investments in digital health innovations create an environment supportive of HIE and facilitate the development of the technological and sociopolitical components that make HIE possible for clinicians and researchers.

31.3 Origins of health information exchange in Israel

Like many HIE efforts, interoperability in Israel was born when two phenomena were present at the same time within the health system: technical prowess and necessity. In the early 2000s, more than 95% of ambulatory providers documented care in electronic medical record (EMR) systems [8]. However, hospitals only used EMRs for admission and discharge. Communication between inpatient and outpatient settings was, therefore, primarily on paper, rendering the patient to serve as intermediary between health providers.

The electronic exchange of data between settings was pioneered by Clalit Health Services (Clalit), the nation's then-and-now largest HMO, that owns 14 hospitals as well as around 1400 community clinics all across the country. Beginning around 2002, the IT division within Clalit created a vision in which the disparate health information systems could integrate data and provide a comprehensive view of the patient's medical record to clinicians across care settings. This vision, which continues to exist now, focuses principally on integrating clinical data to support patient care. Over the next 3 years, Clalit created an enterprise HIE, connecting its eight general hospitals with its primary care clinics and laboratories. Fig. 31.1 is a timeline highlighting the development and expansion of the enterprise HIE network.

Beginning in 2005, the enterprise HIE initiative began to expand beyond Clalit to include hospitals outside of the HMO. The network became known as Ofek, which translates in Hebrew to horizon [9]. Hospitals outside the Clalit HMO voluntarily joined the HIE network to facilitate interoperable data sharing for patient care. As the outside effort gained traction, some in the nation championed the idea of transitioning the enterprise HIE into an Israeli National HIE platform that would interconnect all health facilities [8].

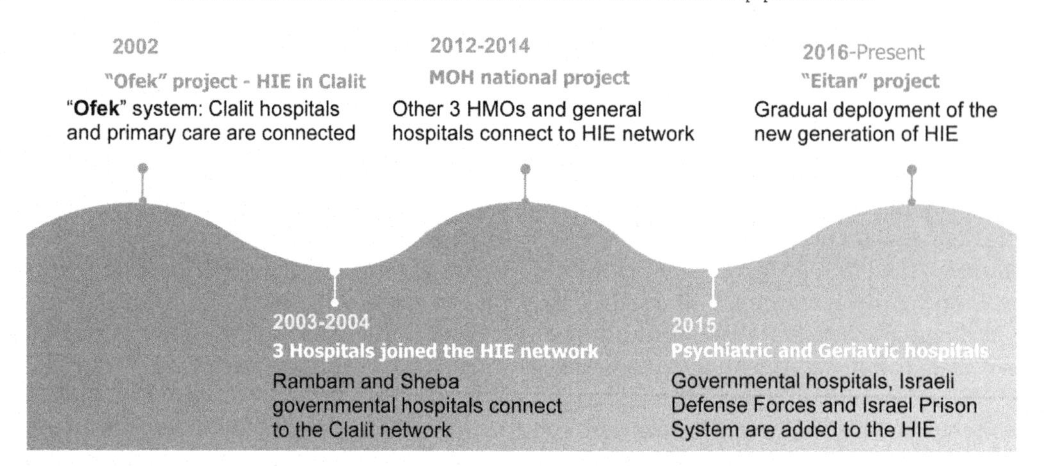
2002
"Ofek" project - HIE in Clalit
"Ofek" system: Clalit hospitals and primary care are connected
2012-2014
MOH national project
Other 3 HMOs and general hospitals connect to HIE network
2016-Present
"Eitan" project
Gradual deployment of the new generation of HIE
2003-2004
3 Hospitals joined the HIE network
Rambam and Sheba governmental hospitals connect to the Clalit network
2015
Psychiatric and Geriatric hospitals
Governmental hospitals, Israeli Defense Forces and Israel Prison System are added to the HIE

FIGURE 31.1 Evolution of HIE in Israel over time. Source: *Used with permission from the Information and Computing Division of the Israeli Ministry of Health.*

Achieving a national HIE infrastructure, however, required governance and governmental leadership. Although the other HMOs were willing to work toward the vision of a national HIE network, the Ministry of Health (MOH) needed time to develop the sociopolitical structure in which a formal, government-facilitated HIE network could be developed. The MOH initially provided support for the idea of a national network and organized four working groups [8]:

- Steering Committee: Leaders from across the health system worked to define the vision, mission, and goals of the HIE network. This group agreed upon the concept of a virtual medical record, explained below.
- Technological Committee: This committee of independent IT professionals made recommendations for the architecture of the HIE network.
- Content and terminology: This committee defined the minimum data set (MDS) for exchange and spearheaded efforts and national terminology standards.
- Ethics and Legislation: This committee examined existing national laws and regulations then made recommendations for new policies that would build trust in HIE while ensuring privacy and security of health information.

These working groups created technical, governance, and policy guidelines for a national HIE infrastructure. Although Ofek existed, the working groups sought to work across the health system to discuss and reach consensus on what a national system might entail. This system might be similar to Ofek, but leaders wanted other options explored. Furthermore, the group needed time to establish minimum data requirements, rules for data usage, and agree upon security protocols and information standards. It is important to note that the nontechnical aspects of HIE take significant time to develop for any HIE network, especially national networks. Therefore the working groups required several years to develop consensus around the technical, governance, privacy, and security components that would become codified into the now national-level Ofek.

The MOH released a formal request for proposal in 2011 to construct the national HIE network [10]. This document detailed the technical and nontechnical requirements of the network as well as the entity leading the implementation. During the following year, the MOH selected Clalit's model to be the national HIE network. The largest HMO's Ofek platform was selected, because it was operational and included other hospitals outside of the Clalit HMO. The MOH ultimately decided that expanding Ofek nationally would be better than developing or purchasing a novel HIE platform.

In 2012, the MOH actively encouraged hospitals to adopt Ofek. Technically, the national HIE network was a directive from the ministry, not a requirement (e.g., there was no law requiring participation). Hospitals had to voluntarily connect to Ofek. Clalit took the position they would support any hospital when that hospital was ready to join. The ministry and working groups provided guidance to Clalit on how to expand Ofek. Clalit provided guidance, technical support, and other forms of assistance to HMOs and hospitals that volunteered to join the network.

Hospitals began going live with the national Ofek network in February 2013. To encourage more hospitals to join Ofek, the ministry created monthly adoption and usage reports [10]. These reports were sent to hospitals, putting peer pressure on them to either join the network or increase their utilization of Ofek. In an analysis of HIE participation following the distribution of reports from the ministry, adoption of Ofek by non-Clalit hospitals steadily increased through the beginning of 2016. As of 2016, 30 (71%) of the nation's 42 hospitals were connected to Ofek [10]. At the time of writing this case study, nearly all of the nation's hospitals (exclusions are some private hospitals not affiliated with any HMO) are connected to and using the national HIE network.

In addition to hospitals, all of Clalit's ambulatory care sites used Ofek as of the writing of this case study. The nation is currently in the process of migrating from Ofek to the next generation of its HIE network, described toward the end of this case study.

31.4 Technical infrastructure of Ofek

Using the definitions from Chapter 1, the Israeli national HIE system (Ofek) can be classified as a *government-facilitated HIE network.* The network connects nodes together to exchange information, yet there is no centralized database. The network operates on top of a software-oriented architecture (SOA) platform in which web services call out to each member of the network to retrieve information when it is needed. Although the network does possess some push capabilities (described later), the network operates primarily as a pull HIE system in which clinicians retrieve data *on demand.*

Each participant—the four HMOs plus public and private hospitals—implements a common database within its environment that mirrors the data in its EHR system. As data are loaded into the edge database, they are normalized to a common data model. Once loaded, data are primed and ready for querying when needed by other sites across the network. Each edge data repository operates similarly to an enterprise data warehouse, which is modern terminology for a centralized database of information normalized across an organization. The initial concept was conceived by computer science professionals who sought to solve a health care problem using a template from the IT world known as Enterprise Resource Planning, which integrates and shares information about an organization's financial, supply chain, commerce, inventory, operations, manufacturing, and human resources into a single, integrated IT system.

The participants in Ofek are depicted in Fig. 31.2, which suggests the architecture used for the HIE network. Each HMO, hospital, or participant loads its data into an edge database deployed behind its own firewall. Middleware, provided by dbMotion, is then used to securely connect each node of the network so that users at Point of Care A can query for data from the other network participants. The middleware searches across the network for the patient

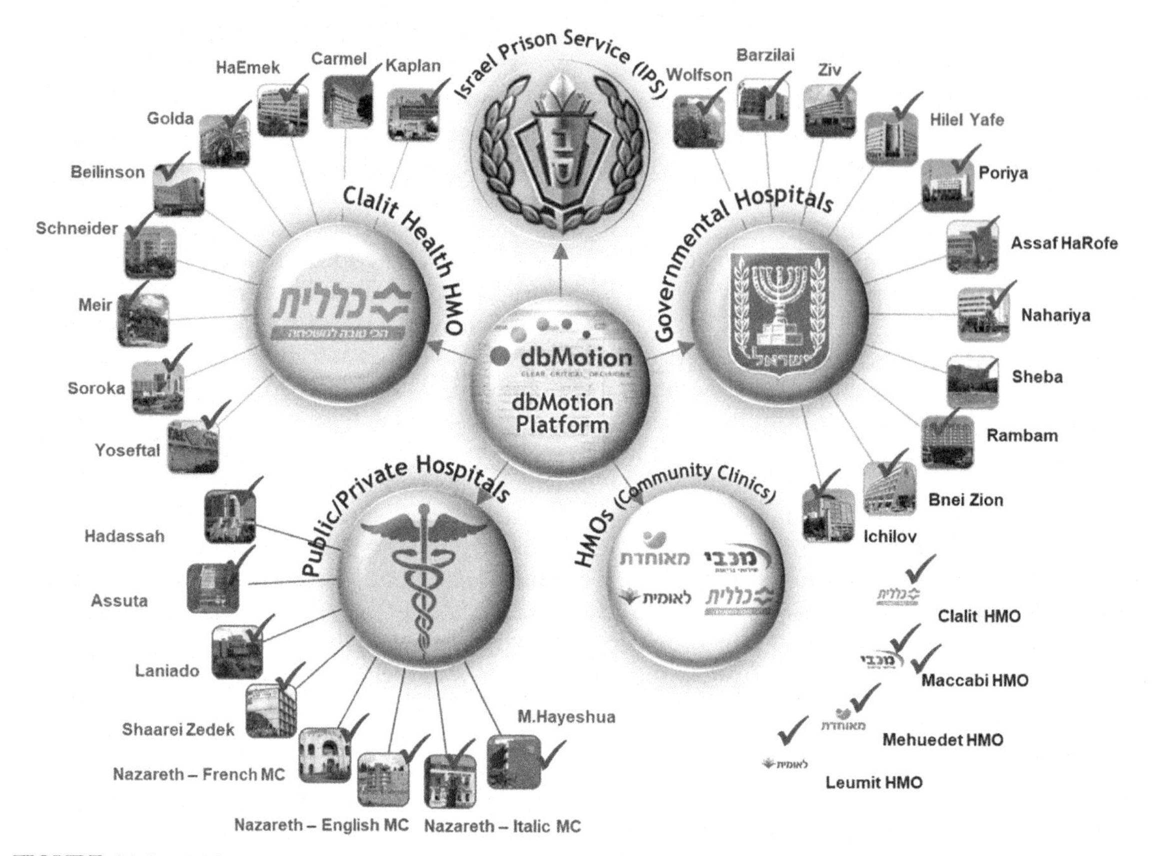

FIGURE 31.2 Ofek participants and major HIE hubs connecting hospitals and community clinics across Israel, pioneered by the Clalit HMO. The middleware is powered by the dbMotion platform. *HMO*, Health Maintenance Organization. Source: *Used with permission from the Information and Computing Division of the Israeli Ministry of Health.*

identified by Point of Care A and retrieves the common, defined data set for the patient. Once the information is gathered, it is loaded into a **virtual patient object (VPO)**. The middleware can then perform a number of tasks with the VPO, including (1) presentation of the data to a user via the Viewer Layer or (2) execution of decision support algorithms [8].

Some sites can elect to have the Ofek system deliver (or push) discharge summaries and other documents directly into its own enterprise EHR/HIE system. Two HMOs elect to do this, which allows them to display the information directly within their own enterprise systems rather than taking users to an interface hosted by the MOH for viewing Ofek information. Each night, clinical data summaries for recently discharged patients are structured into a custom XML document (called a capsule). This deep integration between the HIE and local EHR system is something many larger health systems are capable of supporting, yet such integration remains challenging for small hospitals and most ambulatory providers. Most interaction with Ofek requires the clinician to request information, via a button displayed within the local EHR system, that is retrieved in that moment from the edge servers then virtualized for the clinician to review. When the clinician is done viewing the information in the VPO, he or she closes the object, and the data disappear from the presentation layer. Momentary integration means that data are typically not duplicated across nodes on the network. This model facilitates better security as well as governance of clinical data at the heart of the exchange.

There exist a wide range of data in Ofek. In Table 31.1, the various categories of data contained within the HIE network are described. The available data are quite similar to most other HIE efforts around the globe. Furthermore, these categories are all commonplace in C-CDA documents, although many of these data are not required for a MDS.

31.4.1 Security Protocols

Although security was important when Ofek operated within Clalit as an enterprise HIE, security became critical to the expansion of Ofek into a national HIE network. There are two key security protocols that help Ofek ensure only authorized, appropriate individuals access patient records. First, the network employs a role-based access rule that enables individuals to access records for patients only while they are under their care. For example, a clinician at a department in Hospital X can only access the VPO for a patient while that patient is admitted to that department in Hospital X. Upon admission to the hospital, the patient's records can be queried by staff at that facility. Similarly, the patient's general practitioner (GP) can only access patient for whom the GP is attributed. This limits access to a subset of network users that are more likely to have a business relationship with the patient (i.e., providing active care to the patient). Other individuals whose relationship cannot be determined are not allowed to request the VPO for the given patient.

A second security feature is automatic log-out after 30 minutes of inactivity. This feature likely frustrates some clinicians. However, the feature helps to prevent accidental breaches of data because a clinician was interrupted and walked away from a computer. Interruptions happen all the time in health care delivery. When the clinician wishes to return to viewing the VPO, he or she would need to log back into Ofek and query again for the records. This feature is common in many HIE networks where the clinicians log into a portal to view centralized records for a patient.

Any patient who wants may opt-out from the Ofek although it is very rare [12].

31.4.2 Commercial connection

The Ofek system was developed and piloted within Clalit in collaboration with dbMotion, an

TABLE 31.1 Categories and descriptions of data in the Israeli national HIE network (Ofek).

Category	Description
Demographics	Patient data summary, demographic details
Diagnostic results	Laboratory results summary, imaging tests summary
Procedures	Past procedures (surgeries, cardiac catheterizations) summary; procedure notes
Encounters	Outpatient and community clinic visits summary, previous ED and hospital visits; diagnostic codes from visits
Documents	Discharge summaries from hospitals
Medications	Prescribed medications, medication allergies

Derived from published literature including Politi L, Codish S, Sagy I, Fink L. Use patterns of health information exchange systems and admission decisions: reductionistic and configurational approaches. Int J Med Inform 2015;84(12):1029–1038 [11].

Israeli company. The company dbMotion was founded in 1996 and incubated within Ness, one of the earliest and largest Information Systems and Technology services companies in Israel [13]. The Ofek system helped launch dbMotion as an independent company in 2004. In 2013, Allscripts Healthcare Solutions purchased dbMotion, although dbMotion continues to operate as a separate division of the large EHR company.

At the time of writing, Allscripts continued to offer a dbMotion Solution that enables enterprise HIE for health systems [14]. Furthermore, dbMotion continues to support the nation's HIE efforts. According to an Allscripts company blog post from late 2021 [15], dbMotion continues to operate the national HIE network in cooperation with the MOH. Moreover, according to Allscripts, "dbMotion is replacing the Ofek legacy system with new technology that will enable advanced data analysis and semantic-level interoperability." [15].

Based on speeches given by the MOH in 2019 shortly before the COVID-19 pandemic, national interoperability efforts are now focused on supporting the fully continuum of care. This indicates a shift from a primary focus on hospital and GP settings to the full spectrum of places where patients receive care, including long-term and specialty care practices.

In addition, these days the MOH also talks about leveraging the national HIE infrastructure to support research and other secondary uses. There exists a strict process by which researchers can request information from Ofek. Researchers must adhere to the Declaration of Helsinki principles and submit appropriate documentation to an ethics committee for review and approval. The HIE network uses a standard process for reviewing requests and validating the ethics approval documentation. Data are typically provided as de-identified datasets to researchers.

31.5 Utility and use of HIE in Israel

31.5.1 Functions and services

From its beginning, Ofek has been focused on a single, primary directive: support better clinical decisions with timely, relevant clinical information. Initially, the HIE network focused on hospital-based care delivery, bringing information to hospitalists, emergency department (ED) personnel, and internal medicine physicians. Currently, the network supports all hospital departments plus ambulatory clinics as well. Clinicians in all of these settings use the information to support patient care. This remains the focus of the network. Moreover, as one informant put it, Ofek is simply a part of patient care in Israel. Most clinicians, at least those in Clalit, use it on a regular daily basis to access information, although it is not used necessarily for every patient.

31.5.2 Critical HIE research by Israel

An important contribution of Ofek beyond supporting patient care in Israel is its role as a platform for studying the development, implementation, and use of HIE networks. Since its inception, Israeli researchers have used Ofek as a living laboratory for studying EHRs and HIE services. This is unique among HIE networks in the world as few have any publications about their development or operations, and just a small handful have as many publications as Ofek.

Early research papers on Ofek described the emerging landscape of EHR systems in Israel and the efforts of Clalit to connect its hospitals with an enterprise HIE [8]. Several papers, prior to the expansion of Ofek beyond Clalit, examined the benefits of integrated EHRs using HIE methods to facilitate better care delivery and patient outcomes [16–20]. Nirel et al. [20] found that after implementing Ofek in hospitals, the internal medicine department decreased the number of laboratory tests and computerized tomography (CT) tests ordered. These reductions were considered to be both "financially and medically significant." Ben-Assuli et al. [17] found a negative relationship between clinicians in the ED using their EHR system and/or Ofek led to a reduction in 7-day readmissions. The researchers further observed that when clinicians used the HIE network, or "external medical history" (e.g., Ofek), the number of redundant (or unnecessary) admissions to the hospital also decreased [17]. Studies like these are critical to establishing the value proposition for HIE (see Chapter 17).

Over time, research from Israel shifted to focus on the adoption and impact of OEFK beyond the Clalit HMO. Gefen et al. [10] used an interrupted time series analysis to examine the adoption of Ofek as non-Clalit hospitals connected to the HIE network and the MOH encouraged adoption. The researchers found that as adoption of HIE network by non-Clalit facilities increased, use of Ofek grew within Clalit in parallel. This suggests that as data from outside facilities are more available, clinicians are more likely to use the system to retrieve information that does not exist in their system. The researchers further concluded that HIE adoption follows the Bass model of adoption [10], a theoretical model that explains the diffusion of an innovation over time [21].

In another study, Bahous and Shadmi [22] compared the information available on pediatric patients who required care in the (ED.) The ED was located in a non-Clalit hospital. The researchers compared three information sources: the patient's own account of their medical history, the referral letter sent from the GP, and Ofek. In Israel, patients are referred to the ED under a hospitalist model with a letter that contains the patient's medical history, medication list, and lab test results, as well as the current reason for referral [22,23]. Looking across all three information sources for 170 ED encounters, researchers concluded that Ofek was more complete than the referral letter from the GP [22] demonstrating the high degree of information coverage using the HIE. The HIE was significantly more complete with respect to documented allergies (11% vs 5%), prior diagnoses (96% vs 32%), and medications (91% vs 52%). However, it should be noted that the patient's direct accounting of their information was most accurate and complete overall.

In addition to demonstrating the impact of HIE on care delivery processes and outcomes, Israeli researchers pioneered studies on the use of HIE systems by clinicians. Most studies on HIE use compare clinical settings where HIE is available to those where HIE is not available. Early research on Ofek used this approach [9]. This method of comparison provides a reasonable proxy, yet it is not as accurate as observing actual use of the HIE by clinicians. Very few studies accurately measure whether, for a given encounter or visit, the clinician treating the patient used the HIE network to lookup information or accessed information from the HIE [24,25]. Israeli researchers have conducted numerous studies in which the access log files from the HIE were leveraged to examine whether use of HIE makes a difference in care delivery and/or outcomes [10,11,16,25–28].

One example involved an examination of nearly 1 million adult ED referrals across Clalit using the earliest version of Ofek from Ben-Assuli et al. [16]. Encounters where data from the HIE network were viewed were compared to those in which data were not accessed. The researchers found that utilization of HIE significantly influenced ED clinicians' admission decisions, which were driven by the clinicians' viewing previous hospitalizations, laboratory results, and imaging data [16]. The study underscored the importance of clinician access to comprehensive, integrated medical records.

A later study [11] confirmed that availability of information in the HIE is positively associated with admission, including admission to intensive care unit (ICU). Furthermore, the more recent study further examined the length of time clinicians spent viewing the information, and they controlled for external factors such as patient and provider characteristics. The researchers observed that "quick and dirty" views of the HIE data are not associated with ICU admission, but more extensive time by the clinician interacting with HIE-based information increases the likelihood of ICU admission. In other words, more complete medical history information, when thoughtfully viewed by clinicians, reduces uncertainty, which enhances clinical decision-making.

31.5.3 Ofek facilitated national COVID-19 pandemic response

Within days of the first cases of COVID-19 identified in Israel, Ofek offered clinicians in Israel a new dashboard that contained a list of COVID-19 patents in their facility along with key clinical data relevant to COVID-19 for those patients. The dashboard also provided clinicians with population level statistics [15], such as:

- total patients tested;
- total confirmed cases;
- total new daily cases;
- total patients converted negative;
- total currently hospitalized patients;
- total and percent confirmed from high-risk populations;
- gender and age distribution;
- distribution of cases by ZIP code;
- incidence of related clinical presentations, such as cough, wheezing, and fever; and
- incidence of reasons for high risk for severe illness, such as asthma and being older than 65.

Applications used at the point-of-care in Israeli facilities were also updated to indicate in the corner of the screen the COVID-19 status (e.g., positive, recovered, negative) of each patient [15]. In December 2020, when vaccination efforts began in Israel, the clinical applications were updated to display the vaccination status for each patient.

Israel also leveraged its national HIE network to support epidemiological investigations of new cases of COVID-19 by MOH district clinicians [15]. The HIE provided these MOH investigators with access to patient records, enabling them to gain insights on COVID-19 clinical pathways. The MOH also integrated its nationwide vaccine registry into the national HIE so all providers could access vaccination information regardless of where a patient received the vaccine or care. The MOH further supported those providers in motivating the patients that were not vaccinated. The efforts in Israel to support COVID-19 pandemic response are extremely similar to those of the Indiana HIE [29] and other HIE networks around the globe, demonstrating the power of a statewide or national infrastructure for use during emergencies and emerging health threats.

31.6 Facilitators and barriers to HIE in Israel

31.6.1 Facilitators of HIE

The Ofek system began as a vision by a leader who directed enterprising IT professionals to solve a problem using their technical prowess, but a vision of HIE is only part of the equation that leads to success. Israel possesses several factors that facilitated the development, implementation, and use of HIE within Clalit and now across the nation. In this section, we briefly summarize those factors.

31.6.1.1 The Israel national identity number

Like other nations (see Chapter 28), Israel uses a national identifier (ID) to uniquely distinguish citizens across public and private services. The same ID number is used by individuals to subscribe and use mobile phone services, secure credit to purchase a vehicle, and enroll in health care benefits with one of the four HMOs. That same ID is used by health care providers to record health care services when rendered to the patient. Therefore all EMRs for a person are stored using the same unique ID number. As data are loaded into the edge servers for Ofek, patient ID numbers are stored with records, which facilitates record linkage (see Chapter 12). Deterministic methods can be used to accurately retrieve all medical records for the same person. This condition facilitates development and implementation of HIE, and it facilitates accurate retrieval of information during regular, ongoing use of HIE services.

31.6.1.2 *Opt out consent model*

Culturally, roadside checkpoints routinely scrutinize the identification of the individuals as well as the contents of their car trunks, purses, and backpacks. Israelis expect and embrace a communal culture in which anonymity and privacy often yield to security and safety of the population. This is not to say that citizens are comfortable with their private information being freely available to anyone, but they defer to HMOs, hospitals, and government agencies to manage their private information in exchange for the services they receive.

Israel uses an opt out consent model to govern the data in Ofek. Citizens have a right to opt out of the HIE network, meaning their data would not be shared across HMOs and providers. However, very few individuals have opted out to date [12].

Instead of opting out, some informants for this case study suggested that, due to cultural norms, patients are satisfied with their passive system of HIE in which data are shared between their providers without the patient needing to actively carry files to appointments or push a button to send information to their next care provider. Moreover, health information technology is ubiquitous in Israel. Citizens can logon to apps provided by the HMOs to schedule appointments, view lab results, etc. They see technology and the sharing of their information seamlessly behind the scenes as a perk of their health care system, not an affront to their privacy. Another reason might be the obscurity of OEFK as well as the opt out option. It is nearly impossible to find information on how to opt out of the HIE network, yet community clinics should know how to direct patients who request to opt-out. Furthermore, few patients understand HIE or its role. These factors may contribute to few people following through with removing their data from the HIE network.

31.6.1.3 *The virtual patient object*

The federated network approach used in Israel in which data are integrated at run-time for view by clinicians who are actively caring for patients is another important facilitator to national HIE. Multiple informants, news articles, and published studies herald the VPO as an important facilitator of HIE (with security), because the temporary nature of the integrated record protects patient privacy and confidentiality of medical records.

Medical records are retained at the source, within the edge server connected to the HIE network. There is no centralized, national database of medical records that could be compromised by a hacker or accidentally breached by a government employee. Data are only brought together temporarily in an EHR system or HIE portal for immediate use by individuals who are authorized to view clinical information for patients in care.

This approach preserves confidentiality and builds trust in the system by the participants. This model is likely one reason that the competitive HMOs are willing to participate in the network. Data from each HMO remain within the firewall of the HMO, and it is only shared for a short period of time for the specific patients under care by a provider from another HMO. This scenario is much easier for an organization to support rather than carte blanche access to all records by someone working in a competitor's hospital. Moreover, the simplicity of this approach makes it easy to explain to stakeholders (including lawmakers) and the public how the system works while protecting privacy. The VPO, therefore, contributes to the wide support from health care and governmental stakeholders as well as the public.

31.6.1.4 *Strong support from the Israeli Ministry of Health*

Another facilitator of HIE in Israel is the strong executive support for Ofek within the MOH as well as the nation's HMOs. Over the past decade, the MOH established a bold vision for making Israel a leader in digital health. In each iteration of the nation's eHealth/Digital Health strategy, HIE has been featured as a key enabler of the Israeli digital health ecosystem. The MOH encouraged non-Clalit providers to join Ofek, and the MOH worked to ensure all governmental hospitals became part of the HIE network. By cultivating a strong digital health ecosystem in the country and openly advocating for HIE, the MOH helped create a culture of HIE. This advocacy at the national level brings awareness to the HIE network and, more importantly, creates opportunities and resources for the network. Over the past decade, the MOH has increasingly taken ownership of the HIE and today manages the network. Therefore, what was a Clalit initiative is now a robust, MOH-led initiative. This means that public funding from the Digital Health Division of the MOH is used to manage operations and invest in innovative functions and services for the future. Executive support as well as public resources are vital to the sustainability of the Israeli national HIE network.

31.6.2 Barriers to national HIE adoption and use

Although Israel has a comprehensive, national HIE infrastructure, the nation does not have 100% adoption of HIE across all of its hospitals and clinics. Despite the fact that Ofek is used extensively within the nation's largest HMO and to a great extent by the other HMOs, the national HIE network remains a work in progress. In this section, we review historical barriers to achieving the goal of widespread adoption and use of HIE. Some of these barriers are being addressed by the evolving new HIE platform or could be addressed through future policy and regulations from the MOH.

31.6.2.1 *HIE remains a directive, not a requirement*

Current regulations in Israel encourage HMOs, hospitals, and ambulatory care providers to adopt and use the national HIE network. While adoption is high, adoption and use are not mandatory. Therefore some providers are not yet connected or contributing information to Ofek. This includes some private hospitals and clinics as well as a small handful of public facilities.

Informants suggested that, several years prior to writing this case study, there were efforts to legally mandate national adoption of HIE. It failed to pass because of concerns over regulations. Legislators wanted to regulate the HIE network, especially with respect to privacy and security. According to one informant, this remains the largest barrier to true nationwide adoption of HIE in Israel.

31.6.2.2 *Separate but equal edge servers*

The federated model used by Ofek normalizes data into edge servers that are queried using a common data model when information is needed. Technically each node in the network hosts two separate edge servers: one for inpatient EHR data and one for ambulatory EHR data. Therefore inpatient and ambulatory data are not truly integrated within the HMOs. They remain distinct EHR data sources that require technical workarounds so that Ofek can seamlessly query them in the background.

The same is true with the newer HIE platform. In fact, the barrier is greater, because each node on the network must support interfaces to legacy Ofek nodes as well as newer platform nodes that use a different data model.

This design is not known to end users, so it is not a barrier, per se, to use of the system by clinicians. However, it is a barrier to more advanced uses of Ofek, including population health analytics. Many population health studies conducted in Israel (think about all the COVID-19 cohort studies featured in news stories) use data from only one HMO, perhaps due to this technical barrier. The nation hopes to address this in the future, perhaps through the emerging, next-generation HIE network.

31.6.2.3 *No* lingua franca

Each HMO uses its own terminology. Governmental health facilities use a separate terminology. Historically, Ofek has not required the use of semantic standards, and the nation has not previously mapped the disparate terminologies used into a common *lingua franca* (a language adopted broadly by all speakers whose native languages are different). Edge servers that use a common data model can force, for example, laboratory results to generally be structured the same way. However, it is not easy to interpret all HbA1c test names used by the various HMOs and public hospitals. Therefore, while large volumes of data are exchanged each day, it is difficult to conduct population-level summary statistics on diabetes screenings.

Lacking a common set of terminologies at the national level is a major barrier to true interoperability. Many nations establish common, required terminologies ahead of their HIE technical integrations as part of their overall digital health strategy. Because Israel's HIE network emerged as a grassroots effort within one HMO that later expanded nationally, the nation did not follow this pathway, which is now recommended as a best practice. Moreover, in the early 2000s when Ofek emerged, many of today's internationally recognized semantic standards were not mature and were sparsely adopted. Sometimes being a first mover in the market means you must learn some lessons the hard way.

31.6.2.4 *Limited patient experience*

Despite broad use of health IT and HIE in Israel, it should be noted that patient-facing technologies remain limited at the national level. Although patients can view a significant amount of their clinical information including lab results via a portal from the HMO, patients do not have access to their complete medical records. In addition, patients cannot edit or amend medical records through the portals offered by the HMOs. Even more important is that the information displayed to patients via the portals is not actionable. The data are not put into context supporting patient-centered health care decision-making [30,31]. Therefore, while the socio-political and technical environments facilitate data sharing, there is more work ahead for Israel to transform its health system and the patient experience with technologies including its national HIE network.

31.6.2.5 *Investments in other technologies and maintenance of legacy systems*

One of the barriers for other HMOs or their facilities (points of care) to promote full adoption of the information existing in Ofek and/or connecting to Ofek is the HMO obligations to support other existing and new technologies that are getting the attention of the information and communications technology (ICT) managers at the HMO. This is especially true during the COVID-19 pandemic when a lot of focus is devoted to support real-time medical care, distance medicine, and telehealth. For instance, in Israel, TytoCare's telehealth solutions are used to remotely monitor patients by the TytoHome kit [32]. This modular medical kit is designed to observe the heart, lungs, stomach, skin, throat, ears, and body temperature, using dedicated technology for orientation, navigation, and quality analysis. This kit enables physicians to extract vital medical data to remotely monitor the patient, make the diagnosis in many cases, and reduce the heavy workload at clinics. Other future technologies might be also in focus in these years including internet of things, devices (wearable devices), and investing in telehealth solutions' implementations. These technologies and their required resources may delay or even suspend the HMOs efforts to fully implement their two-way connection to Ofek. HIE efforts in other nations, including the United States, have also identified competing priorities as a challenge to interoperability as ICT divisions often have a long "punch list" of projects.

31.7 The next generation of HIE in Israel—Eitan

In 2016, the nation began charting its course for the evolution of its national HIE infrastructure. According to Allscripts, the MOH signed a new agreement with dbMotion to replace the "Ofek legacy system" [15]. The new national HIE network [33], referred to as *Eitan* (meaning strong or firm in Hebrew), has a broad vision to improve the national infrastructure and enable advanced capabilities such as machine learning and artificial intelligence [34]. An initial focus of Eitan is on common clinical terminologies (e.g., SNOMED, ICD-11) that will support data analysis as well as semantic interoperability (see Chapter 10). Another goal is to interconnect medical records in the HMOs with those from the Ministry of Defense, enabling a comprehensive birth-to-adulthood medical record. During compulsory service in the military, medical records are managed outside the HMOs. At the time of writing, there are no published studies on Eitan.

Although there are no reports on Eitan, the national HIE network is operational and gradually increasing in adoption. Most private hospitals and clinics (only one is fully connected) are not using Eitan, but the MOH is working on a plan for HIE with these entities in the future.

Currently, the MOH manages a technical architecture to accommodate parallel HIE across facilities that use either Ofek or Eitan, which is called Ofakim at Clalit. As depicted in Fig. 31.3, Eitan queries across micro-HIE environments that exist at each node on the network. These HIE environments contain either Ofek or Eitan end points that interface with the underlying EMR systems. This allows distributed queries to pull back data from all nodes and present the data either in Ofek or Eitan. The HIE environments hosted at each node are updated daily with data on patients admitted and/or discharged within the last 24 hours. Unfortunately, the current situation exacerbates the separate but equal edge server challenge, which will exist until Ofek can be sunset and the entire nation is on the Eitan platform.

The user experience (UX) for Eitan is significantly different from Ofek. As opposed to a button in the EMR, which takes the clinician out to an Ofek web application through which they can view the VPO, Eitan is implemented as a layer on top of the EMR system. As depicted in Fig. 31.4, the Eitan "Agent" application hovers in the upper left-hand corner of the screen. The Agent displays summary information about the patient, including their COVID-19 status (e.g., vaccinated, infected, recovered). To interact with the VPO, clinicians drop down menus and select the information they wish to view. The data are then presented on screen, on top of the EMR application. In other words, it is not a separate application or screen, but Eitan is seamlessly integrated on top of the EMR system. As the clinician navigates to a new patient's local medical record, the distributed query in the background fetches data from the HIE network so it is readily accessible on demand.

According to MOH informants, Eitan will play a major role in helping Israel achieve its next national digital health strategy, which is

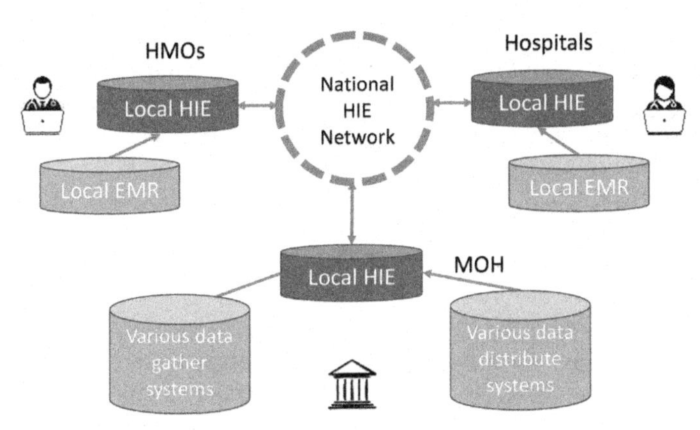

FIGURE 31.3 Architecture of the Israeli national HIE network. Source: *Used with permission from the Information and Computing Division of the Israeli Ministry of Health.*

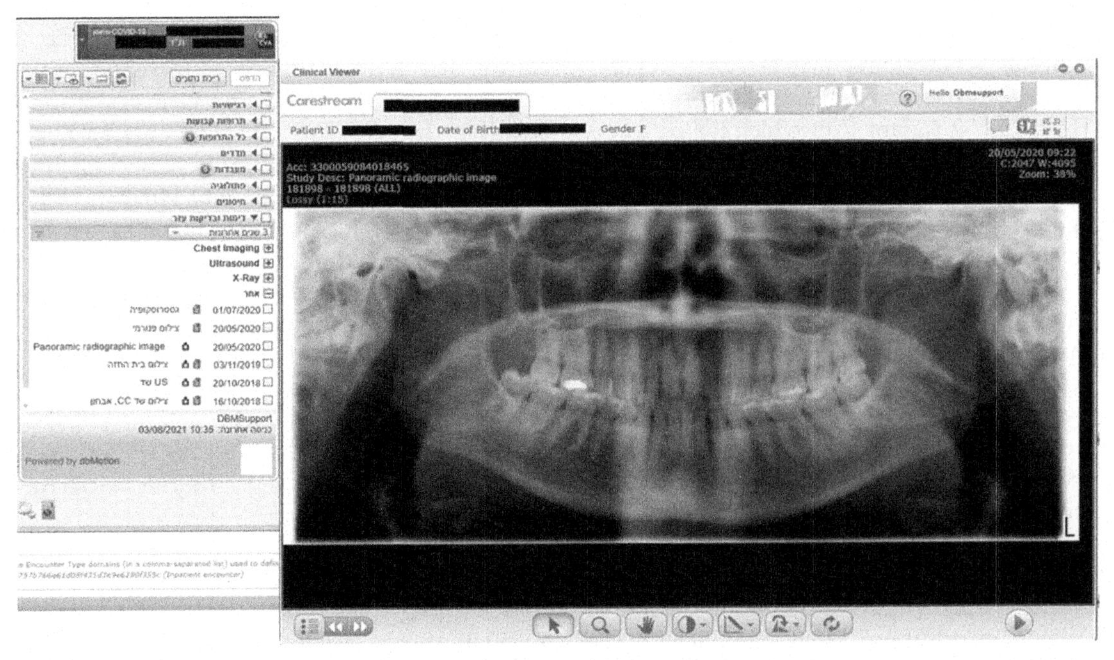

FIGURE 31.4 Screenshot of the Eitan "Agent," an application embedded within the electronic medical record system that provides access to records outside the current facility. The agent is on the left and displays information from the HIE network on the right, in the context of the EHR system used by the clinician. Source: *Used with permission from the Information and Computing Division of the Israeli Ministry of Health.*

currently under development. The initial focus of Eitan is to achieve the goal of a unifying medical terminology as well as incorporate imaging from all points of care. Through policy and regulations as well as mapping (see Chapter 10), Israel hopes to see the HMOs as well as the governmental and private health facilities move toward use of standard terminologies, including

SNOMED, ICD-11, and LOINC. This will help the nation achieve its semantic interoperability goals and enable advanced, population health capabilities including analytics.

Using a commercial image sharing solution, Eitan is making images (e.g., CT, X-Ray) available to clinicians (see Fig. 31.4) beyond the existing textual reports, such as structured notes from radiologists. The images are not transferred from their source into the VPO. Instead, clinicians can temporarily view the image via the commercial solution integrated into Eitan, saving significant network bandwidth.

In the future, Eitan will include additional data types not available today. Social determinant data are on the priority list (see Chapter 19). The nation also plans to add more clinical data, such as retinal screenings, including images, for glaucoma prevention. Furthermore, Eitan will add details on the SARS-CoV-2 variant with which the patient is actively infected to the Agent. More broadly, the MOH plans to focus more on data quality, developing ongoing, systematic analyses to improve completeness of the data in the edge servers.

The MOH has several innovative, technical enhancements for Eitan planned as well. First, Eitan will evolve to use a FHIR-based structure to replace the current SOA-based distributed query model. The network further plans to improve the UX/UI (user experience/user interface) for clinicians who interact with the Agent. Moreover, Israel plans to develop a mobile platform for Eitan, allowing clinicians to access Eitan using a mobile app on smartphones or other devices, which is essential in the age of telehealth. In addition, Eitan will include the ability for clinicians to request and manage consults with specialists or colleagues who may be in other facilities outside their HMO.

31.8 Summary

The story of the national HIE network in Israel highlights several important aspects of HIE. First, it demonstrates how a grassroots effort to facilitate access to "outside records" can mature into a national HIE infrastructure. This evolution took 15 years and required the socio-political aspects of HIE in the nation to catch up to the vision of Clalit, which demonstrated the value of HIE not only to the rest of the Israeli health system but also the world. Second, the story highlights a working example of a federated HIE architecture across an entire health system, enabling comparison with the centralized models seen in other nations. Third, the story of Israel's HIE network revels the importance of a focus on delivering value to clinicians, patients, and HMOs. The network involved clinical leaders early on in its development, and health system leaders guide its future. The central mission to focus on clinical care has remained front and center. Although steadfast in its focus, the HIE network also pivots as necessary to adapt to new challenges, like the COVID-19 pandemic. Finally, Israel's story demonstrates how HIE is facilitated by a strong, unique national identifier.

Upon a solid foundation of HIE within Clalit, Israel implemented one of the most robust national HIE networks in the world. A future in which Eitan can build upon this legacy and facilitate advanced functions like those described in Chapters 10, 18, and 19 is an exciting prospect for Israel and HIE as a discipline.

Questions for discussion

1. What are the strengths and limitations to a national person identifier (ID) like the one used in Israel? Does your nation have a national ID or universal health ID? Is this required for HIE success?
2. The HIE network in Israel has served as a platform for conducting cutting edge research on HIE. Yet, data from the HIE network is not allowed to be used for biomedical research. Is this a paradox?

Should data in HIE networks be available for uses beyond patient care? To what extent can the MDCLONE solution can be used?

3. What makes the national HIE network in Israel sustainable? What, if anything, would cause the government, health system, or citizens to stop supporting the HIE network?
4. What are the main three barriers to national HIE adoption in Israel and globally, using Israel's barriers as case studies? What efforts can be made to moderate the barriers in Israel and worldwide?
5. What are the key factors that enabled the national HIE network in Israel to succeed?

Acknowledgments

The authors gratefully acknowledge the time and information shared from a number of individuals interviewed for background on this case study. These individuals include:

1. Shabtai Itamar, MBA, PhD, Dean, School of Economics, College of Management Academic Studies
2. Tsipi Heart, MBA, PhD, Head of the Computer Science and Information Systems School at Ono Academic College
3. Talya Miron-Shatz, PhD, Professor, Ono Academic College and Visiting Researcher, University of Cambridge
4. Shlomi Codish, MD, MPH, Director General, Soroka Medical Center
5. Mali Shapira, Directorate of Medical Technologies, Informatics & Research, Ministry of Health
6. Milka Margalit-Weissman, Directorate of Medical Technologies, Informatics & Research, Ministry of Health

References

[1] Israel's technology industry: punching above its weight: The Economist; 2005 [cited 2022 Apr 9]. Nov 12. Available from: https://www.economist.com/business/2005/11/10/punching-above-its-weight.

[2] OECD. Gross domestic spending on R&D: Organisation for Economic Co-operation and Development; [cited 2022 Apr 9]. Available from: https://data.oecd.org/rd/gross-domestic-spending-on-r-d.htm.

[3] Summary report on health file management in September–November 2021 and calculation of the distribution key for 1.1.2022: State of Israel Social Security; 2021 [updated Dec; cited 2022 Apr 8]. Available from: https://www.btl.gov.il/Mediniyut/Situation/haveruth1/2022/Pages/capitatia_012022.aspx.

[4] Bar Siman-Tov M. How Israel turned decades of medical data into digital health gold. *Forbes* [Internet]. 2019 [cited 2022 Apr 9]. Available from: https://www.forbes.com/sites/startupnationcentral/2019/03/26/how-israel-turned-decades-of-medical-data-into-digital-health-gold/?sh=3665f6743ee4.

[5] MDClone. Homepage: MDClone; [cited 2022 Apr 9]. Available from: https://www.mdclone.com/.

[6] NC3. National COVID cohort collaborative: CTSA Program National Center for Data to Health (CD2H); [cited 2022 Apr 9]. Available from: https://covid.cd2h.org/.

[7] MDClone. MDClone and National Institutes of Health (NIH) to Support National Scientific Exploration for COVID-19 Efforts 2020 [cited 2022 Apr 9]. Available from: https://www.mdclone.com/news-press/articles/mdclone-and-national-institutes-of-health.

[8] Saiag E. The Israeli virtual national health record: a robust national health information infrastructure based on a firm foundation of trust. Stud Health Technol Inform 2005;116:427–32.

[9] Flaks-Manov N, Shadmi E, Hoshen M, Balicer RD. Health information exchange systems and length of stay in readmissions to a different hospital. J Hosp Med 2016;11(6):401–6.

[10] Gefen D, Ben-Assuli O, Stehr M, Rosen B, Denekamp Y. Governmental intervention in Hospital Information Exchange (HIE) diffusion: a quasi-experimental ARIMA interrupted time series analysis of monthly HIE patient penetration rates. Eur J Inf Syst 2019;28(6):627–45.

[11] Politi L, Codish S, Sagy I, Fink L. Use patterns of health information exchange systems and admission decisions: reductionistic and configurational approaches. Int J Med Inform 2015;84(12):1029–38.

[12] Rosen B. Healthcare in Israel for us audiences: Myers-JDC-Brookdale Institute; 2011 Available from: http://brookdale-web.s3.amazonaws.com/uploads/2011/01/133-11-Israel-Healthcare-US-Audiences-2-REP-ENG.pdf.

[13] Ness. About Ness: Ness Digital; [cited 2022 Apr 9]. Available from: https://www.ness-tech.co.il/en/.

[14] Allscripts. The dbMotion solution: Allscripts Healthcare, LLC; [cited 2022 Apr 9]. Available from: https://www.allscripts.com/solution/dbmotion/.

[15] Gorodischer E. Powering Israel's pandemic response with a nationwide interoperability platform: Allscripts Healthcare, LLC; 2021 [cited 2022 Apr 9]. Available from: https://www.allscripts.com/2021/10/powering-israels-pandemic-response-with-a-nationwide-interoperability-platform/.

[16] Ben-Assuli O, Shabtai I, Leshno M, Hill S. EHR in emergency rooms: exploring the effect of key information components on main complaints. J Med Syst 2014;38(4):36.

[17] Ben-Assuli O, Shabtai I, Leshno M. The impact of EHR and HIE on reducing avoidable admissions: controlling main differential diagnoses. BMC Med Inf Decis Mak 2013;13:49.

[18] Nirel N, Rosen B, Sharon A, Blondheim O, Sherf M, Cohen AD. OFEK virtual medical records: an evaluation of an integrated hospital-community system. Harefuah. 2011;150(2):72–8 209.

[19] Nirel N, Rosen B, Sharon A, Samuel H, Cohen AD. The impact of an integrated hospital-community medical information system on quality of care and medical service utilisation in primary-care clinics. Inf Health Soc Care 2011;36(2):63–74.

[20] Nirel N, Rosen B, Sharon A, Blondheim O, Sherf M, Samuel H, et al. The impact of an integrated hospital-community medical information system on quality and service utilization in hospital departments. Int J Med Inform 2010;79(9):649–57.

[21] Bass FM. A new product growth for model consumer durables. Manage Sci 1969;15(5):215–27.

[22] Bahous MC, Shadmi E. Health information exchange and information gaps in referrals to a pediatric emergency department. Int J Med Inform 2016;87:68–74.

[23] Tabenkin H, Gross R. The role of the primary care physician in the Israeli health care system as a 'gatekeeper'—the viewpoint of health care policy makers. Health Policy 2000;52(2):73–85.

[24] Rahurkar S, Vest JR, Finnell JT, Dixon BE. Trends in user-initiated health information exchange in the inpatient, outpatient, and emergency settings. J Am Med Inform Assoc 2021;28(3):622–7.

[25] Politi L, Codish S, Sagy I, Fink L. Use patterns of health information exchange through a multidimensional lens: conceptual framework and empirical validation. J Biomed Inform 2014;52:212–21.

[26] Ben-Assuli O, Padman R. Analysing repeated hospital readmissions using data mining techniques. Health Syst (Basingstoke) 2018;7(3):166–80.

[27] Politi L, Codish S, Sagy I, Fink L. Substitution and complementarity in the use of health information exchange and electronic medical records. Eur J Inf Syst 2020;1–19.

[28] Politi L, Codish S, Sagy I, Fink L. Balancing volume and duration of information consumption by physicians: the case of health information exchange in critical care. J Biomed Inform 2017;71:1–15.

[29] Dixon BE, Grannis SJ, McAndrews C, Broyles AA, Mikels-Carrasco W, Wiensch A, et al. Leveraging data visualization and a statewide health information exchange to support COVID-19 surveillance and response: application of public health informatics. J Am Med Inform Assoc 2021;28(7):1363–73.

[30] Miron-Shatz T. Your life depends on it: what you can do to make better choices about your health. Basic Books; 2021. p. 272.

[31] Pandita D. Consumer health informatics: engaging and empowering patients and families. In: Finnell JT, Dixon BE, editors. Clinical informatics study guide: text and review. 2nd ed. Cham: Springer; 2022. p. 351–74.

[32] tytocare. How does TytoCare work?: TytoCare Ltd; [cited 2022 Apr 9]. Available from: https://www.tytocare.com/how-tyto-works/.

[33] Ministry of Health. Health information exchange: state of Israel; [cited 2022 Apr 9]. Available from: https://www.health.gov.il/English/About/projects/shared_medical_info/Pages/default.aspx.

[34] Kostera T. For better care: Israel bets on big data: Bertelsmann Stiftung; 2018 [cited 2022 Apr 9]. Available from: https://blog.der-digitale-patient.de/en/israel-big-data/.

CHAPTER

32

Bringing health information exchange to the Middle East and North Africa: the case of Malaffi in Abu Dhabi

Ahmed Deeb[1], Bisera Lakinska[2], Rahul Goyal[2], Atif Al Braiki[2] and Hamed Al Hashemi[3]

[1]Earlham College, Richmond, IN, USA [2]Malaffi, Abu Dhabi, United Arab Emirates [3]Department of Health – Abu Dhabi, Abu Dhabi, United Arab Emirates

Major themes

- Using a private–public partnership (PPP) model to implement a health information exchange system in Abu Dhabi, United Arab Emirates.
- Driving digital transformation through the exchange of health-care data.
- Leveraging a health information exchange to support COVID-19 response.
- The role of standardized data in a health-care ecosystem as an enabler of information exchange and improved data quality.

32.1 Introduction

Planning for health information exchange (HIE) began in the United Arab Emirates (UAE) in 2016. A few years later, the Emirate of Abu Dhabi launched the first HIE platform in the UAE as well as the Middle East and North Africa region. In a brief span of just a few years, the HIE network has been rapidly implemented and adopted.

This case study tells the story of Malaffi, the HIE network based in Abu Dhabi. The case highlights its origins, its relationship to newer HIE initiatives in the UAE, and the challenges it faced. The case further describes its architecture and its future directions.

32.2 The United Arab Emirates

The UAE (Fig. 32.1) is a constitutional federation of seven emirates: Abu Dhabi, Dubai, Sharjah, Ajman, Umm Al Quwain, Ras Al Khaimah, and Fujairah. Abu Dhabi is the largest of the seven emirates in the United Arab Emirates (UAE), with a population of around 3 million residents.

Health Information Exchange
DOI: https://doi.org/10.1016/B978-0-323-90802-3.00020-4

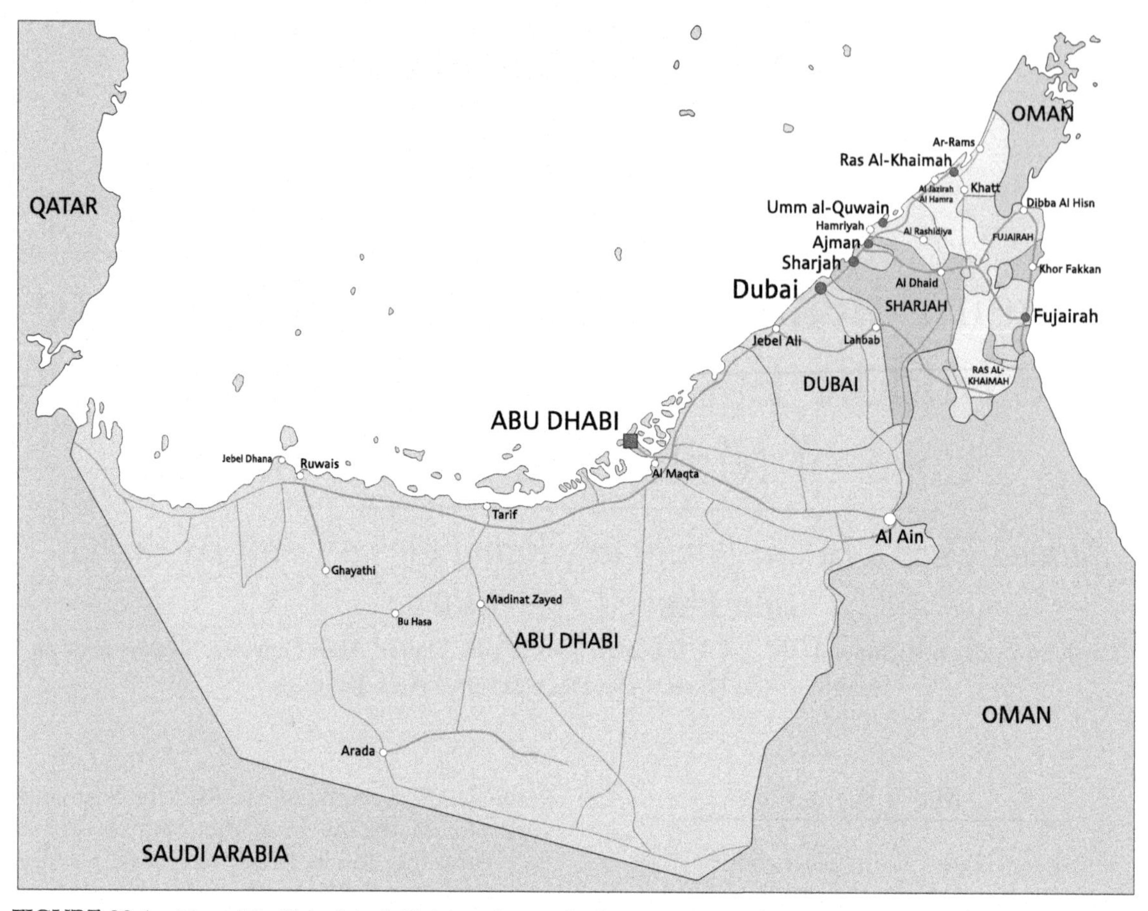

FIGURE 32.1 Map of the United Arab Emirates. Source: *Bardocz Peter, Licensed via Shutterstock.*

In 2014, His Highness Sheikh Mohammed bin Rashid Al Maktoum, Vice-President and Prime Minister of the UAE and Ruler of Dubai, launched a seven-year UAE National Agenda leading to the UAE Vision 2021 which also coincides with the UAE's 50th National Day [1].

One of the agenda items was the achievement of world-class healthcare, through a set of goals that emphasize the importance of preventive medicine and seeks to reduce cancer and lifestyle-related diseases such as diabetes and cardiovascular diseases to ensure a longer, healthy life for citizens. In addition, the agenda aims to reduce the prevalence of smoking and increase the healthcare system's readiness to deal with epidemics and health risks [2].

The UAE Ministry of Health and Promotion (MOHAP) oversees the implementation of government policy in relation to the provision of healthcare for all UAE citizens and residents and provides both healthcare services and regulatory oversight in the Northern Emirates, including Ras Al Khaimah, Ajman, Umm al Quwain, Sharjah, and Fujairah. However, some of the emirates and free zones also have their own regulatory authorities, most notably the Department of Health – Abu Dhabi (DOH) and Dubai Health Authority (DHA), in the Emirates of Abu Dhabi and Dubai, respectively.

In 2018, according to the World Bank, healthcare expenditures in the UAE reached $18.2 billion and were expected to rise to $21.3 billion by 2021. Overall, healthcare spending was projected to account for 4.6% of the country's Gross Domestic Product by 2026, up from 4.27% in 2018. The long-term trend lines for the UAE's healthcare sector are positive [3].

As a result of the problematic lifestyle habits, such as a sedentary lifestyle and use of tobacco, chronic conditions such as cardiovascular diseases, cancer, and diabetes are prevalent [4]. Cardiovascular disease remains the leading cause of fatalities in the UAE, accounting for over two-thirds of all deaths [4]. Strokes are the main cause of disability in the UAE and the third-greatest cause of death. From zero stroke management centers in 2014, the UAE had opened 12 centers by the end of 2019 [4]. Cancer is also a big issue in the country, accounting for 15% of deaths [3]. In 2020, 4807 new cases of cancer in the UAE were diagnosed [3]. However, this figure is still relatively low in comparison to eight other countries of the same size, such as Austria, where the number of new cases diagnosed in 2020 was 48,241 [3]. Diabetes remains widespread in the UAE, although its prevalence dropped to 16.3% of the total population in 2019 from 19.3% in 2013 [3]. According to an UN-backed report, the UAE is lagging behind the rest of the world in its diabetes care, despite having the highest rates of internationally accredited hospitals in the world [5].

32.3 The healthcare system in Abu Dhabi

The UAE has an insurance-based healthcare system. The Emirate of Abu Dhabi first made healthcare insurance mandatory for all residents and citizens in 2006 [6], with more than 2000 public and private healthcare provider facilities. The introduction of mandatory health insurance was a turning point for Abu Dhabi that ensured a minimum level of coverage and was designed to improve health outcomes across the Emirate. This opened the doors for the participation of the private sector and brought tremendous changes to the industry. The increased granularity of the providers also posed challenges with coordination of care, overutilization of services, and increased the financial burden to the cost of the payers. This, coupled with the aging population and the prevalence of chronic diseases, caused a steep rise in the per capita cost of care.

The health insurance regulatory system was divided between two regulators, the DOH, which is responsible for regulating the health sector and the Abu Dhabi Health Services Company (SEHA), responsible for managing government-owned healthcare facilities in Abu Dhabi.

In December of 2014, the DOH released the Abu Dhabi Healthcare Strategic Plan (Fig. 32.2) that included the introduction of an E-Health program as a facilitator for the other priorities [7]. This signified the start of the digital transformation of the healthcare system in the Emirate.

One of the main initiatives to support this strategic priority was the establishment of an HIE platform called Malaffi. The platform aims to connect the Abu Dhabi healthcare ecosystem via a common information infrastructure and allow the real-time sharing of healthcare information among all private and public healthcare entities to support care coordination and, ultimately, improve the quality of care and patient outcomes.

The drivers of this decision included multiple regional challenges, somewhat similar to the global ones. The steep rise of the cost of healthcare in the region [3], particularly in the UAE, presents a significant burden for the healthcare system, along with the underlying issue of overutilization of services and unethical practices. The above-mentioned sedentary lifestyle and tobacco use fuel the prevalence and incidence of chronic disease and put additional strain on the healthcare system (up to 27.8% of adults are

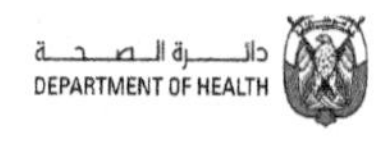

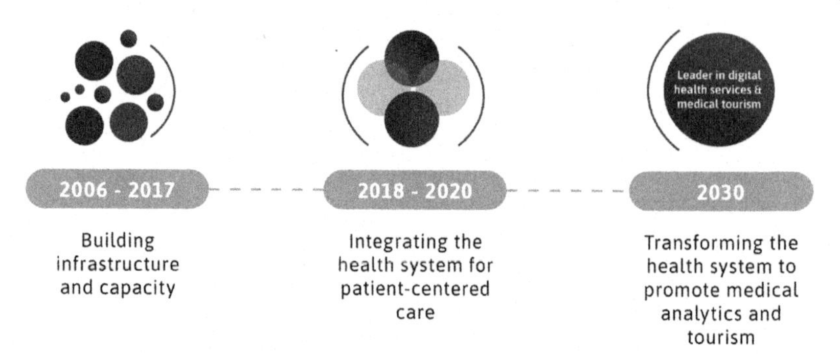

FIGURE 32.2 The digital transformation of the Abu Dhabi healthcare sector. Source: *The Department of Health – Abu Dhabi.*

obese, 25%–30% of men smoke; 16.3% of adults with diabetes in 2019) [3].

The DOH was also facing challenges in controlling the quality of care and getting real-time insights to enable better planning for the healthcare sector. A review of global case studies provided evidence that HIE systems yield multiple benefits in terms of reducing healthcare spending, overutilization, readmissions, and other important quality and cost indicators.

With a vision to establish world-class healthcare and reduce the need for Emiratis to travel abroad for treatment, the Abu Dhabi Government has formed partnerships with many renowned international healthcare institutions such as Cleveland Clinic, Mayo, Imperial College London, King's College London, LabCorp, and others. According to the 2017 statistics issued by the Federal Statistics and Competitive Authority, there were 45 hospitals, 8322 physicians and 20,480 nurses in the government sector, and 98 hospitals, 14,785 physicians and 33,435 nurses in the private sector [8].

32.4 Health information exchange initiatives in the UAE

Malaffi was launched in 2019 as the first HIE in the Middle East and North Africa region as a strategic initiative of the DOH and key to the digital transformation of the healthcare system in the Emirate. The mandate of Malaffi was to connect all more than 2000 healthcare facilities in Abu Dhabi, within a very ambitious timeline of three years. The main guiding document, the Policy on the Abu Dhabi Health Information Exchange [9] was published by the DOH in late 2018, prescribing the main principles of universal provider and patient participation, as well as defining the roles, responsibilities, and strategies around data management and data quality.

Further, in 2019, the DOH started mapping the journey of transforming the care model in Abu Dhabi using digital health and created a 10-year strategy.

Central to the strategy is the notion of creating a Centre of Digital Health and a data lake to collate all sources of information. The availability of the financial and clinical data from the DOH's claims management system, and the clinical data from the HIE Malaffi form the basis for this strategy.

Meanwhile, the DHA established the Dubai HIE, Nabidh, and the MOHAP announced the federal HIE, Riayati, that will connect all healthcare facilities in the Northern Emirates, and integrate with Malaffi in Abu Dhabi and Nabidh in Dubai [10]. These entities are represented in Fig. 32.3.

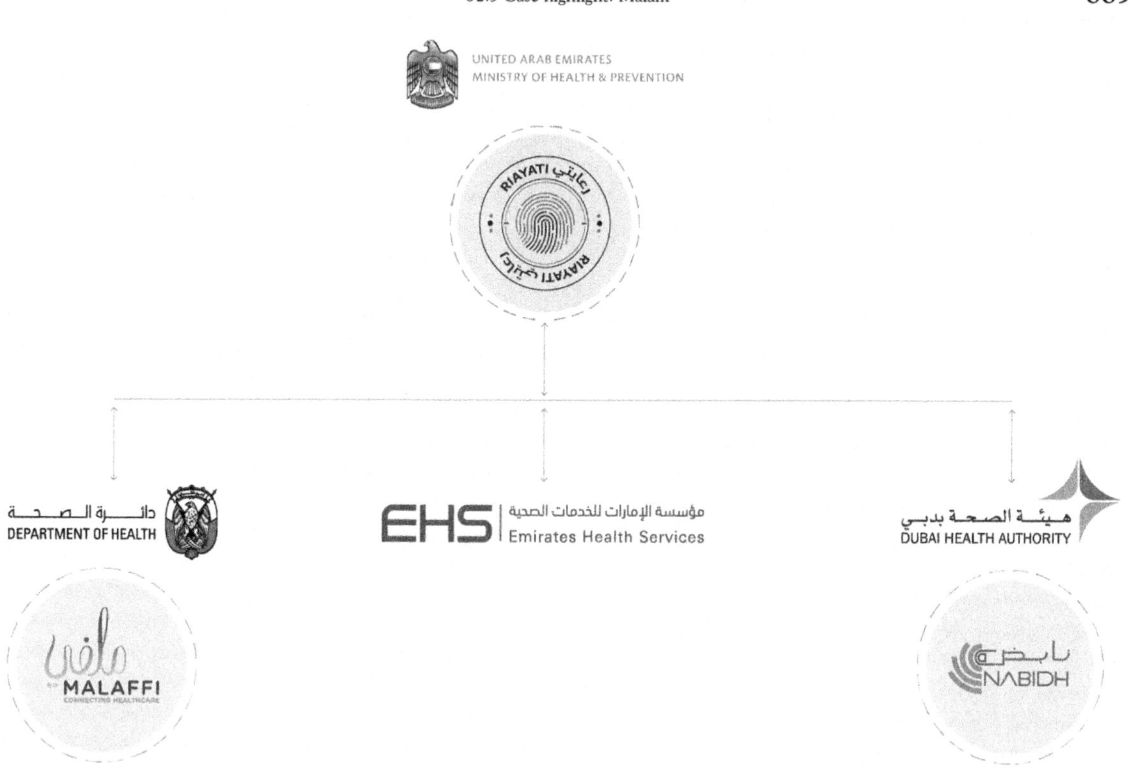

FIGURE 32.3 UAE Ministry of Health and Promotion's National Unified Medical Record Structure, conceptualization by Dr. Bisera Lakinska, based on \ Ref. [10].

32.5 Case highlight: Malaffi

32.5.1 Background

The planning for Malaffi started in 2016. To define the basics of the operational and business model, the planning team examined selected case studies of implementation of HIEs globally, that highlighted major challenges in the models and implementation, which were used to avoid repeating the same errors. Interviews and consultations were conducted with major players and stakeholders to develop a full understanding of the complexities of the market and establish the basic use cases that will drive value, including the providers, technology companies, and government officials.

Further, decisions were made around the three core components of an HIE: business model (government funding in the short term, with a mid- to long-term plan of having the HIE sustainable through payers contribution), technology platform (centralized model), and the operating model (public–private partnership, PPP). The PPP model is widely adopted by the UAE Government to stimulate economic activity and innovation.

The centralized model for the technology platform (Fig. 32.4) was selected primarily because, compared to the other models, it ensures a central repository of clinical data that will be available for population health analytics. There were several models considered, including a centralized, federated, and a hybrid model [11,12].

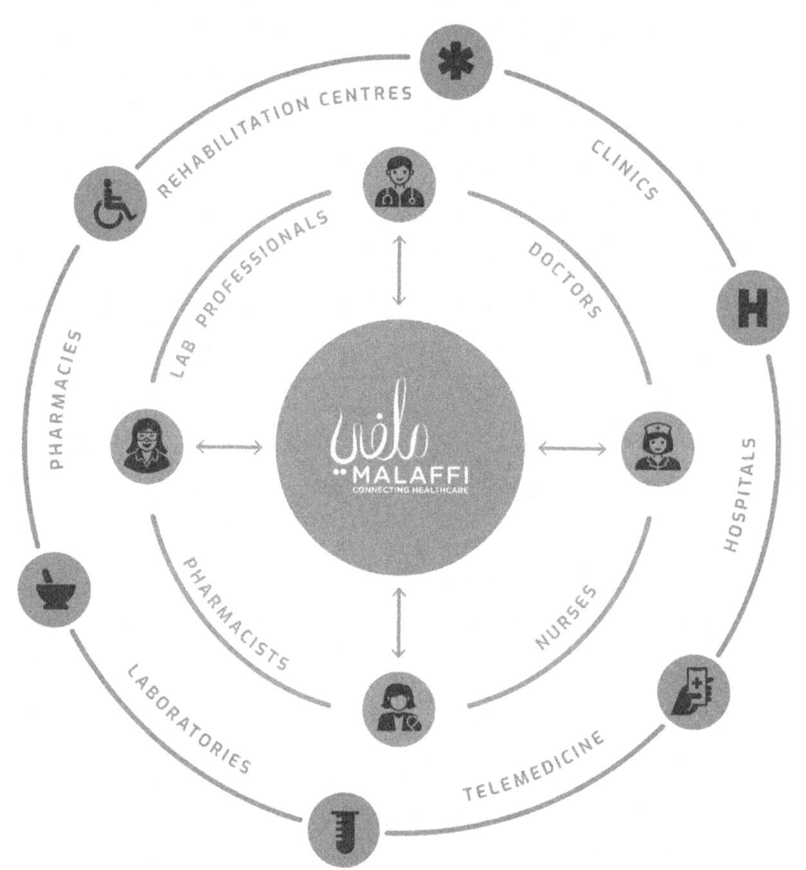

FIGURE 32.4 The Abu Dhabi Health Information Exchange system. Source: *Malaffi HIE.*

Based on those three core components, a detailed study was put in place to start the implementation. Strategic alignment was reached with other government institutions such as the Department of Finance, the Abu Dhabi Digital Authority, and the MOHAP. In addition, alignment with the plans for HIEs of the other emirates was reached in order to ensure the ultimate exchange of information at the federal level.

Malaffi (meaning "my file" in Arabic), was formally established in August 2018 with the signing of the PPP agreement between the DOH and Injazat Data Systems, a company then owned by Mubadala Investment Company, the investment arm of the Government of Abu Dhabi. To facilitate the development, implementation, and adoption of Malaffi, the Emirate established a new company called Abu Dhabi Health Data Services.

32.5.2 Goals

By providing instant access to the patient's longitudinal medical records, Malaffi facilitates better-informed and more efficient clinical decisions, enhances coordination and transition of care, reduces unnecessary duplication of tests and procedures, reduces the risk of medical errors, and improves patient safety and experience. Instant access to real-time, important patient health information plays a vital role in improving the quality of healthcare and patient outcomes.

It facilitates better care coordination and informed decision making, has a significant impact on the delivery of healthcare, and is supporting more efficient, safe, and effective care.

Malaffi reduces the administrative burden on providers and patients as less time is spent searching for historic information and managing other administrative tasks, allowing them to spend more time focused on patient care and improving their experience. Malaffi addresses the strain on the healthcare system caused by an increase in chronic diseases and an aging population.

Access to past test results and reports reduces the need to repeat investigative tests and procedures which can be invasive, costly, and unnecessary. As a centralized database of robust population health information, Malaffi will inform and drive the DOH's public health initiatives for a healthier Abu Dhabi.

32.5.3 History and milestones

The history and major milestones for Malaffi are depicted in Fig. 32.5. Following the launch in January 2019, the first providers were connected in October 2019 [13]. The ambitious launch schedule was planned in phases, based on the digital maturity and size of the providers. To ensure critical clinical value and drive early adoption, the largest providers, including the public system (SEHA) were connected first, that made up to 70% of the inpatient admissions in the Emirate. In addition, data from previous years were ingested to provide instant clinical value.

32.5.4 Mission, vision, and values

Mission: Malaffi promises the safe and secure exchange of patient health information to enhance quality healthcare and patient outcomes [14].

Vision: Connecting healthcare in Abu Dhabi to support communities on their journey to good health, happiness and prosperity.

Values: Malaffi believes in Integrity, Collaboration, Dedication, and Innovation.

32.5.5 Policies, technologies, and process

The main guiding document, the Policy on the Abu Dhabi Health Information Exchange [9] was published by the Department of Health in late 2018, prescribing the main principles of universal provider and patient participation, as well as defining the roles, responsibilities, and strategies around data management and data quality.

In 2019 the DOH also published the Abu Dhabi Healthcare Information and Cyber Security Standard [15] to ensure that healthcare entities will uphold good industry practice for data privacy and security and ensure the safe and secure information exchange through Malaffi.

32.5.6 Project scope

Malaffi was designed as a scalable platform with the future in mind—built with the ability to add on feature service capabilities and functions. The platform featured four main functionalities: Clinical Data Exchange, Provider Portal, Patient Portal, and Population Health Analytics (Malaffi Insights).

The Provider Portal is embedded within the electronic medical record (EMR) systems of the providers as a single-sign-on (SSO) functionality and ensures seamless access and utilization of the HIE through the EMR system of the facility. It allows user to access the HIE file of the patient in one click and avoids the need for clinicians to manage different systems that saves time. The principle behind this design philosophy is to make the Malaffi tool accessible within clinicians' workflows as we know that increased workload, poor EMR usability, and admin tasks have been connected to clinicians' burnout [16,17].

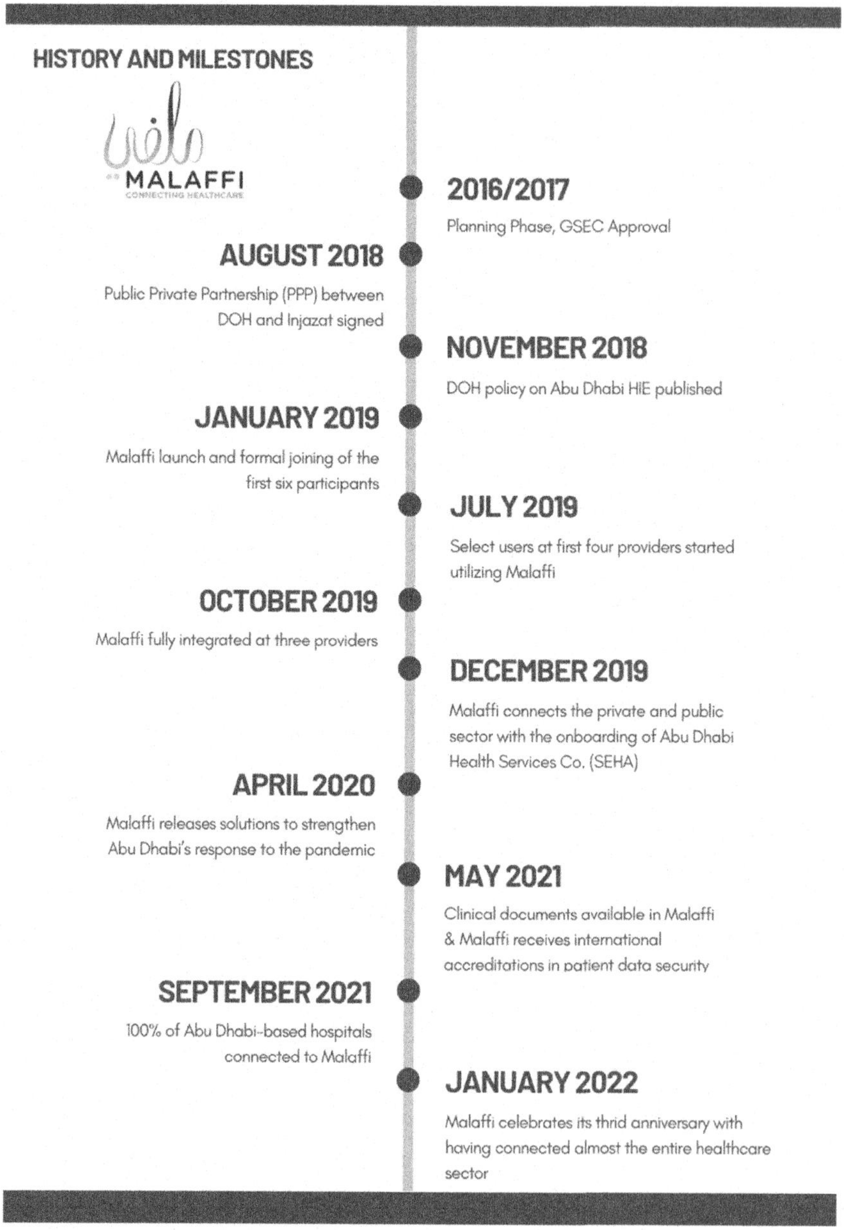

HISTORY AND MILESTONES

MALAFFI
CONNECTING HEALTHCARE

2016/2017
Planning Phase, GSEC Approval

AUGUST 2018
Public Private Partnership (PPP) between DOH and Injazat signed

NOVEMBER 2018
DOH policy on Abu Dhabi HIE published

JANUARY 2019
Malaffi launch and formal joining of the first six participants

JULY 2019
Select users at first four providers started utilizing Malaffi

OCTOBER 2019
Malaffi fully integrated at three providers

DECEMBER 2019
Malaffi connects the private and public sector with the onboarding of Abu Dhabi Health Services Co. (SEHA)

APRIL 2020
Malaffi releases solutions to strengthen Abu Dhabi's response to the pandemic

MAY 2021
Clinical documents available in Malaffi & Malaffi receives international accreditations in patient data security

SEPTEMBER 2021
100% of Abu Dhabi-based hospitals connected to Malaffi

JANUARY 2022
Malaffi celebrates its thrid anniversary with having connected almost the entire healthcare sector

FIGURE 32.5 Malaffi HIE history and milestones. Source: *Ahmed Deeb, adapted from Malaffi. History and milestones. n.d. [cited 2022 Apr 4]. Available from: https://malaffi.ae/what-is-malaffi/history-and-milestones/.*

The New Zealand-based Orion Health was selected as the main technology partner to provide the HIE system with the Amadeus platform for data aggregation and presentation to clinicians, Rhapsody as the integration engine, and NextGate for the Enterprise Master Patient Index (EMPI) solution. Patient demographics are aggregated and managed through the EMPI and the clinical data repository ingested data from the different providers, including demographics, encounters, problems and diagnosis, allergies, laboratory and radiology results, and medication.

The team of Malaffi constantly works to expand the core platform, the scope, and to enhance the functionalities in order to ensure it delivers value to the end-users and the DOH. Value is defined based on user feedback and requirements.

For example, in 2021, new data points were added including clinical documents, immunization history, and vital signs, and the HIE will be adding radiology images among other data points in the future.

Malaffi Insights provides the DOH with population health data and critical insights that help better regulate the sector and manage public and population health programs. It also provides population risk management insights to support care management, improve population health, and assist in ensuring continuity of care. The Malaffi team works closely with the DOH and the stakeholders to maximize the value of the centralized information for improving the overall health and well-being of the people in the Emirate.

The Patient Portal, to be launched in 2022 as a web-based portal and a smartphone app, seeks to provide access to citizens and residents in Abu Dhabi to their medical history in Malaffi with the goal to improve their engagement in managing their own health. Patient data privacy and security were highlighted as a priority for Malaffi and the DOH [18].

In 2021 Malaffi received recognition from two international organizations for excellence in data security and privacy: (1) ISO 27001 certification and (2) accreditation from the Electronic Healthcare Network Accreditation Commission with the Health Information Exchange Accreditation Programme, awarded to Malaffi for the first time outside of the United States. Additionally, Malaffi was awarded with the ISO 22301:2019 Certificate, the International Standard for business continuity management systems.

32.5.7 Organization

Abu Dhabi Health Data Services is a special project company established in 2018 to design, develop, implement, maintain, and operate Malaffi, the Abu Dhabi Health Information Exchange. Under the build/own/operate/transfer model, after 10 years of operation (referred to as the concession period), Malaffi is to be transferred back to the Government of Abu Dhabi.

The company currently employs around 70 staff members across different departments. The core Malaffi team consists of IT, HIE development, clinical, and project management teams that work together on the system rollout and the onboarding of providers. A full in-house team provides the support functions in order to ensure independence and agility of the organization and fast implementation.

32.5.8 Community engagement/providers

To ensure alignment with the providers' community on the main decisions related to the platform, its implementation and road map, Malaffi's team works closely with several Healthcare Advisory Committees composed of representatives from the healthcare providers, including a Clinical, Technical, and Security Committee.

Malaffi also works very closely with a dedicated team at the DOH to ensure alignment, guidance, and government oversight.

The onboarding of the providers was carried out in a phased approach, according to a published launch schedule. To achieve instant value for the early users, historical data from the last five years were ingested from SEHA, the largest public healthcare network consisting of 13 hospitals and 46 clinics.

To join Malaffi, each participant needs to sign a Participation Agreement and go through a series of security reviews to ensure their systems meet all applicable privacy and security laws to ultimately be allowed to connect to Malaffi. This includes a self-review of the Abu Dhabi Health Information Cyber Security policy and a questionnaire. Malaffi is implemented as a SSO function embedded within around 71 EMR systems to ensure that only those that have a relationship with the patient can access their Malaffi file and to enable seamless access without the need to use and sign-in to another system. Malaffi has implemented privacy and security guidelines for authorization and accessibility of the platform. As part of the guidelines, Malaffi maintains activity logs of the authorized users who view patient files and access information and receives notifications in case of misuse of the platform.

There are three levels of access defined for primary, secondary users, and front desk staff. Only the highest level of authorized users (primary) who are clinically treating the patient may "Break the Privacy Seal" meaning they can access patient's sensitive health information (e.g., HIV/AIDS, sexually transmitted diseases, substance abuse, mental health issues). This is on the condition that, in the professional judgment of that clinician, access to such sensitive health information is strictly necessary to ensure optimal treatment of the patient. These activities are monitored to ensure proper usage of the platform.

32.5.9 Finances

Research by the planning team found that ensuring financial sustainability has been a main challenge for global HIE networks, and a factor that determined their success. To ensure the sustainability of the project, the UAE Government is funding the HIE, while it is free for healthcare providers to connect. The providers bear the internal costs incurred during the onboarding, including any costs incurred by the EMR vendors to develop interfaces, SSO, etc., and the secure connection provided by Etisalat, a state-owned telecom operator and the telecom partner of Malaffi [19].

32.6 Usage and impact of health information exchange

In order to stay close to the users' community, different teams at Malaffi continuously gather feedback from the Malaffi users and providers' leadership teams, including an annual user satisfaction survey. The feedback is used for ongoing improvements.

32.6.1 Progress statistics

In a short period of time of about two years since the first connected providers, as of September 2021, Malaffi connected 100% of the Abu Dhabi Hospitals and 99% of all patient episodes. As of February 2022, more than 45,500 end-users have access to Malaffi and around 2000 facilities have been connected. Connected providers include the largest public healthcare network SEHA and the largest private providers groups, medical centers, clinics, and laboratories [20].

32.6.2 Surveys and testimonials

Malaffi ensures constant feedback from the users and the providers community.

> Malaffi has helped us reduce chest x-rays by around 30% in suspected COVID-19 patients, meaning less radiation, quicker diagnosis and reduced cost of care. (Dr. Maria Oliva, General Medicine Doctor, NMC Healthcare, June 2020)

> Through Malaffi, we are able to build the whole picture of our patient's medical history in a click of a button. When dealing with pediatric emergencies, this is even more important and can be life-saving. (Dr. Mohammed Ibrahim, Head of Pediatrics, Danat Al Emarat Hospital for Women & Children, August 2020)

> Because we have instant access to the summary of the medical information in Malaffi, our new patients are particularly satisfied and happy, as they feel that we already know them, even if we see them for the first time. It allows us to spend more face-time with them since we can review their past information prior to their appointment. (Dr. Mujgan Jamil, Consultant Internal Medicine, Imperial College London Diabetes Centre, June 2021)

Through an anonymous survey run during October 2021, feedback was collected from a sample of more than 450 users of the system, as measures on the impact of the system.

- Nine out of ten respondents agreed or strongly agreed that Malaffi improves patient safety and quality of care. Eight in ten also felt that it improves patient outcomes and coordination of care.
- Similarly, users agreed that Malaffi has helped reduce medical errors and prevention of drug-to-drug interaction, the making of better-informed clinical decisions, improved patient experience and satisfaction.
- On average, consulting a patient's Malaffi file halves the time clinicians spend searching for past medical information during consultations and reduces duplication of laboratory test orders by 60%.
- 87% agreed and strongly agreed Malaffi helped them provide better care to their COVID19 patients.

In a 2020 survey of healthcare providers by KLAS Research, a company which engages with end-users to gather insights aimed at improving healthcare delivery, Malaffi stakeholders were universally satisfied with the system.

- They reported seeing positive outcomes in terms of prevention of repetitive testing, higher quality and more accurate care, and easy access to patient data from other providers.
- Almost 25% reported noticing immediate outcomes and over 50% have seen outcomes within just six months.
- Organizations confirmed that the data they have access to provide real value and are looking forward to continued feature developments.

32.6.3 Clinical adoption results

Currently, Malaffi is constantly seeing more than 30% unique logins monthly, expressed as a percentage of the total unique user population with access, which compares favorably to averages of other global HIE networks.

32.7 Challenges

The implementation of such a robust and complex system was inevitably faced with challenges. Below is a list of the most important ones, as well as the recommended tried-and-tested mitigation strategies.

32.7.1 Challenge 1—business case sustainability

- Develop the HIE core services scope in a phased approach while keeping economic impact in mind.
- Design a sustainable revenue model that best aligns with all stakeholders.

- Ensure alignment and buy-in from all stakeholders based on their priorities.
- Backload data to provide instant clinical value to users and ensure early adoption.

32.7.2 Challenge 2—aggressive connection timeliness

- Ensure early engagement and change management of providers through awareness sessions and consistent communication.
- Apply a bulk onboarding approach through cooperation with the major EMR vendors to ensure accuracy and efficiency in connecting clinics and centers that are using their system.
- Built standardized interfaces for all facilities in scope under DOH to ensure market alignment and efficiency in connecting to Malaffi.
- Align adoption execution with onboarding activities—phased approach.

32.7.3 Challenge 3—provider readiness to connect

Providers had to manage competing priorities, especially during the first months of the pandemic, in addition to the cost that needed to be incurred to ensure the secure connection, and potential loss of revenue due to reduced overutilization.

- Ensure strong value statement (use cases with evidence) and understanding of the implications for all stakeholders.
- Define incentives for providers to connect with the right balance of enforcement.
- Balance between the privacy aspects and ensuring that providers are getting onboard and utilizing the HIE.

32.7.4 Challenge 4—electronic medical record data quality and digital maturity

- Ensure early market survey of readiness/capability to connect with detailed awareness sessions.
- Engage a strong team with expertise in clinical data exchange to help walk providers through workflows.

32.7.5 Challenge 5—interoperability and data standardization

- Implement a unified specification and terminology services to normalize data for analytics.

32.7.6 Challenge 6—mutual responsibilities of participants

- Define a robust policy and legal framework that lays out obligations, responsibilities, and expectations of participants with each other.
- Define a strong governance structure and committees which ensure clinical engagement.

32.8 COVID-19 and Malaffi

32.8.1 Background

When the pandemic started in early 2020, mass testing for COVID-19 was one of the first strategies to help manage the dire situation. At that time, in parallel with the rollout of the testing capacities, the DOH mandated Malaffi to provide solutions to manage COVID-19 laboratory results in the Emirate centrally. Even though Malaffi was still quite a young system, based on the existing infrastructure, and the established EPMI, it swiftly scaled to capture more than 90% of total COVID-19 testing, provided databases that are quick and easy to search, multiple dashboards for public health decision-making, and access to test results to the front-line workers, therefore becoming an essential factor in the successful pandemic response of the Emirate.

Further to the testing, Malaffi supported the massive vaccination operation via expanded searchable databases and expansion of public health dashboards, which placed the UAE among the countries with the highest vaccinated population rates and Abu Dhabi on top of the list of the world's leading cities for their response to the COVID-19 pandemic, according to the published report by the London-based Deep Knowledge Group in 2021 [21].

32.8.2 Solutions deployed

32.8.2.1 *Urgent access to Malaffi to frontline workers*

Urgent secure access to the Malaffi Provider Portal was granted to those that are not connected to Malaffi and are part of Abu Dhabi's COVID-19 response. Patients with underlying medical conditions are at higher risk of experiencing severe symptoms from COVID-19, so by having access to real-time COVID-19 test results and the relevant information from the medical history, front-line medical workers are empowered to make quicker and more effective first-response decisions, whether it is for the patient to be released, isolated, or hospitalized. Having access to medical history also helps doctors treat patients more efficiently when a patient visits an Emergency Room for urgent care.

32.8.2.2 *Malaffi COVID-19 Module*

The customized system, Malaffi COVID-19 Module, consists of a tool to capture lab results and enables EID (Emirates ID) and phone number search for patient results and immunization details. The system uses a series of near-real-time dashboards to support the tracking of patient statuses and lab capacity/turnaround times.

Based on the centralized testing information and integration of other sources of clinical data, the Module features dashboards with accurate near-real-time key pandemic indicators that allow the DOH to monitor the spread of the disease and evaluate the effectiveness of the preventive measures. It further enables the authorities to better plan the testing and healthcare capacities and to coordinate the distribution of the critical resources in the Emirate.

In order to improve interoperability, Malaffi worked with the DOH to mandate the collection of core patient demographics to enhance unique identification and matching. It also enforced the use of COVID-19 CPT codes for PCR (laboratory) orders and standardized result codes/formats to enable reports.

32.8.2.3 *Vaccination Module*

In parallel with the rollout of the vaccination campaign and in coordination with the DOH, Malaffi developed a custom Vaccination Module that enables the collecting and sharing of vaccination information from more than 100 facilities in Abu Dhabi that are part of the program. Due to the vaccination information being centralized in Malaffi, the DOH and the government have real-time insights into the Emirate's vaccination status. Having access to this information enables the authorities to generate operational reports, plan vaccination capacities, streamline logistics and supply chain, and inform public outreach programs. Healthcare professionals in Abu Dhabi have access to the COVID-19 vaccination information in Malaffi, which improves clinical decision making, enhances safety and the efficiency of the vaccination program.

The COVID-19 Malaffi solutions enable the centralized management of COVID-19 information that was key to the successful management of the pandemic.

32.9 Improving interoperability and data standardization

Ensuring that healthcare providers capture high-quality and standardized data is a basic premise for enabling interoperability and the use of digital technology to transform healthcare. The COVID-19 pandemic—when the need to centralize, share, and analyze clinical data became paramount—further accelerated the efforts to improve interoperability and develop processes to monitor and improve data standardization and quality.

While examining the collated data, the Malaffi team found that while some data domains were consistently coded (e.g., diagnoses, procedures) there were significant gaps in others (e.g., allergies, chronic conditions), as well as issues with data quality (e.g., lack of coded allergies, inconsistent demographic data, etc.).

To enhance data quality, the DOH has issued guidance on coding standards and minimum data sets to healthcare providers in Abu Dhabi. The universal adoption of these standards, such as Systematized Nomenclature of Medicine—Clinical Terms (SNOMED CT) and Logical Observation Identifiers Names and Codes (LOINC), is expected to significantly improve interoperability, increase the clinical value of the data, and improve the accuracy and scope of population health insights.

32.10 New frontiers in population health management

Malaffi enables the DOH, for the first time, to draw population health insights in near real-time, based on the analysis of the consolidated clinical data of the entire population. For example, in 2021, Malaffi premiered a demonstration of a population risk management platform that will, once live, empower the healthcare sector to support care management, improve population health, and assist in ensuring continuity of care.

The platform uses advanced artificial intelligence analytic technologies, such as machine learning, to build predictive models based on the clinical data and run algorithms to predict future hospital admissions, emergency department visits, readmissions, disease complications such as diabetes, and other risks. These insights will be used to action targeted measures that will reduce the risk of groups or individual patients developing certain conditions, improve overall efficiencies among providers, and reduce costs.

Malaffi will contribute significantly to creating advanced systems tailored for syndromic and pandemic surveillance and response. Such systems will be of the utmost value for early alerts and increased readiness to handle any potential future outbreak, ensuring Abu Dhabi remains at the forefront of public health and safety. Other solutions will also be developed to take advantage of advanced analytics of the robust population health data in Malaffi, to improve the quality of care and health outcomes for everyone in the Emirate.

32.11 Summary and the next chapter for Malaffi

Malaffi has started to transform healthcare in the Emirate of Abu Dhabi and will undoubtedly continue to do so as the data quality and capabilities of the platform increase.

Having established itself firmly in the healthcare infrastructure of the Emirate, Malaffi now enters the next phase of its development. The remaining healthcare facilities will be connected by the end of 2022 and Malaffi will continue to complete the data sources contributed by the different providers to create a more comprehensive patient record (data patching).

During the pandemic, the people of Abu Dhabi witnessed first-hand how connected healthcare, through Malaffi, plays a significant role in protecting the health and safety of the community. Soon, patients will have access to their records in Malaffi, which will enable them to be better engaged in managing their health.

As the healthcare system matures, Malaffi will become increasingly important for the realization of strategic initiatives of the DOH toward establishing a primary care model, transition to value-based care and the practice of precision medicine. Integration with the federal HIE network, Riayati, will enhance connectedness beyond Abu Dhabi, into the other emirates.

The benefits of HIE platforms are endless. As a hallmark of the UAE, the team is committed to innovating and discovering new capabilities to improve the health and well-being of the population.

Questions for discussion

1. Why does it matter to engage end-users in technology transformation projects?
2. What role does executive leadership and regulation play in digital transformation?
3. How can HIEs support healthcare resource utilization?
4. How can HIEs support healthcare systems transformation towards primary care or value-based models?
5. How can HIEs enable the practice of personalized medicine?
6. How can we improve interoperability and avoid the problem with different/or lack of healthcare data standards?

References

[1] UAE Vision 2021. National agenda. Dubai; 2018 [cited 2022 Apr 4]. Available from: <https://www.vision2021.ae/en/national-agenda-2021>.

[2] UAE Vision 2021. World-class healthcare. Dubai; 2018 [cited 2022 Apr 4]. Available from: <https://www.vision2021.ae/en/national-agenda-2021/list/world-class-circle>.

[3] U.S.-U.A.E. Business Council. The U.A.E. healthcare sector. Washington, D.C.; 2021 [cited 2022 Apr 4]. Available from: <http://usuaebusiness.org/wp-content/uploads/2019/01/2021-U.A.E.-Healthcare-Report.pdf>.

[4] Alvarez & Marsal. UAE health sector pulse. 2021 [cited 2022 Apr 4]. Available from: <https://www.alvarezandmarsal.com/sites/default/files/uae_-health_sector_pulse_q1_2021_final.pdf>.

[5] Webster N. UAE spend on diabetes care falls well short of US and UK, study shows. 2018 [cited 2022 Apr 4]. Available from: <https://www.thenationalnews.com/uae/uae-spend-on-diabetes-care-falls-well-short-of-us-and-uk-study-shows-1.737321>.

[6] Kennedys Law LLP. The evolving face of health insurance in the UAE. 2017 [cited 2022 Apr 4]. Available from: <https://kennedyslaw.com/thought-leadership/article/the-evolving-face-of-health-insurance-in-the-uae/>.

[7] TDRA. Abu Dhabi healthcare strategic plan. 2014 [updated 2021 Apr 20; cited 2022 Apr 4]. Available from: <https://u.ae/en/about-the-uae/strategies-initiatives-and-awards/local-governments-strategies-and-plans/abu-dhabi-healthcare-strategic-plan>.

[8] TDRA. Healthcare providers. 2022 [cited 2022 Apr 4]. Available from: <https://u.ae/en/information-and-services/health-and-fitness/healthcare-providers>.

[9] Health Authority Abu Dhabi. Policy on the Abu Dhabi Health Information Exchange (HIE). 2020 [cited 2022 Apr 4]. Available from: <https://www.doh. gov.ae/-/media/A78104416DF2440E89AC90FB75F11055.ashx>.

[10] Emirates News Agency. Ministry of Health, local health authorities consolidate medical data on 'Riayati' platform. 2021 [cited 2022 Apr 4]. Available from: <https://www.wam.ae/en/details/1395302999628>.

[11] McGee MK. HIE models: security pros and cons. 2012 [cited 2022 Apr 4]. Available from: <https://www.govinfosecurity.com/hie-models-security-pros-cons-a-5079>.

[12] Dixon BE. What is health information exchange? In: Dixon BE, editor. Health information exchange: navigating and managing a network of health information systems. Waltham: Academic Press; 2016. p. 3–20.

[13] Malaffi. History and milestones. n.d. [cited 2022 Apr 4]. Available from: <https://malaffi.ae/what-is-malaffi/history-and-milestones/>.

[14] Malaffi. Mission, vision and values. n.d. [cited 2022 Apr 4]. Available from: <https://malaffi.ae/what-is-malaffi/mission-vision-values/>.

[15] Health Authority Abu Dhabi. Abu Dhabi – Healthcare Information and Cyber Security Standard. 2019 [cited 2022 Apr 4]. Available from: <https://malaffi.ae/wp-content/uploads/2019/11/ADHICS_Standard-Final.pdf>.

[16] National Academies of Sciences, Engineering, and Medicine; National Academy of Medicine; Committee on Systems Approaches to Improve Patient Care by Supporting Clinician Well-Being. Factors contributing to clinician burnout and professional well-being. In: Taking action against clinician burnout: a systems approach to professional well-being. Washington DC: National Academies Press (US); 2019 [cited 2022 Apr 4]. Available from: <https://www.ncbi.nlm.nih.gov/books/NBK552615/>.

[17] Melnick ER, Harry E, Sinsky CA, Dyrbye LN, Wang H, Trockel MT, et al. Perceived electronic health record usability as a predictor of task load and burnout among US physicians: mediation analysis. J Med Internet Res 2020;22(12):e23382.

[18] Malaffi. Health information security & privacy. n.d. [cited 2022 Apr 4]. Available from: <https://malaffi.ae/providers/data-security/>.

[19] Etisalat. About us. [cited 2022 Apr 4]. Available from: <https://www.etisalat.ae/en/footer/about-us.jsp>.

[20] Malaffi. Malaffi progress report. 2022 [cited 2022 Apr 4]. Available from: <https://malaffi.ae/malaffi-progress-report/>.

[21] Available from: https://wam.ae/en/details/1395302968353.

Index

Note: Page numbers followed by "*b*," "*f*," and "*t*" refer to boxes, figures, and tables, respectively.

D

O

P

T

Printed in the United States
by Baker & Taylor Publisher Services